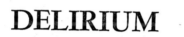

DELIRIUM

Publication Number 1028

AMERICAN LECTURE SERIES®

A Monograph in

The BANNERSTONE DIVISION *of*
AMERICAN LECTURES IN LIVING CHEMISTRY

Edited by

I. NEWTON KUGELMASS, M.D., Ph.D., ScD.
Consultant to the Departments of Health and Hospitals
New York City

DELIRIUM

Acute Brain Failure In Man

By

Z. J. LIPOWSKI, M.D.

Professor of Psychiatry
Dartmouth Medical School
Hanover, New Hampshire

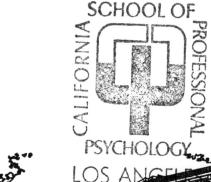

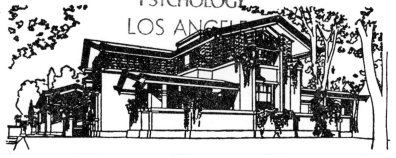

CHARLES C THOMAS · PUBLISHER
Springfield · Illinois · U.S.A.

Published and Distributed Throughout the World by
CHARLES C THOMAS • PUBLISHER
Bannerstone House
301-327 East Lawrence Avenue, Springfield, Illinois, U.S.A.

© *1980, by* CHARLES C THOMAS • PUBLISHER
ISBN 0-398-03909-7
Library of Congress Catalog Card Number: 79-633

With THOMAS BOOKS *careful attention is given to all details of manufacturing and design. It is the Publisher's desire to present books that are satisfactory as to their physical qualities and artistic possibilities and appropriate for their particular use.* THOMAS BOOKS *will be true to those laws of quality that assure a good name and good will.*

Library of Congress Cataloging in Publication Data

Lipowski, Zbigniew Jerzy.
    Delirium: acute brain failure in man.

    (American lecture series; no. 1028)
    Bibliography
    Includes index.
    1. Delirium.   I.   Title.   [DNLM: 1.   Delirium.
WM204   L764d]
RC106.L53   616.8'4   79-633
ISBN 0-398-03909-7

Printed in the United States of America
W-2

PREFACE

DELIRIUM, ONE OF the first mental disorders to be described in the Western medical literature, is probably more prevalent today than ever before. It is most frequent among people aged sixty years and older, and their number is steadily growing. In these elderly persons, delirium constitutes a ubiquitous and thus clinically important sign of cerebral functional decompensation caused by physical illness. Any medical or surgical ward, or emergency department of a general hospital, provides a setting in which delirium is seen daily and is frequently misdiagnosed, or even overlooked, by the medical staff. Lack of generally accepted diagnostic criteria and terminology has no doubt contributed to this nonrecognition. It is one of the curious paradoxes of modern medicine that acute failure of the essential functions of the human brain, those necessary for knowing, remembering, understanding, problem-solving and deciding, has been totally neglected by researchers and ignored by physicians. Apart from its ubiquity and clinical importance, delirium poses questions for every student of brain-behavior relationships, consciousness, sleep-wakefulness cycle, hallucinations, and organization of the mind. Yet, oddly enough, students of all these fields have largely bypassed delirium, an experiment of nature that may be observed daily on any medical or surgical ward. Delirium is excellently described in English medical texts as far back as the sixteenth century, yet not a single book solely about delirium has been published in this language to date. This is the first such monograph, and the writer hopes that it will stimulate research on delirium and aid in its recognition and treatment.

An English surgeon, Gallway, wrote in 1838: "The subject of delirium is generally looked upon by the practical physician as one of the most obscure in the chain of morbid phenomena he has to deal with; whilst the frequency of its occurrence under various diseased conditions of the system renders the affection not a little familiar to his eye. My object in approaching so acknowledged a terra incognita is not, I regret to say, that I have any fresh contribution towards its elucidation to bring into the field, but rather to awaken a more lively inquiry amongst the profession as to its real nature and causes" (1). Today, 140 years later, the subject remains as "obscure" as it is frequent and almost as much a terra incognita as in Gallway's times. Perhaps this writer's attempt to awaken interest in it will prove to be less futile than that of the other authors.

The writer acknowledges with gratitude the receipt of a grant-in-aid from the Commonwealth Fund which has helped him greatly in preparing the material for this book. Relevant references had to be collated from several thousand books and articles bearing titles not even remotely alluding to delirium. I also wish to thank Dr. Layton McCurdy, Chairman of the Department of Psychiatry, at the Medical University of South Carolina in Charleston, S.C., who offered me a visiting professorship and ideal conditions under which to write the bulk of this book. One could hardly wish for a more delightful setting in which to write than that of historical Charleston.

---

(1) Gallway, M. D.: Nature and treatment of delirium. *London Medical Gazette* 1:46-49, 1838.

CONTENTS

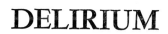

DELIRIUM

PART I

CHAPTER 1

HISTORY OF DELIRIUM

ETYMOLOGY OF DELIRIUM

THE TERM "DELIRIUM" stems from the Latin word "delirare," which literally means to go out of the furrow ("lira," Latin for furrow), but whose figurative meaning is to be deranged, crazy, out of one's wits (1). From this root was derived the now obsolete English verb "delire," meaning to go wrong, to go astray from reason, to rave, to wander in mind, to be delirious or mad (1). "Delirium" has been used in English in two senses: first, to denote a mental disorder due to disturbance of brain functions and featuring incoherent speech, hallucinations, frenzied excitement, and restlessness; and second, as a figure of speech connoting uncontrollable excitement or emotion, "frenzied rapture," or "wildly absurd thought or speech" (1) The word was probably first used in English in the late sixteenth century (1).

The adjective "delirious" has been used to refer to a person affected with delirium, particularly as a consequence or symptom of disease, or to one temporarily insane. It could also mean a characteristic attribute of delirium, or refer to a person, thing, action, etc., featuring wild excitement, or one that is frantic, crazy, or mad (1).

The word "delirium" was probably introduced into medical literature by Celsus (2) in the first century A.D., but its meaning remained ambiguous until the end of the nineteenth century. The ambiguity resulted from the fact that the term was used by medical and psychiatric writers in one of two ways: either in a general sense as a synonym for derangement of the mind or insanity, or, more specifically, to refer to a transient, acute mental disorder associated with many somatic, especially febrile, diseases (3). This inconsistent usage of the term lingered on despite attempts by many writers over the centuries to assign to it precise meaning as a distinct psychiatric syndrome always associated with a primary or secondary brain disorder.

The medical usage of the word "delirium" has influenced, and been in turn influenced by, the popular connotation of the term as reflected in its definitions in the *Oxford Dictionary* just quoted. Thus, delirium has come to connote a psychological state marked by striking excitement and restlessness accompanied by hallucinations. True, often delirious patients do exhibit these dramatic features but many do not: they may be quiet, listless, and sleepy, and may not hallucinate.

The roots of this semantic confusion may be traced back to antiquity. Roman writers, from Celsus on, used the word "delirium" more or less interchangeably with a Greek-derived term "phrenesis," "phrenitis," or "frenzy," which designated a temporary mental disorder occurring in the course of a physical, usually febrile, illness, and featuring excitement and restlessness. The Greek word "phrenitikos" means frantic. The ancient Greek and Roman medical writers distinguished phrenitis from a clinically related but outwardly diametrically opposite condition named "lethargus" or "lethargia," derived from Greek "lethe," forgetfulness. Lethargus was consistently described as a contrast to phrenitis since it featured sleepiness and inertia. We will see in the next Section how these two terms were confused with the term "delirium" over the centuries.

Gowers (4) was perhaps the first English medical writer to state explicitly that delirium could be "quiet" or "active," implying that a delirious patient could exhibit either reduced or increased psychomotor activity and general arousal. Nevertheless the ambiguity has persisted as many nineteenth century authors gradually replaced the term "lethargy" with "simple mental confusion" and thus perpetuated the division. I shall argue later on that a unified modern concept of delirium should encompass both phrenitis and lethargy of the ancients and their followers.

Many qualifying adjectives have been attached to the word "delirium" over the ages. A standard psychiatric dictionary (5) lists over forty variants of the term, nearly all of them both redundant and obsolete. It would be tedious and pointless to review all the vagaries in the usage of "delirium," but it is worthwhile to trace the history of its development as a clinical concept so as to extract its constant and essential features.

HISTORY OF DELIRIUM AS A MENTAL DISORDER

The development of the concept of delirium as a psychiatric syndrome is closely related to the history of psychiatry in general. It reflects changing conceptions about the nature, causes, and pathogenesis of mental disorders. To follow the shifts in the usage of the term has proved an arduous, but rewarding, task. The most striking finding was the recurrent discrepancy between accurate clinical observations of delirium on the one hand, and the inconsistency and ambiguity in its use as a medical term to this day, on the other. It appears that clinicians by and large excel in observing and describing natural phenomena, but often display deplorable looseness in the use of words that are indispensable for labeling, classifying, and explaining what is observed and recorded.

To trace back the history of delirium as a syndrome involved scanning several hundred books and articles covering a period of some 400 years. Some of the best descriptions were found not in psychiatric but in the general medical literature. This is not surprising since delirium is a relatively short-lived mental disorder complicating a wide range of cerebral disorders, both primary and secondary to systemic diseases. Thus, it was bound to be encountered, reported, and treated by general physicians and surgeons rather than by psychiatrists. The standard textbooks of the history of psychiatry have proved to be of little help in the search. Not a single book on delirium in English has been found. The most helpful psychiatric source has been a scholarly work by Hunter and Macalpine (6) that provided useful clues of where to look for relevant information. The works by Whitwell (7) and Mettler (8) also proved valuable.

It would be both pedantic and of little practical value to record all the shifting meanings of the term "delirium" over the ages. Only the more salient contributions will be noted and arranged chronologically.

The Ancients

There are many references to delirium in the extant works of Hippocrates (9) (460-377 B.C.). He did not, of course, use the word "delirium," which is of Latin and not of Greek origin. He did not offer a classification of mental disorders but described those which were named by his translators melancholia, mania, epilepsy, paranoia, hysteria, delirium, and stupor. What Hippocrates called "phrenitis" has been usually translated as "delirium." According to Mettler (8) in the early Greek times the word "phrenes" referred to the region of the diaphragm, but later lost this literal meaning and came to connote the "intellectual complex," or the mind. The word "phrenitis" was used in the medical literature until about the middle of the nineteenth century. It was either synonymous with delirium in general or denoted that due to inflammation of the brain and its covers.

Sprengell (10), who translated into English and interpreted the aphorisms of Hippocrates in the early eighteenth century, uses the term "delirium" several times and quite cogently. Two of the aphorisms are worth quoting: "When a delirium or raving is appeased by sleep, it is a good sign" (10, p. 21). Sprengell interprets this statement as implying that lack of sleep can cause delirium and that the latter may be cured if sleep is restored. This is a striking clinical observation that has been made repeatedly by physicians over the centuries. The second aphorism reads: "Difficulty of breathing and a delirium in continual fevers, are mortal" (10, p. 112). This statement indicates that Hippocrates was aware of the common association between delirium and terminal illness.

A recent English translation of the medical works of Hippocrates by Chadwick and Mann (9) contains numerous references to delirium. The Books of Epidemics are a particularly rich source of them. Many clinical features of the syndrome are referred to: association with physical illnesses, especially febrile ones; unpredictable lucid intervals; nocturnal exacerbation; insomnia; visual hallucinations; shifting mood; restlessness; and "wandering of the wits." Hippocrates noted that delirium in a generally weakened patient was a bad prognostic sign. The seat of the disorder was the brain. Its outward manifestations could vary. Hippocrates describes a patient, for example, who fell ill as a result of drinking and became "delirious without excitement, being well-behaved and silent" (9, p. 80). A few days later, however, he "went mad," with "much tossing about" (9, p. 80). Hippocrates was well aware that if a delirious patient became very quiet and "insensible," the prognosis became grave: "Cases of silent delirium, with restlessness, a changing gaze . . . are likely to prove fatal" (9, p. 261).

As this brief account indicates, Hippocrates was not only a precursor of modern medicine but also lay the ground for psychiatry of somatic diseases. The immense influence of his teaching, of his method of approach to clinical phenomena, and of his empirical observations is still discernible today.

Medical writers who followed Hippocrates used terms such as phrenitis, phrenesis, phrenzy, phrenizy, frenzy, frenesie, frenisie, etc. to denote more or less clearly a transient psychiatric disorder occurring in the course of various physical illnesses. Lethargus, lethargie, or lethargy was the term applied to a condition that also complicated acute organic diseases, but was an opposite of phrenitis in that it featured somnolence, inertia, and reduced responsivity to stimuli. It is not always clear to what extent lethargy was synonymous with stupor and coma, but it appears that these three conditions were viewed as a complex of states of reduced awareness, with a bad prognosis. The word "delirium" was used quite inconsistently: at times as a synonym for phrenitis or phrenesis, at other times as a symptom of the latter, and occasionally as an independent syndrome with manifestations overlapping those of both phrenitis and lethargy, and caused by secondary effects on the brain of systemic diseases.

Delirium was probably introduced into the medical literature by Celsus (2) in the first century A.D. Celsus (25 B.C.-A.D. 50) was a Roman aristocrat, not a physician, who compiled the first great medical work since Hippocrates. His "De medicina," written about A.D. 30, consisted of eight books and offered the first grouping of neuropsychiatric disorders, which influenced psychiatric nosology for centuries. He distinguished phrenitis, lethargy, hysteria, melancholia, and mania. Phrenesis or phrenitis was considered roughly equivalent to febrile insania or delirium. Celsus used the term delirium inconsistently. He listed it among the signs of approaching death and claimed that it was a bad prognostic omen in the disease of the "smaller intestine." These scattered references to delirium hardly amount to a clear definition of it. Lethargy referred to any febrile condition in which there was slowing down of psychic functions associated with somnolence: it was the opposite of phrenesis. The latter was a form of acute insanity that commonly accompanied fever and required no treatment other than that for the latter. Celsus noted that phrenesis could be followed by a "continuous dementia," a chronic insanity. Mettler (8) points out, however, that most terms with psychiatric connotation used in Roman times had no clear-cut meaning and overlapped a great deal.

Aretaeus of Cappadocia (11), active in the second century A.D., proposed a more explicit classification of neuropsychiatric disorders than Celsus. He divided diseases into acute and chronic. Among the former he included phrenitis and lethargy. Melancholia, mania, and senile dementia ("dotage") exemplified the chronic diseases. Phrenitis was roughly equivalent to delirium and could result not only from fever but also from other causes, such as drunkenness and poisoning by mandragora and hyoscyamus. Delirium was clearly distinct from mania because it was a transient condition and usually accompanied by fever. Aretaeus recommended putting a phrenitic patient in a dark place if he was disturbed by light, and in the light if he was afraid of the dark. The patient was to have rest and sleep, the latter best secured by "poppy boiled in oil." Aretaeus clearly distinguished senile dementia or "dotage," which started in old age, accompanied the patient until death, and was marked by "a torpor of the senses, and a stupefaction of the gnostic and intellectual faculties" (11, p. 103). This was probably the first distinction between acute and chronic organic mental disorders recorded in the medical literature. Lethargy referred to another acute mental disorder, featuring symptoms opposite to those of phrenitis or delirium, and requiring different therapy, viz. stimulation instead of sedation.

Galen (7), one of the most influential medical writers of

all times, active c. A.D. 129-199, used the term "delirium" freely but rather ambiguously. His main contribution was to recognize that delirium was secondary to and symptomatic of many physical illnesses and resulted from a disorder of the brain by "consensus" or "sympathetically" in diseases such as pneumonia. He ascribed it to excess of yellow bile in the brain. He considered phrenitis and lethargus as conditions related to delirium, but caused by primary disease of the brain. This distinction had therapeutic relevance; treatment of delirium had to be directed at the underlying systemic disease and not at the brain itself.

Cassius Felix, active in the fifth century A.D., is credited by some authors with being the first author to explicitly link drunkenness with delirium (12). The *Talmud,* compiled mostly in the fourth and fifth centuries A.D., was marked by its enlightened attitude towards mental disorders which, in contrast to the *Bible,* were considered as any other diseases amenable to treatment and recovery. Hankoff (13) maintains that a disorder described in the *Talmud* and called "kordiakos" represents delirium, i.e. a temporary mental derangement with a good prognosis. Its etiology appeared to be excessive drinking of wine. In modern translations of the *Talmud,* kordiakos is usually rendered as delirium (13).

After the death of Galen, the centers of medical thought moved to Byzantium. Paulus Aegineta (A.D. 625-700) was a major medical writer of that period (7). His psychiatric writings are mere elaborations of the views of his illustrious predecessors. He considered phrenitis an inflammation of the meninges or the brain. Delirium was a subspecies of phrenitis brought about as a result of the brain's "sympathizing" with the diaphragm. Phrenitis could cause either excitement or coma vigil. In the former the patient was watchful, sleepless, restless, and forgetful. Lethargy was also considered a disorder of the brain, one caused by humid and cold phlegm. Lethargy could pass into coma vigil or catochus. Clearly, in these descriptions, the symptoms of delirium, stupor, coma, and catalepsy overlap and intermingle. Since all these disorders may occur in the course of a febrile illness even in the same patient, it is understandable that medical observers had great difficulty in distinguishing them as separate syndromes.

The Middle Ages

From Byzantium the focus of medical writing shifted to the Arabs, who held the lead for some five centuries, i.e. from the seventh to the twelfth. Their contributions to neuropsychiatry were meager, but they translated and transmitted the great medical works of the Greco-Roman period. Two of the most outstanding Arab writers, worth mentioning in the present context, came from Persia: Rhazes (A.D. 865-925) and Avicenna (980-1037). The former is credited with distinguishing smallpox from measles (8). He described a condition called "sirsen," which corresponded to both lethargus and phrenitis, and which was associated with fever and indulgence in wine (7). This was a possible precursor of a unified concept of delirium.

Avicenna's most famous and influential work "Canon of Medicine" (7) contained many references to mental disorders. He distinguished phrenitis, lethargus, delirium, amentia or fatuity, disorders of memory and of imagination, mania, melancholia, and lycanthropy (7, p. 95). Whitwell (7) points out, however, that these divisions overlapped; it is difficult from the descriptions to separate, for example, delirium and phrenitis or lethargy and coma vigil. Delirium was mentioned as both a symptom of phrenitis and a separate disorder. It was viewed as a symptom of brain disease caused by black, yellow, or red bile, or by hot and burning blood reaching the organ, or at times had its origin in the brain itself (7, p. 181).

With the decline of the Arabic medicine in the twelfth century the interest in mental disorders waned. Bartholomeus Anglicus, who lived in the thirteenth century, provided a notable exception. His influential encyclopedia "De proprietatibus rerum," was first published in 1470 and translated into English in 1495 (6). It enjoyed great popularity and presented authoritative teaching on mental disorders. Following the ancient writers, Bartholomeus recognized four classes of mental disorders: melancholie, mania, dementia, and frenesie or delirium. Frenesie he believed to be due to disease of the brain and its membranes, and distinguished it from perafrenesi or delirium, secondary to febrile and other systemic diseases. His description of frenesie is quite vivid: anguish, frequent waking, restlessness, laughing, singing, weeping, attempting to get out of bed, etc. As treatment Anglicus recommended bleeding the patient and restoring sleep. Clearly, both frenesie and perafrenesi represented delirium.

The Sixteenth Century

Some striking new developments in the concept of delirium took place during this time. Fracastoro (8, p. 368) gave a good description of delirium appearing in the course of typhus. He noted disorientation and observed that some patients displayed vigilance, others torpor. These two states could occur in the same patient on a single day or some days apart. Mercurialis (8) insisted that phrenitis was invariably a disease of the brain. Yet, as Mettler (8) points out, distinctions between mania, phrenzy, and delirium were far from clear.

An excellent summary of the prevailing views on delirium and related conditions was offered in an influential textbook of medicine by Barrough (14), first published in London in 1583. He explicitly separated frenisie from mania or madness and from melancholia, since the latter two conditions were not accompanied by fever. Frenisie was further distinguished from lethargie. The former was due to inflammation of the brain or its covers, and associated with fever. In its fully developed form it featured disorders of imagination, cogitation, memory, and reason. The symptoms included insomnia and "troublesome" sleep, from which patients woke up agitated, shouting, and babbling "without order or sense." Barrough noted behavior suggesting visual hallucinations and marked recent memory impairment (14, p. 22). He believed that prognosis was serious. For treatment he recommended a light room for those afraid of darkness, and a dark one for those "offended at the light." He advised that the patient's friends should be allowed to stay with him and speak softly and gently. Sleep should be induced with "stupefactive medicines," which had to be used sparingly lest the patient's frenisie turn into lethargie and he be made "sleep so, that you can awake him no more" (14, p. 24). Anything that might make the patient angry or sad should be avoided. To make him more comfortable one could apply to his nose odors of roses and violets. By contrast, lethargie was characterized by sluggishness, forgetfulness, dullness, and sleepiness; it was "nothing else but dull oblivion." Like frenisie, however, it was always associated with fever. It ought to be treated by bleeding and all kinds of stimulants. Lethargie might on occasion clear up to be followed by loss of memory, either alone or with concurrent loss of reasoning power. Barrough also described "vigilans sopor" or "the watching drowsiness," which combined features of both frenisie and lethargie.

Barrough's is one of the best, if not the best, early descriptions of delirium, even though he chose the terms "frenisie" and "lethargie," instead. He was one of the first writers to spell out in modern terms the core psychopathology of the syndrome. Shortly after the appearance of his textbook, the first known book on delirium was published: it was Haunoldt's (15) "De delirio," printed in 1593. In England, the word "delirium," defined as "that weakness of conceite and consideration, which we call dotage," was used by Cosin in 1592 (6). This was probably the first time the term was used in English to refer to a mental disorder.

One other sixteenth century contribution is worth mentioning. Ambroise Paré (1510-1590), a famous French surgeon, discussed delirium complicating surgical conditions and procedures. His works, translated into English in 1634 (16), referred to delirium as a perturbation of the fantasy, marked by "raving, talking idly or doting." It was a transient disturbance that commonly occurred in association with fever and pain accompanying wounds, following surgery attended by excessive bleeding, and in gangrene.

The Seventeenth Century

Not surprisingly, the most important contribution to the evolution of the concept of delirium in the seventeenth century came from the pen of a great physician, neuroanatomist, and neurophysiologist, Thomas Willis (17). In his treatise devoted to mental disorders "De anima brutorum," published in 1672 and translated into English in 1683, he gave an excellent description of delirium and discussed its etiology. He observed that delirium was not a disease but a "symptom," which could complicate a variety of physical illnesses of toxic, nutritional, infectious, and visceral origin. Its main manifestations included "incongruous conceptions and confused thoughts," or what we would today call cognitive impairment. Fatigue, fasting, and sleep deprivation predisposed one to delirium. Its prognosis was generally good, and it typically cleared up rather rapidly.

Thus, Willis described the essential features of the syndrome. It is worth noting that he recognized that delirium was not just a concomitant of fever, a view held by his contemporaries. For example, Morton (8, p. 552) explained the occurrence of delirium as due to fever, which caused increased velocity of the flow of blood; this in turn interfered with the secretions of the brain glands needed for activation of the nerves by means of the vital fluid circulating along them. Delirium occurred as a result of this interference and represented a *waking dream*. In both dreams and delirium incoherent ideas were excited by irregular fluctuation of the animal spirits.

The Eighteenth Century

As Barrough and Willis gave us clear descriptions of delirium in the sixteenth and seventeenth centuries respectively, so Hartley (18) performed this task admirably in the eighteenth century. An English philosopher and physician, he formulated a psychophysical theory of "alienation." He noted that the insane or "mad" persons differ from the normal people only relatively, by displaying failures and abnormalities of memory, judgment, emotions, reasoning, consciousness, and actions. He distinguished in his classification of mental disorders "The deliriums attending acute or other distempers." His description of delirium was superb: "disgustful" associations; distortion of reasoning; "a vivid train of visible images" forcing itself on the eyes; incoherent speech; and disorientation for place. Hartley noted that the patient is most likely to be delirious while going to or waking from sleep, or when placed in a dark room. When one brings light to the room, the patient tends to recover and talk rationally until the candle is removed again. Hartley commented that in the dark internally derived images and associations overpower "impressions from real objects."

Another medical writer of that period, Cheyne (19), stressed the importance of sleep in delirium, a theme which runs through the writings on the subject over the centuries. Cheyne stated that "Sleep in Phrenzies and all Deliria is a main Intention Physicians aim at" (19, p. 369) If delirious patients manage to sleep soundly, they become "perfectly restored to their Intellects." On the other hand, while the "Fury of the Spirits continues, Sleep is utterly banished" (19, p. 369).

A number of works, mostly written in Latin, devoted to delirium appeared in the eighteenth century. Frings (20) wrote the only known dissertation on phrenitis in English. None of these contributions, however, could match the excellence of clinical description by Hartley or the intriguing theoretical conceptions of Erasmus Darwin and John Hunter.

Erasmus Darwin (21), a great physician and the grandfather of Charles Darwin, distinguished delirium from madness on the basis of salient clinical features and was probably the first writer to propose that it was a manifestation of impaired or reduced consciousness. Darwin compared delirium to a dream and speculated that dreaming might protect one against developing it. He asserted that in fevers dreaming was somehow interfered with; thus a protection against the syndrome was lost. In both dreams and delirium the capacity for attention to external objects was absent. Darwin claimed that delirium could result from two different causes: from putrid and malignant fevers on the one hand, and from the intake of fermented liquors or opium on the other. In the latter case the syndrome was due to too much pleasurable sensation, and resembled madness or reverie: senses were not "precluded from external stimulation" and the capacity for attention to the surroundings was present. This was an attempt to offer an explanatory hypothesis for delirium as a syndrome caused in part by disordered sleep and representing a breakthrough of dreaming into waking life.

A famous contemporary of Darwin, John Hunter (22), developed this line of thought further. He spoke of delirium as a "diseased dream arising from what may be called diseased sleep" (22, p. 33). In delirium, as in sleep, the consciousness of the connection and relationship between body and mind is cut off, with the result that "what the mind thinks appears to be real." Furthermore, in both sleep and delirium there is reduced susceptibility to external impressions. The two conditions differ from insanity in that by using a strong stimulus one may rouse the person who is asleep or delirious and make him aware of his situation. In insanity, however, "truth and error are inextricably blended together" (22, p. 335).

Benjamin Rush (23), the author of the first American textbook on mental diseases, shared the views on delirium of his English contemporaries. He claimed that dreaming was the effect of unsound sleep and shared with delirium the incoherence of thought; thus "a dream may be considered as a transient paroxysm of delirium, and delirium as a permanent dream" (23, p. 300). Fordyce (24), an authority on fevers, asserted that loss of sleep could actually cause delirium.

Thus, by the end of the eighteenth century a fairly sophisticated conception of delirium had been developed. Hartley provided an excellent descriptive account of it, while Darwin, Hunter, and others developed an explanatory hypothesis linking sleep, dreaming, and delirium. They spelled out this relation, which has been noted in passing by many medical writers from Hippocrates on. We will develop this important theme in the light of present knowledge in the later chapters.

The Nineteenth Century

The main development of the early nineteenth century was the description of *delirium tremens,* a term coined by Sutton (25) in 1813. Romano (26) points out that writers such as Lettsom, Pearson, and Armstrong had provided earlier and even more detailed descriptions of delirium tremens than Sutton. For example, Pearson wrote "Observations on brain fever" in 1801 and had it published in 1813 (27). He offered an accurate description of delirium tremens and stressed its main features: confusion of thoughts, illusions and hallucinations, restlessness, fear, disorientation, and brief lucid intervals. Pearson distinguished brain fever related to alcohol (presumably delirium tremens) from that of "putrid fever," which accompanied infections. Sutton (25) coined the term "delirium tremens" and separated it from phrenitis because he found that it required different treatment: it responded to large and repeated doses of opium, but was made worse by bloodletting. Delirium tremens was also distinguished by marked tremor of the hands. Sutton was convinced that the syndrome was causally related to excessive drinking, or at least to a person's constitutional sensitivity to alcohol. He noted that both delirium tremens and phrenitis were, at the height of the disorder, clinically similar, but differed in that the former did not follow exacerbation of fever, had a less sudden onset, and was accompanied by tremors.

Within twenty years of Sutton's seminal work many writers in England and America published observations on delirium tremens. Hayward (26) proposed a change of name to delirium vigilans, since watchfulness struck him as a characteristic symptom. Coates (26) noted that delirium tremens was produced by cessation of habitual intake of alcohol as well as of narcotics.

Meanwhile, an Irish contemporary of Sutton, Hallaran (28), made distinction between "mental" insanity and that due to primary or secondary disease of the brain. He urged physicians to learn to distinguish mental disorders due to primary or secondary disease of the brain for the purpose of choosing proper treatment. He stressed that delirium was a condition marked by excitement, maniacal symptoms, and hallucinations not unlike those of mental insanity, but was associated with and readily traceable to a bodily disease. Thus, in the early nineteenth century delirium became once more explicitly linked to organic etiology.

Febrile, toxic, alcoholic, and nocturnal senile delirium were all known by the early nineteenth century. In 1834 Dupuytren (29) published in the *Lancet* a translation of his lecture on nervous or traumatic delirium occurring after injury or surgery. He describes seven patients suffering from this disorder and gives an excellent clinical account of it. He notes "confusion of things, places, and persons," insomnia, preoccupation with personally important matters, insensitivity to pain, restlessness, the flushed and animated face, the bright eyes. Dupuytren believed that delirium was transient and its prognosis generally good, but that death could occur for no obvious reason. He was puzzled by lack of fever and of tachycardia in his patients. His favored treatment was a laudanum enema. It should be noted, however, that delirium related to surgical procedures was already mentioned by Paré (16) in the sixteenth century.

Some nineteenth century writers advanced a *unified concept* of delirium, one encompassing the features of delirium, phrenitis, and lethargy of the ancients and their followers. For example, Quain's Dictionary of Medicine (30) presents delirium as a common symptom in many fevers, brain lesions, poisonings, and after epileptic attacks; he describes its three distinct types: low or muttering; delirium tremens; and wild or raving. These three variants represent gradations of psychomotor activity ranging from lethargy to overactivity. Delirium tremens is used in this context to denote an intermediate form, one featuring restlessness, hallucinations, fears, and tremors. Salter (31) and Fothergill (32) wrote excellent clinical papers on the management of delirium based on this modern conception of it.

Three French writers, active in the second half of the nineteenth century, made important contributions to the concept of delirium and allied states. Delasiauve (33) and Chaslin (34) elaborated the concept of "confusion mentale," which the former writer compared to sleep, a basic state on which were superimposed mental phenomena: dreams on sleep, hallucinations on mental confusion. Regis (35) carried the analogy further and coined the term "delire onirique" to underscore the dream-like character of certain confusional states, especially those due to infections and intoxications. The concept of mental confusion implied a core psychological impairment featuring inability to think coherently and logically, reduced perceptual discrimination, spatiotemporal disorientation, and defective memory. Superimposed on this picture one could find hallucinations and dreamlike mentation, which constituted the oneiric features, seen in many delirious patients and typically in delirium tremens. The confusional oneiric syndrome, developed by the French school, could be idiopathic, or secondary to a whole range of organic disorders, or psychogenic. It obviously overlaps but is not coterminous with what we call "delirium." In Germany, Meynert introduced the term "amentia" to designate confusional states

(36). The concept of "acute delirium," introduced in 1845, will be discussed in Chapter 3.

By the end of the nineteenth century the concept of delirium had become well established. This is clearly reflected in an excellent discussion of it in *Tuke's Dictionary of Psychological Medicine* (3), published in 1892. For Tuke the main impairment of delirium lay in the area of intellectual or cognitive functions. Around this basic psychopathological core were clustered the common symptoms: disturbances of attention and perception, restlessness, incoherent speech, and delusions. Delirium was to be viewed as a transient complication of a wide range of somatic disorders. Thus, in contrast to France and Germany, in the English-speaking countries the term "delirium" prevailed.

Worcester (37), an American psychiatrist, gave an exceptionally clear account of delirium in 1889. He lamented that the syndrome was taken for granted by most medical writers who made no effort to differentiate it symptomatically, rather than etiologically, from other forms of insanity. Worcester tried to separate the "essential" from the "accidental" symptoms of delirium. He concluded that the essential abnormalities encompassed sensory disturbances, i.e. illusions and hallucinations, and mental bewilderment or confusion, "with failure to identify surrounding persons and objects." Either one or both of these core abnormalities were invariably present. The accidental symptoms included abnormal emotions, reduced or increased psychomotor activity, delusions, etc. Worcester noted the lucid intervals during which the patient could be "momentarily recalled to consciousness." He found that the emotional state of the delirious patient was often influenced by hallucinations and delusions, and could vary widely from case to case. Some patients were hilarious, some anxious and even terrified, still others displayed despair. They could sustain and inflict injuries in attempts to attack or escape imaginary foes. The patient had as a rule an incomplete, if any, recall of the whole delirious experience, but occasionally could remember the more vivid fragments of it after recovery and refuse to accept that they were not actual happenings. Worcester, like many before him, compared delirium to dreaming and expressed doubt that this was merely a superficial resemblance. He maintained that the term "delirium" referred to a well-defined and constant set of symptoms which distinguished it from most other forms of insanity, such as mania, melancholia, dementia, and delusional states. The differential diagnosis of delirium was the subject of an excellent paper by Hirsch (38).

Thus, by the end of the nineteenth century the clinical syndrome of delirium had been clearly delineated. A few writers ventured beyond the descriptive stage and put forth hypotheses to try to explain the psychopathology of the syndrome. The most prominent such theoretical contribution was made by the famous English neurologist, Hughlings Jackson (39). His work has had a lasting influence on neuropsychiatry in general, and on the interpretation of delirium in particular, and deserves a more thorough discussion.

Jackson viewed mental disorders as the most complex examples of diseases of the nervous system. They resulted from afflictions of the highest nervous centers, those which constitute the physical basis of the mind or consciousness, terms used by Jackson synonymously. The main principles of his theoretical system may be summarized as follows:

In accordance with the theory of evolution, the functional organization of the central nervous system—the "nervous centers" —is arranged hierarchically in three layers or levels: highest, middle, and lowest. The highest centers are the most complex and voluntary, the least organized, and the most susceptible to disorganization and loss. They represent the "climax of nervous evolution" (39, v. 2, p. 46). The mind, or consciousness, is a concomitant of the activity of the highest nervous centers. In every nervous and mental disorder there are two components: the negative and the positive, respectively. The former reflect dissolution, i.e. the reverse of evolution. They represent local or uniform losses of function of the nervous centers. The positive components, or symptoms, represent activity of the intact lower centers. In uniform dissolution there is reversal of the whole nervous system towards the more organized, automatic, and primitive functioning.

Jackson chose delirium to illustrate the application of his

theoretical views to mental disorders. The condition of a delirious patient may be viewed as partly negative and partly positive. The negative part results from some degree of loss of function of the "topmost" layer of the highest centers. Defective orientation, impairment of memory and thinking, and confusion are all negative symptoms, or deficits of consciousness. Misidentification of people and surroundings, illusions, hallucinations, delusions, abnormal emotions, and "extravagant conduct" represent activity of the second layer of the highest centers which has been released from the control of the topmost layer; they reflect the remaining consciousness. The latter is, of course, defective: to be confused implies that one has a defect of consciousness. One may encounter clinically all degrees of defective or reduced consciousness, ranging from "slightest confusion of thought to deepest coma" (39, v. 1, p. 187). Jackson compared the three degrees of defective consciousness to sleep with dreams, deeper sleep with somnambulism, and deep sleep without dreams, respectively. Delirium corresponds to the first two of these levels of reduced consciousness. The less dissolution occasioned by disease, the less negative mentation and the more elaborate the mental state that is remaining. Furthermore, the shallower the dissolution, or the less defective the consciousness, the more evident is the influence on the symptoms of the rate of dissolution, of the patient's personality, and of bodily states and external circumstances. The latter three factors exert a pathoplastic influence on the symptoms of the disorder.

Jackson's theoretical conceptions provided a schema with which to interpret the symptoms of delirium. His concept of the levels or degrees of consciousness became tied closely to acute organic brain syndromes, and especially to delirium. The lower the level, the closer is a patient's state to stupor and coma. The higher the degree of consciousness, the more rich and differentiated are the patient's symptoms and the more expressive of his or her personality, conflicts, wishes, etc. These concepts provide a theoretical basis for a unified view of delirium, whose core abnormality is some degree of reduced consciousness, and in which the relative contribution of positive symptoms varies greatly. One must remember, however, that Jackson applied his hypotheses to *all* mental disorders and not just delirium, which he considered a rather simple example of insanity. Furthermore, he used the terms "consciousness," "mind," and "mentation" synonymously and thus blurred the concept of consciousness. French psychiatrists, such as Ey (40), have applied Jackson's views to psychiatric disorders in general and thus weakened their explanatory power. It seems preferable to confine the concepts of dissolution and of levels of consciousness to delirium.

Twentieth Century

Early in this century a German psychiatrist, Bonhoeffer (41, 42), made the most influential contributions to the whole area of psychopathology due to acute somatic diseases. On the basis of painstaking clinical observations he proposed that such diseases could give rise to one or more of five overlapping psychiatric syndromes which he called "acute exogenous psychic reaction types." They included *delirium, epileptiform excitement, twilight state, hallucinosis,* and *amentia.* "Exogenous" in this context implied origin of the disorder in the body outside the brain, a concept, incidentally, not unlike that advanced by Galen and his later followers. Bonhoeffer observed that the exogenous reaction types differed symptomatically from the so-called endogenous, or functional, mental disorders, and that to diagnose one of them offered presumptive evidence of the presence of a cerebral disorder secondary to a systemic disease. The type of the exogenous syndrome encountered was not diagnostic of any particular physical disease. To put it differently, no organic disease gave rise to a uniquely specific mental disorder. The main common characteristic of the exogenous reactions was a disorder, a clouding, of consciousness. In other words, most exogenous reactions, including delirium, represented disorders of consciousness.

Bonhoeffer's work was a turning point in the history of psychiatry of somatic diseases. His adherence to the clinical method and the ingenuity of his generalizations helped advance this whole area. As Hoch (43) wrote, he had "greatly advanced our knowledge of delirium tremens and of deliria in general." Hoch himself followed Bonhoeffer's lead and investigated delirium produced by drugs (43). He concluded that both delirium tremens and the drug deliria shared the same nucleus despite certain differences: "a constant tendency to dip down to a lower level of consciousness" or "a condition of mental dissociation analogous to dreaming or to the hypnagogic state, in which hallucinations are also present" (43, p. 86).

During the sixty or so years since Bonhoeffer's pioneering work some of his conceptions have been modified and his terminology changed. As Bleuler (44) noted recently, it became clear that not only acute systemic diseases but also cerebral ones, as well as intoxication by drugs and poisons, could give rise to one of the exogenous reaction types. Their list has been modified. The term "amentia" has been dropped by most psychiatrists (36). Bleuler has proposed that the clinical state that this term originally designated should be classified as either delirium or a confusional state. The latter differs from delirium, according to Bleuler, by predominance of incoherent thinking and absence of perceptual abnormalities. The present writer sees no need for such a distinction and will discuss the problem in the section on definition of delirium.

In the United States, Adolf Meyer (45) proposed his own classification of mental disorders, or "mental reaction types," which included the so-called dysergastic reaction. Its prototype was delirium, with hallucinosis as its variant. This class of reactions referred to mental disorders due to "impaired nutritive and circulatory support" of the brain. Meyer's term embraced and replaced "exogenic psychoses," "symptomatic psychoses," "acute delirious mania," delirium due to fever and drugs, "toxic-infectious psychoses," and "infective-exhaustive psychoses" (45). The terms "delirium" and "dysergastic reaction" became synonymous, but the latter term never took hold and delirium remained as the main designation for the acute organic mental disorders.

A classic clinical study, quoted in many textbooks to this day, was that by Wolff and Curran (46), published in 1935. It is a fine example of meticulous description of clinical phenomena of delirium, but it has obvious flaws. The study was done on a group of patients who had been admitted to psychiatric wards presumably because of their severely disturbed and disturbing behavior. Furthermore, nearly one-third of these patients had abused alcohol, which was considered causally related to the delirium. Thus, the sample was highly skewed and could hardly be regarded as representative of the average delirious patients encountered in medical and surgical settings. While the description of the patients' symptoms was no doubt accurate, it was inevitably heavily biased in favor of the more flamboyant features of delirium, such as hallucinations, restlessness, excitement, incoherence, etc. These symptoms have been uncritically quoted from the Wolff and Curran study in textbook after textbook and helped create an unbalanced conception of the syndrome. As a result, the quiet delirious patient who disturbs nobody tends to be overlooked and undiagnosed. Engel and Romano (47) deserve credit for having tried to correct this misconception, but it takes decades before new findings, which are at variance with the popular notions, find their place in the textbooks.

Between about 1940 and 1946 a group of American investigators, led by Engel and Romano, carried out pioneering research on delirium. This work was published in a series of papers and summarized in an article which appeared in 1959, and it has been a standard reference on the subject since (47). These researchers attempted to correlate clinical, psychological, and encephalographic data in patients with delirium due to various physical illnesses. Their approach combined clinical and experimental methods on a scale not attempted in the studies of delirium before. Their findings, first summarized in 1945 (48), led them to the following main conclusions: delirium is a disturbance in the level of consciousness and depends on the presence of a cerebral disorder. The level of consciousness, established clinically by responses to tests of cognitive functions, corresponds with the degree of slowing of the EEG. A derangement of cerebral metabolism underlies delirium in all cases and is reflected in cognitive impairment and EEG slowing, both of which tend to vary simultaneously. Psychiatric symptomatology of delirium is related to the increased fluctuation in the level of awareness. Psychologic variables correlating best with the slowing of the EEG frequency are attention, memory, and comprehension. The most significant EEG change in delirium is a relative shift to the lower frequencies of the background activity as compared to the subject's premorbid mean frequency. And finally, manifest behavior of a delirious patient may range from overactivity to underactivity and stupor.

The above studies were a breakthrough in that they went beyond the purely descriptive approach and initiated a scientific inquiry into the pathophysiological mechanisms underlying delirium, and on their measurable indicators which could have diagnostic applications. Furthermore, these studies reaffirmed a *unified concept* of the syndrome of delirium, one which transcends superficial variability of its behavioral manifestations, such as the level of psychomotor activity, and is based on essential psychopathological characteristics (47). Unfortunately, the investigators soon abandoned this field of research and have found relatively few successors who would extend their findings. In fact, no comparably extensive studies of the syndrome have been reported in the English literature in the past thirty years.

The last few decades have seen studies of delirium of various specific etiologies, such as drugs, withdrawal from alcohol, sedatives and hypnotics, metabolic disorders, etc. Yet there have been remarkably few investigations of the syndrome as a whole. Trends in psychiatric theory and research, especially in the United States, have bypassed mental disorders due to somatic diseases. This situation is changing as a result of the growing interest in geriatric psychiatry and liaison work with medicine, that is two areas of clinical psychiatry which have to deal with the diagnostic and therapeutic problems posed by delirium of many etiologies. A great deal of information relevant to delirium has accumulated in the last thirty years. One need only mention psychopharmacology, psychophysiology of sleep, sensory deprivation, and the knowledge about brain-behavior relationships. Some of this more recent work as it pertains to delirium was reviewed by this writer in 1967 (49).

Progress in the knowledge about delirium has been slow and hampered to a large extent by the inconsistent terminology and unclear diagnostic criteria. Despite its frequency and clinical importance, it has attracted relatively few investigators. This issue was eloquently stated by Gallway (50) in 1838:

> The subject of delirium is generally looked upon by the practical physician as one of the most obscure in the chain of morbid

phenomena he has to deal with; whilst the frequency of its occurrence under various diseased conditions of the system renders the affection not a little familiar to his eye. My object in approaching so acknowledged a terra incognita is not, I regret to say, that I have any fresh contribution towards its elucidation to bring into the field, but rather to awaken a more lively inquiry amongst the profession as to its real nature and causes.

This quotation sums up well the purpose of this book, which has been written in the hope that it will stimulate interest and research in a syndrome that illustrates the inseparable relationship of brain and mind, of soma and psyche.

REFERENCES

1. Murray, J.A.H., Ed.: *A New English Dictionary on Historical Principles.* Vol. 3, p. 165. Oxford, Clarendon Press, 1897.
2. Celsus: *De Medicina.* 3 vols. Translated by W.G. Spencer. London, Heinemann, 1938.
3. Tuke, D.H.: *A Dictionary of Psychological Medicine.* Philadelphia, Blakiston, 1892.
4. Gowers, W.R.: *A Manual of Diseases of the Nervous System.* Philadelphia, Blakiston, 1888.
5. Hinsie, L.E. and Campbell, R.J.: *Psychiatric Dictionary.* 3rd edition. New York, Oxford University Press, 1960.
6. Hunter, R. and Macalpine, I.: *Three Hundred Years of Psychiatry, 1535-1860.* London, Oxford University Press, 1963.
7. Whitwell, J.R.: *Historical Notes on Psychiatry.* Philadelphia, Blakiston, 1937.
8. Mettler, C.C.: *History of Medicine; A Correlative Text, Arranged According to Subjects.* Philadelphia, Blakiston, 1947.
9. *The Medical Works of Hippocrates.* Translated by J. Chadwick and W.N. Mann. Oxford, Blackwell, 1950.
10. Sprengell, C.: *The Aphorisms of Hippocrates, and the Sentences of Celsus.* 2nd edition. London, Wilkin, Bonwick, Birt, et al., 1735.
11. *The Extant Works of Aretaeus, the Cappadocian.* Edited by F. Adams. London, Sydenham Society, 1861.
12. Liebowitz, J.O.: Studies in the history of alcoholism. II: Acute alcoholism in ancient Greek and Roman medicine. *Br J Addict* 62:83-86, 1967.
13. Hankoff, L.D.: Ancient descriptions of organic brain syndrome: The "Kordiakos" of the Talmud. *Am J Psychiatry* 129:147-150, 1972.

14. Barrough, P.: *The Method of Physick.* 3rd edition. London, Field, 1596.

15. Haunoldt, A.: *De Delirio.* Witerbergae, Gronenbergii, 1593.

16. *The Works of That Famous Chirurgion Ambrose Parey.* Translated by T. Johnson. London, Cotes and Young, 1634.

17. Willis, T.: *Two Discourses Concerning the Soul of Brutes.* London, Bring, Harper and Leigh, 1683.

18. Hartley, D.: *Observations on Man, His Duty, and His Expectations.* London, Leake and Frederick, 1749.

19. Cheyne, G.: *An Essay on Health and Long Life.* London, Strahan, 1725.

20. Frings, P.: *A Treatise on Phrensy.* London, Gardner, 1746.

21. Darwin, E.: *Zoonomia; or, the Laws of Organic Life.* Vol. 1. London, Johnson, 1794.

22. Hunter, J.: *The Work of John Hunter, F.R.S.* Vol. 1. Edited by J.F. Palmer. London, Longman, Rees, Orme, Brown, Green, and Longman, 1835.

23. Rush, B.: *Medical Inquiries and Observations upon the Diseases of the Mind.* Philadelphia, Kimber & Richardson, 1812.

24. Fordyce, G.: *Five Dissertations on Fever.* 2nd American edition. Boston, Bedlington and Ewer, 1823.

25. Sutton, T.: *Tracts on Delirium Tremens, on Peritonitis and on Some Other Inflammatory Affections.* London, Underwood, 1813.

26. Romano, J.: Early contributions to the study of delirium tremens. *The Annals of Medical History, Third Series, 3*:128-139, 1941.

27. Pearson, S.B.: Observations on brain fever. *Edinburgh M & SJ*: 9:326-332, 1813.

28. Hallaran, W.S.: *Practical Observations on the Causes and Cure of Insanity.* Cork, Hodges & M'Arthur, 1818.

29. Dupuytren, B.G.: On nervous delirium (traumatic delirium)—Successful employment of laudanum lavements. *Lancet 1*:919-923, 1834.

30. Quain, R., Editor: *A Dictionary of Medicine.* 7th edition. New York, Appleton, 1884.

31. Salter, T.: Practical observations on delirium. *Prov Med & Surg J 1*:677-784, 1850.

32. Fothergill, J.M.: The management of delirium. *The Practitioner 13*: 400-408, 1874.

33. Delasiauve, from Chaslin, P.: *La Confusion Mentale Primitive.* Paris, Asselin et Houzeau, 1895.
34. Chaslin, P.: *La Confusion Mentale Primitive.* Paris, Asselin et Houzeau, 1895.
35. Regis, E.: *Précis de Psychiatrie.* 6th edition. Paris, Doin, 1923, pp. 383-387.
36. Pappenheim, E.: On Meynert's amentia. *Int J Neurol* 9:310-326, 1975.
37. Worcester, W.L.: Delirium. *Am J Insanity* 46:22-27, 1889.
38. Hirsch, W.: A Study of Delirium. *The New York Med J* 70:109-115, 1899.
39. Jackson, J.H.: *Selected Writings.* 2 vols. Edited by J. Taylor. London, Hodder and Stoughton, 1932.
40. Ey, H.: "Disorders of Consciousness in Psychiatry," in P.J. Vinken and G.W. Bruyn, Eds., *Handbook of Neurology*, Vol. 3. Amsterdam, North Holland Publishing Co., 1969, pp. 112-136.
41. Bonhoeffer, K.: *Die Geistesstorungen der Gewonheitstrinker.* Jena, Fischer, 1901.
42. Bonhoeffer, K.: "Die Psychosen im Gefolge von akuten Infektionen, Allgemeinerkrankungen und inneren Erkrankungen." In Aschaffenburg, G.L., Ed. *Handbuch der Psychiatrie*, Spez. Teil 3, pp. 1-60. Leipzig, Deuticke, 1912.
43. Hoch, A.: A study of some cases of delirium produced by drugs. *Studies in Psychiatry, 1*:75-93, 1912.
44. Bleuler, M.: "Acute Mental Concomitants of Physical Disease." In Benson, D.F. and Blumer, D., Eds. *Psychiatric Aspects of Neurological Disease.* New York, Grune & Stratton, 1975, pp. 37-61.
45. Meyer, A.: *Collected Papers*, Vol. 3, pp. 304-305. Winters, E.E., Ed. Baltimore, Johns Hopkins Press, 1951.
46. Wolff, H.G., and Curran, D.: Nature of delirium and allied states. The dysergastic reaction. *AMA Arch Neurol Psychiatry* 33:1175-1215, 1935.
47. Engel, G.L., and Romano, J.: Delirium, a syndrome of cerebral insufficiency. *J Chron Dis* 9:260-277, 1959.
48. Romano, J., and Engel, G.L.: Physiologic and psychologic considerations of delirium. *Med Clin N Am* 28:629-638, 1944.
49. Lipowski, Z.J.: Delirium, clouding of consciousness and confusion. *J Nerv Ment Dis 145*:227-255, 1967.
50. Gallway, M.B.: Nature and treatment of delirium. *Lond Med Gazette 1*:46-49, 1838.

Additional References

Aurelianus, C. *On Acute Diseases and on Chronic Diseases.* Edited by I.E. Drabkin. Chicago, University of Chicago Press, 1950.

Diethelm, O. *Medical Dissertations of Psychiatric Interest Printed Before 1750.* Basel, Karger, 1971.

Greiner, F.C. *Der Traum und das Fieberhafte Irreseyn.* Altenburg, F.A. Brockhaus, 1817.

Mickle, J. Mental wandering. *Brain 24*:1-26, 1901.

Müller, F.C. *Psychopathologie des Bewusstseins.* Leipzig, A. Abel, 1889.

Orschansky, J. Ueber Bewusstseinsstörungen und deren Beziehungen zur Verrücktheit und Dementia. *Arch Psychiatr 20*:309-353, 1889.

Quincy, J. *Lexicon Physico-Medicum: or, A New Medical Dictionary,* 7th Edition. London, Longman, 1757.

Rees, A. *The Cyclopedia; or Universal Dictionary of Arts, Sciences, and Literature.* First American Edition. Vol. 12. Philadelphia, S.F. Bradford, 1818.

Verco, A. Delirium. *St. Bart Hosp Rep (Lond) 13*:332-342, 1877.

Winslow, F. *On Obscure Diseases of the Brain and Disorders of the Mind.* Philadelphia, Blanchard & Lea, 1860.

CHAPTER 2

DEFINITION OF DELIRIUM

DELIRIUM AS AN ORGANIC MENTAL DISORDER
(ORGANIC BRAIN SYNDROME)

In Chapter 1 the evolution of the concept of delirium was traced back to its earliest recorded descriptions over 2,000 years ago. It became evident that despite shifting meanings and resulting ambiguity of the term the cluster of symptoms which it has come to designate has been consistently described over the ages and represents a clear-cut syndrome. Furthermore, this syndrome has been linked from the beginning with physical illness and is usually considered to represent behavioral manifestations of acute cerebral dysfunction due to primary brain disease, or one secondary to systemic. Thus, delirium has been regarded as an organic mental disorder par excellence. This view prevailed despite repeated failure to find gross cerebral pathology in many cases of delirium that came to autopsy. Fordyce (1), for example, writing in the early nineteenth century, marvelled at the commonly normal appearance of the brain in patients dying in febrile delirium and wondered if the condition might arise in these cases as an "affection of the mind only."

Since the beginning of this century it has been customary to divide mental disorders into organic and functional, respectively. This nosological approach has some obvious practical advantages in that it influences diagnostic procedures and treatment. To identify a psychiatric disorder as "organic" directs attention of the clinician to the presumed underlying physical illness and its treatment, if such be currently available. It is assumed that an organic mental disorder arises as a result of a direct insult or injury, physical or chemical, to the cerebral substrate of the mental or psychological processes and functions, namely cognition, motivation, emotion, and psychomotor activity.

31

The resulting psychopathology could not be accounted for by using explanations involving psychological and social concepts and hypotheses (2). To express it differently, a disorder of cerebral function due to a physical, chemical, or biological noxious agent is a necessary, if not always sufficient, condition for the occurrence of an organic mental disorder. By contrast, the so-called functional psychiatric disorders may be at least in part cogently explained by invoking the personal meaning for the individual of the internal and external information inputs, and the resulting strivings, conflicts, emotions, and other consequences expressed in psychological terms (2).

A definition of delirium rests on the above assumptions and nosological concepts. To define it clearly involves establishing its place in the whole class of organic mental disorders or, as they are currently called, organic brain syndromes. A discussion of this classification follows.

CLASSIFICATION OF ORGANIC MENTAL DISORDERS (ORGANIC BRAIN SYNDROMES)

The current official classification of mental disorders of the American Psychiatric Association (3) contains a separate class named "Organic Brain Syndromes." They are said to be manifested by the following psychological characteristics: impairment of orientation, memory, all intellectual functions, and judgment, and lability and shallowness of affect. These so-called basic symptoms are stated to be present to some degree regardless of the level of severity of the syndrome. In fact, the above set of symptoms is referred to as "the organic brain syndrome," one which usually arises from diffuse impairment of cerebral function of any cause. Psychotic symptoms and disturbed behavior may be associated with the basic syndrome.

The official classification makes a distinction between "acute" and "chronic" brain disorders, respectively. The former term implies reversibility; the latter implies irreversibility of the brain pathology and its concomitant brain syndrome. Although delirium is not mentioned in this classification, it is roughly equivalent to the acute organic brain syndrome, since it contains the basic defining features and is reversible.

The present classification is currently in the process of revision and will be replaced by a new edition, DSM-III, which is expected to come into effect in 1979. A draft of the new classification, which the present writer has coauthored, contains a thorough revision of the class of organic brain syndromes (4). The present classification of these syndromes has serious flaws discussed in detail elsewhere (5, 6). The proposed revision is worth presenting here in the anticipation that it will become official.

The whole class of disorders under discussion will be referred to as "Organic Mental Disorders." Within this class it is proposed to distinguish seven Organic Brain Syndromes (OBS) to be grouped as follows:

1. OBS with relatively *global cognitive* impairment
   (a) Delirium
   (b) Dementia
2. OBS with relatively *selective cognitive* deficit or abnormality
   (a) Amnestic Syndrome
   (b) Organic Hallucinosis
3. OBS with predominantly *noncognitive* psychopathological features
   (a) Organic Delusional Syndrome
   (b) Organic Affective Syndrome
   (c) Organic Personality Syndrome

The foregoing classification has advantages, on logical and clinical grounds, over the current one in that it gives justice to the undeniable differences in psychopathological manifestations of cerebral disorders of different extent and localization. There is no uniform, invariable "organic brain syndrome" as the current official classification would have us believe. Psychiatric manifestations of cerebral disorders are not homogeneous, but on the contrary, display considerable heterogeneity which needs to be acknowledged in any system of classification to be used for diagnosis, treatment, communication, and research.

The organic mental disorders are separated from other classes of psychiatric conditions on logical and pragmatic grounds: logical, since the organic disorders may not be diagnosed unless a concurrent cerebral dysfunction can be demonstrated by the use of medical diagnostic techniques, or the patient is known to have been exposed to a cerebral insult prior to the onset of the psychiatric disorder. In both instances a causal relationship between the cerebral dysfunction or damage and the psychiatric disturbance is assumed. The so-called functional mental disorders cannot be shown at present to be caused by a cerebral disorder. Pragmatically, organic disorders imply that a brain disorder is present and needs to be identified if the concurrent organic brain syndrome is to be treated effectively.

Delirium is an organic mental disorder par excellence. It comprises all the psychological deficits and abnormalities which have been for centuries recognized as due to disturbed brain function. These psychopathological features reflect defective information processing or impaired cognitive functioning. Unfortunately, semantic problems have long beset the whole area of organic mental disorders, including delirium. A terminological muddle has partly impeded progress in the elucidation of the pathophysiology of delirium. Thus, the issues of terminology and definition have to be addressed.

DEFINITION OF DELIRIUM

Delirium is defined here as a *psychiatric syndrome characterized by a transient disorganization of a wide range of cognitive functions due to widespread derangement of cerebral metabolism.* The disorganization is manifested by an impaired ability to receive, select, process, and retain ongoing internal and external information inputs, and to integrate them meaningfully with one's previous knowledge for the purpose of sustained goal-directed activity. This impairment usually fluctuates over the course of a day and is most marked at night or in a darkened room (5, 6).

The above definition has three major components which need to be made explicit. Delirium designates a cluster of psychological symptoms which tend to occur together. These symptoms are purely descriptive and refer to the core psychological abnormalities in delirium, namely those pertaining to cognitive function, to remembering, thinking, and perceiving.

Thus, delirium is in this sense a descriptive psychiatric term. The word "transient" in the definition refers to the all-important time dimension of the syndrome. Delirium is never a chronic disorder going on for years. This is a defining characteristic noted from the time the term was first used in the literature. Finally, the definition contains a reference to etiology by linking delirium to disturbance of cerebral metabolism. This reference implies that it should be possible to demonstrate by independent means, biochemical, electrophysiological, etc., that is to say by nonpsychological techniques, that a derangement of cerebral metabolism closely antedates and/or coexists with the clinical syndrome of delirium.

Thus, delirium is an acute psychiatric syndrome characterized by global cognitive dysfunction and caused by a cerebral disorder, either primary or secondary to systemic.

Since the term "delirium" is still used quite inconsistently in the psychiatric and medical literature, it is essential to spell out its diagnostic features as clearly as possible. This will be done in Chapter 3, in which the key clinical features of the syndrome will be discussed in detail and its diagnostic criteria will be operationally defined. It is still necessary at this point to review briefly the various terms that have been used by contemporary writers to designate syndromes identical or overlapping with delirium.

CONFUSIONAL STATES

Several terms overlapping, if not synonymous, with delirium have been used in the psychiatric and medical English-language literature: acute organic brain syndrome, acute confusional state, toxic psychosis, infective-exhaustive psychosis, exogenous or symptomatic psychosis, encephalopathy. These are but the most popular terms still encountered. They have contributed to the semantic muddle plaguing the area of psychopathology of acute cerebral disorders. Historically, delirium is by far the oldest term, as was amply documented in Chapter 1. The other terms need to be discussed briefly to indicate their relation to delirium as here defined.

Acute confusional state is a term most often substituted for delirium. An authoritative recent monograph on stupor and coma (7) speaks of acute or subacute confusional state as a manifestation of moderately advanced clouding of consciousness, that is, a state of reduced wakefulness or awareness. The confusional state is said to feature reduced attention span, misinterpretation of stimuli, bewilderment, disorientation and defective memory (7, p. 4). Delirium is defined as a more florid expression of clouded consciousness than a confusional state. Thus the difference between the two syndromes is presented as being one of degree, a distinction which is quite vague and arbitrary. Adams and Victor (8, p. 149) proposed a somewhat different terminology. For them "confusion" designates a person's incapacity to think with his or her accustomed speed and clarity. They define a confusional state as one characterized by reduced alertness and psychomotor activity. They refer to delirium as a special type of confusional state featuring gross disorientation, misperceptions, and psychomotor and autonomic nervous system hyperactivity. Thus delirium is viewed by these authors as a *variant* of acute confusional states, which in addition comprise the confusional state and beclouded dementia. These three syndromes are said to be characterized mainly by clouding of consciousness. It is of note that other authorities consider the confusional state and delirium to be manifestations of such clouding (7). Adams and Victor acknowledge that delirium and acute confusional state do overlap and may be difficult to tell apart, but should be distinguished since they involve different pathogenic mechanisms and pathways.

This distinction reflects a long tradition, one going back to Celsus in the first century A.D. We saw in Chapter 1, how the medical writers from antiquity and until the last century tended to distinguish between phrenitis or delirium on the one hand, and lethargus on the other. It appears that what contemporary authorities, such as Adams and Victor (8) or Bleuler (9), call "confusional state" is a modern derivative of lethargus. To compound the problem further, some European authors, especially French and Scandinavian, use the term "confusional state" or "simple confusion" in regard to certain *psychogenic* mental disorders. A Russian psychiatrist, Orschansky (10), published in 1889 an excellent description of what he called "clouding of consciousness," the clinical manifestations of which he referred to as "geistige Verwirrtheit," i.e. mental confusion. He stated that this symptom complex usually followed a strong affect and represented a phase or stadium of an acute or chronic psychosis, especially one occurring on the basis of hysteria, neurasthenia, or epilepsy. Many writers have since applied the term "confusional state" to a mental disorder bearing a resemblance to delirium but lacking objective evidence of concurrent cerebral disorder and usually assigned to psychic causes, such as a personal calamity, a terrifying experience occasioned by various natural catastrophes, etc. (11, 12, 13, 14). French authors use the term "bouffées délirantes" to refer to such states (15).

To avoid semantic confusion the present writer has advocated a unified concept of delirium, previously advanced by Engel and Romano (16). He proposes that the term delirium should encompass what others have called organic acute confusional states. There is no logical reason to distinguish those states from delirium since they all share certain core psychopathological features. The latter include impairment of a broad spectrum of cognitive functions as well as abnormalities of psychomotor behavior, alertness, and vigilance; an acute onset; a tendency of the symptoms to fluctuate over the course of a day; a relatively brief duration; and medical, i.e. nonpsychological, evidence of disordered brain function. Delirium is a syndrome reflecting a disorganization of activating and integrative cerebral processes. It is proposed that the ancient term "delirium" be used to designate this psychopathological syndrome.

To resolve the controversy, it is proposed to distinguish within the syndrome of delirium two major subtypes: *hyperactive* and *hypoactive*, respectively (6). The latter features reduced alertness, vigilance, and psychomotor activity. The former is characterized by hypervigilance, psychomotor overactivity, hyperresponsitivity to stimuli, increased cortical excitation, and sympathetic nervous system arousal. The two variants represent opposite ends of a spectrum of behavioral manifestations of dissolution of highest nervous activity in Hughlings Jackson's sense. They share a crucial core of psychopathology, namely disruption of normal cognitive processes, or information processing. They differ in regard to the level of psychomotor activity and cerebral cortical excitation or arousal. One may postulate that these differences reflect distinct pathophysiological changes in the brain. This whole issue will be taken up again in the later chapters. For the time being it may suffice to use an analogy. There are two behaviorally distinct forms of depressive psychosis: retarded and agitated, respectively. One could hardly imagine more different clinical pictures than those of depressive stupor on the one hand, and of severely agitated depression on the other. Yet they are both considered manifestations of the same basic disorder, a depressive psychosis. Unless and until research results force us to modify our views, we propose to view the two variants of delirium analogously to the two forms of psychotic depression.

The other related terms need to be dealt with only briefly. *Toxic psychosis* is a term most often used in reference to organic mental disorders caused by drugs and poisons. The use of this ambiguous term should be discouraged since it does not refer to any particular descriptive or etiologic class of disorders, but conceals several syndromes, including delirium, of various etiologies. *Infective-exhaustive psychosis* is an obsolete term which used to refer to organic mental disorders due to systemic infections (17). *Encephalopathy* is a word used mostly by neurologists and not consistently by anybody. It means literally "brain disease" and is used most often in reference to metabolic, infectious, and toxic disorders of the brain in which the latter is diffusely involved and the clinical manifestations typically include a disorder of consciousness or awareness, such as delirium, stupor, or coma, a variety of focal neurological signs, and symptoms such as convulsions. *Exogenous* or *symptomatic* psychoses are terms used mostly by German-speaking writers and designate organic mental disorders due to acute physical illnesses.

In summary, the term "delirium" is used here to designate an organic brain syndrome of acute onset and transient duration, characterized by global cognitive impairment, and due to widespread disturbance of cerebral metabolism. The term encompasses "acute confusional states" and "simple confusion" of other authors, provided that they use these terms to designate organic mental disorders. Diagnostic criteria for the syndrome are given in Chapter 3.

REFERENCES

1. Fordyce, G.: *Five Dissertations on Fever.* 2nd American edition. Boston, Bedlington and Ewes, 1823.
2. Lipowski, Z.J.: Psychiatry of somatic diseases: epidemiology, pathogenesis, classification. *Compr Psychiatry 16*:105-124, 1975.
3. *Diagnostic and Statistical Manual of Mental Disorders.* 2nd edition. Washington, D.C., American Psychiatric Association, 1968.
4. *DSM-111 Draft.* Task Force on Nomenclature and Statistics. American Psychiatric Association. January, 1978.
5. Lipowski, Z.J.: Organic brain syndromes: A reformulation. *Compr Psychiatry, 19*:309-322, 1978.
6. Lipowski, Z.J.: "Organic Brain Syndromes: Overview and Classification." In Benson, D.F., and Blumer, D., Eds. *Psychiatric Aspects of Neurological Disease.* New York, Grune and Stratton, 1975, pp. 11-35.
7. Plum, F. and Posner, J.B.: *Diagnosis of Stupor and Coma.* 2nd edition. Philadelphia, Davis, 1972.
8. Adams, R.D. and Victor, M.: "Delirium and Other Acute Confusional States." In Harrison's *Principles of Internal Medicine.* 7th edition. Wintrobe, M.M., Thorn, G.W., Adams, R.D., et al., Eds. New York, McGraw-Hill, 1974, pp. 149-156.
9. Bleuler, M.: "Acute Mental Concomitants of Physical Disease." In Benson, D.F. and Blumer, D., Eds. *Psychiatric Aspects of Neurological Disease.* New York, Grune & Stratton, 1975, pp. 37-61.
10. Orschansky, J.: Ueber Bewusstseins-stoerungen und deren Beziehungen zur Verruecktheit und Dementia. *Arch f Psychiatr 20*:309-353, 1889.
11. Carlson, H.B.: The relationship of the acute confusional state to ego development. *Int J Psychoanal 42*:517-536, 1961.
12. Carlson, H.B.: Identity-confusion (acute confusional state): Research design for identification of the syndrome and analysis of preliminary results. *Int J Neuropsychiatry 1*:452-465, 1965.
13. Kasanin, J.: The syndrome of episodic confusions. *Am J Psychiatry 93*:625-638, 1936.
14. Skoog, G.: The course of acute confusional states. *Acta Psychiatr Scand, Suppl 203*:29-32, 1968.
15. Ey, H.: *Etudes Psychiatriques 3.* Paris, Désclées de Brouwer, 1952, pp. 323-348.
16. Engel, G.L. and Romano, J.: Delirium, a syndrome of cerebral in-

sufficiency. *J Chronic Dis.* 9:260-277, 1959.

17. Hinsie, L.E. and Campbell, R.J.: *Psychiatric Dictionary.* 3rd edition. New York, Oxford University Press, 1960, p. 606.

Additional References

Lipowski, Z.J. "Organic Mental Disorders: Introduction and Review of Syndromes." In Freedman, A.M., Kaplan, H.I., and Sadock, B.J., Eds., *Comprehensive Textbook of Psychiatry,* 3rd Edition. Baltimore, Williams & Wilkins, in press.

Lishman, W.A. *Organic Psychiatry.* Oxford, Blackwell Scientific Publ., 1978.

Livesley, B. The pathogenesis of brain failure in the aged. *Age Ageing* (Suppl) 6:9-19, 1977.

CHAPTER 3

CLINICAL FEATURES

T HE HISTORICAL OUTLINE in Chapter 1 has traced the evolution of the concept of delirium as a clinical syndrome. Recurrent ambiguity in the usage of the term over the centuries has been highlighted. The shifting meaning has likely reflected the rather bewildering variability in the clinical manifestations of delirium summed up so well by Fothergill (1) 100 years ago: ". . . each case differs somewhat from every other case, and there are peculiarities in each and every one. In order, then, to meet such cases with a fair attention to their needs, the first thing requisite is a pretty clear comprehension of delirium as a whole." The purpose of this chapter is to try and achieve just that by means of a composite description of the syndrome, stress on its essential features, and attention to its clinical variants.

ESSENTIAL CHARACTERISTICS

The following features of delirium are considered essential:
1. Impaired awareness of self and surroundings and their relationships.
2. Impairment of memory.
3. Disturbance of attention.
4. Impairment of directed thinking.
5. Diminished perceptual discrimination with a tendency to illusions and hallucinations.
6. Impairment of spatiotemporal orientation.
7. Increased or decreased alertness.
8. Sleep disturbance, usually drowsiness during the day, or insomnia at night, or both.
9. Relatively rapid fluctuations in awareness and severity of symptoms (2) through (7) during daytime and tendency

to their exacerbation at night or in the dark.
10. Acute onset and relatively short duration.
11. Laboratory evidence of cerebral dysfunction, especially
     diffuse changes of background activity in the electro-
     encephalogram.

The above list of essential features reflects the core psychological abnormality in delirium, viz. *defective ability to extract,
process, retain, and retrieve information about oneself and one's
environment.* As there are multiple cognitive deficits and abnormalities in delirium, i.e. those involving perceiving, remembering, and thinking, one may speak of global cognitive impairment (2) or reduced level of cognition (3). As a result of these
core deficits the patient finds it difficult, if not impossible, to
integrate ongoing stimulus input with previously acquired knowledge and experience, or learning, and thus to act rationally.
Thus, the patient is to some extent disabled by his or her cognitive impairment and in need of protection. The following account
of the symptoms and course of delirium will flesh out the rather
abstract concepts discussed so far.

SYMPTOMS AND COURSE

The onset of delirium is typically rapid, usually a matter of
hours or a few days. The mode of onset depends to some extent
on the cause. Delirium resulting from a concussion or acute
intoxication will come on suddenly while that occurring in the
course of an infection or metabolic encephalopathy may have a
more gradual onset. In the latter case, one may usually distinguish a *prodromal phase* during which the patient tends to
have difficulty in concentration and thinking clearly, feels anxious
and restless, and may complain of irritability, fatigue, hypersensitivity to lights and sounds, drowsiness, insomnia and vivid
dreams, or nightmares, or even transient hallucinations. Many of
us have experienced such symptoms in the course of a febrile
illness and can attest to their unpleasantness. Every mental
effort is unwelcome and one tends to drift from reverie to sleep
and back. At night one is apt to wake up startled, sometimes
remembering a vivid and likely an unpleasant dream, and wonder
where one is.

The patient may never progress beyond the prodromal symptoms, or the latter may increase in intensity and the patient grows more restless or drowsy, awareness of time becomes blurred, thinking increasingly escapes attempts at controlling it, attention waxes and wanes, and illusions and hallucinations may now appear. Full-blown delirium may first become manifest at night. The patient wakes up and finds it difficult to tell if he or she is still dreaming. The dreams may now continue as hallucinations, and the patient tends to respond to their content with appropriate emotion, often fear, and actions, such as an attempt to get out of bed and run away. This is particularly likely to happen if the person is in an unfamiliar place, such as a hospital, and tries desperately to leave and find a familiar environment. As Fothergill (1) put it so well, "Every sick person craves ardently to be at home amidst relatives and friends; and in delirium the craving commonly takes the direction of an attempt to get away home by immediate escape. . . ." If such behavior occurs on a hospital ward, the night nurse becomes alarmed, notes in the chart that the patient is confused, and asks the doctor on call to prescribe a sedative. If the patient tries to resist attempts to get him or her back to bed, a wild struggle and a hefty dose of parenteral sedation are liable to follow. The patient is likely to wake up the next morning being relatively lucid and cooperative, and the whole nocturnal episode is apt to be forgotten unless it recurs during the next night or the patient shows evidence of being grossly disturbed on awakening.

A mildly delirious patient may be aware of and alarmed by the increasing difficulty in controlling his or her thoughts, perceptions, and memory, and react to the awareness of these difficulties with anxiety, embarrassment, and attempts at giving appearance of being normal. When spoken to, the patient may try to conceal his or her confusion by answering questions briefly and avoiding topics which might expose faulty memory and grasp. Some patients try more actively to cover up their cognitive deficits by voicing physical complaints or grumbling about the hospital. When an examiner tries to assess such a patient's mental state by asking questions on orientation, memory, etc., the patient often evades the issue by trying to change the

subject or return the questions, by jokes or sarcasms, by embark-
ing on a rambling account of some familiar topic, and occasionally
by an outburst of anger and abusive language. Other patients
answer questions slowly and hesitantly and may actually complain about being forgetful and confused. People vary markedly
in their reactions, emotional and behavioral, and in their coping
strategies evoked by subjective awareness of cognitive impairment. These individual differences in response contribute to
the striking variability of the clinical manifestations of delirium.

As delirium progresses in severity a number of symptoms
appear that increase the subjective sense and objective evidence
of confusion. The word "confusion" is commonly used in this
context by both doctors and patients. It is a term devoid of
precise meaning, one which usually implies a combination of
muddled thinking, difficulty in grasping one's situation, forgetfulness, and some degree of disorientation for time, place, and
person. The patient becomes disoriented for time before being
unable to identify his whereabouts and people around him. At
first there is difficulty in naming the correct day of the week and
the date, and this can progress to an inability to identify the
month, the season, and the year. The patient either admits not
knowing these things or confabulates, i.e. gives grossly incorrect
answers but insists, with varying degrees of conviction, that
they are accurate. Orientation for place is liable to be impaired
once that for time is unequivocally faulty. The patient thinks
he or she is at home instead of in the hospital, or in a hotel, or
in a hospital with which he or she is most familiar. This tendency
to misidentify the unfamiliar for the familiar surroundings is
quite characteristic of delirium. As delirum becomes severe,
not only the place but also the surroundng people become
misidentified. Nurses and doctors are mistaken for relatives or
friends, or are viewed as strangers engaged in other than their
true occupations: a doctor may be thought to be a chef because
of his white coat, while nurses are not uncommonly misidentified
as maids or waitresses. Sometimes the patient includes members
of the staff into his or her dream-like, hallucinatory, and delusional experience and refers to the doctors as butchers and the
nurses as prostitutes, for example. Such errors offend some

members of the clinical staff even though they obviously reflect the patient's inner experience and are not likely to be intentionally offensive. In the most severe delirium the patient cannot recognize his or her next-of-kin and close friends, and rarely indeed loses the sense of his or her own identity.

As delirium worsens, the patient becomes increasingly distractible and either drowsy or, on the contrary, hyperalert and excited. In either case, however, he or she has difficulty in deploying, fixing, holding, and shifting attention. This is obvious to the examiner who finds that the patient cannot sustain a train of thought for more than a brief period. Uncontrolled thoughts or hallucinations may intrude, the question or the beginning of the sentence is forgotten, or the patient may simply doze off. Concurrently, thinking becomes increasingly labored and slow, or rapid but incoherent. Perceptual discrimination is affected and the patient's capacity to integrate percepts and make sense of them wanes. Perceptual abnormalities in the form of illusions and hallucinations, most commonly visual but often mixed with auditory and other misperceptions, are apt to appear at this stage, especially at night when they may merge with dreams. The patient may be aware of hallucinating and frightened or embarrassed by the fact, or accept the hallucinations as real happenings and react to them accordingly, namely try to speak to, call, or shout at hallucinated figures, follow them with the eyes, reach out to them, or try to escape them. Fear, anger, helplessness, longing may all be experienced in response to the hallucinated images and be reflected in the patient's facial expression, gestures, motions, and speech.

To an observer the patient may display a gamut of behaviors. One type of behavior may predominate, and the patient looks inert, sleepy, and withdrawn or, on the contrary, restless, fidgety, and hypervigilant. The predominant behavior shifts in some patients unpredictably to its opposite. A drowsy, or alert but hypoactive, patient tends to respond to questions slowly, with a bewildered or indifferent facial expression, and often with long pauses between words. Such a patient may ask to be left alone or otherwise indicate a wish to be undisturbed. This may be expressed in a groaning, pleading, or irritated voice. It requires persistance on the part of the examiner to engage the patient in a verbal exchange long enough to allow assessment of the mental status.

Other patients may be observed to scan their surroundings and suddenly exclaim, cringe as if frightened, speak excitedly to an invisible person or animal, or strike as if in self-defense or attack. The patient may seem to search for something on or under the bed, pick at bedclothes, mutter, laugh, sing, call for help, curse, or wail. Attempts to get out of bed are common in the more restless and frightened patients, and injuries may easily result. When approached, the hyperactive and excitable patient looks bewildered, fearful, or annoyed. He or she may start to answer a question and then suddenly look away, point to a corner of the room and shout that "they" must be thrown out. Noisy expressions of fear or anger, or of pleas to be allowed to go home, may be repeated loudly and monotonously for hours on end. They may be interrupted by bursts of low muttering, moaning, whining, screams for help, etc.

At any time, unpredictably, a raving and obviously hallucinating patient may calm down, ask about his or her whereabouts, the time, the family or doctor, and answer questions relatively coherently and to the point. These so-called *lucid intervals,* i.e. rather brief and irregular episodes of relative normalization of the patient's thinking and behavior, are quite characteristic of delirium. The waxing and waning of the intensity of the patient's symptoms during a twenty-four-hour period are usually referred to as *fluctuations* in the level of awareness and, if present, strongly suggest the diagnosis of delirium. The lucid intervals may last minutes to hours, and the longer they are the more normal is the patient's mental state liable to be. He or she may exhibit only some recent memory loss and mild disorientation, i.e. symptoms readily ignored by those in attendance. As a rule, the patient is liable to have longest and most frequent lucid intervals during daylight hours and become more disturbed and less accessible in the evening and at night.

The behavior of a delirious patient may be quite different from his or her habitual one. Personality traits, as expressed in observable behavior, may be accentuated or else altered. In the former case, the patient speaks and acts in a manner reflecting enhanced mistrust, timidity, boisterousness, or withdrawal. Rather than accentuation of habitual traits, however, the patient may display unaccustomed tendencies. Thus, a shy and retiring person may become loud and combative, or a placid individual may exhibit a frankly paranoid attitude and act in a belligerent and accusatory manner. Patients with predominantly schizoid, hypomanic, cyclothymic, paranoid, or impulsive premorbid personalities are liable to exhibit any of these personality styles in bold relief, and actually in the form of psychotic symptoms, such as persecutory delusions. Such symptoms may accompany relatively mild cognitive impairment and create a false diagnostic impression of a schizophrenic or affective psychosis.

A patient's verbal productions reflecting his or her inner experience during an episode of delirium may strike an observer as bland and impoverished, or fearful, or depressed, or dreamlike and bizarre. It is the latter patients, those reporting complex hallucinations and other strikingly irrational and deviant experiences and thoughts, who are most liable to be misdiagnosed. For the patient such experiences are usually intensely real in the same way that a dream is usually experienced as real by the sleeper. The patient may have unaccustomed and bizarre thoughts, images, and fantasies, which at times intermingle with illusions and hallucinations to result in an experience not unlike a waking dream or nightmare. Hidden or conscious wishes, conflicts, guilty feelings, and fears may be reflected in the delirious patient's inner productions. Intense emotions of fear, anger, shame, depression, pleasure, or craving may accompany the imagery. External stimuli are readily incorporated into the whole experience and the normally automatic distinctions between dream and fantasy and reality become blurred or even abolished.

A woman delirious in the course of uremia provided a good example of this merging of boundaries between fantasies and hallucinations on the one hand, and veridical perceptions on the other. She reported that she awoke after a nightmare whose nature she could not recall, and immediately saw a young man with a red moustache who proceeded to massage her breasts until they became flat, then tried to push a thermometer into her breasts but stopped since she yelled for help. The patient recounted this experience seriously as a fact and would not accept the suggestion that her experience was partly a hallucination and partly the perception of a nurse's taking her temperature. Merging of the dream contents, waking hallucinations, and fragments of true perceptions is common in delirium and accounts for its often weird and unpleasant subjective quality. Darkness, shadows, unexpected noises, monotonous sounds of recording apparatus in an intensive care unit, voices beaming from an intercom system—all these factors tend to aid and abet the delirious patient's psychotic productions and experiences.

Delirium may begin to subside at any stage, and its maximum intensity will vary depending on its cause, the patient's physical condition, timely treatment, and other factors. Its worsening may take the form of either gradual reduction of alertness and transition into stupor, or of increasing excitement and restlessness ending in cardiovascular collapse. A severely delirious patient may just mutter to himself, oblivious of his surroundings and unresponsive to verbal stimuli. Involuntary movements, such as coarse tremor, flapping motions of the hands and arms, groping, jerking, or persistent tossing about (jactitation) are exhibited by some patients. Incontinence of urine, and less often of feces, is usual at an advanced stage. Speech may vary from mutism to almost uninterrupted flow of incoherent and apparently unrelated words. Signs of sympathetic nervous system overactivity with flushing of the face, sweating, tachycardia, dry mouth, and dilated pupils occur in some patients. Others show pallor, dry and dehydrated skin, coated tongue, and normal pulse rate or even bradycardia. The patient's cognitive processes are now almost totally disrupted and largely uninfluenced by the environment. From this point on there must be progression either towards death, or to more or less full recovery, the latter being the usual course. Severe delirium lasts no more than several days, rarely weeks. Episodes of delirium, especially at night, may recur for many weeks if the underlying condition persists. On the average, however, delirium tends to be short-lived, lasting about one week.

CLINICAL VARIANTS

Delirium is characterized by marked *variability* of its clinical manifestations both between cases and often in the same case over time. This variability reflects several factors, or dimensions, which will be discussed in more detail in Chapter 4. These dimensions are: *level of awareness* or degree of cognitive disorganization; *psychomotor activity; alertness* or arousal or responsivity to stimuli; and *psychotism* or degree of abnormal cognitive activity, that is, hallucinations and delusions. Reduced level of awareness is the basic dimension and equivalent to dissolution of consciousness in Hughlings Jackson's sense. It varies in degree relatively independent of the other three dimensions and determines the severity of delirium. It is the three remaining dimensions that provide a basis for distinguishing clinical variants of delirium. We shall call these variants the *hyperactive,* the *hypoactive,* and the *mixed,* respectively. Their description follows.

The Hyperactive Variant

This clinical subtype is characterized by psychomotor overactivity, both verbal and nonverbal. The patient is visibly restless, shows a great deal of more or less purposive movement, gets out of bed, screams, talks incessantly, etc. Alertness or responsivity to stimuli is enhanced, and the patient displays what may be called hypervigilance. Any type of sensory stimulation is responded to promptly and generally excessively. In the early stages of this form of delirium the patient may complain of being hypersensitive to light, sound, and tactile stimuli, all of which tend to evoke an unpleasantly intense response. As cognitive disorganization progresses, this type of patient no longer complains, but rather responds motorically, vocally, and usually autonomically in a manner indicating increased general arousal of the nervous system. Coupled with the increased psychomotor activity and alertness is a tendency to psychotism, i.e. to the development of complex illusions and hallucinations, delusions, and misinterpretations of the situation.

Delirium Tremens. The most important and best known example of the hyperactive variant is delirium tremens. It shows all of the characteristics of the latter developed to a high degree. This fact has prompted some observers to view it as a syndrome in its own right, one distinct from delirium as a whole. Others have tended to regard it as a prototype of delirium in general and to set it apart from the confusional states. In this book we shall consider delirium tremens to be no more than a typical example of the hyperactive variant of delirium as a whole, a position which Hoch (4) adopted on the grounds of a careful clinical analysis.

The most extreme form of the hyperactive variant is a rare condition which has been described by different writers under a variety of labels, such as "acute delirium," "acute pernicious psychosis" (5), "Bell's delirious mania," etc. This semantic confusion should not obscure the fact that the various labels conceal valid clinical observations. For this reason it is appropriate to examine the original works that contain descriptions of the cases of this form of delirium.

Brièrre de Boismont (6) described in 1845 a condition which he called "délire aigu" or "acute delirium." This disorder, which he related to phrenitis of the ancients, was characterized by incoherence of thought, severe disturbance of attention, extreme excitement and restlessness, muscle spasms, lucid intervals, hallucination and illusions, fear, aversion to food and drink, severe insomnia, and a tendency to collapse. He noted that some patients showed only intermittent excitement and were stuporous most of the time. Indeed, a few of his patients were said to remain mute and motionless and to show no excitement. Nevertheless, striking psychomotor overactivity was a hallmark of most cases. The disorder was acute in onset and of short duration, and usually resulted either in full recovery or in death.

In 1849, Luther Bell (7), the superintendent of the McLean Asylum near Boston, described a similar condition which his followers named "Bell's disease" or "Bell's delirious mania" or "typhomania." Bell found 40 cases of it among some 1,700 patients admitted to the Asylum over 12 years. Their main features included sudden onset, tremulousness, severe insomnia, "intellectual wandering" with lucid intervals, hallucinations, delusions, extreme excitement and restlessness, anxiety, and either complete recovery or death in two to three weeks. Bell emphasized that this new disorder was, despite marked similarities, distinct from mania, delirium tremens, and inflammatory diseases of the brain and meninges. The few cases on which he carried out an autopsy showed only "slight cerebral and meningeal engorgements." Bell stated clearly that "the mental disturbance is rather delirium than mania." Careful reading of his nine case histories leaves little doubt that they represent severe hyperactive delirium.

Bell considered the syndrome idiopathic. Some of his contemporaries, however, ascribed it to typhus. Williams (8), for example, claimed to have seen many cases similar to Bell's among the newly arrived Irish immigrants and maintained that "the exciting cause was typhus poison." This conclusion led him to call the syndrome "typho-mania." In the subsequent decades many more cases of acute delirium came to be reported and a protracted debate about the nature and etiology of this condition ensued. A lengthy editorial in the *American Journal of Insanity* in 1864 summarized the views of de Boismont and Calmeil, respectively (9). The former believed that the disorder was secondary to noncerebral disease, while the latter ascribed it to active disease in the brain itself.

Today, the term "delirious mania" is used in representative American textbooks of psychiatry to designate the most extreme stage of mania (10, 11). "Acute delirium" has lost its separate nosological status, but some writers (2) still use the term to refer to the syndrome originally described by Brierre de Boismont. Recent authors have added neurogenic hyperthermia to the clinical picture (12). If inadequately treated, the disorder is fatal. It has been observed to complicate the course of a whole range of organic diseases: epilepsy, encephalitis, multiple sclerosis, systemic infections, and brain tumor; as well as of schizophrenic, manic, and depressive psychoses. An identical syndrome has been described under the name "acute pernicious psychosis" and observed to occur during puerperium and with thyrotoxicosis (5). This form of delirium is distinctly rare, its etiology and pathophysiolgy are still obscure. Its clinical features, however, are clearly consonant with those of an extremely severe hyperactive delirium.

The Hypoactive Variant

This variant provides a contrast to the preceding one. It features a generally reduced level of psychomotor activity and alertness. Psychotic symptoms, i.e. hallucinations and delusions, are less pronounced than in the hyperactive variant and may be absent. The hypoactive variant corresponds roughly to the "lethargus" of the old writers, and to "simple mental confusion" of many contemporary authors.

The patient is quiet, speaks little and may even be mute, tends to drift off into sleep in the course of an examination, responds slowly to questions and other stimuli, and displays generally diminished mental and psychomotor activity. This appearance may be misleading since an occasional patient may appear lethargic and yet report intense fantasy life. Some patients are catatonic and may be mistaken for being schizophrenic. Others lie with open eyes but appear oblivious to what goes on around them. They may mutter more or less incoherently and gesture incongruously. Some of these patients do hallucinate but show few or no outward emotional and behavioral expressions of their inner experiences. Such patients are sometimes considered depressed by the staff and may actually feel dejected, but many are merely lethargic. Cases of the so-called coma vigil belong to this variant.

The hypoactive type of delirium has been traditionally viewed as a state of clouded consciousness interposed between full alertness on the one hand, and stupor and coma on the other. The subject of clouded consciousness will be discussed in Chapter 4 dealing with psychopathology of delirium. It is in the hypoactive variant that one is most likely to find EEG changes in the direction of generalized slowing of the background frequencies.

It is currently a matter of controversy if the hypoactive and the hyperactive variants should be considered different forms of a single psychiatric syndrome, namely delirium, or as two distinct syndromes with different underlying pathophysiological mechanisms. The present writer has opted for the former alternative and views the two clinical patterns as variants of the same psychopathological syndrome. This does not, of course, preclude the probability that the two variants represent behavioral expressions of different pathophysiological processes in the brain. This matter will be further discussed in the later chapters.

The Mixed Variant

This clinical pattern is characterized by features of both the hypoactive and the hyperactive variants. The patient's behavior alternates irregularly between states of lethargy verging on stupor and of marked excitement. Such striking changes in the patient's behavior tend to occur unpredictably during the same day or on different days in the course of a single delirious episode. Such patients may be particularly difficult to manage since their behavior may change relatively suddenly and unexpectedly, and thus create problems and crises for the medical staff. It is easy to either oversedate or insufficiently sedate a patient of this type. While relevant statistics are lacking, it is this writer's clinical impression that the mixed variant is very common. It provides one more reason to consider delirium a unified syndrome with a wide spectrum of overt behaviors, alertness, arousal, and psychotism.

INCIDENCE

Delirium can occur at any age but appears to be most frequent in children and in people over sixty years of age. Information about its prevalence and incidence is almost nonexistent. All we have are rough estimates and a few data on the incidence and prevalence of the condition in selected populations, such as alcoholics or surgical patients. Engel (13) estimates that 10 to 15 percent of inpatients on acute medical and surgical wards are likely to suffer from delirium of some degree of severity. Swiss investigators (14) offer a lower estimate for the same type of population, namely 5 to 10 percent. Among geriatric patients the incidence is much higher. Forty-five percent of the patients aged sixty-five years or over who were admitted to the psychiatric wards of the San Francisco General Hospital suffered from an acute organic brain syndrome (15). A study of sixty-five consecutive admissions to a general medical ward at the Royal Victoria Hospital in Montreal did not find a single patient with delirium (16). It is true, however, that several patients were too sick to be examined and that patients with such conditions as uremia and myocardial infarction were admitted to special units. These factors may have resulted in negative findings because the patient population was relatively selected and less likely to have compromised cerebral function.

Anesthetists have reported postoperative "emergence" delirium in 5 to 6 percent of a large sample of surgical patients (17). In a random sample of 200 surgical patients, delirium was found in 7.8 percent (18). The incidence of delirium in surgical intensive care units has been reported to be in the range of 2 to 30 percent (19, 20, 21). The incidence in coronary and general medical intensive care units varies considerably and ranges, according to different writers, from 2 to 20 percent (22, 23, 24, 25). Open heart surgery has been followed by delirium in about 20 to 30 percent of patients (26).

In general, data on the incidence and prevalence of delirium are few and of questionable validity. This is not surprising in view of the relatively short duration of the syndrome, its being notoriously frequently undiagnosed on the medical and surgical wards, and the semantic muddle surrounding the term "delirium." No official statistics on the frequency of the acute organic brain syndromes are available in this country. It is likely that the incidence of delirium is underestimated since only cases of it that have attracted somebody's attention due to disturbed behavior are likely to be reported. Furthermore, the population known to be at risk for developing delirium is large and includes those aged over sixty years; the alcoholics and drug addicts; those suffering head injuries in traffic accidents; people intoxicated by prescribed and illicit drugs; those suffering from chronic metabolic, cardiovascular, and respiratory disorders; and those undergoing major surgery. An estimate that 5 *to 10 percent* of an average hospitalized medical and surgical population displays symptoms of delirium reflects the impression of experienced liaison psychiatrists. In a similar population aged over sixty years, the prevalence of delirium is estimated at about 40 percent (27).

PROGNOSIS

The outcome of delirium includes the following possibilities:

1. Full recovery, usually within a week or so, but sometimes after several weeks or even months;

2. Progression to stupor and coma, or sudden cardiovascular collapse and death;
3. A transitional cognitive, affective, behavioral, or mixed, abnormality in a state of full alertness, and gradual full recovery;
4. Progression to an irreversible organic brain syndrome with global or selective cognitive deficits and/or organic personality disturbance;
5. A functional psychosis.

Delirium as such is never a long-lasting or permanent condition. This statement refers to delirium as a clinical syndrome and not to the patient's overall psychological functioning and well-being or even survival. "Delirium" designates a cluster of psychopathological symptoms indicative of a temporary cerebral dysfunction. It is the cause of the latter which determines whether the patient will survive the illness, return to the premorbid condition, or display some form and degree of permanent psychological impairment or abnormality absent prior to the onset of delirium. If the latter occurs in the course of an irreversible dementia, the metabolic derangement underlying delirium may result in more cerebral damage and thus in an increase or acceleration of the dementing process.

The most common outcome of delirium is *full recovery*. Sometimes, the patient may experience recurrent episodes of it over a period of months or even years. This is most likely to happen in someone suffering from a progressive cerebral disease of any type, or from a metabolic disease punctuated by recurrent exacerbations and concomitant cerebral decompensation. Chronic renal, hepatic, or pulmonary diseases offer relevant examples.

Data on mortality rate of patients suffering from delirium are scant. Study of a group of 122 patients diagnosed "acute brain syndrome" of various etiologies found that 12 percent died (28). An investigation of 262 patients with an "organic brain syndrome" referred for psychiatric consultation from the medical and surgical wards showed that twice as many (11%) of them died during the index admission than of control patients matched for age, sex, and medical diagnosis. Thus, the presence of delirium in the course of a medical hospitalization indicates greater severity of the underlying physical illness and a more serious prognosis (29, 30). Delirium arising in the course of senile dementia points to increased probability of death during the first year of the disease. Delirium is often a terminal event in cancer and other diseases (14, 31).

Some patients pass through a *subacute* organic syndrome before recovering. This syndrome may take several forms: subacute dementia; amnestic syndrome; a depressive or anxiety disorder with marked fatigue, poor concentration, lack of initiative, impaired ability for sustained intellectual effort, insomnia or hypersomnia, irritability, etc.; or a frontal lobe syndrome with impaired action planning and social judgment. An amnestic syndrome occurs most often after delirium due to Wernicke's encephalopathy, head injury, encephalitis, and tuberculous meningitis.

An unknown percentage of patients who display delirium will subsequently show a permanent, or chronic, organic brain syndrome of some type, usually dementia or amnestic syndrome. A patient who sustains a severe head injury, for example, will be comatose at first, then delirious for a period more or less directly proportionate to the duration of coma, and may then show some form and degree of cognitive impairment, or of personality disturbance, or both, and gradual but *incomplete* recovery. Such a course may also be observed in patients with Wernicke's encephalopathy (32).

Rarely, delirium of any etiology may trigger off a schizophrenic, paranoid, or affective psychosis. Delirium may occur at a time of intense psychological stress for the person and allow intrusion into consciousness of previously repressed wishes and impulses in the form of uncontrolled imagery, hallucinations, and delusions. This whole constellation of factors may be sufficient to result in a breakdown of defense mechanisms and a psychosis. It is remarkable that such a sequence is so relatively uncommon. Schizophrenic patients who become delirious may show subsequently a temporary lessening or remission of their chronic psychosis (14).

There is a striking paucity of studies on the effects of delirium in children on their subsequent development and psychiatric history. In one of the few articles on this subject Bollea (33) distinguishes seven disorders of consciousness, including confusional state, oneiric state, and acute febrile delirium. The latter, he states, is very frequent in childhood up to the age of ten or eleven years, tends to occur at the height of fever and during its fall, and has a good prognosis. If the picture of delirium is complicated by signs of oneirism and outlasts the febrile period, then the prognosis is less favorable. About 3 percent of adult schizophrenics are said to have suffered one or more delirious episodes in childhood (33). Bender (34) asserts that terrifying hallucinations and panic occurring in children in the course of acute infection or intoxication may be followed by schizophrenic decompensation. Some of these children display psychological vulnerability in subsequent development. Finally, circumstantial evidence suggests that delirium in the course of one of the common non-neurotropic viral infections in childhood is often accompanied by EEG abnormalities and subsequent learning problems and behavior disorders (35). There is an obvious need for firm data on these important issues.

REFERENCES

1. Fothergill, J.M.: The management of delirium. *The Practitioner 13*: 400-408, 1874.
2. Lipowski, Z.J.: Delirium, clouding of consciousness and confusion. *J Nerv Ment Dis 145*:227-255, 1967.
3. Engel, G.L. and Romano, J.: Delirium, a syndrome of cerebral insufficiency. *J Chronic Dis 9*:260-277, 1959.
4. Hoch, A.: The problem of toxic-infectious psychoses. *New York State Hospital Bull 5*:384-392, 1912.
5. Tolsma, F.J.: The syndrome of acute pernicious psychosis. *Psychiatr Neurol Neurochir 70*:1-21, 1967.
6. Brierre de Boismont, A.: Du délire aigu observé dans les établissements d'aliénés. *Mém Acad de Méd, Par. 11*:477-595, 1845.
7. Bell, L.V.: On a form of disease resembling some advanced stages of mania and fever, but so contradistinguished from any ordinarily observed or described combination of symptoms, as to render it probable that it may be an overlooked and hitherto unrecorded malady. *Am J Insanity 6*:97-127, 1849.
8. Williams, A.V.: Typho-mania. *Am J Insanity 8*:146-149, 1851-2.
9. Acute delirium, in 1845 and 1860. *Am J Insanity 21*:181-200, 1864.

10. *American Handbook of Psychiatry.* 2nd edition. Vol. 3. Arieti, S. and Brody, E.B., Eds., p. 461. New York, Basic Books, 1974.

11. Freedman, A.M., Kaplan, H.I., Sadock, B.J.: *Comprehensive Textbook of Psychiatry.* 2nd edition. Vol. 1, p. 1018. Baltimore, Williams & Wilkins, 1975.

12. Christoffels, J. and Thiel, J.H.: Delirium acutum, a potentially fatal condition in the psychiatric hospital. *Psychiatr Neurol Neurochir* 73:177-187, 1970.

13. Engel, G.L.: "Delirium." In Freedman, A.M. and Kaplan, H.S., Eds. *Comprehensive Textbook of Psychiatry.* Baltimore, Williams & Wilkins, 1967.

14. Bleuler, M., Willi, J. and Buhler, H.R.: *Akute psychische Begleiterscheinungen korperlicher Krankheiten.* Stuttgart, Thieme, 1966.

15. Freedman, D.K., Troll, L., Mills, A.B., and Baker, P.: *Acute Organic Disorder Accompanied by Mental Symptoms.* Sacramento, Calif., California Department of Mental Hygiene, 1965.

16. Lowy, F.H., Engelsmann, F., and Lipowski, Z.J.: Study of cognitive functioning in a medical population. *Compr Psychiatr* 14:331-338, 1973.

17. Coppolino, G.A.: Incidence of post-anesthetic delirium in a community hospital: A statistical study. *Milit Med* 128:238-241, 1963.

18. Titchener, J.L., Zwerling, I., Gottschalk, L., et al.: Psychosis in surgical patients. *Surg Gynecol Obstet* 102:59-65, 1956.

19. Hale, M., Koss, N., Kerstein, M., et al.: Psychiatric complications in a surgical ICU. *Crit Care Med* 5:199-203, 1977.

20. Katz, N.M., Agle, D.P., De Palma, R.G., De Cosse, J.J.: Delirium in surgical patients under intensive care. *Arch Surg* 104:310-314, 1972.

21. Wilson, L.M.: Intensive care delirium. *Arch Intern Med* 130:225-226, 1972.

22. Holland, J., Sgroi, S.M., Marwit, S.J., and Solkoff, N.: The ICU syndrome: Fact or fancy? *Psychiatr Med* 4:241-249, 1973.

23. Cay, E. L., Vetter, N., Philip, A.E., Dugard, P.: Psychological reactions to a coronary care unit. *J Psychosom Res* 16:437-447, 1972.

24. Parker, D.L. and Hodge, J.R.: Delirium in a coronary care unit. *JAMA* 201:702-703, 1967.

25. Hackett, T.P., Cassem, N.H., and Wishnie, H.A.: The coronary-care unit. An appraisal of its psychologic hazards. *N Engl J Med* 279:1365-1370, 1968.

26. Editorial: Delirium after surgery. *Br Med J* 2:702-703, 1974.

27. Robinson, W.G., Jr.: "The Toxic Delirious Reactions of Old Age." In Kaplan, O.J., Ed. *Mental Disorders in Later Life,* pp. 332-351. Stanford, Stanford University Press, 1956.

28. Farber, I.J.: Acute brain syndrome. *Dis Nerv Syst* 20:296-299, 1959.

29. Guze, S.B. and Daengsurisri, S.: Organic brain syndrome. *Arch Gen Psychiatry 17*:365-366, 1967.
30. Guze, S.B. and Cantwell, D.P.: The prognosis in "organic brain" syndromes. *Am J Psychiatry 120*:878-881, 1964.
31. Levine, P., Silberfarb, P.M., Lipowski, Z.J.: Mental disorders in cancer patients. A study of 100 psychiatric referrals. *Cancer 42*: 1385-1391, 1978.
32. Victor, M., Adams, R.D., and Collins, G.H.: *The Wernicke-Korsakoff Syndrome*. Philadelphia, Davis, 1971.
33. Bollea, G.: "Acute Organic Psychoses in Childhood." In Howells, J.G., ed. *Modern Perspectives in International Child Psychiatry*, pp. 706-732, New York, Brunner & Mazel, 1971.
34. Bender, L.: "The Maturation Process and Hallucinations in Children." In Keup, W., Ed. *Origin and Mechanisms of Hallucinations*. New York, Plenum Press, 1970.
35. Weinman, H.M.: EEG changes in acute viral disease in infancy and childhood. *Electroencephalogr Clin Neurophysiol 22*:93, 1967.

Additional References

Lipowski, Z.J. "Organic Mental Disorders: Introduction and Review of Syndromes." In Freedman, A.M., Kaplan, H.I., and Sadock, B.J., Eds., *Comprehensive Textbook of Psychiatry*, 3rd Edition. Baltimore, Williams & Wilkins, in press.

Stedeford, A. Understanding confusional states. *Br J Hosp Med 20*:694-704, 1978.

CHAPTER 4

PSYCHOPATHOLOGY OF DELIRIUM

I_N C_{HAPTER} 3 _{THE} clinical features, both essential and associated, of delirium were described. In this chapter the psychopathology of the syndrome will be discussed in more detail. It will become apparent that while many excellent descriptions of delirium can be found in psychiatric literature, there are relatively few reports of systematic studies of the various psychological abnormalities which comprise it. The purpose of this chapter is to review these abnormalities, to point out the gaps in our understanding of them, and thus to suggest areas for future research.

DELIRIUM AS DISORDER OF COGNITION

It is generally accepted that the core abnormality in delirium involves cognitive processes. There is less agreement, however, in what specific ways these processes are deranged. To some extent these disagreements are problems of semantics, of the meaning of the explanatory terms. The term "cognition" will be used in this discussion to connote all the processes involving symbolic operations, namely perceiving, remembering, creating imagery, and thinking. In delirium one observes *disorganization and global impairment of cognitive functions.*

The above statement has several implications. First, it implies that, under normal conditions, cognitive processes are organized and that in delirium this organization is to a greater or lesser extent disrupted. This disruption is particularly marked in the train of thought of a delirious patient, and in his manner of responding to and processing information inputs. Second, there is observable impairment of performance in *all* the major aspects or phases of cognition. And third, this impairment represents a decrement from the individual's habitual level of performance.

Clinicians have attempted to account for the cognitive impairment in delirium by invoking a quasi-explanatory concept of "clouding of consciousness." It first appeared in the American psychiatric literature at the end of the nineteenth century, when Hirsch (1) defined delirium as a "psychical state characterized by an abolition of self-consciousness, by an incoherence in the chain of conceptions, and by the appearance of symptoms of sensory and motor irritation." The abolition of self-consciousness was manifested, according to Hirsch, by disorientation for place, disturbances of perception, and subsequent partial or total amnesia for the experience of delirium. Hirsch spoke of "cloudiness of self-consciousness." Hoch (2), influenced by Bonhoeffer's work on delirium tremens, asserted that the most specific and cardinal feature of delirium in general was a "constant tendency to dip down to a lower level of consciousness." Hoch used the term "clouding of consciousness" and asserted that this state was a condition analogous to sleep; there was in it a "general dissociation" of thought processes and external reality not unlike dreaming. Disorientation, hallucinations, impairment of recent and remote memory, and attention disorder were all to be viewed as consequences and manifestations of the general clouding of consciousness.

Thus, since the beginning of this century the concepts of delirium, confusion, and clouding of consciousness have become inextricably linked. Their usage, however, has been very inconsistent and muddled. For some authors delirium implies a manifestation of clouded consciousness, while for others the latter represents a cardinal feature of the former. A recent article, describing a patient suffering from an acute brain syndrome due to lithium toxicity, provides a typical example of the semantic confusion in this area: "He was distractable, withdrawn and showed progressive degradation of personal habits. He developed visual illusions and became totally disoriented as to time, place, and person. Despite the similarity of this illness to an acute delirium with occasional lucid intervals, the patient had no clouding of consciousness" (3). Here is a good description of delirium with a typically muddled diagnostic conclusion.

To clarify the psychopathology of delirium it should be useful to try to identify those clinical observations that have given rise to the concept "clouding of consciousness." Such an inquiry may throw some light on the core psychopathological features of delirium and help delimit this syndrome from dementia in which global impairment of cognitive functions is also a defining characteristic. Once these features have been abstracted they could serve as criteria for the diagnosis of delirium, and the term "clouding of consciousness" might then be either more explicitly defined than is usually the case, or it could be abandoned.

DELIRIUM AND CLOUDING OF CONSCIOUSNESS

There is no generally accepted definition of consciousness and the connotations of this term have grown in number in the last decade or so (4, 5, 6). It would be quite beyond the scope of this book to include a review of this subject. Yet some discussion of it is needed to clarify the issue of the clouding of consciousness.

Hebb (7) regards consciousness as the state of being normally awake and responsive, and of being capable of engaging in complex thought processes to guide behavior. Insight, purpose, and immediate memory are, in Hebb's view, the key features of consciousness. Kleitman (8) points out that consciousness and wakefulness are not synonymous: a person asleep but dreaming displays a mode of conscious experience. Psychiatrists and neurologists have traditionally viewed consciousness as a continuum of states of being aware of one's self and one's environment, and of being able to respond to the latter. In this usage, consciousness has a *quantitative* connotation: one may be more or less conscious.

A different way to conceptualize consciousness is to talk of its *contents*, which may be altered by drugs, hypnosis, drowsiness, etc., and thus result in *qualitatively* different inner experiential states. These two overlapping and yet distinct ways of referring to consciousness, the quantitative and the qualitative, have contributed to the current semantic confusion surrounding this concept. We actually have three frequently confused pairs of polarities to consider: consciousness versus unconsciousness, wakefulness versus sleep, and normal versus altered consciousness.

Clouding of consciousness cuts across all of the above polarities and implies presence of the following characteristics:

1. The person is awake;
2. Awareness is reduced;
3. Both immediate and recent memory are impaired;
4. Attention is disordered;
5. Thinking is more or less disorganized and thus altered;
6. Ability to match current information inputs against stored information resulting from past learning is diminished;
7. The person is unable to overcome this state by deliberate effort.

The foregoing characteristics have been extracted from the descriptions of clouding of consciousness to be found in the literature (9-15). They may be viewed as manifestations of the dissolution of the nervous system and as negative symptoms in Hughlings Jackson's (16) terminology. It is worth noting, however, that the concept of clouding of consciousness represents no more than a designation for a cluster of psychological abnormalities characterizing delirium. The word "consciousness" in this context is misleading in that it implies the existence of a defined psychological attribute which becomes changed or "clouded." The term "clouding of consciousness" has been applied at times as if it were an explanatory concept, but this implication is illusory and misleading: it is merely a descriptive term devoid of explanatory power. In the writer's opinion it is obsolete, ambiguous, and redundant. It is high time to drop it from scientific discourse and psychiatric terminology, as Peters (15) has recently advocated. To abandon it may open the way to a fresh and unbiased look at the clinical phenomena that it has served to label and obscure. Advances in our understanding of the underlying pathophysiological cerebral processes should result from such an inquiry.

In conclusion, "clouding of consciousness" refers to a set of psychological deficits and abnormalities that constitute the core of the syndrome of delirium. They include not only decrements in cognitive functioning but also disturbances of the sleep-wakefulness cycle, and of arousal, vigilance, and attention. These latter disturbances tend to fluctuate in intensity irregularly and unpredictably in the course of a day. They accompany, and possibly underlie, the readily observable cognitive deficits. Rather than link all these pathological changes to the vague and controversial concept "consciousness," or its "clouding," it may be more profitable to view them as a disturbance of the sleep-wakefulness cycle.

DELIRIUM—A DISORDER OF WAKEFULNESS

In keeping with the preceding discussion it is proposed to refer to delirium from now on as a *disorder of wakefulness*. This designation expresses a hypothesis which will require empirical support, yet its choice is neither arbitrary nor devoid of cogent supporting arguments. The following discussion should make this point clear.

The term "wakefulness" has been at times equated incorrectly with "consciousness." The two terms refer to distinct although obviously overlapping states. The sleep-wakefulness dichotomy is absent in consciousness since dreaming represents a mode of conscious experience during sleep (8). In contrast to consciousness, both wakefulness and sleep are psychophysiological states that can be objectively observed and to some extent measured (8). They have measurable physiological correlates or indicators and comprise definable stages. In both these states certain cyclic or rhythmic events have been described which in wakefulness appear to be related to gradation of alertness (17). To link delirium with wakefulness offers the advantage of relating it to a rather well-defined psychophysiological concept, one not mired in ambiguity and controversy as is consciousness.

One may cite some cogent reasons to support the contention that delirium represents a form of pathology of wakefulness. The syndrome has been frequently linked with the concepts of alertness, arousal, activation, vigilance, and attention, all of which refer to integral aspects or properties of wakefulness, although some of them may pertain to sleep as well. Abnormalities of all of these aspects of the waking state are among the disturbances characteristic of delirium. It is possible to view these abnormalities as intervening variables between acute cerebral dysfunction on the one hand, and the impairments of cognition on the other.

A close relation between disordered sleep and delirium has been postulated by many observers since Hippocrates. The reader can find relevant quotations in Chapter 1. One could argue that statements to the effect that delirium is a waking dream, for example, are merely metaphors or analogies. Yet such claims were derived from clinical observations which need to be thoroughly reviewed and the hypotheses based on them carefully examined in the light of present knowledge.

Numerous writers over the centuries advanced hypotheses that delirium reflects pathology of sleep. Hunter, Darwin, and many others were quite explicit in this regard. Heinroth (18) published a dissertation in 1842 in which he argued that delirium was an intermediate state between sleep and wakefulness ("status medius est inter somnum atque vigiliam").

Other writers postulated a relationship between delirium and dreaming. Hunter (19) spoke of delirium as a "diseased dream." A century later, Lasegue (20) wrote an article titled "Alcoholic delirium is not a delirium but a dream." In recent years this theme has been revived by some sleep researchers who proposed that delirium tremens represents an intrusion of dreaming state into wakefulness (21, 22).

The relations between sleep and delirium will be discussed in detail in Chapters 5 and 6. They are brought up at this point only to underscore their relevance to the hypothesis that the syndrome represents a disorder of wakefulness. Recent studies of the latter have shown that it is not a homogeneous state, but rather one in which distinct stages or levels may be distinguished. Continuous polygraphic studies of normal waking subjects have resulted in the definition of six such stages (23). Similar research carried out over twenty-four hours revealed the presence of recurrent periods of rapid eye movement (REM), not only during sleep but also during wakefulness (24). These waking REM periods do not correlate, however, with the periods of the most intense daydreaming. On the contrary, Kripke and Sonnenschein (25, 26) have demonstrated a negative correlation between them. These investigators have found that the peaks of fantasy or daydreaming tend to show a ninety-minute cycle that is positively correlated with EEG alpha frequency. These peaks appear to occur in a drowsy state resembling hypnagogic reverie and display a rhythm similar to that of REM sleep, but physiologically distinct from it.

What, if any, relevance for delirium the above findings may have one cannot say with assurance at this time. Research continues and its results necessitate frequent revisions of the hypotheses that have been put forth to account for various observations of the sleep-wakefulness cycle. For example, the most recent studies have challenged Kleitman's hypothesis that a basic rest-activity cycle (BRAC) exists during wakefulness (27). It appears now that the REM cycle is sleep-dependent and that the ninety-minute rhythm found in some waking activities is not an expression of REM cycle found during sleep (27). As Johnson (28) observed recently, the relation of sleep stages to waking behavior and performance is still a mystery. Yet the disruption of the sleep-waking cycle, as well as that of the REM-NREM cycle in sleep, will probably prove to influence psychological functioning during wakefulness. Studies of sleep deprivation provide a key methodological approach in this area (29-32).

The concept of a disorder of wakefulness is not new. Guilleminault et al. (33) have recently described a syndrome of hypersomnia with automatic behavior and proposed that it might be related to an impairment of the structures of wakefulness rather than of those subserving sleep. These investigators postulate that the patients suffering from this syndrome display a tendency to "micro-sleep" episodes during the daytime and are never wide awake. A related disorder has been referred to as the "sub-wakefulness syndrome" and ascribed to catecholamine deficiency (34, 35).

Particularly relevant are the studies by Ey et al. (36) of the sleep patterns of patients suffering from certain confusional states, such as confusional episodes and acute delirious episodes or "bouffées délirantes." (One should keep in mind that this terminology cannot be readily translated into English diagnostic terms, and this calls for caution in interpreting the results of these interesting studies.) These investigators observed striking disturbances of the sleep-wakefulness cycle in the confused patients, namely severe insomnia at night coupled with a difficulty to remain awake during daytime. EEG tracings obtained during the day showed fluctuations and transitions between wakefulness, somnolence, and light sleep, respectively, as well as episodes of "micro-sleep." Night recordings documented not only shortening of the total sleep time, but also relative loss of modulation and orderly progression of the stages of sleep. Discrimination of the "rapid" and slow sleep was less easy than in normal controls because of the marked increase in intermediate (not associated with rapid eye movements) phases of rapid sleep. REM sleep appeared in some cases shortly after sleep onset. The investigators assert that in confusional states one observes disorganization of the normal structure of sleep and its various constituents or, more to the point, of the total sleep-wakefulness cycle.

There is obviously a need for more research on the relations between sleep and dreaming, on the one hand, and delirium due to a whole range of etiological factors, such as intoxication with drugs, metabolic encephalopathies, infections, etc., on the other. Explorations of the pathology of wakefulness, a concept basic to the present discussion, have only begun. Yet, as Luria (37) claims, study of "varied symptoms of *disorders of wakefulness* has become a most important clinical task" (emphasis added).

To hypothesize that delirium is a disorder of wakefulness is likely to prove methodologically more fruitful than to view it as a syndrome of clouded consciousness. The latter concept has been methodologically sterile. The focus on the sleep-wakefulness and the REM-NREM sleep cycles, respectively, and on various patterns of their disruption, may be expected to revive interest in research on delirium. Such a focus should help clarify the relation of the syndrome to sleep and dreaming, to activation and arousal, and to the neurophysiological and biochemical processes regulating these various states and functions. To underscore this shift in emphasis the following discussion of the psychopathology of delirium will begin with disturbances of attention, a psychological function invariably affected in delirium and one whose control involves arousal and activation.

DISORDERS OF ATTENTION IN DELIRIUM

Attention refers to the directivity and selectivity of mental processes (38, p. 256). Hebb (7) defines it as selectivity in that aspect of the environment the subject responds to, or as an activity of central mediating processes that enhances the effects of a sensory stimulus while other such stimuli are inhibited or ignored. Studies on human attention have distinguished three components of it: *alertness*, that is, the ability to develop and maintain an optimal sensitivity to external stimulation; *selectivity*, that is, the ability to select information from one source or of one kind rather than another; and *processing capacity*, which refers to the concept of a limited ability to process information inputs (39).

Hernandez-Peon (40) regards attention as the primary process underlying perception, memory, and thinking, and relates it to the vigilance system, i.e. arousing neurons in the brain stem, which can be activated by the specific sensory pathways and by descending projections from the cortex. Luria's (38) discussion of attention impresses one as being particularly useful for the study and understanding of its disorders in delirium. He points out that some degree of attention is indispensable for organized mental activity. Elementary or involuntary forms of attention need to be distinguished from the higher or voluntary ones. The former may be observed during the first few months after birth as the so-called orienting reaction, which consists of turning the eyes and the head towards an external stimulus. This motor response is accompanied by autonomic responses, namely a psychogalvanic reflex, changes in respiratory rate, and constriction of peripheral vasculature while the blood vessels in the head are dilated. As the brain matures, additional physiological components of the orienting reaction may be distinguished: inhibition of the alpha rhythm in the electroencephalogram, or strengthening of the evoked potentials in response to an appropriate stimulus. The orienting reaction is evoked selectively by a change in the stimulus input. Voluntary attention, argues Luria, develops as a result of the child's relations with adults and is thus of social, and not of biological, origin.

Of crucial importance is the central organization of attention. Pribram and McGuinness (41) have distinguished three inter-acting neural systems involved in the control of attention: 1. The amygdala circuits for the control of the core brain arousal systems and thus of *arousal*, defined in terms of phasic physio-logical responses to an input change; 2. the basal ganglia-cen-tered system for the control of *activation*, that is tonic physio-logical readiness to respond; and 3. The hippocampal system, which coordinates arousal and activation—an operation which calls for *effort*.

One of the essential conditions for attention is the activity of the ascending reticular system of the brain stem which sub-serves wakefulness and arousal (42). This system extends into the hypothalamus and has diffuse connections with the forebrain whereby it can effect widespread arousal response. Reciprocal facilitatory and inhibitory circuits centered on the amygdala and the related frontal cortical areas control the onset and dura-tion of arousal (41). This whole system can change the level of activity of cerebral cortical neurons, and it is in turn modu-lated by changes occurring in the cortex. Further, it subserves the orienting reaction to incoming sensory stimuli and the voluntary, complex attention. A second system, centered on the basal ganglia, appears to control activation of the perceptual expectancy and the motor readiness. The third system, one involving hippocampal circuits, appears to exert control over the relationship between arousal and activation and is necessary for the effort of voluntary attention (41).

Lesions of the upper brain stem and the ascending reticular system result in disturbances of wakefulness and of capacity for attention. Lesions of the limbic system (amygdala, hippocampus) lead to instability of selective attention, fatigability, distract-ibility, and unselective responses to different stimuli (38). Ir-relevant stimuli readily evoke associations and thus tend to disrupt the train of thought. Finally, in massive lesions of the frontal lobes involuntary attention may be indiscriminately enhanced, but the ability to maintain voluntary attention is impaired (38).

Disorders of attention constitute fundamental manifestations of disorders of wakefulness. The normal waking state in man is characterized by the capacity to mobilize, focus, maintain, and shift attention not only in response to significant internal and external stimuli, but also voluntarily or intentionally. In delirium this capacity is impaired in all its aspects, and the selectivity of mental processes is compromised. Luria (38) points out that the principal feature of oneiroid states is "loss of the selectivity of mental processes affecting all spheres of mental activity" (38, p. 63). Significant and insignificant stimuli tend to evoke the same type of response—the train of thought becomes disorganized, and incidental associations are elicited by common words.

From the clinical viewpoint, pathological changes of attention in delirium include:

1. Impaired ability to mobilize active attention;
2. Impaired ability to select information inputs;
3. Impaired ability to maintain attention, i.e. distractibility;
4. Impaired ability to shift attention;
5. Abnormal spontaneous fluctuations of attention;
6. Decreased capacity to process incoming information.

All these disturbances of attention may be observed in delirious patients. They occur in various degrees and patterns dependent on the severity of delirium and on the level of arousal. In the predominantly hypoactive variant of delirium, for example, the levels of arousal, activation, and alertness are reduced to some extent and the patient is more likely to display general difficulty in mobilizing, maintaining, and shifting attention. In the hyperactive variant, exemplified by delirium tremens and withdrawal delirium from barbiturates, arousal and alertness are heightened; and the patient attends readily, if indiscriminately, to all kinds of stimuli. At the same time, he is highly distractible. In both variants the ability to maintain attention and to select and process information is impaired. Further, in many cases of delirium one may observe characteristic and apparently spontaneous, that is, internally generated, fluctuations in the general capacity for attention. One may speculate that these fluctuations are brought about by changes in the activity of the ascending reticular system occasioned by the metabolic processes rather than by arrival of external stimuli.

It should be acknowledged that the above account of attentional deficits in delirium is based on clinical impressions and not on systematic studies using standardized tests of attention. This is an obvious drawback, but clinical observations and hypotheses derived from them constitute the bulk of our knowledge of delirium today and are being presented here for critical scrutiny.

It is hypothesized that the disorders of attention in delirium are directly related to the disorganization of the cerebral systems and mechanisms subserving it. This implies the loss of coordinated activity of the reticular activating system, limbic system, basal ganglia, and frontal lobes. Disturbance of attention is viewed by some observers as the psychological deficit underlying the disorganization of cognitive processes in delirium and resulting in global cognitive impairment. The main aspects of the latter will now be examined.

DISORDERS OF THINKING

Disturbances of thinking processes have always been viewed as an integral component of delirium. Barrough (43) wrote of disordered imagination, cogitation, and reason. Willis (44) noted "incongruous conceptions and confused thoughts." Hartley (45) spoke of disgustful associations, vivid imagery, and distortion of reasoning. More recently, Hirsch (1) considered "incoherence in the chain of conceptions" to be one of the defining characteristics of the syndrome. Terms such as "confusion" and "clouding of consciousness," which have been frequently used to describe the core psychopathology of delirium, both carry the connotation of a disturbance of normal thought processes (46).

One may distinguish two main modes of thinking: *associative*, as in reverie, dreams; and *directed*, that is, critical and creative

(47). One of the features of thought pathology in delirium consists of some degree of *disorganization of directed thinking coupled with a relative preponderance of associative thinking.* It is this feature that has encouraged comparisons between delirium and dreaming, and given rise to the concept of "oneirism" or dream-like mode of mentation which is often encountered in delirium. Levin (48) maintains, in what is probably the only article in English devoted to thinking disturbances in delirium, that the main characteristics of thought pathology in this syndrome include disorientation, disturbances of association, illogical thinking, inability to grasp new and complex information, and unawareness of faulty and inconsistent reasoning or "morbid lack of perplexity."

Systematic studies of thinking in delirium are lacking in the English psychiatric literature. As with all the other aspects of the psychopathology of the syndrome one is forced to rely on clinical impressions—an unsatisfactory situation from a scientific viewpoint. To present this clinical material in an organized way it will be discussed under the following headings representing interrelated aspects of thinking:

1. Organization, i.e. selective ordering of ideas for the purpose of problem solving, action planning, decision making, and meaningful communication;
2. Dynamics, i.e. evolution and rate of progression of thoughts over time sequences;
3. Concept formation; and
4. Content.

Clinical observations allow one to postulate that all of the above aspects of thinking are disturbed in delirium. Organization of thoughts is disrupted to a varying extent, that is, thinking is more or less incoherent, fragmented, illogical, and undirected. Logical contradictions are overlooked or unrecognized by the patient. For example, he or she may greet the physician by calling him or her "Doctor" and yet, on direct questioning, deny the knowledge of his or her occupation (48). Sustained, directed train of thought is difficult and may be impossible. It is liable to be disrupted by both internal and external factors. Internally, there is a tendency to experience more or less dis-

jointed images, fantasies, and thoughts, not unlike a free flow
of associations. Externally, the patient tends to respond indiscriminately to environmental stimuli that elicit unaccustomed
or irrelevant associations. The latter contribute to the disorganized train of thought and make any thinking effort more difficult
to accomplish. Capacity to select thoughts and maintain their
orderly sequence for the purpose of solving problems, planning,
and grasping the meaning of stimuli and the whole situation is
reduced. As a result of these impairments the patient is less
able to match incoming information against stored memories,
and thus to relate meaningfully what goes on around him or her
to past experience and knowledge. Consequently the judgment
is also faulty, and the capacity for purposive and adaptive
behavior reduced.

The flow of thoughts may be retarded or accelerated, as
reflected in the patient's either slow and hesitant, or hasty yet
incoherent, speech. In the prodromal stage of delirium patients
may actually complain of an uncontrollable slowness or speed
of the train of thought. This disturbed dynamic of thinking
contributes to its overall disorganization.

Concept formation is impaired, with a tendency to an
increased difficulty in thinking abstractly. Romano and Engel
(49) have stated that their data documented the "loss of ability
to think in the abstract." This deficit can be elicited at the
bedside by asking the patient to define words, find synonyms,
list words belonging to a certain category, synthesize and differentiate properties of objects, interpret proverbs, etc. All these
various operations are performed by the patient with more
difficulty and errors than one could expect on the basis of his
or her level of education and, by inference, intelligence.

Content of thought may simply be impoverished, few thoughts
being available. Uncontrolled images and fantasies may dominate
thinking, or the patient may engage in intense reverie and
ignore the environment. This thinking activity may reflect the
person's unique preoccupations, conflicts, wishes, guilt feelings,
fears, etc., both past and current. There is often a dream-like
quality to the thought content and related unconscious symbolism.
The patient may find it difficult to separate fact from fantasy,
dream from waking imagery. Yet, as Fothergill (50) observed

a century ago, delirium should not be viewed as an "upheaval of hidden thoughts"; that is to say, delirious thinking does not regularly consist of conflictual, emotionally charged, unconscious material. Fothergill wrote that "all that is carefully hidden does not ordinarily escape in delirious raving," and on the contrary, much of the patient's thought is focused on everyday concerns related to job, family, recent experiences, and ongoing environmental stimuli. Willi (51) has recently reported that a delirious patient's thought content tends to reflect his or her concerns about the impact of the physical illness underlying the delirium on the personal life situation and future prospects. Thus, much of the symbolism of the imagery and fantasies can express, in a disguised form, preoccupation with disability, mutilation, or death.

Delusions, false beliefs incongruous with the patient's cultural and educational background, may develop. They are typically unsystematized, fleeting, and environment-bound, that is, elicited and modified by current stimuli. Wolff and Curran (52) noted in their classic study that feelings of perplexity, strangeness, mistrust, and suspicion were invariably present in their delirious cases. In the majority of them these vague feelings and apprehensions crystalized into a delusional belief. The ease with which this happened seemed to be influenced by the patient's personality. Once formed, however, the delusions usually remained unstable and were readily abandoned only to be replaced by new ones. Delusions of persecution are the most common type. Wolff and Curran (52) found that every patient in their sample believed to some extent and at some time that he or she was being persecuted. Some believed they would be killed, tortured, or abducted. Others insisted that they had been robbed; or that they were the object of plotting, harassment, or annoyance. Some patients develop delusions that their family members or friends are dead, in danger, or persecuted. Transient delusions of guilt may be encountered.

Delusions merge imperceptibly with illusions and hallucinations, and separation of these phenomena in clinical practice may be impossible, pointless, and arbitrary. In fact, perhaps the most common delusion in delirium is the belief in the reality of one's hallucinations. Patients differ, however, in the degree to which they elaborate upon their hallucinations and misinterpret events in their surroundings.

The incidence of delusions in delirium has been variously reported as ranging from 40 to 100 percent of cases (52, 53, 54). The patient population studied and the investigator's definitions of delirium and delusion are likely responsible for this discrepancy. It is rather arbitrary, for example, to separate delusions not only from hallucinations but also from confabulations, which are not uncommon in delirium. A patient may insist, for instance, that a deceased person is alive and has just visited him or her. A delirious woman had her eyes examined and when seen again an hour or so later stated that a doctor had looked into her eyes and told her that he saw in them gold, which he would remove by performing an operation. It is purely arbitrary if one labels such a statement a delusion or a confabulation. In any case, these transient and shifting delusional ideas, readily influenced by events in the surroundings and by suggestion, stand in sharp contrast to the relatively stable and systematized delusions common in functional psychoses. They are frequent in delirium but not diagnostic of it. They are in part a reflection of the patient's personality and past experience and in part a manifestation of the disturbance of information processing.

In summary, thinking is invariably disorganized in delirium, and characterized by impairment of the capacity for directed and abstract thought, by predominance of associative thinking uninfluenced by logic and fact, and by frequent emergence of normally unconscious imagery. As a result of these cognitive disturbances the patient's ability to evaluate his or her situation rationally, exercise judgment, and act purposefully is to some degree impaired. Frequent occurrence of transient delusions is a manifestation of disorganized information processing.

DISORDERS OF PERCEPTION

Perception has been defined as the activity of the mediating processes to which sensation gives rise directly. It implies incorporation of sensory information into thought process (7). Perception may also be viewed as the process of extracting information about one's body and external environment (55).

It is linked inextricably to thinking, remembering, and learning and is influenced by the person's motives and emotions. The brain subserves two functions in perception: *reception* and *selection*. The reticular formation plays an important part in perceptual processes. It is open to the greatest diversity of afferent channels (55). It appears to facilitate reception of stimuli by activating the cerebral cortex and bringing about a state of arousal and alertness. It may also, aided by the limbic system, influence selection of information which signals physiological needs as well as of external sensory input of particular significance to the person because of its novel, threatening, attractive, or aversive meaning.

Deficient or excessive cortical arousal resulting from fluctuations in the activity of the ascending reticular system may impair perceptual discrimination, as is the case in delirium. There, perceptual processes appear to be impaired as a result of a disorganization of cerebral activity secondary to a metabolic derangement involving both the neocortex, and the limbic and the ascending reticular systems. The brain receives patterns of impulses and also functions in their selection, integration and modification, operations influenced by the stored information or memories against which the incoming stimuli are matched. These selective, integrative, and modifying processes are invariably impaired in delirium. As a result, one observes not only defective perceptual discrimination but also distortions and misinterpretations of perceived objects, situations, and events; as well as hallucinations of varying degrees of complexity.

Drowsiness and other levels of reduced alertness are common in delirium. A drowsy or hypoalert patient tends to display absence of expectancy and perceptual searching as well as difficulty in integrating percepts (56). Hyperalert patients show increased responsiveness to stimuli, but they too exhibit impaired perceptual discrimination and integration. Some patients seem unable to maintain their habitual anticipatory and supporting attitudes (set) in the presence of competing and discordant stimulation (57). In the prodromal phase of delirium the patient is often hypersensitive to auditory, visual, and other sensory stimuli. He or she may complain that lights are too bright and glaring, sounds unpleasantly loud.

Perceptual abnormalities in delirium may affect all sensory modalities, exteroceptive, proprioceptive, and interoceptive. There may be impairment of the subjective perception of the passage of time (time sense), spatiotemporal relationships, and people's intentions and expressive behavior. Disturbances of the body image, that is, alteration in perception of the size, shape, position, weight, texture, etc., of one's body and its parts, as well as reduplication of the body, limbs, or head may occur (58). Visual perceptual distortions involving perceived and/or hallucinated objects are not uncommon. They may include: polyopsia (multiplication of a single perceived object); metamorphopsia (alteration of the size of object—micropsia, macropsia); alteration of position in space, such as tilting; waviness of linear components; fragmentation of lines and gaps in the contours of objects seen; apparent movement of stationary objects or subjective acceleration or slowing of moving ones; dysmorphopsia (alteration or distortion of shape); and autoscopy (visual hallucination of the self) (58-61).

Perceptual abnormalities in delirium include illusions and hallucinations, which are frequently but not invariably encountered. Impairment of attention and of information processing seems to facilitate their occurrence.

ILLUSIONS. Illusions have been defined as premature or improper labeling of aspects of the perceptual field (56). They are common in delirium, especially the visual ones. Misinterpretations of visual, auditory, tactile, kinesthetic, somesthetic, and other sensory stimuli may occur. They range from relatively simple to highly elaborate and symbolic misidentifications of the sensory input. Most commonly the patient mistakes spots on a wall for crawling insects, folds in the bedcovers for snakes, or the sound of a falling object for a pistol shot. More complex illusions may be regarded as projections of personally meaningful symbols and fantasies onto environmental stimuli (52, 56). For example, a female barbiturate addict, delirious as a result of withdrawal from the drug, misidentified her hospital room as a prison cell from which she would be taken for execution. She mistook a window for a door and was caught in the act of opening it in order to escape. She was mistakenly thought by the staff to be suicidal, although a subsequent psychiatric interview uncovered feelings of guilt over her addiction and related fears of punishment but failed to elicit suicidal impulses. Such illusions merge with delusions and may lead to inadvertent accidents or even death. Darkness, shadows, sounds of the hospital intercom system, and other unaccustomed stimuli from ward activities foster misperceptions and misinterpretations. Both excessive and deficient sensory inputs may do so and are to be avoided.

HALLUCINATIONS. In any sensory modality hallucinations may occur in delirium, but visual ones are the most common. In only one reported study did auditory hallucinations predominate. Farber (53) studied 122 patients with delirium of various etiologies and found that 54 percent of them experienced hallucinations: 21 percent auditory, 14 percent visual, 16 percent both auditory and visual. One notes that 13 percent of all the patients in that series had a history of alcohol addiction, and some of them had previously been admitted for delirium tremens or acute alcoholic hallucinosis. Farber admits that in some of his cases it was impossible to distinguish the latter condition from "acute brain syndrome" or delirium. This problem may have influenced the reported incidence of the various hallucinations. Wolff and Curran (52) found visual hallucinations to be the most common type experienced by their patients: they occurred in 66 percent of them, while auditory hallucinations were observed in 41 percent. A Swiss study of 300 patients with "exogenous psychosis," roughly equivalent to what is here called delirium, revealed the following incidence: visual hallucinations in 73 percent, auditory in 23 percent, and both types combined in 17 percent of the patients (51).

The overall incidence of hallucinations in delirium is practically unknown. Farber (53) found them in 54 percent of his patients. Other investigators are silent on this point. Some authors include hallucinations in their operational definition of delirium and thus imply that 100 percent of their reported subjects had them. The incidence of all types of hallucinations in cases meeting the criteria for delirium used in this book is estimated to be in the range of 40 to 75 percent. The reported frequency of hallucinations in delirium may be expected to be influenced by the characteristics of the patient population studied as well as by the investigator's definition of delirium and hallucination. Patients aged sixty or older have a relatively low reported incidence of hallucinations, about 40 percent (54). It has been claimed that the younger delirious patients hallucinate more readily than the older ones (62). Patients suffering from delirium related to hepatic, pulmonary, or cardiac decompensation experience hallucinations less often than subjects going through a withdrawal from alcohol or barbiturate-type drugs, for example. About 40 percent of those delirious patients who hallucinate tend to do so only at night (63). It is common to observe hallucinations in one or two modalities occurring simultaneously, but a combination of three or more modalities appears to be much less frequent. In this respect as well as in the predilection for visual rather than auditory misperceptions, delirium differs from schizophrenia. Proprioceptive and interoceptive hallucinations may occur in addition to exteroceptive. Tactile ones usually take the form of crawling, creeping, burning, and other sensations which are difficult to separate from paresthesiae. Delusions of infestation or parasitosis and sexual interference tend to accompany tactile hallucinations. Vivid kinesthetic hallucinations of floating in the air, flying, or falling from heights have been described, for example, in typhus (64) and poliomyelitis (65).

Hallucinations may be viewed from two related perspectives: *formal features* and *content*, respectively. The formal attributes of visual hallucinations include duration and other temporal characteristics: size, intensity, distinctness, color, shape, motion, etc., of the hallucinated objects; the reality or true-to-life quality of the vision; their projection into and placement in space; and the degree of the subject's belief in their veridical nature, personal reference, source, etc., which is to say the extent of delusional interpretation by the patient of the experienced misperceptions (63).

Visual hallucinations in delirium are interpreted by most patients as real. They are usually projected to the nearby space and are experienced as bright, colored, and clear three-dimensional pictures, whose elements frequently change in shape, size, or number and move about in the visual field (63). Lilliputian hallucinations may occur and usually consist of brightly colored and distinct little people (66). Frieske and Wilson (63) compared visual hallucinations in patients with delirium, schizophrenia, and affective psychoses. Delirious patients' hallucinations were distinguished by being relatively brief, often nocturnal, less complex, less often involved with personal meaning, and more often involving objects in motion. These hallucinations may be fleeting and intermittent or more or less continuous like a movie film. In the latter case the pictures may vary in the degree to which they are thematically connected, that is to say they may or may not show a discernible theme. Some patients hallucinate only with their eyes closed, especially when they try to go to sleep. These hallucinations are probably hypnagogic and may make the patient afraid of falling asleep.

The contents of visual hallucinations in delirium are highly variable. They vary greatly with regard to the degree of their organization, complexity, and symbolic elaboration. Lowe (67) has distinguished three aspects of hallucinatory contents: *noun,* that is, the predominant thing hallucinated: *verb,* that is, the action within the hallucination in regard to the patient; and *reaction,* that is, the patient's attitude to such action. Visual hallucination in delirium may comprise a wide range of things, from relatively simple and unformed colored spots, stars, balls, dust specks, flakes of light, geometric figures, whorls, etc., at one end of the spectrum, to inanimate objects, animals, human figures, mythological or ghost-like apparitions, monsters, and complex panoramic scenes, at the other end. Wolff and Curran (52) reported that patients in their series experienced visual hallucinations of figures in motion; all kinds of animals, ranging from cockroaches to elephants; vividly colored objects, some of which seemed to have symbolic significance such as coffins and hearses; and ghost-like forms. Head (68) found that patients suffering from pulmonary and cardiac diseases experienced visions consisting of white, black, or gray stationary figures. The visions of alcoholics in delirium tremens typically teem with small animals such as mice or rats, insects, or snakes in vivid color and constant motion. Young children, aged three to six years, may hallucinate being attacked by snakes, and other animals, and react with panic (69).

Actions of these hallucinated objects with regard to the patient vary. They may appear indifferent and unrelated or attacking, engulfing, pursuing, etc. The patient's reactions are correspondingly variable. They may range from amused detachment to panic, from a tendency to approach the visions to frantic attempts at fleeing from them. Frieske and Wilson (63) found that 67 percent of their delirious patients responded to their visual hallucinations by taking some action such as hitting at or trying to run away from the visions. Farber's (53) subjects reacted to these hallucinations with fear and so did over 60 percent of those reported by Frieske and Wilson (63). The fear is a typical response of patients suffering from delirium tremens. In general, unpleasant emotions of fear, anger, and despair appear to be the most common affective responses to hallucinations in delirium. Some patients are aware that they are hallucinating, feel ashamed, and tend to conceal and deny their misperceptions. Pleasurable and amusing hallucinations seem to be relatively uncommon in delirium unless the latter has been deliberately self-induced by taking a deliriogenic drug for the purpose of experiencing an altered state of awareness. Most people become delirious in the course of an illness that they have not wished for and that has aroused fear and other disturbing emotions. Delirium is liable to enhance the patient's distress, and hallucinatory experiences are likely to do the same, as well as to reflect the distress, fear, helplessness, and wishes to get away from one's predicament. The patient's inner conflicts and guilt may also influence the contents of the hallucinations.

Visual hallucinations are neither pathognomonic nor diagnostic of delirium. Auditory hallucinations, alone or combined with visual ones, occur in about 30 percent to 50 percent of cases (51, 52, 53, 63). They display as much variability as the visual misperceptions. They may be relatively simple, such as shooting, or involve hearing whole conversations, music, singing, screams, etc. There is nothing characteristic about auditory hallucinations in delirium. Tactile hallucinations are the third most common type of misperception encountered in delirium. It is difficult to distinguish them from pains and paresthesiae. They are estimated to occur in 10 to 20 percent of the patients. In one study they were found to be combined with visual hallucinations in 23 percent of the cases (63). Olfactory misperceptions are even less common. Only about 10 percent of patients (52, 63) report hallucinating odors, which are nearly always unpleasant (63). Gustatory hallucinations are very uncommon in delirium in contrast to schizophrenia (52, 63, 70).

In summary, the frequency of hallucinations in delirium is unknown but estimated to be about 40 to 75 percent. Hallucinations are neither invariably present in, nor necessary for, the diagnosis of delirium. Visual illusions and hallucinations are the misperceptions most often encountered. Tactile, kinesthetic, olfactory, gustatory, and interoceptive hallucinations may occur but are less frequent than either visual or auditory ones. The latter two types occur together in about 20 percent of the cases.

One may raise several questions regarding hallucinatory experiences in delirium: first, why do delirious patients tend to hallucinate? Second, why is it that some do and some do not? Third, why do visual misperceptions predominate? Fourth, what determines the form and contents of hallucinations in delirium?

These questions touch upon important theoretical issues concerned with the organization of human information processing and the consequences of its disruption. Satisfactory answers cannot be offered at this stage of our knowledge and one may only attempt to formulate hypotheses based on diverse and indirect lines of evidence. It is the author's hope that the following discussion will stimulate badly needed research in this area. Even though hallucinations have attracted much attention lately, their occurrence in delirium has been largely ignored by investigators. The most recent monograph on hallucinations barely mentions delirium (71). Considering that this syndrome is likely to be the most common mental disorder in which hallucinations occur, its neglect by the students of perceptual abnormalities is difficult to explain.

Recent research on hallucinations has gone beyond description and reached the stage of validation of explanatory hypotheses, which hypotheses have been formulated from several vantage points: biochemical, neurophysiological, psychological, and sociocultural (71, 72, 73, 74). Methodological approaches to the study of hallucinations have included the use of hallucinogenic drugs, cerebral stimulation, sensory and sleep deprivation, hypnosis, and observations of people with cerebral lesions caused by disease. All of this research is relevant to the problem of hallucinations in delirium but cannot be discussed here. Furthermore, hallucinations need to be considered in relation to other perceptual phenomena such as imagery, daydreams, illusions, dreams, etc. Klüver (75) has pointed out that all these subjective phenomena, including visual hallucinations, may have the same content and that there may be transitions from one kind of subjective experience to another: "for instance, a negative after-image may be followed by, or transform itself into, a pseudo-hallucination; a pseudo-hallucination into a hallucination; and a memory-image into an eidetic image" (75, p. 19). Such transitions are facilitated in many pathological states which give rise to delirium with the result that the person is increasingly unable to control vivid daydreaming and to distinguish internally derived imagery from external stimulus objects. There is thus a postulated continuity among the various perceptual phenomena both in health and delirium. In the latter one observes pathological accentuation of the "endogenous stream of perceptual imaginings" seen in normal relaxed wakefulness (76).

To return to the questions posed above—first, the occurrence of hallucinations in delirium appears to be co-determined by a constellation of factors which may be hypothesized to include the following: 1. disruption of the normal sleep-wakefulness cycle; 2. reduced or excessive cerebral cortical activation and arousal; 3. fluctuating level of alertness and attention; 4. stimulation or disinhibition of the temporal cortex and limbic structures; and 5. disorganization of thought processes with consequent impairment of reality testing.

West (77) has proposed a "perceptual release" theory of hallucinations which is of some value in explaining their occurrence in delirium. Briefly, this theory asserts that an optimal sensory input is needed to keep currently irrelevant memory traces derived from past percepts out of awareness. Thus during normal wakefulness the information input to the brain enables the person to maintain a scanning and screening activity. When the sensory input is reduced or impaired for any reason, and at the same time adequate cerebral cortical arousal is maintained, perceptual or memory traces may be released and re-experienced with varying degrees of vividness. The higher the level of arousal, the greater the vividness of the released percepts will be. The latter may appear in awareness as fantasies, images, illusions, dreams, or hallucinations.

In delirium the above conditions are present. The usual sensory or information input is reduced and/or impaired as a result of the patient's lowered receptivity to it, decreased capacity to process it, or both. Normal sleep-wakefulness cycle is disrupted and mental phenomena which are usually associated with sleep, drowsiness, and daydreaming dominate waking awareness. Alertness and attention fluctuate so that maintenance of screening and inhibition of percepts, memories, and images becomes difficult or impossible. Cortical arousal is sufficient for awareness and may actually be enhanced. At the same time there is either stimulation of the temporal lobe structures or their disinhibition, or both, and this allows uncontrolled intrusion of stored percepts into awareness. Concurrent disorganization of thought processes impairs reality testing and discrimination of percepts derived from sensory stimulation from those released from memory storage, respectively. Reduced, ambiguous, discordant, novel, or excessive external sensory input tends to facilitate perceptual release and the hallucinatory experiences.

It is hypothesized that a confluence of synergistically acting factors accounts for the frequent occurrence of hallucinations in delirium. They are most pronounced in the hyperactive variant of the syndrome exemplified by delirium tremens and other withdrawal deliria as well as in states of intoxication with anticholinergic drugs, for example. In the hypoactive variant, the cerebral cortical arousal, or activity of the limbic system, or both, appear to be reduced, and hallucinations are less frequent.

Much attention has been given in recent years to the hypothesis that dreams and hallucinations are related phenomena, a hypothesis which may be relevant to delirium. It has been postulated that the same basic neurophysical mechanisms may underlie both dreams and hallucinations. Dement et al. (78) have proposed that the malfunction or failure of the serotonergic system could result in waking dreams, that is, hallucinations. In delirium induced experimentally by Ditran®, atropine, and other anticholinergic agents, there are reduced wakefulness and hallucinations, as well as slow and very fast activity in the EEG similar to that of REM sleep (79). Inhibition of a central cholinergic mechanism has been invoked to account for these findings. Yet this hypothesis should be critically examined. It has been reported that physostigmine can reverse delirium due to a variety of agents having anticholinergic properties, but it fails to suppress delirium tremens (80). This suggests that more than one mechanism is likely to be involved in bringing about both delirium and hallucinations.

Some investigators have postulated that in delirium tremens and the withdrawal syndromes from hypnotics and sedatives there is a combination of increase of REM sleep coupled with reduced stage four sleep, as well as increased cortical arousal, which together enable intrusion of dreams into waking life in the form of hallucinations. More recent studies, however, have failed to replicate earlier findings of increased REM activity in delirium tremens (81). It has been suggested that a dissociation of the phasic and the tonic features of REM sleep, with an increase in stage 1-REM (mixed-frequency EEG activity, REM burst and tonic mental EMG) was somehow responsible for the occurrence of hallucinations in delirium tremens (81). Clearly, this issue is still open and one should avoid its premature closure. It does appear, however, that a combination of reduced wakefulness or awareness and enhanced cortical arousal favors the emergence of hallucinations.

To conclude, the hypothesis of equivalence or identity of dreams and hallucinations appears to be inadequately supported by empirical evidence. This writer is inclined to view both dreams and hallucinations as related perceptual phenomena but occurring in different states of the organism. To postulate their identity may only serve to obscure their distinct features. The occurrence of hallucinations in delirium may be viewed as a derangement of normal waking mentation, which encompasses imagery of hallucinatory vividness (76). In delirium, this imagery becomes predominant and intensified, and the person is no longer able to control and suppress it.

The remaining questions concerning hallucinations in delirium permit only brief comments for lack of relevant information. Why do only some delirious patients hallucinate? We do not know the answer. One may postulate that on the one hand there are individual differences in susceptibility to both delirium and hallucinations, and on the other hand different conditions that cause delirium have unequal potential for eliciting hallucinatory experiences. Why do visual misperceptions predominate in delirium? Several possible factors may be suggested to account for this fact. Studies of waking mentation show that about 70 percent of imagery in relaxed wakefulness is visual in nature (76). It is remarkable how closely this percentage corresponds to the reported proportion of visual hallucinations in delirium (51, 52). This close correspondence seems to support the author's hypothesis that delirium represents a disorder of wakefulness. By contrast, auditory hallucinations occur in about 74 percent of schizophrenic patients diagnosed by strict WHO criteria (74). Furthermore, about 80 percent of nocturnal REM sleep reports refer to visual imagery (76). It has been proposed that there is a greater storage of visual than other memories, and this may account for the predominance of visual misperceptions in the sensory deprivation experiments (56). Hypnagogic hallucinations and sleep mentation of narcoleptics which may be closely related to, or even identical with, those in delirium nearly always involve vision (82, 83). All this admittedly circumstantial evidence suggests that in states of reduced wakefulness and of sleep *visual* imagery and hallucinations predominate.

This observation seems to support two notions: first, that hallucinatory experiences in delirium reflect, at least in part, intensified and more or less uncontrollable visual imagery; and second, that delirium is a disorder of wakefulness in which mentation characteristic of drowsiness and sleep intrudes in varying degrees. Furthermore, there is an implied basic difference between delirium and schizophrenia. It is interesting that hallucinating schizophrenic patients, in contrast to the delirious ones, distinguish clearly between dreams and hallucinations (84).

Finally, what are the determinants of the form and contents of delirious hallucinations? It is not known what determines their form, but there are some observations regarding the factors influencing contents. They include psychodynamic variables, illness-related variables, and the current sensory input. It has been suggested that the delirious patient's illusions and hallucinations reflect his or her remote and recent life-history as well as unconscious conflicts, impulses, and defenses (52, 65, 85, 86). These psychodynamic hypotheses are plausible but lack empirical studies to support them. Clinical impressions suggest that delirious hallucinations cover a whole spectrum of personally meaningless elementary hallucinations, of released past memories, as well as of rather elaborate symbolic expressions of currently dominant intrapsychic and interpersonal conflicts. Furthermore, such hallucinations may express the patient's concerns about his or her illness and its prognosis and personal consequences. They are also readily influenced by the ongoing internal and external sensory stimulation.

MEMORY DISORDERS IN DELIRIUM

Impairment of memory is one of the essential components of delirium. There is disturbance of registration, retention, and retrieval of memories to some degree in every delirious patient. Recent memory tends to be more markedly affected than that for remote events and "crystallized" knowledge. Impairment of registration is probably secondary to reduced alertness and to disorders of attention. It may be inferred retrospectively from the presence of some degree of permanent amnesia for delirium after it has cleared up. The patient may recall practically nothing of the whole experience, but more often the amnesia is only partial. Some patients remember delirium spottily as a "chaotic dream." Wolff and Curran (52) state that clear memory of the hallucinations is the rule. The persistent retrograde amnesic gap is strong presumptive evidence that delirium has taken place.

RETENTION. Usually retention is impaired to some extent. Immediate recall is faulty, as manifested by the reduced digit span (87). Generalizability of this statement is open to question, however, in view of recent studies on the effects on memory of scopolamine and physostigmine, respectively. The former appears to impair the acquisition of new information but not

immediate memory (88). Physostigmine, an antagonist of scopolamine and other anticholinergic agents, has the opposite effect;
that is, it impairs short-term memory as tested by the digit span
(89). Considering that scopolamine in contrast to physostigmine
is strongly deliriogenic, caution is advised in making general
statements about the impairment of various aspects of memory
function in delirium. Systematic studies are needed to establish
if memory is affected in the same way regardless of the etiology
of the syndrome, or if some relatively cause-specific constellations of memory disorders can be distinguished. It is likely,
however, that once a given drug or other noxious factor has
affected cerebral function to an extent sufficient to be manifested by delirium, then the memory function in all its aspects
will to some extent be defective.

RECENT MEMORY IMPAIRMENT. One of the necessary diagnostic features of delirium is recent memory impairment. Romano
and Engel (49) reported that the serial subtraction of numbers
was the most valuable bedside diagnostic test for delirium. In a
later paper (87), these authors claim that this procedure tests
not only attention but also retention of memories. Mesulam
and Geschwind (90) maintain that the patient with the acute
confusional state (delirium) displays a "generally sluggish recall
with no consistent temporal gradient" and a "defective ability
to memorize." These deficits are most pronounced and consistently present with respect to the events occurring just prior
to and since the onset of delirium. Thus one observes some
degree of both anterograde and retrograde amnesia. The former
is equivalent to defective capacity for new learning. In some
conditions, such as tuberculous meningitis, herpes simplex encephalitis, and Wernicke's encephalopathy, memory is affected
with disproportionate severity, indicating pathology of the diencephalic or temporal structures, or both (91). In such cases one
could speak of concurrent amnestic syndrome and delirium.

Confabulation has been observed in about 15 percent of
delirious patients (52). It connotes a tendency to fill gaps in
memory with invented imaginary happenings which are elaborated to varying degrees (92). In delirium, confabulations are
usually relatively simple, shifting, and merge imperceptibly with

delusions. Wolff and Curran (52) found that the most frequent confabulations in their delirious patients concerned familiar everyday activities such as visits from and conversations with relatives. Another common type of confabulation was insistence on the part of the patients that they had to keep important appointments and for this reason ought to leave the hospital. Confabulations may be expressed by the patient spontaneously, or in response to questions about his or her recent activities and other facts, or both. The presence of a tendency to confabulate may be elicited by asking the patient to repeat a story.

It should be emphasized that this account of memory disturbances in delirium is based on clinical reports and observations. Systematic studies remain to be done.

DISORDERS OF SPATIOTEMPORAL ORIENTATION

ORIENTATION. As the term is used in psychiatry, orientation refers to correct knowledge of one's temporal, spatial, and personal relationships (93). Orientation as to time implies the ability to state correctly the day of the week, the date, and time of day. Orientation in space includes correct knowledge of the identity of the place one is in, the ability to follow some normally familiar route, and the appreciation of the topographical arrangements of one's familiar surroundings such as one's house. Orientation for person refers to correct identification, by name and occupation, of familiar people in one's surroundings. The term is also applied sometimes to the awareness of one's personal identity. To avoid ambiguity it is recommended that this usage of the term should be avoided.

Orientation is not usually included among cognitive functions such as memory, thinking, and perception. The reason for discussing it here in a separate section is its clinical importance in delirium. Furthermore, orientation cannot be reduced to any single and more basic cognitive function. On the contrary, it may be viewed as a product of integrated cognitive processes.

DISORIENTATION. It is customary to refer to disturbances of spatiotemporal orientation as "disorientation," which may occur in reference to time, place, space, and person. Disorientation is considered by some authorities as an essential feature of delirium. Levin (94) states clearly: "Every delirious patient is disoriented." In another article he asserts that disorientation is the basic thinking disturbance in delirium (48). A representative textbook of psychiatry includes disorientation among the defining characteristics of the syndrome (95, p. 2582). This view is not universally accepted. For example, Romano and Engel (96) observe that when the disturbance of awareness is mild the delirious patient is usually correctly oriented. This writer proposes that some degree of disorientation, at least for time, at some period during a day is necessary for the diagnosis of delirium.

Disorientation is often equated with "confusion." For example, a standard psychiatric dictionary defines the latter as a state of disordered orientation (93). The textbook just quoted offers the same definition of confusion and yet includes both it *and* disorientation among the defining criteria of delirium (95). This type of semantic muddle is unfortunately all too common in this area.

Temporal disorientation varies in severity, which fluctuates with degree of cognitive disorganization as a whole. It is the first disorder of orientation to appear in delirium, the one invariably associated with, and the last to recover. In its mildest form disorientation for time involves an inability to state correctly the date and the day of the week. It is to some extent arbitrary what degree of error should be considered evidence of disorientation and thus a pathological sign. Mistakes in giving the date and day of the week are quite common among well people. A study of presumably normal passersby at the Hebrew University showed that about 12 percent of the subjects made an error in response to the question "What day of the week is today?" The mistakes involved mostly one day in the middle of the week and were readily corrected by the subjects (97). Clinically, one may regard an error of three days on the date or the day of the week as abnormal. Furthermore, mistaking a week day for the weekend may be viewed as significant. Errors concerning the month, season, and year are abnormal. Mistakes in giving the time of the day may be considered significant if they involve a period of four or more hours. A more objective and less arbitrary way of assessing temporal orientation has been described by Benton et al. (98, 99). It involves scoring the answers to a set of five questions concerning day of week, day of month, month, year, time of day. Mistakes result in points being taken off from an assigned perfect score of 100. Moderate and severe disorientation are defined operationally in terms of the attained score.

In mild delirium, only temporal disorientation is likely to be present at some time during the day. Disorientation as to place and for the people around the patient, i.e. as to person, appears as delirium increases in severity and it recovers before temporal disorientation. Levin (100, 101) has pointed out a characteristic feature of delirious disorientation: *the patient tends to mistake the unfamiliar for the familiar.* Thus, the hospital may be misidentified as home, or a hotel, or place of work, or a more familiar hospital. The patient mistakes the city or other location he is in for one with which he is more familiar. Similarly, doctors and nurses may be misidentified as friends or relatives. As delirium becomes severe, members of the family may no longer be recognized. Rarely does the patient lose awareness of his or her own identity. Spatial disorientation is manifested by the patient's inability to find his or her own room, or to describe how to reach home or some other familiar point, or to follow some normally known route, or to indicate spatial relations of the various components of a familiar place (102).

Disorientation has been accounted for in terms of Hughlings Jackson's (16) concept of dissolution. Loss of orientation represents a negative symptom indicative of dissolution; misidentification or confabulation are positive symptoms reflecting activity of the intact lower centers of the brain and a reduction to a more automatic condition of the organism (101). Other investigators have postulated that disorientation as to place and time is an expression of denial of illness and wish to leave the hospital, rather than a manifestation of disordered memory, perception, and thought (103). This hypothesis makes no distinction between negative and positive aspects of disorientation, respectively. The former amount to not knowing the facts as a result of a cerebral disorder and some loss of function of the brain.

The latter include misinterpretations and confabulations which may at times be influenced by the patient's wishes to avoid some aspect of the present painful reality or by the tendency to express negative feelings, for example. When a disoriented patient calls a physician "butcher" and mistakes the hospital for a slaughterhouse, then such misinterpretations may be viewed as expressions of negative attitudes. Other misidentifications and confabulations, on the other hand, may represent wish fulfilling attempts to minimize a threatening unfamiliarity of surroundings and to reduce ambiguity, anxiety, and a sense of helplessness.

Disorientation is a clinically important sign of delirium. It is not, however, pathognomonic of it. A patient suffering from dementia, amnestic syndrome, severe anxiety or depression, or schizophrenia, or one mentally retarded, may be disoriented to some degree, especially to time, without being delirious. Further, disorientation may clear up temporarily during lucid intervals and reappear when delirium intensifies once more. It is not diagnostic in the absence of other features of delirium. It may be regarded as a manifestation of disorganization of cognitive processes and resulting impairment of the ability to integrate current percepts and thoughts with memories, which provide points of reference for the identification of temporal relations, surroundings, and people.

NONCOGNITIVE PSYCHOLOGICAL DISORDERS

We have discussed the core psychopathology of delirium on which its diagnosis rests. It must be emphasized, however, that delirium involves changes in the patient's overall *subjective experience* and *observable behavior*. These changes may be regarded as nonspecific and as "accessory" to the essential attentional and cognitive disorders. Nevertheless, they are crucially important to the patient and need to be appreciated by the doctor. Complications of delirium such as accidents may result from the nonspecific symptoms such as panic and hyperactivity. Further, these symptoms may cause difficulties in differential diagnosis, for example, in distinguishing delirium from acute schizophrenia. For these reasons the noncognitive disorders in delirium need to be discussed as part of the account of its psychopathology. The following disturbances will be considered: *subjective experience; psychomotor behavior; mood and emotions; and psychophysiological arousal.*

Subjective Experience

Fothergill's (50) remarks made 100 years ago are still valid today: "Very few care to analyse their sensations or their remembrances of a delirious past, and consequently there is but little in our literature which tells us of the attitude of delirium from the patient's point of view." Levin (104), the author of many clinical papers on delirium, has given us a description of his own encounter with the syndrome in the course of a bout of pneumococcal meningitis. He insists that throughout his delirium he was preoccupied with his work; it was, as he states, an "occupational delirium." Guttman (64) reports that while suffering from typhus he experienced an "oneiric delirium," in the course of which he relived in a picture-like mode, a sequence of impressive events of his life. Thomson (105), a nurse, describes vividly her experiences during delirium: "Birds and stars floated around my head. I was in the bottom of a whirlpool, peering out at the faces of the doctors and nurses calling to me at the top. I whirled and whirled, wanting to call out, to tell them I was coming, but I couldn't." Wilbourn (106), delirious during an attack of meningoencephalitis, describes intense irritability, distressing nightmares, seeing the outside world through a "haze," and general hypersensitivity. He sums up his subjective state as one of "unpleasant twilight state between sleep and wakefulness."

Clearly, as these few and fragmentary personal accounts by physicians and a nurse suggest, the subjective experience of delirium is highly variable but almost invariably unpleasant. It may be rich in personally significant and disturbing thoughts and hallucinations which can remain in the patient's memory long after the delirium is over. Or it may be predominantly an episode of unaccustomed sleepiness, dullness, and indifference. Certainly not all the patients experience a vivid, dream-like "oneiric" delirium. Conrad (107) has paid particular attention to the totality of subjective experience in delirium. He maintains that the delirious patient suffers a breakdown or change of Gestalten—an imaginative phrase which applies to only some episodes of delirium. Wolff and Curran (52) report that all of the patients in their study experienced various combinations of uncertainty, perplexity, strangeness, and mistrust. Unconscious conflicts were sometimes activated during a delirious episode. Patients tended to have similar experiences from episode to episode, regardless of etiology of the delirium.

All in all, from the subjective point of view, delirium is usually an unpleasant experience, one that may be quite distressing and disturbing. For some patients it has the character of a more or less chaotic, frightening dream or nightmare. For others, it is a period of sleepy and dull lethargy.

PSYCHOMOTOR BEHAVIOR (PSYCHOMOTILITY)

This aspect of behavior includes such variables as reaction time (speed of initiating movement), speed in continued movement such as tapping, and speed in controlled movement (finger dexterity) (108). In clinical practice the term "psychomotor" usually refers to observed verbal and nonverbal behavior of a person in a given situation. It encompasses the flow of speech, but not its content; and the kinds and tempo of both voluntary and involuntary movements and handwriting. Our knowledge of psychomotor behavior in delirium is based entirely on clinical descriptions and this is reflected in the imprecise terminology used by the clinician.

A delirious patient may display a whole spectrum of motor speed, ranging from *hypoactivity* to *hyperactivity*. In the former the patient displays reduced speed in initiating and continuing movements, both spontaneous and those produced on command. Furthermore, there is reduction in the number of spontaneously performed voluntary movements throughout the waking state. On the contrary, the hyperactive patient shows an increase in the rate of spontaneous movements as well as an increased speed in initiating and continuing them. The cardinal feature of this hyperactive psychomotor behavior is its largely purposeless, uncontrollable, and inefficient quality. Either the hypoactive or the hyperactive mode of psychomotor behavior may predominate in a given delirious episode, or the same patient may display both in varying and unpredictable sequences. Certain etiological factors predispose toward increased or decreased psychomotor activity. Syndromes of withdrawal from alcohol, sedatives, and hypnotics, as well as intoxication with certain drugs, such as Artane®, are typically accompanied by hyperactivity and increased excitability. Conditions like Wernicke's encephalopathy and hepatic encephalopathy are usually marked by hypoactivity unless delirium tremens supervenes. In uremia, for example, dramatic shifts in the level of psychomotor activity tend to occur: "The entire course of the illness may shift rapidly from states of overactivity with aggressiveness, crying, laughing, singing, dancing, and swearing to states of lethargy" (109). Similar observations have been reported on many other diseases.

It must be emphasized that the usual definitions of delirium found in medical and psychiatric textbooks frequently include hyperactivity as an essential feature. Freedman et al. (95), for example, include in their definition such characteristics as restlessness and agitation (95, p. 2582). Brain's textbook of neurology states that "Delirium has been defined as confusion with an overlay of excitement" (110, p. 1177). Harrison's textbook of medicine includes overactivity of psychomotor functions in the definition of delirium (111, p. 149). These statements are misleading in that they do not reflect clinical observations on a sufficiently wide range of delirious subjects, or else represent an overly narrow concept of the syndrome. Romano and Engel (96) report that while many delirious patients display motor excitement, many more show varying degrees of somnolence and stupor. Engel (112) distinguishes several typical clinical patterns of delirium, two of which underscore hypoactivity: the quiet and torpid, and the blandly confused types, respectively. Wolff and Curran (52) noted that restlessness was invariably present in their patient series. It is obvious that if an investigator includes restlessness and overactivity in the definition of delirium, then all hypoactive patients will be excluded from the study. If, however, delirium is defined as in this book, then hyperactive and hypoactive behavior will likely be found in about equal percentages of patients. This statement would not hold, of course, if one studied a selected sample of delirious patients, such as those with delirium tremens, which is marked by hyperactivity.

HYPOACTIVITY. Hypoactivity may range from stupor to simple slowness of motor response and reduced frequency of spontaneous movements, including speech. Catatonic, cataleptic, and mute patients may be encountered. Patients suffering from typhus, for example, may display so-called coma vigil, which is characterized by marked inhibition of speech and muscular movements (64). Some patients suffering from encephalitis lethargica displayed prominent lethargy, catatonia, catalepsy, and marked slowness of motor responses and movement. Others, by contrast, were hyperkinetic, and showed unpredictable shifts from hyperactivity to lethargy or vice versa (113). Actually, the manifestations of delirium associated with encephalitis lethargica provide one of the most compelling arguments in favor of a unified concept of the syndrome as one which encompasses the whole spectrum of psychomotor activity from wild excitement to stupor. The majority of hypoactive patients do not show extreme slowing of reaction and catatonic immobility; they are simply underactive, unspontaneous, somnolent, indifferent, and hypokinetic rather than akinetic. Such patients may be roused, or rouse themselves, to answer a few simple questions, exchange greetings, and state that they feel well. Left alone, they tend to remain quiet or drift into sleep. Willi (51) reports that some patients who appear markedly quiet and indifferent may still experience intense feelings, hallucinations, etc. In other words, one must not jump to the conclusion that when a patient appears lethargic, or even stuporous, he or she is necessarily oblivious of surroundings or devoid of lively inner experience. It is practically important that such hypoactive patients tend to be overlooked by doctors and nurses; their cognitive impairment may be unrecognized, and their anguish not even surmised.

HYPERACTIVITY. This is manifested by increased speed of motor responses and by heightened frequency of movements of all kinds. Typically, however, the responses are indiscriminate, that is, they are elicited by a wide range of random environmental stimuli. This heightened motor responsivity must not be mistaken for vigilance, which connotes deliberate and selective attention to inconspicuous signals maintained for fairly long periods (114). Furthermore, the increased frequency of spontaneous movements in a hyperactive delirious patient may range from involuntary tremor and other nonpurposive movements to relatively complex and goal-directed but unplanned and inefficient actions. Clinically, one speaks of excitement and restlessness to denote this type of psychomotor behavior.

Hyperactivity may be manifested in many ways. On a simple level it features coarse tremor of the hands and other parts of the body; choreiform movements; groping, flapping, tossing, squirming, grasping, picking, jerking, flailing, etc.; moaning, laughing, crying, and similar movements. Older authors used special terms for some of these movements. Carphology, for example, was used to denote aimless picking or plucking at bedclothes and other objects. Jactitation referred to tossing about and similar whole-body movements. At a more organized and purposeful plane, the patient may strike, dress or undress, get out of bed, explore the surroundings, and so forth. Some patients mimic their various familiar or occupational activities such as sewing, filling a glass, driving, taking measurements, etc. If these activities are well organized and sustained and reflect the patient's job or hobby, one may speak of "occupational delirium" —a purely descriptive and redundant term. A delirious patient may occasionally carry out acts of violence, usually in the course of an attempted attack against or escape from hallucinated persecutors or other imaginary dangers. Verbal overactivity is also part of an enhanced psychomotility: the patient speaks fast, under pressure, and may switch from topic to topic without rhyme or reason to the point of complete incoherence. Shouted commands, calling for relatives, wailing for help or mercy, screamed obscenities, and loud singing are all common features of a hyperactive patient's vocal expression. All the verbal and nonverbal movements may be repeated by the patient to the point of exhaustion. Delirium tremens and the so-called delirium acutum, described in Chapter 3, provide classical examples of severe hyperactivity.

SPEECH. In delirium speech has already been mentioned. It may be increased or decreased in reaction time and tempo. It is often hesitant and slurred. It may range from mutism to verbigeration, that is, ceaseless repetition of disjointed, and usually the same, words and phrases. Intensity of the speech may vary from whisper and low muttering (delirium mite or mussitans) to loud vocalizations. Dysphasia and paraphasia may be present. Chedru and Geschwind (115) have studied speech and writing in confused (delirious) patients. They found such abnormalities as hesitation, repetitions, circumlocution, and frequent slips of tongue in spontaneous language; poorly organized structure of speech; and some verbal paraphasias, that is, inappropriate substitutions of words or misnaming. Writing of the patients was nearly always defective. It included: poorly drawn letters, neographisms, improper spatial alignment of letters, and spelling errors (116). The investigators conclude that dysgraphia is the most constant linguistic disorder in the confused patient and clears up as the confusional state abates.

PERSEVERATION. A common feature of the delirious patient's psychomotor behavior is perseveration. Allison (117) defines it as the continuation or recurrence of a purposeful response which is more appropriate to a preceding stimulus than to the succeeding one which has just been given, and which is necessary to elicit it. It is an involuntary phenomenon which can be readily provoked and demonstrated by first asking the patient to shut his eyes and then to put out the tongue. If the patient responds correctly to the first request and then continues to repeat the response after a new command has been given, perseveration is judged to be present. Other relevant tests involve verbal responses, such as counting from 1 to 20, giving the days of the week and the months of the year, both forwards and backwards. The perseverating patient will carry out the first request correctly but when asked to switch to the next task will tend to continue with the preceding one (117, 118). The observer may suspect that the patient perseverates if the latter repeats in an apparently purposeless manner certain words, phrases, and gestures.

In summary, the level and form of psychomotor activity in delirium are highly variable and of limited diagnostic importance. They may range from almost total immobility to frantic hyperkinesia, which may result in cardiovascular collapse. The predominant level of activity underlies the distinction between hyperactive and hypoactive delirium. Most patients display some degree of one or the other type of abnormal psychomotor behavior either as the predominant mode or as a mixture of both.

MOOD AND EMOTIONAL DISORDERS

Lability of emotional expression is common in delirium. Depression, anxiety, irritability, and anger are often observed in various combinations and time sequences. It is a common experience, recently documented experimentally (119) that unpleasant changes of mood preceed and accompany fever. They are not confined to febrile illnesses. A patient's irritability may be manifested by a lowered threshold of tolerance for all sensory stimuli. Bright lights and loud noises may provoke displeasure and annoyance.

The majority of patients experience anxiety, apathy, anger, or sadness. These emotions tend to vary in intensity and duration throughout a delirious episode, and even during a single day, which justifies the phrase "lability of mood and emotions." Emotional arousal may range from panic to apathy. Either state may predominate or there may be shifts between them. Some patients show no abnormal emotions regardless of the degree of severity of delirium. Others display morbid fear, euphoria, elation, or rage. On the whole, unpleasant mood and emotions tend to predominate. One should make a distinction, however, between delirium arising in the course of an unwanted illness and that which is deliberately self-induced with deliriogenic agents for the purpose of experiencing hallucinations and an altered state of awareness. In the former case the delirium is rarely a pleasant experience; in the latter, it may be.

Autonomic arousal is a usual concomitant of emotions, such as anxiety or fear, anger, and elation. When these emotions occur in delirium, one notes tachycardia, sweating, dilated pupils, increased blood pressure, low grade fever, pallor or flushing of the skin, etc. These and other autonomic changes may, of course, be brought about by direct pharmacological action of the agents responsible for the delirium, such as anticholinergic drugs. Stimulation or disinhibition of either central or peripheral parts of the autonomic nervous system, or direct interference with the neurotransmitters in the sympathetic or parasympathetic components of the autonomic system, may bring about different patterns of autonomic arousal in a given delirious patient. The resulting symptoms may serve to enhance emotional arousal such as fear.

Emotional responses of a delirious patient have many potential determinants. They reflect personality; nature of the underlying illness and its symptoms; presence and content of released thoughts, images, and hallucinations; and the characteristics of the sensory environment in which delirium is lived through (120). Field-dependent individuals seem to react with intense anxiety to the blurred and often distorted perception occasioned by the illness. People whose sense of security depends on cognitive and perceptual clarity are particularly liable to experience cognitive disorganization as an overwhelming threat of loss of control, and respond with anxiety to the point of panic. Others may, for the same reasons, experience shame, depression, or anger. Paranoid trends in the personality are readily brought to the fore by cognitive disorganization and the associated sense of danger and helplessness. Persecutory delusions may then arise out of the heightened mistrust, anxiety, and a tendency to misinterpret stimuli. If, as often happens, delirium complicates a severe, painful, debilitating, or terminal illness, the objective discomfort and realistic sense of danger or loss are liable to evoke and enhance unpleasant emotions. Onset of the underlying disease, or its exacerbation, at a time when the patient is experiencing intensified inner or interpersonal conflicts, or both, or has suffered a recent personally meaningful loss, is likely to facilitate the development of delirium and influence adversely the patient's emotional state. In such cases, the psychological stress of the illness itself and that related to external events reinforce each other and bring about some degree of failure of the patient's defense and coping mechanisms. This results in the emergence of distressing emotions, which facilitate the onset of, and are in turn enhanced by, disturbing thoughts, imagery, and perceptual distortions. Apart from psychosocial factors, other variables related to the etiology of a given delirious episode may influence the quality and intensity of the emotions experienced by the patient. One may postulate that selective affinity of a given pathogen for the various components of the limbic system is likely to play a role in determining the patient's emotional state.

Emotional disturbances in delirium are of both theoretical and practical interest. Intense fear, depression, or anger may lead to behavior endangering the safety of the patient and people around him or her. High degree of emotional and autonomic arousal may have an adverse effect on the patient's capacity to recover from the underlying disease, particularly if the cardiovascular system is compromised. Depression may occasionally lead to a suicide attempt. Panic can result in accidental and sometimes even fatal injury if the patient attempts a wild flight. A frightened, delirious patient, who was ineffectively sedated, ran out of the hospital and fell onto the street, sustaining fatal cerebral hemorrhage. The hospital was subsequently sued for damages and lost the case. Clearly, a delirious patient's emotional state and related behavior must be assessed and adequately managed if injury or even death and medicolegal complications are to be prevented.

In summary, emotional abnormalities are common in delirium but none of them can be considered to be an invariable component of the syndrome. Definitions of delirium that include fear among the diagnostic criteria are misleading. Many delirious patients do experience fear of some degree of intensity and may act accordingly with flight or fight. Many other patients, however, are mildly depressed, embarrassed, angry, or just apathetic and indifferent. These emotional states may shift rapidly and unpredictably as do other symptoms. Emotional lability is common. The quality of the emotions in delirium has multiple determinants, colors the subjective experience of the illness, and must be assessed for proper management and prevention of serious complications.

REFERENCES

1. Hirsch, W.: A study of delirium. *NY Med J* 70:109-115, 1899.
2. Hoch, A.: A study of some cases of delirium produced by drugs. *Studies in Psychiatry* 1:75-93, 1912.
3. Agulnik, P.L., DiMascio, A., and Moore, P.: Acute brain syndrome

associated with lithium therapy. *Am J Psychiatr 129*:621-623, 1972.

4. Deikman, A.J.: Bi-modal consciousness. *Arch Gen Psychiatr 25*:481-489, 1971.

5. Globus, G.G., Maxwell, G., and Savodnik, I., Eds.: *Consciousness and the Brain.* New York, Plenum Publ. Corpor., 1976.

6. Tart, C.T.: States of consciousness and state-specific sciences. *Science 176*:1203-1210, 1972.

7. Hebb, D.O.: *Textbook of Psychology.* 3rd edition. Philadelphia, Saunders, 1972, p. 250.

8. Kleitman, N.: Sleep, wakefulness, and consciousness. *Psychol Bull 54*:354-359, 1957.

9. Adams, A.E.: Über Grundlagen und Störungen des Bewusstseins. *Fortschr Neurol Psychiatr 40*:308-322, 1972.

10. Aggernaes, A., Myschetzky, A., Paikin, H., and Vitger, J.: Empirical investigations on the reliability and the value for differential diagnosis of 21 clinical symptoms of disturbed states of consciousness. *Acta Psychiatr Scand 51*:51-66, 1975.

11. Boor, W. de: *Bewusstsein und Bewusstseinsstörungen.* Berlin, Springer, 1966.

12. Ey, H.: "Disorders of Consciousness in Psychiatry." In Vinken, P.J. and Bruyn, G.W., Eds. *Handbook of Clinical Neurology,* Vol. 3, pp. 112-136. Amsterdam, North-Holland Publ. Co., 1969.

13. Fischer, S.: Die sogenannten Bewusstseinsstörungen. *Arch Psychiatr Nervenkrank 67*:537-568, 1923.

14. Orschansky, J.: Uber Bewusstseinsstörungen und deren Beziehungen zur Verrücktheit und Dementia. *Arch f Psychiatr 20*:309-353, 1889.

15. Peters, U.H.: Bewusstseinstrübung-Vigilität-Vigilanz. *Nervenarzt 47*:173-175, 1976.

16. Jackson, J.H.: *Selected Writings.* Taylor, J., Ed. 2 vols. London, Hodder and Stoughton, 1932.

17. Kleitman, N.: Not only sleep—wakefulness as well! *Waking and Sleeping 1*:121, 1977.

18. Heinroth, A.: *De Delirio Inter Somnum et Vigiliam.* Lipsiae, Typis Guil. Staritzii, 1842.

19. Hunter, J.: *The Works of John Hunter, F.R.S.* Vol. 1 Palmer, J.F., Ed. London, Longman, Rees, Orme, Brown, Green, and Longman, 1835.

20. Lasègue, C.: Le délire alcoolique n'est pas un délire, mais un rêve. *Arch Gen Med 88*:513-536, 1881.

21. Greenberg, R. and Pearlman, C.: Delirium tremens and dreaming. *Am J Psychiatry, 124*:133-142, 1967.

22. Maxion, H. and Schneider, E.: Alkohol-delir und Traumschlaf. *Arch Psychiatr Nervenkr 214*:116-126, 1971.

23. Simon, O., Schulz, H., and Rassmann, W.: The definition of waking stages on the basis of continuous polygraphic recordings in normal subjects. *Electroencephalogr Clin Neurophysiol* 42:48-56, 1977.
24. Othmer, E., Hayden, M.P., and Segelbaum, R.: Encephalic cycles during sleep and wakefulness in humans: A 24-hour pattern. *Science 164*:447-449, 1969.
25. Kripke, D.F. and Sonnenschein, D.: A 90 minute daydream cycle. *Sleep Res 2*:187, 1973.
26. Kripke, D.F. and Sonnenschein, D.: *A biologic rhythm in waking fantasy.* Personal communication, 1977.
27. Moses, J., Lubin, A., Johnson, L.C., and Naitoh, P.: Rapid eye movement cycle in a sleep-dependent rhythm. *Nature 265*:360-361, 1977.
28. Johnson, L.C.: Are stages of sleep related to waking behavior? *Am Sci 61*:326-338, 1973.
29. Kjellberg, A.: Sleep deprivation and some aspects of performance. *Waking and Sleeping 1*:139-143, 1977.
30. Johnson, L.C.: "The Effect of Total, Partial, and Stage Sleep Deprivation on EEG Patterns and Performance." In *Behavior and Brain Electrical Activity.* Burch, N. and Altschuler, H.L., Eds. New York, Plenum Publishing Company, 1975.
31. Naitoh, P.: Sleep deprivation in human subjects: A reappraisal. *Waking and Sleeping 1*:53-60, 1976.
32. Vogel, G.W.: A review of REM sleep deprivation. *Arch Gen Psychiatr 32*:749-761, 1975.
33. Guilleminault, C., Philips, R., and Dement, W.: A syndrome of hypersomnia with automatic behavior. *Electroencephalogr Clin Neurophysiol 38*:403-413, 1975.
34. Jouvet, M. and Pujol, J.F.: Role des monoamines dans la regulation de la vigilance. *Rev Neurol 127*:115-138, 1972.
35. Livrea, P., Puca, F.M., Barnaba, A., and Di Reda, L.: Abnormal central monoamine metabolism in humans with "true hypersomnia" and "sub-wakefulness." *Eur Neurol 15*:71-76, 1977.
36. Ey, H., Lairy, G.C., de Barros-Ferreira, M., and Goldsteinas, L.: *Psychophysiologie du Sommeil et Psychiatrie.* Paris, Masson, 1975.
37. Luria, A.R.: The quantitative assessment of levels of wakefulness. *Soviet Psychology 12*:73-84, 1973.
38. Luria, A.R.: *The Working Brain.* London, Penguin Books, 1973.
39. Posner, M.I. and Boies, S.J.: Components of attention. *Psychol Rev 78*:391-408, 1971.
40. Hernandez-Peon, R.: "Physiological Mechanisms in Attention." In Russell, R.W., Ed. *Frontiers in Physiological Psychology,* pp. 121-147. New York, Academic Press, 1966.

104   *Delirium: Acute Brain Failure in Man*

41. Pribram, K.H. and McGuinness, D.: Arousal, activation, and effort in the control of attention. *Psychol Rev 82*:116-149, 1975.
42. Magoun, H.W.: *The Waking Brain.* Springfield, Ill., Charles C Thomas, 1958.
43. Barrough, P.: *The Method of Physick.* 3rd edition. London, Field, 1596.
44. Willis, T.: *Two Discourses Concerning the Soul of Brutes.* London, Bring, Harper and Leigh, 1683.
45. Hartley, D.: *Observations on Man, His Duty, and His Expectations.* London, Leake and Frederick, 1749.
46. Jaspers, K.: *General Psychopathology.* Chicago, Univ. of Chicago Press, 1963, pp. 137-154.
47. Hilgard, E.R.: *Introduction to Psychology.* 2nd edition. New York, Harcourt, Brace, 1957.
48. Levin, M.: Thinking disturbances in delirium. *AMA Arch Neurol Psychiatr 75*:62-66, 1956.
49. Romano, J. and Engel, G.L.: Delirium. 1. Electroencephalographic data. *AMA Arch Neurol Psychiatr 51*:356-377, 1944.
50. Fothergill, J.M.: The management of delirium. *The Practitioner 13*:400-408, 1874.
51. Willi, J.: "Delir, Dämmerzustand und Vervirrtheit bei Körperlich Kranken." In *Akute psychische Begleiterscheinungen korperlicher Krankheiten.* Bleuler, M., Willi, J., and Buhler, H.R., Eds. Stuttgart, Thieme, 1966, pp. 27-158.
52. Wolff, H.G. and Curran, D.: Nature of delirium and allied states. *AMA Arch Neurol Psychiatr 33*:1175-1215, 1935.
53. Farber, I. J.: Acute brain syndrome. *Dis Nerv Syst 20*:296-299, 1959.
54. Simon, A. and Cahan, R.B.: The acute brain syndrome in geriatric patients. *Psychiatr Res Rep 16*:8-21, 1963.
55. Forgus, R.H.: *Perception.* New York, McGraw-Hill, 1966.
56. Morris, G.O. and Singer, M.T.: Sleep deprivation: The context of consciousness. *J Nerv Ment Dis 143*:291-304, 1966.
57. Cameron, N. and Margaret, A.: *Behavior Pathology.* Boston, Houghton Mifflin, 1951.
58. Lunn, V.: On body hallucinations. *Acta Psychiatr Scand 41*:387-399, 1965.
59. Dewhurst, K. and Pearson, J.: Visual hallucinations of the self in organic disease. *J Neurol Neurosurg Psychiatry 18*:53-57, 1955.
60. Lunn, V.: Autoscopic phenomena. *Acta Psychiatr Scand 46, Suppl. 219*:118-125, 1970.
61. Willanger, R. and Klee, A.: Metamorphopsia and other visual disturbances with latency occurring in patients with diffuse cerebral lesions. *Acta Neurol Scand 42*:1-18, 1966.

62. Robinson, W.G., Jr.: "The Toxic Delirious Reactions of Old Age." In Kaplan, O.J., Ed. *Mental Disorders in Later Life*, pp. 332-351. Stanford, Stanford University Press, 1956.

63. Frieske, D.A. and Wilson, W.P.: "Formal Qualities of Hallucinations: A Comparative Study of the Visual Hallucinations in Patients with Schizophrenic, Organic and Affective Psychoses." In Hoch, P.H. and Zubin, J., Eds. *Psychopathology of Schizophrenia*. New York, Grune & Stratton, 1966, pp. 49-62.

64. Guttman, O.: Psychic disturbances in typhus fever. *Psychiatr Quart* 26:478-491, 1952.

65. Mendelson, J., Solomon, P. and Lindemann, E.: Hallucinations of poliomyelitis patients during treatment in a respirator. *J Nerv Ment Dis 126*:421-428, 1958.

66. Lewis, D.J.: Lilliputian hallucinations in the functional psychoses. *Can Psychiatr Assn J 6*:177-201, 1961.

67. Lowe, G.R.: The phenomenology of hallucinations as an aid to differential diagnosis. *Br J Psychiatr 123*:621-633, 1973.

68. Head, H.: Certain mental changes that accompany visceral disease. *Brain 24*:344-356, 1901.

69. Bender, L.: "The Maturation Process and Hallucinations in Children." In Keup, W., Ed. *Origins and Mechanisms of Hallucinations*. New York, Plenum Press, 1970, pp. 95-101.

70. Goodwin, D.W., Alderson, P. and Rosenthal, R.: Clinical significance of hallucinations in psychiatric disorders. *Arch Gen Psychiatry* 24:76-80, 1971.

71. Siegel, R.K. and West, L.J., Eds.: *Hallucinations*. New York, Wiley, 1975.

72. Keup, W., Ed.: *Origin and Mechanisms of Hallucinations*. New York, Plenum Press, 1970.

73. Siegel, R. K.: Hallucinations. *Sci Am 237*:132-140, 1977.

74. Slade, P.: Hallucinations. *Psychol Med 6*:7-13, 1976.

75. Klüver, H.: "Neurobiology of Normal and Abnormal Perception." In Hoch, P.H. and Zubin, J., Eds. *Psychopathology of Perception*. New York, Grune & Stratton, 1965, pp. 1-40.

76. Foulkes, D., Fleisher, S. and Trupin, E.: Thought-sampling in relaxed wakefulness. In Levin, P. and Koella, W.P., Eds. *Sleep 1974*. Basel, Karger, 1975, pp. 142-145.

77. West, L.J.: "A Clinical and Theoretical Overview of Hallucinatory Phenomena." In Siegel, R.K. and West, L.J., Eds. *Hallucinations*. New York, Wiley, 1975, pp. 287-311.

78. Dement, W., Halper, C., Pivik, T., et al.: "Hallucinations and Dreaming." In Hamburg, D., Ed. *Perception and Its Disorders*. Baltimore, Williams & Wilkins, 1970, pp. 335-359.

79. Itil, T.M.: Anticholinergic drug-induced sleep-like EEG pattern in man. *Psychopharmacologia (Berlin) 14*:383-393, 1969.

80. Modestin, J.: Zur Pathogenese deliranter Zustände. *Confinia Psychiatr 17*:42-52, 1974.
81. Tachibana, M., Tanaka, K., Hishikawa, Y. and Kaneko, Z.: A sleep study of acute psychotic states due to alcohol and meprobamate addiction. *Adv Sleep Res 2*:177-205, 1975.
82. Ribstein, M.: Hypnagogic hallucinations. *Adv Sleep Res 3*:145-160, 1976.
83. Vogel, G.W.: Mentation reported from naps of narcoleptics. *Adv Sleep Res 3*:161-168, 1976.
84. Kass, W., Preiser, G. and Jenkins, A.H.: Inter-relationship of hallucinations and dreams in spontaneously hallucinating patients. *Psychiatr Q 44*:488-499, 1970.
85. Kubie, L.S.: "The Psychodynamic Position on Etiology." In Kruse, H.D., Ed. *Integrating the Approaches to Mental Disease*, p. 24. New York, Hoeber-Harper, 1957.
86. Tausk, V.: Alcoholic occupation delirium. *J Nerv Ment Dis 56*:537-539, 1922.
87. Engel, G.L. and Romano, J.: Delirium, a syndrome of cerebral insufficiency. *J Chron Dis 9*:260-277, 1959.
88. Petersen, R.C.: Scopolamine induced learning failures in man. *Psychopharmacology 52*:283-289, 1977.
89. Davis, K.L., Hollister, L.E., Overall, J., et al.: Physostigmine: Effects on cognition and affect in normal subjects. *Psychopharmacology 51*:23-27, 1976.
90. Mesulam, M.M. and Geschwind, N.: Disordered mental states in the postoperative period. *Urol Clin N Am 3*:199-215, 1976.
91. Whitty, W.C.M. and Zangwill, O.L., Eds.: *Amnesia*. London, Butterworths, 1966.
92. Mercer, B., Wapner, W., Gardner, H. and Benson, F.: A study of confabulation. *Arch Neurol 34*:429-433, 1977.
93. Hinsie, L.E. and Campbell, R.J.: *Psychiatric Dictionary*. 3rd edition. New York, Oxford University Press, 1960.
94. Levin, M.: Delirium: A gap in psychiatric teaching. *Am J Psychiatry 107*:689-694, 1951.
95. Freedman, A.M., Kaplan, H.I. and Sadock, B.J., Eds.: *Comprehensive Textbook of Psychiatry*. 2nd edition, Vol. 2, p. 2582. Baltimore, Williams & Wilkins, 1975.
96. Romano, J. and Engel, G.L.: Physiologic and psychologic considerations of delirium. *Med Clin N Am 28*:629-638, 1944.
97. Koriat, A. and Fischhoff, B.: What day is today? An inquiry into the process of time orientation. *Memory & Cognition 2*:201-205, 1974.
98. Benton, A.L., Allen, M.W., van and Fogel, M.L.: Temporal orientation in cerebral disease. *J Nerv Ment Dis 139*:110-119, 1964.

99. Levin, H.S. and Benton, A.L.: Temporal orientation in patients with brain disease. *Appl Neurophysiol 38*:56-60, 1975.
100. Levin, M.: Varieties of disorientation. *J Ment Sci 102*:619-623, 1956.
101. Levin, M.: Delirious disorientation: The law of the unfamiilar mistaken for the familiar. *J Ment Sci 91*:447-450, 1945.
102. Levin, M.: Spatial disorientation in delirium. *Am J Psychiatry 113*:174-175, 1956.
103. Weinstein, E.A. and Kahn, R.L.: *Denial of Illness*. Springfield, Ill., Charles C Thomas, 1955.
104. Levin, M.: Delirium: An experience and some reflections. *Am J Psychiatr 124*:1120-1123, 1968.
105. Thomson, L.R.: Sensory deprivation: A personal experience. *Am J Nurs 73*:266-268, 1973.
106. Wilbourn, A.J.: A report on the infection inside my head. *Hosp Phys 3*:38-64, 1972.
107. Conrad, K.: "Die symptomatischen Psychosen." In Gruhle, H.W., Jung, R., Mayer-Gross, W. and Mueller, M., Eds. *Psychiatrie der Gegenwart*, Band 2, pp. 369-436. Berlin, Springer, 1960.
108. King, H.E.: "Psychomotor Correlates of Behavior Disorder." In Kietzman, M.L., Sutton, S. and Zubin, J., Eds.: *Experimental Approaches to Psychopathology*. New York, Academic Press, 1975, pp. 421-450.
109. Baker, A.B. and Knutson, J.: Psychiatric aspects of uremia. *Am J Psychiatr 102*:683-687, 1946.
110. *Brain's Diseases of the Nervous System*. 8th edition. Revised by Walton, J.N. Oxford, Oxford University Press, 1977, p. 1177.
111. *Harrison's Principles of Internal Medicine*. 7th edition. Wintrobe, M.M., Thorn, G.W., Adams, R.D., et al., Eds. New York, McGraw-Hill, 1974, p. 149.
112. Engel, G.L.: "Delirium." In Freedman, A.M. and Kaplan, H.S., Eds. *Comprehensive Textbook of Psychiatry*. Baltimore, Williams & Wilkins, 1967, pp. 711-716.
113. Walters, J.H.: Encephalitis lethargica revisited. *J Oper Psychiatr 8*:37-46, 1977.
114. Broadbent, D.E.: *Decision and Stress*. New York, Academic Press, 1971, p. 18.
115. Chedru, F. and Geschwind, N.: Disorders of higher cortical functions in acute confusional states. *Cortex 8*:395-411, 1972.
116. Chedru, F. and Geschwind, N.: Writing disturbances in acute confusional states. *Neuropsychologia 10*:343-353, 1972.
117. Allison, R.S.: Perseveration as a sign of diffuse and focal brain damage. *Br Med J 2*:1027-1032, 1966.
118. Levin, M.: Perseveration at various levels of complexity, with comments on delirium. *AMA Arch Neurol Psychiatr 73*:439-444, 1955.

119. Canter, A.: Changes in mood during incubation of acute febrile disease and the effects of pre-exposure psychologic status. *Psychosom Med 34*:424-430, 1972.
120. Lipowski, Z.J.: Delirium, clouding of consciousness and confusion. *J Nerv Ment Dis 145*:227-255, 1967.

Additional References

Cramon, von D. Consciousness and disturbances of consciousness. *J Neurol 219*:1-13, 1978.

Jacobs, B.L. Dreams and hallucinations: A common neurochemical mechanism mediating their phenomenological similarities. *Neurosci Biobehav Rev 2*:59-69, 1978.

Kripke, D.F. and Sonnenschein, D. "A Biologic Rhythm in Waking Fantasy." In Pope, K.S. and Singer, J.L., Eds., *The Stream of Consciousness*. New York, Plenum Press, 1978, pp. 321-332.

Natsoulas, T. Consciousness. *Am J Psychol 33*:906-914, 1978.

Shallice, T. Dual functions of consciousness. *Psychol Rev 79*:383-393, 1972.

Singer, J.L. Navigating the stream of consciousness: Research in day-dreaming and related inner experience. *Am J Psychol 30*:727-738, 1975.

Staub, H. and Thoelen, H., Eds. *Bewusstseinsstörungen*. Stuttgart, Thieme Verlag, 1961.

Zinberg, N.E., Ed. *Alternate States of Consciousness*. London, Collier Macmillan Publishers, 1977.

CHAPTER 5

ETIOLOGY OF DELIRIUM

THE SYNDROME OF delirium can be caused by a wide range of cerebral and systemic diseases. A necessary condition for its development is a *diffuse disturbance of cerebral metabolism*. Such disturbance may result from any factor (or combination of factors) that interferes with the supply, uptake, and/or utilization of glucose, oxygen, or both, by the cerebral neurons. There may be interference with substrate availability, or enzymatic disturbances (lack of enzyme activators, inhibition, or destruction of enzymes), or a combination of these factors. Thus, there is a disturbance of the production or utilization of energy involving cerebral cortex and subcortical structures whose integrated activity is necessary for the maintenance of organized cognitive functioning and awareness. It follows that the range of potential etiological factors is vast. They are listed in Table 5-I. This list is comprehensive but incomplete: to list all of the disorders and agents that may give rise to delirium would be neither feasible nor practically useful. All of the clinically important causes have been included.

The occurrence of delirium as such does not allow identification of the causal noxious agent or disease. In this sense the syndrome may be regarded as a *nonspecific psychopathological* manifestation of cerebral disorder brought about by one or more toxic, infectious, metabolic, or other pathogenic factors or conditions which disrupt to some extent the highest integrative functions of the brain. The pathogenic mechanisms involved are in many cases unknown. There is some evidence, discussed in Chapter 6, that a number of possible pathogenic pathways may intervene between a given etiological factor and the onset of delirium. Furthermore, the probability of the occurrence of the latter may be increased if certain predisposing and facilitating psychobiological and environmental variables are present. All these factors need to be taken into account in a discussion of the etiology of delirium. For the sake of clarity, the etiological factors will be discussed under the following three headings: *organic causes, predisposing factors,* and *facilitating factors.*

TABLE 5-I

ORGANIC CAUSES OF DELIRIUM

1. INTOXICATION BY DRUGS AND POISONS
   a. drugs: anticholinergic agents, sedative-hypnotics, digitalis derivatives, opiates, corticosteroids, salicylates, antibiotics, anticonvulsants, anti-arrhythmic and antihypertensive drugs, antineoplastic agents, cimetidine, lithium, antiparkinsonian agents, disulfiram, indomethacin, bismuth salts, phencyclidine
   b. alcohol: ethyl and methyl
   c. addictive inhalants: gasoline, glue, ether, nitrous oxide, nitrites
   d. industrial poisons: carbon disulphide, organic solvents, methyl chloride and bromide, heavy metals, organophosphorus insecticides, carbon monoxide
   e. snakebite
   f. poisonous plants and mushrooms

2. WITHDRAWAL SYNDROMES
   a. alcohol: delirium tremens
   b. sedatives and hypnotics: barbiturates, chloral hydrate, chlordiazepoxide, diazepam, ethchlorvynol, glutethimide, meprobamate, methyprylon, paraldehyde
   c. amphetamines

3. NUTRITIONAL, HORMONAL AND METABOLIC DISORDERS
   a. hypoxia
   b. hypoglycemia
   c. hepatic, renal, pancreatic, pulmonary insufficiency (encephalopathy)
   d. avitaminosis: nicotinic acid, thiamine, cyanocobalamine (vit. B12), folate, pyridoxine (?)
   e. hypervitaminosis: intoxication by vitamins A and D
   f. hormonal disorders: hyperinsulinism, hyperthyroidism, hypothyroidism, hypopituitarism, Addison's disease, Cushing's syndrome, hypoparathyroidism, hyperparathyroidism
   g. disorders of fluid and electrolyte metabolism:
      i. dehydration, water intoxication
      ii. alkalosis, acidosis
      iii. hypernatremia, hyponatremia, hyperkalemia, hypokalemia, hypercalcemia, hypocalcemia, hypermagnesemia, hypomagnesemia
   h. errors of metabolism:
      i. porphyria
      ii. carcinoid syndrome
      iii. hepatolenticular degeneration (Wilson's disease)

4. INFECTIONS
   a. systemic: pneumonia, typhoid, typhus, acute rheumatic fever, malaria, influenza, mumps, diphtheria, brucellosis, infectious mononucleosis, in-

fectious hepatitis, malaria, subacute bacterial endocarditis, bacteremia, septicemia, Rocky Mountain spotted fever, legionnaires' disease
  b. intracranial: acute, subacute, and chronic
    i. viral encephalitis; aseptic meningitis; rabies
    ii. bacterial meningitis—meningococcal, pneumococcal, Hemophilus influenzae, etc.
    iii. postinfectious and postvaccinial encephalomyelitis
    iv. tuberculous meningitis
    v. neurosyphilis
    vi. fungal infections: cryptococcosis, coccidioidomycosis, histoplasmosis, moniliasis, mucormycosis
    vii. protozoal infections: toxoplasma encephalitis, cerebral malaria
    viii. trichinosis

5. HEAD TRAUMA: concussion, contusion
6. EPILEPSY: ictal and postictal automatism
7. VASCULAR DISORDERS
  a. cerebrovascular disorders:
    i. transient ischemic attacks
    ii. hypertensive encephalopathy
    iii. thrombosis, embolism
    iv. polyarteritis nodosa
    v. systemic lupus erythematosus
    vi. rheumatoid vasculitis
    vii. temporal arteritis
    viii. subarachnoid hemorrhage
    ix. Wegener's granulomatosis
    x. Neuro-Behçet's disease
    xi. pulseless disease
  b. cardiovascular disorders:
    i. myocardial infarction
    ii. congestive heart failure
    iii. cardiac arrhythmias
  c. migraine
8. INTRACRANIAL SPACE-OCCUPYING LESIONS
  a. tumor
  b. abscess
  c. subdural hematoma
  d. aneurysm
  e. parasitic cyst
9. CEREBRAL DEGENERATIVE DISORDERS
  a. multiple sclerosis
  b. Alzheimer's disease and senile dementia
10. EXTRACRANIAL NEOPLASM: e.g. bronchogenic carcinoma
11. DISORDERS OF THE HEMATOPOIETIC SYSTEM
  a. pernicious anemia
  b. erythremia
  c. thrombotic thrombocytopenic purpura
12. INJURY BY PHYSICAL AGENTS
  a. heatstroke
  b. radiation
  c. electrocution
13. DISORDERS DUE TO HYPERSENSITIVITY
  a. serum sickness
  b. food allergy

ORGANIC CAUSES OF DELIRIUM

Table 5-I lists the more common organic causes of delirium. The presence of a cerebral disorder due to at least one of these organic factors is a necessary condition for the occurrence of delirium. The mere presence of a given pathogenic agent need not, however, constitute a *sufficient* condition for the syndrome to occur. Certain characteristics of the organic factors involved as well as those inherent in the patient, in his or her environment, or both, tend to codetermine the onset, severity, and duration of delirium (1). The following characteristics of the organic causal factors influence the probability of the occurrence of delirium in a given individual exposed to one or more of them.

Absolute Strength of the Pathogenic Factor

This variable refers to the quantitative dimension of the etiologic factor. It is a common clinical observation that the degree of deviation from the dynamic steady state of the organism, or homeostasis, tends to influence the probability that a given noxious agent or the deficiency of an essential constituent of cerebral metabolism will result in delirium. Examples are provided by the degree of hypoglycemia or hypoxia; the concentration of the various electrolytes in the body fluids; the quantity in the body of a particular toxin, such as bromide; degree of deviation from the normal blood pH; the force of impact of mechanical trauma to the head; etc. As a general rule, the greater the amount or strength of a toxic or other noxious agent, or the higher degree of deviation from the normal in the concentration of a constituent of cerebral metabolism, the greater the probability that delirium will take place.

Concurrence of Two or More Pathogenic Factors

If more than one etiologic factor is present at a given time, the probability of the onset of delirium increases. For example, in many cases of postoperative delirium there is a combination of several pathogenic factors, such as administration of anesthetic agents, electrolyte imbalance, infection, hypoxia, etc., which have an additive adverse effect on cerebral metabolism and thus increase the probability of the occurrence of delirium. Other common examples of such multifactorial deliriogenic conditions are provided by systemic infections and severe burns. The higher the number of the pathogenic factors present in an individual at one time, the greater the risk that delirium will occur and be severe.

Rate of Change in the Physico-Chemical Milieu of the Brain

The higher the rate of such change, the more likely is delirium to occur. A rapidly rising intracranial pressure, sudden drop in blood sugar or calcium concentration, precipitate withdrawal of alcohol or sedatives from a person addicted to them, rapid onset of hypoxia or hypercapnia—all of these conditions increase the probability of the onset of delirium due to the short time span in which the pathogenic change has occurred. Patients suffering from a chronic disease, say pulmonary or renal insufficiency, have had time to adapt to the changes in the interval brought about by the disease and may show little or no evidence of cognitive dysfunction with concentrations of CO_2 or BUN which would have been high enough to result in delirium had they occurred rapidly.

Duration of Exposure to the Etiologic Agent

It appears that, other factors being equal, a critical duration of exposure to a given pathogenic factor is needed for delirium to occur. If the duration is too brief, the syndrome may not take place; if it is too long, a subacute or chronic organic brain syndrome rather than delirium is more likely to develop.

Degree of Invasiveness of the Etiologic Agent

This variable pertains to the capacity of a given pathogenic factor to bring about *widespread* derangement of cerebral metabolism. It appears that only diffuse involvement of cerebral neurons may result in delirium. In other words, the metabolism of the brain as a whole has to be impaired if the syndrome is to be precipitated. Toxic and metabolic disorders are commonly accompanied by delirium thanks (presumably) to their capacity to bring about widespread derangement of brain metabolism. Delirium may also be caused by focal lesions of the brain, such as neoplasms. One may postulate that in these cases the lesion exerts a widespread effect on cerebral metabolism, either because it leads to increased intracranial pressure or because it inhibits the function of the reticular activating system or of other cerebral structures which can affect the metabolism of the brain as a whole.

In clinical practice, the most common causes of delirium include intoxication by endogenous or exogenous substances, hypoxia, electrolyte imbalance, systemic infections, drug withdrawal syndromes, head trauma, and epilepsy. These and other organic causes of delirium will be discussed in specific detail in Part II.

PREDISPOSING FACTORS

One could postulate that susceptibility to delirium is universal, that is, any person could develop it if exposed to one of the pathogenic factors of sufficient strength and for an adequate period of time. Yet marked *individual differences* in susceptibility to develop delirium in response to any given etiologic agent exist. Some persons become delirious in the course of even a mild infection or after the intake of a small amount of a drug or other chemical substance. It appears that such high susceptibility to delirium may be either *selective* or *general*. In the former case, the person is liable to develop the syndrome on the basis of a selective, or specific, vulnerability to the effects of a particular drug, for example, an anticholinergic compound, or hypoxia, or hypoglycemia. Such differential vulnerability to a given chemical agent or other causative factor is likely to reflect genetic or acquired neurophysiological or neurochemical defect. For example, acute porphyria with delirium may be precipitated by barbiturates, steroids, and other drugs. Hepatic encephalopathy may be triggered by barbiturates, opiates, ammonium chloride, etc. Acute pathologic alcoholic intoxication is liable to occur in a person who has suffered damage to a temporal lobe (2). Idiosyncrasy to a specific drug, such as acetylsalicylic acid, may underlie susceptibility to delirium on taking a therapeutic dose of it.

General susceptibility implies that the person is prone to develop delirium readily in response to a wide range of causative agents. Only three factors have been firmly established to predispose to delirium in general (3):

1. age sixty years or over
2. addiction to alcohol, drugs, or both
3. cerebral damage due to any cause

The fact that the aged are particularly susceptible to the development of delirium has considerable practical importance and is discussed in detail in Chapter 18.

There is not any conclusive evidence for hereditary or personality predisposing factors, although some authors challenge this (4, 5). They point out, for example, that a person who had suffered from a functional psychosis or delirium in the past is more likely to develop the latter after an operation (5, 6). This observation does not throw any light on the issue of inherited or personality predisposing factors. There is suggestive evidence that maladaptive psychological functioning manifested by an abnormal personality style, paranoid or hysterical for instance, may predispose a person to delirium (5, 7). It has been proposed that people characterized by the perceptual-cognitive style designated "field dependence" are more prone to respond with cognitive disorganization to a wide variety of factors, which may impair cerebral functioning (8). Intake of potentially deliriogenic substances, sleep and sensory deprivation, and information overload share the capacity to disorganize the field dependent subject (8, 9). These observations are suggestive and worthy of further investigations, yet it may be stated that so far not a single psychological variable has been conclusively shown to predispose one to delirium.

Willi (10) has found no relationship between predisposition to schizophrenia and to delirium. There was neither an excessive incidence of schizophrenia among relatives of delirious patients nor an unusually high frequency of delirium in schizophrenics and their relatives. These findings are surprising in view of the often encountered clinical opinion that individuals predisposed to or suffering from schizophrenic disorganization of personality are also more likely to display cognitive disorganization of the delirious type when exposed to an appropriate organic insult to the brain. The whole issue of psychological predisposition to delirium is still unresolved and must await results of future clinical and epidemiological studies.

FACILITATING FACTORS

Susser (11) rightly points out that a common type of causal conditions in disease is that which is neither necessary nor sufficient for its occurrence but only contributory. In this section we will discuss a category of causal factors in delirium which in the present state of knowledge should be regarded as facilitating or contributory rather than either necessary or sufficient for the syndrome to occur. Certain psychobiological and environmental variables have been identified which fit into this category. It is not yet clear if any of these factors can bring about delirium in the absence of the so-called organic causative conditions. Some evidence has been accumulated, however, which allows one to postulate that the following variables can facilitate the development of delirium, intensify it, or both:

1. psychological stress
2. sleep deprivation and other disorders of the sleep-wakefulness cycle
3. sensory deprivation and overload
4. immobilization

Psychological Stress

Psychological stress refers to external and internal stimuli that are perceived by the person, are meaningful to him or her, activate emotions, and elicit physiological changes in the organism that make adaptive demands on it (12). So defined, psychological stress may be used to designate a class of etiologic factors that include social and psychological variables whose harmful effects on body functioning result from their subjective meaning for the individual and the consequent emotional arousal. The latter, with its associated neuroendocrine and peripheral physiological changes, can adversely influence health. The most extensively studied response to a stressful event or situation has been that involving the emotions of anxiety and fear. The distinction, if any, between these two emotions is purely psychological; while fear is seen as a reasonable response to a realistic danger, anxiety refers to irrational fear elicited by symbolic and anticipated, rather than current, dangers. This distinction needs to be restated to avoid semantic confusion. Many investigators use the words "anxiety" and "fear" synonymously. In the discussion to follow, anxiety will be used as the only relevant term.

It is hypothesized that intense anxiety experienced by the person in close temporal relation to the exposure to a deliriogenic organic factor may facilitate development of delirium. Chapman et al. (13) claim that life situations that elicit conflict or otherwise constitute psychological stress for the individual and consequently evoke an intense or prolonged emotional arousal may impair higher cortical functions. Anxiety may, in this context, be regarded as an intervening variable or as the "emotional arousal" involved. There is some evidence that intense anxiety may be accompanied by increased blood flow to, and energy consumption by, the brain (14). This appears to be a catecholamine-mediated change. One may speculate that such an increased demand for energy in response to psychological stress could, if coupled with reduced capacity by cerebral neurons to produce energy, facilitate delirium. Impending surgery or a life-threatening illness may be viewed as kinds of situations in which anxiety is readily aroused and potentially contributes to the onset of delirium in the presence of the various organic factors such as exposure to general anesthetics, electrolyte imbalance, blood loss, and so forth. If this hypothesis is valid, appropriate therapy for anxiety, say sedation or supportive psychotherapy, should be considered to be a preventive measure reducing the probability of the onset of delirium.

Can psychological stress and consequent emotional arousal bring about delirium in the absence of physical illness or exposure to exogenous toxic agents? No definitive answer can be given to this question, and it must remain an open one at this time. For over a century many medical writers have claimed that the so-called acute delirium and related acute confusional states may follow a personally calamitous life change, "emotional shock," and similar events of suggestive psychological stress and intense emotional arousal. Levin (15) wrote of "psychogenic delirium" and discussed its differential diagnosis from "organic" delirium. Clouding of consciousness, which since Bonhoeffer (16) has been regarded as a cardinal feature of acute organic psychoses including delirium, is claimed to occur in a substantial proportion of so-called psychogenic or reactive psychoses (17).

All this impressive literature suggests a relationship of similarity, identity, or overlap between delirium as defined in this book and the various acute mental disorders arising in response to overwhelming psychological stress. This whole issue will be discussed in detail in Chapter 8 dealing with the differential diagnosis. Only the much-needed future research may resolve this controversy. In the present stage of our knowledge, or ignorance, it is judicious to avoid premature closure. To include psychological stress among facilitating or contributory factors in delirium underscores its etiological role and yet leaves open the question if it can precipitate the syndrome in an otherwise healthy individual and one not exposed to any potentially deliriogenic substance. One cannot rule out the possibility, however, that intense emotional arousal, especially anxiety, accompanied by sleep deprivation, hyperventilation, and fatigue might precipitate delirium.

Sleep Deprivation

Since the earliest writings on the subject, sleep deprivation has been invoked as a cause of delirium. Clinical descriptions of delirium almost invariably include some reference to insomnia and other sleep disturbances occurring in close temporal relationship to it. Insomnia commonly precedes the onset of delirium and is usually listed among its prodromata. Prolonged sound sleep was regarded by Hippocrates (18) and countless subsequent observers as a welcome sign of recovery from delirium complicating febrile and other illnesses. Fever has recently been shown to be accompanied by frequent awakenings and reduction of stage 4 and 1-REM sleep (19). Many delirious patients are drowsy and may actually sleep during the day but suffer from insomnia at night. Nocturnal worsening of delirium is its common and characteristic feature.

All the above observations and claims of a causal relationship between disordered, particularly deficient, sleep and delirium repeated in the medical literature for over 2,000 years demand a careful if critical scrutiny. This subject was already introduced in Chapter 4, and a hypothesis was advanced that delirium was a disorder of wakefulness, one in which dissolution of the normal sleep-wakefulness cycle and intermingling of the psychophysiological phenomena of both sleep and waking were cardinal features. This hypothesis will be developed further in this and subsequent chapters. Before resuming this discussion, however, let us focus on the evidence that sleep deprivation is a causative factor in delirium. Results of both experimental and clinical research on this subject are relevant and need to be considered.

EXPERIMENTAL STUDIES. Patrick and Gilbert (20) carried out the first known experimental study of sleep deprivation (SD) in 1896. Since then, numerous papers have been published on this subject; the majority of them in the last twenty years. Several comprehensive recent reviews allow a measure of orientation in this complex field (21-25). Only material relevant to delirium will be reviewed here.

Research on SD has had three foci: loss of all sleep (total sleep deprivation), reduction of total sleep time (partial sleep deprivation), and differential sleep deprivation (sleep-stage deprivation) (21, 25). The earlier work involved mostly *total SD*. Tyler (26) studied 350 men deprived of sleep for up to 112 hours. Seventy percent of the subjects reported hallucinations, and 2 percent developed transient psychotic disorganization resembling paranoid schizophrenia. This latter development attracted undue attention and emphasis. Luby and Gottlieb (27) proposed that SD could produce a model psychosis similar to schizophrenia. West et al. (28) likewise focused on the alleged psychotogenic effects of prolonged SD. They asserted that psychosis would inevitably follow total SD continued for more than 100 to 120 hours.

These early dramatic claims have not been supported by subsequent studies. Thus a 17-year-old volunteer was studied during 264 hours of SD, and at no time displayed psychotic behavior (29). He did show, however, transient disorientation for time, "waking dreams," lapses of memory, an occasional illusion, irritability, and suspiciousness. At no time was there evidence of delusions, hallucinations, or delirium. A study of 4 men deprived of sleep for 205 hours failed to demonstrate psychosis (30). The subjects experienced episodes of disorientation for time, visual illusions and hallucinations, and some degree of cognitive disorganization. These psychopathological manifestations occurred episodically and seemed to coincide with periods of drowsiness and brief lapses into sleep with eyes open (microsleeps). Seven medical student volunteers were studied during seventy-two hours of SD (31). Once again, no psychosis developed, but the subjects experienced visual misperceptions, feelings of depersonalization, disturbances in time perception, and mild intellectual impairment. These changes were ascribed to "hypnogogic states." Four of the volunteers received LSD-25 during SD, and all developed hallucinations. The observers proposed that SD enhanced ego disruptive effects of the hallucinogen.

Two important studies have focused on disorientation and other cognitive abnormalities related to drowsiness during SD (32, 33). The investigators claimed that each level of drowsiness, light, moderate, or severe, is accompanied by primary changes in attention, thinking, and interest, and secondary changes in memory, perception, orientation, and affect expression (32). Not all drowsy subjects experience the secondary changes. Primary process thinking, that is to say thoughts governed by unconscious mental mechanisms and relatively uninfluenced by rules of logic and by facts, was readily released during drowsiness. Visual, but not auditory, hallucinations occurred frequently. The degree of cognitive impairment increased with the duration of SD and the related drowsiness. The sleep-deprived subjects were found to exhibit prolonged episodes of drowsiness with intermittent "lapses," or waves of increased drowsiness, the deepest of which ended in sleep lasting several seconds, or "microsleep." Impairment of focal attention appears to be the primary disorder in drowsiness. Fantasy illusions and hallucinations in the drowsy state are believed to be identical to dreams and result from a failure to separate inner images from outer percepts. The investigators suggest that the cognitive changes observed in drowsiness resemble those seen in narcolepsy, sensory deprivation, and bromide intoxication (32). We may conclude that these changes represent a mild delirium in a state of reduced wakefulness. It appears that the abnormal phenomena encountered in total SD are generally associated with drowsiness and microsleep. The latter might be, in part, sleep onset REM and related hallucinations (34). In any case, it is postulated that drowsiness and the "lapses" provide a crucial link between SD and delirium.

In summary, the most consistently reported psychological abnormalities after total SD include irritability, fatigue, visual illusions and hallucinations, depersonalization, and episodes of reduced selective attention accompanied by varying degrees of disorientation, thinking disturbances, and generally deteriorated cognitive performance. The cognitive-perceptual abnormalities seem to be, at least in part, accounted for by drowsiness and microsleeps. Some researchers, however, have proposed that impaired formation of memory traces and information processing could account for at least some of the abnormalities (21). The latter are consistent with the diagnosis of mild delirium.

EEG changes accompany total SD. There is a decrease in voltage and in percentage of waking alpha activity and an increase in percentage of delta and theta (21). These changes have been interpreted to represent a concomitant of drowsiness with increasing lapses into microsleep (35). Following SD, there is an increase in slow-wave sleep on the first recovery night as compared to its pre-SD level. REM sleep may or may not increase; if it does, the increase occurs on the second recovery night (21). All in all, EEG changes during and after SD are slight or moderate in extent.

Johnson (21) points out that a person's response to SD depends on his or her age, physical condition, mental health, experimental situation, environmental support, and use of drugs to stay awake. It has long been known, for example, that SD is a major precipitating factor in seizure disorders, and it has been used as an activating procedure to bring out epileptic discharges in the EEG (36). Chronic schizophrenics exposed to SD for 100 hours exhibited reactivation of acute psychotic symptoms (37). It may be hypothesized that the aged, the brain-damaged, and those suffering from a chronic physical illness would prove to be more vulnerable to the effects of SD than young and healthy subjects. Furthermore, duration of total SD appears to be an important variable: the longer the exposure, the higher the probability that significant cognitive abnormalities will be observed. Sleep loss of less than forty hours does not impair cognitive functions (23).

Partial SD involves abrupt or gradual restriction of the person's habitual sleep time within a twenty-four-hour period (21, 25). Thus, if an individual routinely sleeps seven hours and his sleep is restricted in the laboratory to three hours, he or she is exposed to partial SD. There is no indication so far that this experimental procedure has brought forward findings relevant to delirium.

Differential or sleep stage SD has involved preventing the subject selectively from obtaining REM or stage 4 sleep (21, 25). Dement (38) pioneered the studies on REM deprivation and reported that subjects deprived of REM sleep for five consecutive nights displayed anxiety, irritability, and difficulty in concentration. There was a statistically significant increase in REM sleep, or "rebound," following deprivation. Early workers in this area of SD research hypothesized that REM deprivation, and thus dream deprivation, would result in eruption of the mental contents of the dream cycle into wakeful awareness and result in the development of hallucinations, delusions, and other psychotic symptoms. This hypothesis, which appeared to be highly attractive and plausible, has not been validated. In 1972, Dement (39) provided an anticlimax for his earlier statements when he wrote that "the behavioral change induced by deprivation is trivial compared to the massive effort required to eliminate REM's for long periods of time."

It is generally recognized now that REM deprivation is not coterminous with dream deprivation since mental activity, mostly visual in character, is frequently reported from NREM sleep (24). Furthermore, frequent dreaming occurs during sleep onset in the absence of REM sleep (24, 40). Dreams occurring during stage 1 sleep onset are indistinguishable from those reported on awakening from REM sleep (24). Dreaming occurs in some form in all stages of sleep, and REM deprivation neither prevents it nor causes marked changes in waking behavior (21). These recent insights are only confirmatory of much earlier views such as those expressed by Holland (41) already in 1839: ". . . no part of sleep is without some condition of dreaming" (p. 266). It appears that only total SD could result in dream elimination. Yet even this possibility is open to question since mental activity either similar to or actually identical with dreaming, as reported on awakening from REM sleep, occurs throughout the sleep-wakefulness cycle (24). This continuity was also postulated by Holland (41) when he wrote that if a person closed his eyes and remained quietly resting while retaining enough of waking consciousness to register his inner experiences, then he would notice images and increasingly confused ideas, and would have diminishing control over them. Holland says: "This, carried further, becomes dreaming" (p. 141). Recent research has provided support for the existence of links, similarities, and transitions among waking imagery, hypnagogic phenomena, and dreaming. One thing is clear: many studies of even prolonged REM deprivation have failed to show any marked behavioral effects (21, 23, 24). This research has thrown no new light on delirium. Two related studies, however, are an exception and call for a more detailed discussion. The first of them has focused on a comparison between REM sleep (8, 42) dreaming and delirium induced experimentally by an anticholinergic drug. The second explored individual differences in response to both REM deprivation and the effects of the deliriogenic drug.

Cartwright (42) has succeeded in inducing a dream-like state in wakefulness by administering a small dose (3.5 mg. intramuscularly) of piperidyl benzilate (Ditran®) to a group of young healthy volunteers. She hypothesized that the subjects who were high dream producers (high REM %) would also be high producers of hallucinations under the drug; that the content of dreams and of drug-induced hallucinations would be similar in the degree of "imaginativeness"; that the EEG and behavioral features of the two states would differ; and that the themes of the drug-induced fantasy and the normal dream fantasy in the same subject would be similar. The first two of these hypotheses were not supported; the last two were. EEG characteristics of the drug state were different from both waking and sleep records of the same subjects. REM's were persistent. EEG showed slow wave activity resembling stage 2 or 3 sleep with superimposed fast activity. Thus, under the drug, the EEG records showed a mixture of the signs of wakefulness and those of stages 1, 2, and 3 of sleep. The subjects reported amnesia for most of the drug experience. Behaviorally, they were at first hyperactive; later some appeared stuporous, but most others entered a hallucinatory state and showed intermittent contact. The hallucinations bore a marked similarity to dreams and were referred to as such by the subjects. Total REM time after drug session was significantly reduced. Cartwright concluded that dream fantasy and drug-induced fantasy were similar and presumably derived from the same substrate of ongoing mental life. She also proposed that the subjects who were more dependent on adequate sensory input (field dependent) were also the ones who responded to the drug with more imaginative hallucinations than the field independent subjects. Piperidyl benzilate seems to create a neurophysiological state similar to that of REM sleep. In a subsequent study Cartwright et al. (8) found that REM sleep-deprived subjects who responded with repeated attempts to regain it and with much EEG disturbance (many intrusions of stage 2 signs into stage 1 REM on the first recovery night) were the same ones who were much disturbed in response to Ditran. Cartwright proposed that they were characterized by high anxiety levels and a low tolerance for changes in usual brain states.

These two studies are interesting in that they suggest similarities between delirium and dreaming, and indicate that Ditran, an anticholinergic compound, may cause delirium at least in part as a result of bringing about an intermediate state between wakefulness and sleep, a state which also facilitates hallucinatory activity. Cartwright has also produced some evidence for the existence of individual differences in susceptibility to both delirium, or at least to hallucinations in delirium, and to disruptive effects of SD. Field dependence and trait anxiety seemed to be the relevant variables.

Deprivation of stage 4 sleep has been less fully explored than that of REM sleep. Studies reported to date have not shown any adverse behavioral effects (21, 23, 43). It has been reported that some blind people have no slow wave sleep at all (44). Rebound of stage 4 sleep during recovery following deprivation of this stage has been demonstrated more consistently than rebound of REM sleep (21). So far, stage 4 deprivation studies have contributed nothing to the understanding of delirium.

Johnson (45) concluded that the *disruption* of the sleep-wakefulness cycle and of the REM-NREM cycle might prove more
important for waking behavior than the time spent in specific
sleep stages. Clinical research seems to confirm this and appears
to be more relevant to the problem of delirium than either partial
or sleep stage SD.

CLINICAL STUDIES. In contrast to the experimental studies
the clinical ones involve investigation of "experiments of nature"
in the form of established pathological conditions. At times,
however, a pathogenic agent may be introduced deliberately
in attempt to replicate a spontaneously occurring disorder and
to study its effect on sleep patterns as a dependent variable.
Thus, fever may be induced by administering a pyrogen, or
delirium may be provoked by injection of an anticholinergic
drug.

Clinical observers from Hippocrates on have repeatedly postulated a cause and effect relationship between sleep loss and
delirium. Furthermore, many writers have called attention to
the similarities between dreaming and delirium and claimed that
the latter represented an intrusion of dreams into waking awareness. Holland (41), whom we quoted earlier, maintained 140
years ago that links and gradations existed among waking
imagery, reverie, dreaming, delirium, and chronic "insanity."
He pointed out that especially in old age the phenomena of
dreaming and "waking aberration" are "closely blended together" and the distinction between sleep and waking is often
blurred. Lasegue (46) maintained that delirium tremens was
nothing but a waking dream. Other authors holding such views
were quoted in Chapter 4 and theoretical implications of their
observations and hypotheses were discussed. This whole theme
will be developed further now, with a particular focus on recent
clinical studies exploring the postulated links between sleep disorders and delirium. While the earlier writers had to depend
on clinical observations and indirect evidence to support their
hypotheses, investigators in the past twenty-five years have
enjoyed the advantage of having at their disposal research tools,
such as the electrooculography introduced by Aserinsky and
Kleitman (47) in 1953, allowing more or less precise delineation
of the several sleep stages in health and disease. These methodo-

logical advances have brought about a vast increase in sleep research and allowed the testing of some of the old and intriguing hypotheses linking delirium to the disorders of sleep. The following discussion will focus on these recent studies. No attempt will be made to review current views on the organization and psychophysiology of sleep (48). Readers are referred to recent monographs on the subject.

Recent sleep research relevant to delirium has focused mostly on alcohol and drug withdrawal syndromes. These studies had been inspired by the earlier, experimental work on the effects of SD, and especially on deprivation of REM sleep. Gross et al. (49) postulated that alcohol would suppress REM sleep and that during withdrawal of alcohol in heavy drinkers there would be REM rebound, manifested clinically by dream-like hallucinatory activity. These investigators had heard alcoholics complain of nightmares following heavy bedtime drinking and report that at times they were unsure whether they were asleep and dreaming or awake and hallucinating. If the alcoholic stopped or reduced his alcohol intake at this stage, he would enter a phase marked by sleeplessness and hallucinations. The latter would typically occur at night, when the patients lay awake with the lights off and eyes closed. These clinical reports struck Gross and his colleagues as indicative of initial REM deprivation, followed by REM rebound. This hypothesis was strengthened by the finding of Gresham et al. (50) that a reduction of REM sleep could be induced by a single bedtime dose of alcohol. In 1963, Gross and his co-workers embarked on a series of studies which have thrown new light on the role of sleep disturbances in the alcohol withdrawal syndrome. This, and related work by others, was exhaustively reviewed recently by Gross and Hastey (51). A summary of these studies follows.

Gross et al. (49) advanced a hypothesis that alcohol withdrawal would precipitate in a heavy drinker a marked rebound of REM sleep, which would then intrude into waking awareness in the form of hallucinations, delusions, and other psychotic phenomena. As noted above, this hypothesis was based partly on clinical observations and partly on Dement's claim (38) that REM deprivation could result in psychosis. In their first paper, Gross et al. (49) reported observations on four patients suffering from acute alcoholic psychoses. They found striking elevations of REM sleep and almost complete absence of slow-wave sleep. The patients described vivid dreams that continued into the waking hallucinations. The investigators proposed that heavy alcohol intake had a dual effect: to enhance the propensity for REM and to block its discharge. When alcohol is withdrawn, there is consequently a massive eruption of REM, whose hallucinatory elements appear in the waking state. The researchers concluded that neither REM deprivation nor REM rebound could adequately account for alcohol withdrawal delirium. Yet, Greenberg and Pearlman (52) proposed just that. They studied the effects of alcohol and of withdrawal from alcohol on sleep. They found that withdrawal consistently resulted in increase in stage 1-REM sleep, which reached 100 percent of total sleep time just before delirium tremens developed. The investigators hypothesized that dream deprivation resulted from heavy alcohol intake and that withdrawal of alcohol led to "an overflow of stage 1-REM into the waking state." Clinically, this "overflow" manifested itself as delirium tremens.

The work just described attracted much attention for both theoretical and practical, therapeutic reasons. It seemed to demonstrate a pathogenic role of sleep disturbances in delirium tremens and to endorse Lasegue's (46) claim that delirium tremens was equivalent to a waking dream. Subsequent studies, however, showed that things were more complex. Johnson et al. (53) reported on a study of chronic alcoholics during both intake and withdrawal of alcohol. The most striking findings were the *fragmentation* of sleep and absence of slow-wave sleep. The former was shown by frequent awakenings and stage shifts and a high number of movements. The total REM percentage was reduced during two nights of alcohol intake but soon returned to normal levels. Stage-4 sleep remained absent in most patients over ten days of withdrawal. Johnson and co-workers asserted that changes in sleep characteristics represented the result and not the cause of disturbed behavior, yet it is not clear how they arrived at this conclusion. The fact is that the only patient in the study who developed delirium tremens showed sleep patterns almost identical with those reported by Gross et al. (49) and Greenberg and Pearlman (52). They consisted primarily of stage-1 sleep and showed REM sleep disrupted by frequent awakenings. The relationship between the reported sleep changes and delirium was not clarified by this study.

Vogel (54) has criticized some of the early studies linking the rebound of increased REM pressure with hallucinations and other symptoms of delirium. He pointed out that what some of the investigators regarded as "REM sleep" could have been a confusional state with visual hallucinations occurring during wakefulness. Vogel maintained that Gross et al. (49) and Greenberg and Pearlman (52) had not provided sufficient evidence that the reported hallucinations were a waking REM discharge because of increased REM pressure. He suggested that total sleep deprivation might have accounted for the observed sleep changes and hallucinations. A number of investigators have attempted to settle these issues in the past decade. Maxion and Schneider (55) studied patients during and after alcoholic delirium and reported that during delirium there were no normal alternating sleep stages. Instead, "waking stage-1 REM sleep" predominated. The authors concluded that during delirium tremens penetration of wakefulness by REM sleep occurs. This assertion is challenged by Wolin and Mello (56), who have carried out carefully designed studies of alcoholics in states of both intoxication and withdrawal. They concluded that it would be premature to assume a predictable relationship between hallucinatory episodes and REM activity. The proposed continuum of perceptual changes that progressed from alterations to illusions, vivid dreams, and finally hallucinations could not be confirmed. There was no consistent sequence of alcohol-induced suppression of REM sleep, followed by REM rebound, during alcohol withdrawal. Hallucinations were observed during intoxication and withdrawal, and they showed no invariant relationships to REM activity. The investigators concluded that their data offered no unequivocal support for the hypothesis that hallucinations represent waking dreams.

Reviews by Gross and his associates (51, 57, 58) have underscored the complexity of the relationships between sleep disturbances and delirium of alcohol withdrawal. They emphasize that in order to understand these disturbances it is necessary to appreciate the effects of alcohol on sleep. The level of blood alcohol concentration and its duration are among the key factors affecting the probability of the occurrence of withdrawal delirium. The most prominent sleep disturbances in the alcoholic were noted during prolonged periods of high blood alcohol concentrations (ab. 200-350 mg. per 100 ml.) and the acute withdrawal period that followed. In alcoholics *all aspects of sleep may be disrupted*. The symptoms include insomnia, hypersomnia, poor sleep, increased napping during daytime, increased frequency of awakenings at night, and nightmares. EEG sleep studies reveal the following changes: instability of the circadian and ultradian sleep rhythms, i.e. fragmentation of the normal organization of sleep, respectively; increasing reduction in the quantity of REM sleep with increasing blood alcohol concentrations; and increase followed by reduction of slow-wave sleep. During the acute withdrawal from alcohol one may observe severe insomnia resulting from difficulty staying asleep, returning to sleep after awakening, and falling asleep at the onset of sleep. Total lack of sleep may occur. EEG studies during acute withdrawal show reduced percentage of slow-wave sleep coupled with a tendency to a rebound of REM sleep. Gross and Hastey (51) have proposed that a relationship exists between higher bedtime blood alcohol levels, a greater reduction of REM during alcohol intake, a higher incidence of nightmares during the early phase of withdrawal, a higher probability of REM rebound during the first three days of withdrawal, and increased chance of hallucinations during withdrawal. During the first week of acute withdrawal one may observe several disturbances of REM sleep in addition to its rebound: sleep onset REM, reduced time of REM onset, and fragmentation of the individual REM periods. Reduction of slow wave sleep has been proposed to increase the vulnerability to and the severity of acute withdrawal (58).

Feinberg and Evarts (59) have advanced a hypothesis to account for the occurrence of delirium due to withdrawal of alcohol and drugs. Two factors are postulated to determine if delirium occurs: first, increased REM pressure; and, second, diffuse impairment of brain processes associated with cognitive deficits and disorientation. This alteration of brain function permits intrusion of REM activity into waking awareness. The authors proposed that the nocturnal delirium commonly occurring in patients with chronic brain syndrome could have a similar basis. In a later paper, Feinberg (60) asserts that changes in slow-wave sleep may be "the necessary condition for delirium to occur," since the syndrome has been found to come on in the presence of normal or low REM levels. Gross and Hastey (51) conclude that while the REM disturbances are the most striking feature of acute alcohol withdrawal, the reduction in slow-wave sleep is the most consistent characteristic.

In summary, it appears that neither rebound of REM sleep nor suppression or absence of slow-wave sleep can alone be regarded as a sufficient condition for alcohol withdrawal delirium to occur. Fragmentation or dissolution of normal circadian and ultradian sleep patterns may prove to be more important in this regard. Gross et al. (57) have proposed that sleep disturbances may play a causal role in the development of the delirium. This is still no more than a hypothesis. Rather than to view sleep disturbances as a cause of delirium, it may be more appropriate to regard them as a key *pathogenetic mechanism* in the development of the latter. The cause in this case is alcohol intoxication, followed by withdrawal from alcohol. One also cannot rule out the possibility that the sleep disturbances and delirium are *separate* consequences of the same pathological cerebral process and that their mutual relationship is one of reciprocal reinforcement.

Oswald and Priest (61) have reported REM rebound following *barbiturate withdrawal*. As with alcohol, it was hypothesized that this factor contributed to the delirium occurring as part of the barbiturate withdrawal syndrome. Evans and Lewis (62) reported gross increase in REM sleep in such delirium. More recent work by Tachibana et al. (63) casts some doubt on the REM rebound hypothesis of alcohol and drug withdrawal delirium. These researchers failed to find a uniform increase in REM sleep in delirious patients. What they observed, however, was "a peculiar state of sleep characterized by concomitant appearance of low-voltage, mixed-frequency EEG activity, REM burst and tonic mental EMG." They called this state "stage 1-REM with tonic EMG." The main difference between delirious and nondelirious alcoholics consisted in the quantitative and qualitative changes in stage 1-REM and not in the amount of REM sleep. The investigators proposed that delirium in alcohol and meprobamate withdrawal could result from an increase in the phasic features of REM sleep and their dissociation from its tonic features.

It appears that difficulties in interpreting EEG records in terms of the accepted criteria for the various stages of sleep may have contributed to the contradictory findings reported so far. The issue of the role of REM sleep in the pathogenesis of delirium in acute alcohol and drug withdrawal will only be settled when the investigators agree on how to interpret and label EEG recordings during sleep of delirious subjects. Furthermore, it would be desirable to carry out EEG recordings on a twenty-four-hour basis, to concurrently record EOG and EMG, and to collect subjective reports as well as objective observations of the delirious patients throughout. It is only then that the various hypotheses on the role of specific sleep disturbances in delirium may be tested.

While delirium due to withdrawal of alcohol and barbiturates has attracted particular attention of sleep researchers, sleep disturbances associated with delirium due to other causes has so far been little explored. Karacan et al. (19) have studied the effects of *fever* on sleep and dreaming. Male student volunteers were given injections of a pyrogen, either etiocholanolone or Lipexal®, and their body temperatures and sleep patterns were recorded for four consecutive nights before the injection and two nights after it. The highest mean body temperature was 38.9°C. After the injection, latency of the onset of stages 1 and 1-REM as well as of stage 4 sleep was markedly increased, there were more awakenings, and the amount of stage 1-REM was reduced. There was suppression of both stage 4 and stage 1-REM sleep compared to the baseline nights. These changes were ascribed to fever. There was no rebound of REM sleep during the recovery nights. The investigators speculated that with higher and more prolonged fever the suppression of the two sleep stages would be even more marked and might result in (unspecified) complications. This study appears to be relevant to delirium which may accompany fever of any origin. Ebaugh et al. (64) studied 200 patients treated with induction of high fever in a hypertherm. Fifty-four percent of these subjects developed delirium at least once during the course of pyretotherapy. Fever alone seemed to be the necessary causative factor. More research is obviously needed to clarify the effects of fever on sleep.

An interesting clinical sleep study relevant to delirium has been reported recently. Billiard et al. (65) recorded sleep patterns in three subjects suffering from delirium caused by insoluble salts of *bismuth* (bismuth encephalopathy). The patients showed total sleep loss. The recovery of normal sleep patterns lagged behind clinical recovery.

Studies of sleep disturbances after open heart surgery had been prompted by claims that delirium, which often follows this type of surgery, might be in part due to sleep deprivation related to frequent awakenings and other factors commonly seen in intensive care units (66, 67). Johns et al. (68) reported that two of the patients studied by them developed delirium after open heart surgery, while two did not. The severity of sleep deprivation during the first two postoperative days did not distinguish patients who later developed delirium from those who did not. The delirium was accompanied by absence of REM sleep and a marked reduction of delta wave sleep. There were prolonged periods of drowsiness and stage 1 sleep, which may have contributed to the delirium. The sleep-wakefulness cycle as a whole was disrupted. Orr and Stahl (69) have recently reported similar findings. They found evidence of deprivation and fragmentation of sleep in their patients, yet none of them developed delirium. It appears that sleep disturbance alone is not a sufficient condition for delirium to develop.

Studies of sleep disturbances in metabolic encephalopathies are especially relevant since the latter are commonly accompanied by delirium. Marked sleep abnormalities have been reported in hepatic encephalopathy (70), renal insufficiency (71), cardiac decompensation (72), and respiratory insufficiency (73). These sleep disturbances are generally characterized by reduction of total sleep time, frequent awakenings, disorganization of sleep cycles, and reduction of slow-wave sleep. These abnormalities increase in severity as the encephalopathy worsens and diurnal EEG disturbances increase.

Not only sleep deprivation and fragmentation, but also *hypersomnia* appears to be associated with delirium. Roth et al. (74) described "sleep drunkenness" occurring in certain hypersomniacs and associated with confusion, disorientation, slow responsivity, and some incoordination. This state, which may last from about fifteen minutes to several hours, may occur on awakening in individuals suffering from hypersomnia as well as those suddenly awakened after too little sleep, especially in unfamiliar surroundings, or following the intake of hypnotics, tranquilizers, or alcohol. Rarely a patient may display assaultive and homicidal behavior (75). Sleep drunkenness appears to represent a transient delirious episode related to insufficient wakefulness or arousal in the presence of partial return of motor functions. Guilleminault et al. (76, 77) have described "altered states of consciousness" associated with a syndrome of hypersomnia. These states are related to excessive drowsiness and microsleeps. The patients have an abnormally low amount of slow-wave sleep at night. They tend to display episodes of automatic behavior, apparently accompanying microsleeps. It is unclear if these episodes represent true delirium.

In summary, the results of experimental and clinical studies converge to support a relationship between sleep disturbances and delirium. The precise nature of this relationship, however, remains unclear. Total sleep deprivation appears to be capable of inducing mild delirium in at least some subjects. Clinical studies confirm the ancient observation that sleep disturbances consistently accompany delirium. These disturbances include *insomnia, fragmentation and depatterning of sleep,* and *disruption of the circadian sleep-wakefulness cycle.* Slow-wave sleep is usually reduced or lacking, but REM sleep may be increased, normal, reduced, or absent. Interpenetration of the phenomena of wakefulness and sleep appears to be the rule. Sleep disturbances appear to be related to delirium in four possible ways: 1. they may *facilitate* the onset of delirium due to any etiology. Viewed in this way, sleep disturbances constitute a pathogenetic mechanism intervening between a given etiologic agent and cognitive disorganization; 2. they may *enhance the severity* of cognitive impairment, which is caused independently of them; 3. they may help determine whether the delirious patient will *hallucinate;* and 4. they may, in some cases, actually *cause* cognitive disorganization.

One may hypothesize that some degree of disruption of the normal sleep-wakefulness cycle and of fragmentation of nocturnal sleep is an integral constituent of delirium. Furthermore, it appears that in some cases the sleep disturbances may accompany and enhance, and in other cases bring about, cognitive disorganization or impairment of information processing. These hypotheses, however, must await validation by future studies. It remains to be established which particular relationship between sleep disturbances and cognitive disorganization exists and whether that relationship remains constant for all causes of delirium; it is also unproven if different relationships hold for certain categories of causes, such as alcohol and drug withdrawal or metabolic encephalopathies. These issues are of considerable theoretical interest and may have consequences for the treatment of delirium.

The relationship between dreaming and delirium also remains unclear. For one thing, the definition of dreams is still rather ambiguous: Is dreaming defined only as the mentation which accompanies REM sleep or does it also include hypnagogic hallucinations and hallucinatory activity encountered in non-REM sleep? There is little doubt that not all delirious patients hallucinate, and it would thus be inaccurate to refer to delirium, as herein defined, as a "waking dream." At the turn of the century, Regis (78) coined the term "délire onirique" (óneiros —dream) to describe dream-like mentation experienced by some patients delirious as a result of infection or intoxication. Oneirism was viewed as hallucinatory activity superimposed upon simple mental confusion. It is a common clinical observation that hallucinating delirious patients have difficulty in distinguishing between their dreams, veridical perceptions, and hallucinations. This was dramatically illustrated by a delirious woman who repeatedly asked the author during a clinical interview: "Are you really there or am I dreaming?" It is conceivable that the hallucinations in delirium may be identical with dreams. This, however, appears to be primarily an issue of semantics.

It was proposed in Chapter 4 that delirium was a *disorder of wakefulness*. The material discussed in this section offers some support for this contention. An alternative, and possibly more accurate, formulation would assert that delirium is a disorder of the sleep-wakefulness cycle characterized by irregular appearance of the elements of sleep during wakefulness and of the waking state during sleep. As Heinroth (79) asserted in 1842: delirium is an intermediate state between sleep and wakefulness. This hypothesis will be discussed from different viewpoints, those of neurophysiology and neurochemistry, in Chapter 6.

Sensory Deprivation and Overload

Sensory deprivation and *overload* have been reported to impair cognitive and perceptual functions. Their facilitating role in delirium has been proposed (3). Experimental and clinical studies of sensory deprivation (SD) that are relevant to delirium will be reviewed first.

EXPERIMENTAL SENSORY DEPRIVATION (SD). Hebb and his coworkers at McGill University introduced in 1951 an experimental technique that marked the beginning of studies on the psychophysiological effects of sensory deprivation (80, 81). Volunteer subjects used in the McGill studies were confined to bed, their eyes covered with translucent goggles allowing only formless light to pass through; they carried earphones through which a constant buzzing sound was presented, and their arms and hands were covered with cardboard cuffs and cotton gloves, reducing the amount of tactile stimulation. The subjects exhibited, after varying periods of confinement, such phenomena as decreased intellectual efficiency, vivid imagery, visual and auditory hallucinations, mood shifts, increased suggestibility, impaired directed thinking, and delusions. Most subjects could not tolerate the experiment for more than seventy-two hours; those who remained in the confinement for longer periods usually developed complex hallucinations and delusions. These widely publicized early SD experiments inaugurated two decades of intensive studies using three different techniques: confinement to bed in a soundproof room, confinement in a tank-type respirator, and suspension in a water tank. A distinction has been made between *sensory deprivation* in which the experimental environment provided absolute reduction of intensity of sensory input (darkness, soundproof room) and *perceptual deprivation* in which the sensory input was homogeneous and unpatterned (white noise, diffuse light) (81). The original McGill experiments exemplified the perceptual deprivation technique. Later, however, this whole area of research came to be designated "sensory deprivation." Several reviews of this area provide indispensable guides to the voluminous literature (81-83).

Hebb, the pioneer of SD studies, after reading this writer's review of delirium, commented: "The hallucinatory activity (which I call hallucinatory because the subjects reported that if they didn't know that they were wearing goggles they would have thought that they were looking at a movie screen) in these nonpsychiatric subjects (of perceptual-isolation studies) is obviously closely related to the phenomena of delirium" (84). This impression was strengthened by reports that even relatively brief SD (one-hour session) induced EEG slowing manifested by a decrease in occipital alpha wave frequency (85). Yet, as in the case of sleep deprivation, the dramatic symptoms reported in the early studies of SD were not found as often in the later experiments. Zubek (86), for example, exposed fifteen male volunteers to fourteen days of confinement in an isolation chamber, under conditions of constant, diffuse light and white noise. He observed marked intellectual deficits during isolation, such as inability to concentrate and impaired ability to think and reason. On the other hand, "hallucinatory-like experiences" in the visual sphere were infrequent and mostly of a simple and unstructured type. In the auditory sphere only illusions were reported. Suedfeld (83) has suggested recently that variables other than SD as such could have confounded many of the earlier studies and resulted in reports of psychological stress of a strange and novel experiment. This, coupled with suggestion and other aspects of the experimental situation, could have contributed to the adverse psychological effects of SD reported in the early studies. The question of hallucinations in SD experiments has remained controversial. Suedfeld (83) asserts that it is extremely rare for a subject exposed to SD to report hallucinations of the type seen in psychotics. Rather, illusions and vivid imagery seem to have been mislabeled by some investigators as "hallucinations." Ziskind (87) has reviewed critically the phenomena of SD and proposed that immobilization as well as social isolation are confounding variables in SD experiments and may contribute to their effects. Furthermore, he hypothesized that reduced awareness due to a hypnagogic state occurring in SD subjects could account for pseudo-hallucinations, dream-like perceptual distortions, confusion, anxiety, and restlessness. This "hypnoid syndrome" appears to be identical with that exhibited by subjects of sleep deprivation studies, one ascribed to drowsiness and recurrent microsleeps (32). It has been pointed out that hallucinations in SD are predominantly visual, simple, and transient (81).

Cognitive changes have been reported to occur in SD experiments (81). Complex intellectual functioning is impaired. On the other hand, performance on simple tasks, such as digit span, rote learning, or recall, was seldom impaired and was often improved by SD (82). Other observed abnormalities included impaired directed thinking and facilitation of primary process, or prelogical thinking, distractibility, short attention span, increased suggestibility, and temporal disorientation (81).

In summary, experimental SD studies have demonstrated that subjects exposed to reduced or monotonous sensory input exhibit a variety of cognitive and perceptual abnormalities as well as mild slowing of the EEG. These abnormalities resemble delirium but do not appear to be identical with this syndrome. For one thing, delirium involves some degree of memory impairment, and SD subjects show no consistent deficits of registration, retention, and recall. Their digit span was almost invariably intact in contrast to the typical delirious patients. One may conclude that SD does not induce delirium in a healthy, young subject. This does not, however, rule out the possibility that SD may facilitate delirium in the aged, the brain-damaged, and the physically ill individuals. Clinical studies to be reviewed suggest that this may in fact be the case.

CLINICAL STUDIES. Clinical observations of patients subjected to various forms of sensory and perceptual deprivation suggest that these factors can contribute to and facilitate the onset of delirium. Sichel (88) reported in 1863 the occurrence of delirium in patients aged sixty years or over who had undergone cataract extraction. Schmidt-Rimpler (89) extended these observations and described two patients aged fifty-seven and nineteen years, respectively, who developed severe, transient delirium after being blindfolded and placed in a darkened room. Both these patients suffered from eye disorders: the older one had syphilitic iritis, the younger—bilateral irido-choroiditis. Both had reduced vision and received atropin. Schmidt-Rimpler believed the delirium to be due to the effects of sudden exclusion of accustomed visual stimuli on predisposed individuals. The nature of this predisposition remained unclear. Both patients recovered promptly following discontinuation of treatment. The possible role of atropin was not mentioned and remains unclear.

The foregoing reports are among the first to link reduction in visual sensory input with delirium. Numerous such observations have been published since and were reviewed by Jackson (90). Cameron (91) carried out what was likely the first experimental study of the effects of partial SD on cognitive functioning and delirium. He selected a group of patients suffering from what appears to have been senile dementia and nocturnal delirious episodes and attempted to answer the question if the latter were due to fatigue or to darkness. The patients were blindfolded early in the day and within one hour of the onset of the experiment were unable to locate various objects in the room whose location they had been able to point out with the eyes open. The majority of the patients confabulated and, while blindfolded, described the location of nonexistent objects, such as windows. Cameron concluded that the senile patient could not preserve the "spatial image" after darkness had cut off visual cues. This loss of spatial orientation was postulated to result in anxiety, which increased the confusion. Cameron proposed that the nocturnal delirium in the senile patients might be based on "an inability to maintain a spatial image without the assistance of a repeated visualization." The problem with this hypothesis is that initially, as Sichel (88) had already observed, delirium in patients blindfolded after cataract surgery occurs mostly during the night; secondly, the senile subjects studied by Cameron did not really develop delirium after he blindfolded them. The effects of eye surgery will be discussed in more detail in Chapter 17. Jackson (90) concluded his extensive review of delirium in hospitalized eye-surgery patients with the cautious remark, "the evidence for sensory deprivation has been mixed, and the issue has not been resolved" (p. 372).

SD has been suggested as an explanation for such clinical phenomena as the "break-off phenomenon" of pilots at high altitude (92); delirium in intensive care units (93) and tank-type respirators (94); and psychological disturbances in leukemic patients treated in germ-free isolator units (95, 96). Kornfeld (93) claims that sensory monotony has played a major part in contributing to delirium in patients in the surgical intensive care units. Other observers have made similar claims to account for delirium in intensive care units (97). All these clinical reports call for a critical scrutiny.

A report by Mendelson et al. (94) on the occurrence of hallucinations in patients with poliomyelitis treated in a respirator seems to have stimulated interest in the application of the findings of experimental SD to account for certain psycho-pathological phenomena seen in clinical medicine and surgery. Their patients exhibited not only hallucinations but also dis-orientation, "confusion," and delusions. They were obviously delirious even though the authors do not label them as such. The hallucinations were multiple: visual, auditory, kinesthetic, tactile, gustatory, and olfactory. The last two types were rare. The hallucinatory phenomena were vivid, predominantly visual, and mostly pleasant. The patients had difficulty in telling them apart from their dreams. EEG studies were not done and thus no objective index of brain function was obtained. Effects of immobilization could not be separated from those of postulated SD. Mendelson collaborated in another study which reported on delirium in medical patients (98). The authors claimed that

SD contributed to the development of the syndrome in some patients, such as the elderly, orthopedic cases.

A number of writers echoed the above claims (99, 100). Not only SD but also social isolation has been proposed to contribute to the "isolation stress" thought to play a causative role in some deliria, especially in the aged (99). A florid delirium in a paraplegic man placed on a Striker® frame and in a woman treated by traction for a femoral fracture was also ascribed in part to SD, since no "toxic agent" could be identified to account for the occurrence of the syndrome (100). It was acknowledged that social isolation, immobilization, and sedation could also have played a contributory role.

In recent years the focus on the postulated effects of SD has shifted to the special hospital environments, such as surgical and coronary intensive care units and germ-free isolators. McKegney (101) proposed the name "intensive care syndrome" for delirium occurring in surgical recovery rooms and acclaimed it a "new disease of medical progress." This flamboyant statement seems quite unjustified; obviously delirium is not a new syndrome, and its occurrence in intensive care units does not justify introducing a new label. Holland et al. (102) suggested that the intensive care syndrome was a myth. These investigators found no significant difference in the incidence of delirium between the patients admitted to a general medical intensive care unit and a matched group of patients admitted to a general medical ward. Twelve and one-half percent of the ICU patients became delirious, and in each case the delirium could be sufficiently accounted for by the underlying physical illness. Sensory monotony or deprivation did not seem to play any role in the development of delirium.

Reports from surgical intensive care units seem to provide some evidence that SD may play a contributory role in delirium occurring in those settings. The most convincing study has been reported by Wilson (103), who found the incidence of postoperative delirium to be more than twice as high in a windowless intensive care unit as compared to one possessing windows. The incidence was 40 percent in the former, 18 percent in the latter. The importance of windows in this setting has been recently reemphasized by Keep (104), who did not provide new data, however. In the most recently reported study, only 7 of 322 patients treated in a surgical ICU were diagnosed as suffering from an organic brain syndrome. It is not clear if SD was implicated in any way (105). Katz et al. (106) have failed to implicate SD in their study of delirium in a surgical ICU. The syndrome could be adequately explained by involving organic factors.

Studies of coronary care units (107-109) have not provided much support for the role of SD in delirium. The incidence of the latter was found to be 3, 5, and 10 percent, respectively (107-109). One report refers vaguely to the probable contributory role of "sensory monotony" (109). Another study speaks of "violent fluctuations in sensory input, ranging from monotony to sudden terror" (107). The investigators marvelled at the low incidence of delirium in this unattractive environment.

Several studies have focused on psychological effects of isolator therapy in acute leukemia and other diseases (95, 96, 110, 111, 112). The isolator units or "life islands" are special germ-free glass or plastic enclosures used for the treatment of patients who are markedly susceptible to infection because of severe granulocytopenia. Most patients so treated suffered from acute leukemia and other neoplastic diseases and received cytotoxic drugs. Patients spend up to several months in a life island and despite claims to the contrary do not seem to suffer from SD but rather from "touch deprivation" (111), a form of social isolation. The patients tolerate this type of restricted environment surprisingly well. Delirium was observed infrequently and mostly in terminal patients.

In summary, clinical studies reported here provide some support for the hypothesis that reduction of sensory input and/or sensory monotony facilitate the development of delirium. Such an effect is most likely to occur in the aged and the brain-damaged individual, especially if other conditions which can disorganize cognitive functioning coexist. These factors include immobilization, sleep deprivation, unfamiliarity of the environment, and anxiety. There is insufficient evidence that SD alone can cause delirium.

SENSORY OVERLOAD. Sensory overload has been reported to result in cognitive impairment, illusions, hallucinations, disturbances in time sense, distortions of body image, and delusions (9, 113, 114). McKegney (101) has suggested that sensory overload produced by auditory and visual stimuli emanating from oxygen equipment, monitoring apparatus, fans, etc., may contribute to delirium in intensive care units. Studies of hospital noise show that high noise levels, attributed to various types of mechanical equipment as well as to personnel and patients, exist in recovery rooms and acute care units (115). Such noise levels may be sufficient to stimulate patients' hypophyseal-adrenocortical axis and to interfere with sleep. It is conceivable that sensory overload, rather than deprivation, is a more common feature of special hospital environments, such as intensive care units. This problem awaits documentation and calls for more experimental studies on sensory overload. Such studies have been few to date and involved various designs which make it difficult to interpret the results (9). The effects of sensory overload in terms of facilitating delirium are probable but remain a matter of speculation.

SOCIAL ISOLATION AND UNFAMILIARITY. Other aspects of the sensory environment which have been linked to delirium include social isolation (99, 100) and unfamiliarity of the environment (116, 117). These aspects seem to affect particularly the elderly patients who tend to manifest delirium on transfer to a new environment, such as the hospital (116, 117). It is likely that these patients suffer from some degree of brain damage and decompensate psychologically when they become deprived of familiar social and sensory cues. Clinicians have been aware for some time that allowing members of the patient's family to stay with him and to provide objects with which he is familiar tends to ameliorate confusion.

IMMOBILIZATION. The last factor on which there is some evidence to suggest the facilitation of delirium is immobilization. A series of studies by Zubek and his associates (118) have documented that immobilized subjects display impaired performance on intelligence tests and those of perceptual-motor functions. Some of the subjects reported "visual experience of hallucinatory-like nature," vivid imagery and dreams, inability to concentrate and difficulty in logical thinking, and loss of contact with reality. Furthermore, they also displayed a slowing of the occipital EEG frequencies. Rote learning and digit span were unaffected. Thus, the effects were similar to those induced by sensory deprivation. It has been proposed that immobilization actually represents reduction in the level of kinesthetic and proprioceptive stimulation and, hence, a form of sensory deprivation. These two experimental conditions, however, are usually discussed independently in the literature.

Ryback et al. (119) have investigated the effects of prolonged bed rest on psychological functioning, sleep, and EEG. Healthy volunteers were confined to bed for five weeks. Psychological tests did not reveal any significant cognitive impairment, even though the subjects complained of mental sluggishness. EEG changes were similar to those found in severe sensory deprivation, even though the sensory input was not restricted apart from that due to confinement to bed. It has been suggested that the decrease in motor-muscular input is responsible for the EEG changes in prolonged bed rest. Sleep was affected in that an increase in deep sleep and a decrease in light sleep (stages 1 and 2) were observed.

Clinical implications of the experimental immobilization have been suggested for patients with orthopedic, neurological, cardiac, pulmonary, and other disorders requiring prolonged periods of immobilization and recumbency (118-120). The role of these factors as facilitators of delirium has not yet been sufficiently demonstrated and remains speculative.

SUMMARY. The etiology of delirium is multifactorial (3). A widespread disturbance of cerebral metabolism is a necessary, but not always sufficient, condition for its occurrence. Many physical disorders can induce a diffuse derangement of brain metabolism and thus bring about delirium. Old age, brain damage, and/or addiction to alcohol and drugs predispose a person to the development of the syndrome. Anxiety in the patient as well as the quantity, patterning, and familiarity of the sensory and information inputs he receives from his environment seem to be significant facilitating variables. Deprivation and fragmentation of sleep as well as disruption of the normal sleep-wakefulness cycle are regular components of delirium that facilitate its development and increase its severity. Sleep disturbances, anxiety, and excessive or deficient sensory and information inputs are often combined and have a cumulative effect in facilitating the onset of delirium and increasing its severity. Individuals show considerable differences in susceptibility to delirium in general and to the deliriogenic effects of specific noxious agents in particular.

REFERENCES

1. Lipowski, Z.J.: "Organic Brain Syndromes: Overview and Classification," in D.F. Benson and D. Blumer, Eds., *Psychiatric Aspects of Neurologic Disease.* New York, Grune & Stratton, 1975.
2. Marinacci, A.A. and Hagen, K.O. von: Alcohol and temporal lobe dysfunction. *Behav Neuropsychiatry 3:*2-11, 1972.
3. Lipowski, Z.J.: Delirium, clouding of consciousness and confusion. *J Nerv Ment Dis 145:*227-255, 1967.
4. Bleuler, M., Willi, J., and Buhler, H.R.: *Akute Psychische Begleiterscheinungen Körperlicher Krankheiten.* Stuttgart, Thieme, 1966.
5. Morse, R.M. and Litin, E.M.: Postoperative delirium: A study of etiologic factors. *Am J Psychiatry 126:*388-395, 1969.
6. Morse, R.M. and Litin, E.M.: The anatomy of delirium. *Am J Psychiatry 128:*111-116, 1971.
7. Abse, W.D.: *Hysteria and Related Mental Disorders.* Bristol, Wright, 1966.
8. Cartwright, R.D. and Monroe, L.J.: Individual differences in response to REM deprivation. *Arch Gen Psychiatry 16:*297-303, 1967.
9. Lipowski, Z.J.: Sensory and information inputs overload: behavioral effects. *Compr Psychiatry 16:*199-221, 1975.
10. Willi, J.: "Delir, Dämmerzustand und Verwirrtheit bei körperlich Kranken," in Bleuler, M., Willi, J., and Buhler, H.R., Eds., *Akute Psychische Begleiterscheinungen Körperlicher Krankheiten.* Stuttgart, Thieme, 1966, pp. 27-158.
11. Susser, M.: *Causal Thinking in the Health Sciences.* London, Oxford University Press, 1973.
12. Lipowski, Z.J.: Psychosomatic medicine in the seventies: an overview. *Am J Psychiatry 134:*233-244, 1977.
13. Chapman, L.F., Thetford, W.N., Berlin, L., Guthrie, T.C., and Wolff, H.G.: "Highest integrative functions in man during stress," in Solomon, H.C., Cobb, S., and Penfield, W., Eds., *The Brain and Human Behavior.* Baltimore, Williams & Wilkins, 1958, pp. 491-534.
14. Siesjö, B.K., Carlsson, C., Hagerdal, M., and Nordstrom, C.H.: Brain metabolism in the critically ill. *Crit Care Med 4:*283-294, 1976.

15. Levin, H.L.: Organic and psychogenic delirium; differential diagnosis; analysis of psychogenic delirium. *N York M J* 99:631-633, 1914.

16. Bonhoeffer, K.: "Die Psychosen im Gefolge von akuten Infektionen, Allgemeinerkrankungen, und inneren Erkankungen," in Aschaffenburg, G.L., Ed., *Handbuch der Psychiatrie*, Spez. Teil 3, pp. 1-60. Leipzig, Deuticke, 1912.

17. Faergeman, P.M.: *Psychogenic Psychoses.* London, Butterworths, 1963.

18. *The Medical Works of Hippocrates.* Translated by J. Chadwick and W.N. Mann. Oxford, Blackwell, 1950.

19. Karacan, I., Wolff, S.M., Williams, R.L., Hursch, C.J., and Webb, W.B.: The effects of fever on sleep and dream patterns. *Psychosomatics* 9:331-339, 1968.

20. Patrick, G.T.W. and Gilbert, J.A.: On effects of loss of sleep. *Psychol Rev* 3:469-483, 1896.

21. Johnson, L.C.: "The Effect of Total, Partial, and Stage Sleep Deprivation on EEG Patterns and Performance," in Burch, N. and Altschuler, H.L., *Behavior and Brain Electrical Activity.* New York, Plenum Publishing Co., 1974, pp. 1-30.

22. Kjellberg, A.: Sleep deprivation and some aspects of performance. *Waking and Sleeping* 1:139-143, 1977.

23. Naitoh, P.: Sleep deprivation in human subjects: a reappraisal. *Waking and Sleeping* 1:53-60, 1976.

24. Vogel, G.W.: A review of REM sleep deprivation. *Arch Gen Psychiatry* 32:749-761, 1975.

25. Webb, W.B.: "Partial and Differential Sleep Deprivation," in Kales, A., Ed., *Sleep.* Philadelphia, Lippincott, 1969, pp. 221-231.

26. Tyler, D.: Psychological changes during experimental sleep deprivation. *Dis Nerv Syst* 16:293-299, 1955.

27. Luby, E.D. and Gottlieb, J.S.: "Sleep Deprivation," in Arieti, S., Ed., *American Handbook of Psychiatry*, Vol. 3. New York, Basic Books, 1959, pp. 406-418.

28. West, L.J., Janszen, H., Lester, B., and Cornelison, F.: The psychosis of sleep deprivation. *Ann NY Acad Sci* 96:66-70, 1962.

29. Gulevich, G., Dement, W., and Johnson, L.: Psychiatric and EEG observations on a case of prolonged (264 hours) wakefulness. *Arch Gen Psychiatry* 15:29-35, 1966.

30. Pasnau, R.O., Naitoh, P., Stier, S., and Kollar, E.J.: The psychological effects of 205 hours of sleep deprivation. *Arch Gen Psychiatry* 18:496-505, 1968.

31. Bliss, E.L., Clark, L.D., and West, C.D.: Studies of sleep deprivation—relationship to schizophrenia. *AMA Arch Neurol Psychiatry* 81:348-359, 1959.

32. Morris, G.O. and Singer, M.T.: Sleep deprivation: the context of consciousness. *J Nerv Ment Dis 143*:291-304, 1966.
33. Morris, G.O., Williams, H.L., and Lubin, A.: Misperception and disorientation during sleep deprivation. *Arch Gen Psychiatry 2*:247-254, 1960.
34. Slap, J.W.: On dreaming at sleep onset. *Psychoanal Q 46*:71-81, 1977.
35. Naitoh, P., Kales, A., Kollar, E.J., Smith, J.C., and Jacobson, A.: EEG activity after prolonged sleep loss. *Electroencephalogr Clin Neurophysiol 27*:2-11, 1969.
36. Ritter, G., Becker, A., and Duensing, F.: Zum diagnostischen Wert des EEG's nach Schlafentzug. *Nervenarzt 28*:365-368, 1977.
37. Koranyi, E.K. and Lehmann, H.E.: Experimental sleep deprivation in schizophrenic patients. *Arch Gen Psychiatry 2*:534-544, 1960.
38. Dement, W.C.: The effect of dream deprivation. *Science 131*:1705-1707, 1960.
39. Dement, W.C.: "Sleep Deprivation and the Organization of the Behavioral States," in Clemente, C., Purpura, D., and Mayer, F., Eds., *Sleep and Maturing Nervous System.* New York, Academic Press, 1972, pp. 319-361.
40. Vogel, G., Foulkes, D., and Trosman, H.: Ego functions and dreaming during sleep onset. *Arch Gen Psychiatry 14*:238-248, 1966.
41. Holland, H.: *Medical Notes and Reflections.* Philadelphia, Haswell, Barrington, and Haswell, 1839.
42. Cartwright, R.D.: Dream and drug-induced fantasy behavior. *Arch Gen Psychiatry 15*:7-15, 1966.
43. Moses, J.M., Johnson, L.C., Naitoh, P., and Lubin, A.: Sleep stage deprivation and total sleep loss: effects on sleep behavior. *Psychophysiology 12*:141-146, 1975.
44. Krieger, D.T., and Glick, S.: Absent sleep peak of growth hormone release in blind subjects. *J Clin Endocrinol 33*:847-853, 1971.
45. Johnson, L.C.: Are stages of sleep related to waking behavior? *Am Scientist 61*:326-338, 1973.
46. Lasegue, C.: Le délire alcoolique n'est pas un délire, mais un rêve. *Arch Gen Med 88*:513-536, 1881.
47. Aserinsky, E., and Kleitman, N.: Regularly occurring periods of eye motility, and concomitant phenomena, during sleep. *Science 118*:273-274, 1953.
48. Williams, H.L., Holloway, F.A., and Griffiths, W.J.: Physiological psychology: sleep. *Ann Rev Psychol 24*:279-316, 1973.
49. Gross, M.M., Goodenough, D., Tobin, M., Halpert, E., Lepore, D., Perlstein, A., Sirota M., Dibianco, J., Fuller, R., and Kishner, I.: Sleep disturbances and hallucinations in the acute alcoholic psychoses. *J Nerv Ment Dis 142*:493-514, 1966.

50. Gresham, S.C., Webb, W.B., and Williams, R.L.: Alcohol and caffeine: effects on inferred visual dreaming. *Science 140*:1226-1227, 1963.

51. Gross, M.M. and Hastey, J.M.: "Sleep Disturbances in Alcoholism," in Tarter, R.E., and Sugarman, H.H., Eds., *Alcoholism: Interdisciplinary Approaches to an Enduring Problem*. Reading, Mass., Addison-Wesley Publ. Co., 1977.

52. Greenberg, R., and Pearlman, C.: Delirium tremens and dreaming. *Am J Psychiatry 124*:133-142, 1967.

53. Johnson, L.C., Burdick, J.A., and Smith, J.: Sleep during alcohol intake and withdrawal in the chronic alcoholic. *Arch Gen Psychiatry 22*:406-418, 1970.

54. Vogel, G.W.: REM deprivation. III. Dreaming and psychosis. *Arch Gen Psychiatry 18*:312-329, 1968.

55. Maxion, H., and Schneider, E.: Alkoholdelir und Traumschlaf. *Arch Psychiatr Nervenkr 214*:116-126, 1971.

56. Wolin, S.J., and Mello, N.K.: The effects of alcohol on dreams and hallucinations in alcohol addicts. *Ann NY Acad Sci 215*:266-302, 1973.

57. Gross, M.M., Goodenough, D.R., Hastey, J.M., Rosenblatt, S.M., and Lewis, E.: "Sleep Disturbances in Alcoholic Intoxication and Withdrawal," in Mello, N.K., and Mendelson, J.H., Eds., *Recent Advances in Studies of Alcoholism*. Washington, D.C., U.S. Department of Health, Education and Welfare, 1971, pp. 317-397.

58. Gross, M.M., Lewis, E., and Hastey, J.: "Acute Alcohol Withdrawal Syndrome," in Kissin, B., and Begleiter, H., Eds., *The Biology of Alcoholism*, Vol. III, Clinical Pathology. New York, Plenum Press, 1973, pp. 191-263.

59. Feinberg, I., and Evarts, E.V.: "Some Implications of Sleep Research for Psychiatry," in Zubin, J., and Shagass, C., Eds., *Neurobiological Aspects of Psychopathology*. New York, Grune & Stratton, 1969, pp. 334-393.

60. Feinberg, I.: Changes in sleep cycle patterns with age. *J Psychiatr Res 10*:283-306, 1974.

61. Oswald, I., and Priest, R.G.: Five weeks to escape the sleeping pill habit. *Br Med J 2*:1093-1099, 1965.

62. Evans, J.I., and Lewis, S.A.: Drug withdrawal state. *Arch Gen Psychiatry 19*:631-634, 1968.

63. Tachibana, M., Tanaka, K., Hishikawa, Y., and Kaneko, Z.: A sleep study of acute psychotic states due to alcohol and meprobamate addiction. *Adv Sleep Res 3*:177-205, 1975.

64. Ebaugh, F.G., Barnacle, C.H., and Ewalt, J.R.: Delirious episodes associated with artificial fever: A study of 200 cases. *Am J Psychiatry 23*:191-217, 1936.

65. Billiard, M., Besset, A., Renaud, B., Baldy-Moulinier, M., and Passouant, P: L'insomnie de l'encephalopathie bismutique. *Electroencephalogr Clin Neurophysiol* 7:147-152, 1977.

66 Blachly, P.H., and Starr, A.: Post-cardiotomy delirium. *Am J Psychiatry* 121:371-375, 1964.

67. Dlin, B.M., Rosen, H., Dickstein, K., Lyons, J.W., and Fischer, K.H.: The problems of sleep and rest in the intensive care unit. *Psychosomatics* 12:155-163, 1971.

68. Johns, M.W., Large, A.A., Masterton, J.P., and Dudley, H.A.F.: Sleep and delirium after open heart surgery. *Br J Surg* 61:377-381, 1974.

69. Orr, W.C., and Stahl, M.L.: Sleep disturbances after open heart surgery. *Am J Cardiol* 39:196-201, 1977.

70. Kurtz, D., Zenglein, J.P., Imler, M., Girardel, M., Grinspan, G., Peter, B., and Rohmer, F.: Étude du sommeil nocturne au cours de l'encephalopathie porto-cave. *Electroencephalogr Clin Neurophysiol* 33:167-178, 1972.

71. Passouant, P., Cadilhac, J., Baldy-Moulinier, M., and Mion, C.: Étude de sommeil nocturne chez des uremiques chroniques soumis à une épuration extrarenale. *Electroencephalogr Clin Neurophysiol* 29:441-449, 1970.

72. Rohmer, F., Kurtz, D., Feuerstein, J., Oberling, F., and Mehdaoui, M.: L'EEG de sommeil des cardiaques. *Electroencephalogr Clin Neurophysiol* 22:348-364, 1967.

73. Gastaut, H., Duron, B., Pappy, J.J., Tassinairi, C., and Waltregny, A.: Étude polygraphique du cycle nycthemérique chez les narcoleptiques, les Pickwickiens, les obèses et les insuffisants respiratoires. *Rev Neurol* 115:456-462, 1966.

74. Roth, B., Nevsimalova, S., and Rechtschaffen, A.: Hypersomnia with "sleep drunkenness." *Arch Gen Psychiatry* 26:456-462, 1972.

75. Bonkalo, A.: Impulsive acts and confusional states during incomplete arousal from sleep: Criminological and forensic implications. *Psychiatr Q* 48:1-10, 1974.

76. Guilleminault, C., Billiard, M., Montplaisir, J., and Dement, W.C.: Altered states of consciousness in disorders of daytime sleepiness. *J Neurol Sci* 26:377-393, 1975.

77. Guilleminault, C., Phillips, R., and Dement, W.C.: A syndrome of hypersomnia with automatic behavior. *Electroencephalogr Clin Neurophysiol* 38:403-413, 1975.

78. Regis, E.: *Précis de Psychiatrie.* Paris, Doin, 1923, pp. 345-387.

79. Heinroth, A.: *De Delirio Inter Somnum et Vigiliam.* Lipsiae, Typis Guil. Staritzii, 1842.

80. Bexton, W.H., Heron, W., and Scott, T.H.: Effects of decreased variation in the sensory environment. *Can J Psychol* 8:70-76, 1954.

81. Zubek, J.P., Ed.: *Sensory Deprivation: Fifteen Years of Research.* New York, Appleton-Century-Crofts, 1969.
82. Zubek, J.P.: "Behavioral and Physiological Effects of Prolonged Sensory and Perceptual Deprivation: A Review," in Rasmussen, J., Ed., *Man in Isolation and Confinement.* New York, Aldine, 1973, pp. 9-83.
83. Suedfeld, P.: The benefits of boredom: Sensory deprivation reconsidered. *Am Scientist 63*:60-69, 1975.
84. Hebb, D.O.: Personal communication, February 2, 1968.
85. Marjerrison, G., and Keogh, R.P.: Electroencephalographic changes during brief periods of perceptual deprivation. *Percept Motor Skills 24*:611-615, 1967.
86. Zubek, J.P.: "Behavioral and EEG Changes During and After 14 Days of Perceptual Deprivation and Confinement," in Pressey, A.W., and Zubek, J.P., Eds., *Readings in General Psychology: Canadian Contributions.* Toronto, McClelland and Stewart, 1970, pp. 165-171.
87. Ziskind, E.: A second look at sensory deprivation. *J Nerv Ment Dis 138*:223-232, 1964.
88. Sichel, A.: Sur une espece particulière de délire senile qui survient quelque fois après l'extraction de la cataracte. *Annal d'Oculistique 49*:154-168, 1863.
89. Schmidt-Rimpler, H.: Delirien nach Verschluss der Augen und in Dunkel-Zimmern. *Arch Psychiatr 9*:233-243, 1879.
90. Jackson, C.W., Jr.: "Clinical Sensory Deprivation: A Review of Hospitalized Eye-Surgery Patients," in Zubek, J.P., Ed., *Sensory Deprivation: Fifteen Years of Research.* New York, Appleton-Century-Crofts, 1969, pp. 332-373.
91. Cameron, D.E.: Studies in senile nocturnal delirium. *Psychiatr Q 15*:47-53, 1941.
92. Clark, B., and Graybiel, A.: The break-off phenomenon: a feeling of separation from the earth experienced by pilots at high altitudes. *J Aviation Med 28*:121-126, 1957.
93. Kornfeld, D.S.: The hospital environment: its impact on the patient. *Adv Psychosom Med 8*:252-270, 1972.
94. Mendelson, J., Solomon, P., and Lindemann, E.: Hallucinations of poliomyelitis patients during treatment in a respirator. *J Nerv Ment Dis 126*:421-428, 1958.
95. Gordon, A.M.: Psychological aspects of isolator therapy in acute leukemia. *Br J Psychiatry 127*:588-590, 1975.
96. Haenel, T. and Nagel, G.A.: Das psychologische Verhalten von Tumorkranken mit Agranulozytose unter Isolierbedingungen. *Schweiz Med Wschr 105*:839-843, 1975.
97. Bowden, P.: The psychiatric aspects of cardiac intensive therapy: a review. *Europ J Intensive Care Medicine 1*:85-91, 1975.

98. Leiderman, P.H., Mendelson, J., Wexler, D., and Solomon, P.: Sensory deprivation: clinical aspects. *Arch Intern Med 101*:389-396, 1958.

99. Ziskind, E.: Isolation stress in medical and mental illness. *JAMA 168*:1427-1431, 1958.

100. Jackson, C.W., Jr., Pollard, J.C., and Kansky, E.W.: The application of findings from experimental sensory deprivation to cases of clinical sensory deprivation. *Am J Med Sci 243*:558-563, 1962.

101. McKegney, F.P.: The intensive care syndrome. *Conn Med 30*:633-636, 1966.

102. Holland, J., Sgroi, S.M., Marwit, S.J., and Solkoff, N.: The ICU syndrome: fact or fancy. *Psychiatr Med 4*:241-249, 1973.

103. Wilson, L.M.: Intensive care delirium. *Arch Intern Med 130*:225-226, 1972.

104. Keep, P.J.: Stimulus deprivation in windowless rooms. *Anaesthesia 32*:598-602, 1977.

105. Hale, M., Koss, N., Kerstein, M., Camp, K., and Barash, P.: Psychiatric complications in a surgical ICU. *Crit Care Med 5*:199-203, 1977.

106. Katz, N.M., Agle, D.P., DePalma, R.G., and De Cosse, J.J.: Delirium in surgical patients under intensive care. *Arch Surg 104*:310-313, 1972.

107. Hackett, T.P., Cassem, N.H., and Wishnie, H.A.: The coronary-care unit. *N Engl J Med 279*:1365-1370, 1968.

108. Cay, E.L., Vetter, N., Philip, A.E., and Dugard, P.: Psychological reactions to a coronary care unit. *J Psychosom Res 16*:437-447, 1972.

109. Parker, D.L., and Hodge, J.R.: Delirium in a coronary care unit. *JAMA 201*:702-703, 1967.

110. Graubert, D.N., and Edmonson, J.H.: Psychologic adaptation of patients isolated in protected environments. *NY State J Med 72*:227-228, 1972.

111. Holland, J., Harris, S., Plumb, M., Tuttolomundo, A., and Yates, J.: Psychological aspects of physical barrier isolation: observation of acute leukemia patients in "germ-free" units. Paper presented at 13th International Congress of Hematology, Munich, Germany, August 1-7, 1970.

112. Kohle, K., Simons, C., Weidlich, S., Dietrich, M., and Durner, A.: Psychological aspects in the treatment of leukemia patients in the isolated bed system "life island." *Psychother Psychosom 19*:85-91, 1971.

113. Gottschalk, L.A., Haer, J.L., and Bates, D.E.: Effect of sensory overload on psychological state. *Arch Gen Psychiatry 27*:451-458, 1972.

114. Ludwig, A.: Sensory overload and psychopathology. *Dis Nerv Syst* 36:357-360, 1975.
115. Falk, S.A., and Woods, N.F.: Hospital noise—levels and potential health hazards. *N Engl J Med* 289:774-781, 1973.
116. Litin, E.M.: Mental reaction to trauma and hospitalization in the aged. *JAMA* 162:1522-1524, 1956.
117. Levin, M.: Toxic delirium precipitated by admission to hospital. *J Nerv Ment Dis* 116:210-214, 1952.
118. Zubek, J.P., and MacNeill, M.: Effects of immobilization: behavioural and EEG changes. *Can J Psychol* 20:316-366, 1966.
119. Ryback, R.S., Lewis, O.F., and Lessard, C.S.: Psychobiologic effects of prolonged bed rest (weightlessness) in young, healthy volunteers (study 11). *Aerospace Med* 42:529-535, 1971.
120. Levy, R.: The immobilized patient and his psychologic well-being. *Postgrad Med* 40:73-77, 1966.

Additional References

Arkin, A.M., Antrobus, J.S., and Ellman, S.J., Editors. *The Mind in Sleep: Psychology and Psychopathology.* Hillsdale, N.J., Lawrence Erlbaum Association, 1978.

Horne, J.A. A review of the biological effects of total sleep deprivation in man. *Biol Psychol* 7:55-102, 1978.

Lishman, W.A. *Organic Psychiatry.* Oxford, Blackwell Scientific Publ., 1978.

Williams, R.L., and Karacan, I., Eds. *Pharmacology of Sleep.* New York, John Wiley & Sons, 1976.

Williams, R.L., and Karacan, I., Eds. *Sleep Disorders. Diagnosis and Treatment.* New York, John Wiley & Sons, 1978.

CHAPTER 6

PATHOPHYSIOLOGY AND PATHOGENESIS

Pathogenesis refers to the events that occur between the impact of a given agent on the host and the outcome that follows from that point (1). In Chapter 5, the determinants of delirium were discussed. In the present chapter we shall focus on the pathophysiological mechanisms and processes that are believed to intervene between the impact of a particular noxious agent or disease on the one hand, and the onset of delirium on the other. Our knowledge of this area is very incomplete. Indeed, what Hart (2) wrote in 1936 is still largely true today: "In discussing at the present time the possible pathogenesis of delirium we have therefore to leave the sphere of knowledge and enter that of hypothesis and speculation." Hart postulated that impairment of cerebral function underlying delirium could be produced by a wide range of causal factors whose connection to the syndrome might be no more specific than that existing between hemiplegia and its various causes. This type of relationship, namely one in which a large number of determinants and intervening pathophysiological mechanisms may result in a relatively circumscribed and constant set of clinical manifestations, almost certainly obtains in delirium.

Engel and Romano (3) have developed the influential view of delirium as a "syndrome of cerebral insufficiency" and hypothesized that a derangement of cerebral metabolism underlies all instances of it. This derangement, they argued, is manifested both psychologically and physiologically. Psychologically, cerebral insufficiency is reflected in an impairment of cognitive functions, that is to say in deficits and/or distortions of attention, awareness, thinking, memory, perception, and spatiotemporal orientation. Physiologically, cerebral insufficiency is indicated by generalized slowing of the EEG, which in turn parallels

152

changes in the functional metabolism of cerebral neurons. Engel and Romano observed that the level of cognitive functioning correlated closely with changes in EEG frequency: reduction in the level of cognition was accompanied by slowing of the EEG, while improvement in cognitive functioning was associated with acceleration of the EEG. These authors marshalled impressive evidence from both experimental and clinical studies which supported their hypothesis of the pathogenesis of delirium. More recently, Engel (4) has asserted that the cerebral metabolic insufficiency postulated to underlie delirium may involve such disturbances as deficient supply of substrates, mostly glucose and oxygen, to the brain, damage to the enzyme systems necessary for proper utilization of the substrates, disruption of synaptic transmission, and damage to cell membranes. Jellinger (5) has proposed that acute organic psychoses are usually caused by disorders of the blood-brain barrier, by acute neuronal dysfunction, or by disruption of synaptic transmission.

Much of what has been written about the pathophysiology of delirium is inferential, since relatively few relevant studies have been carried out on delirious subjects. The only major exception to this statement is provided by EEG investigations in both clinical and deliberately induced delirium. Otherwise, the findings of the studies on the biochemical and neurophysiological disturbances which underlie coma (6-9) have been applied to delirium on the assumption that this syndrome represents a disorder of consciousness whose progression would lead to stupor and coma. The generality of this assumption is open to question, however. It applies to many cases of delirium but not to all. A wide range of disorders, best exemplified by metabolic and toxic encephalopathies, may cause both delirium and coma. On the other hand, drug and alcohol withdrawal syndromes are often accompanied by delirium that does not progress to coma unless complications such as infection, seizures, or cardiovascular collapse alter its course. Some writers have proposed that delirium tremens represents a variant of delirium, one more closely related to organic mental disorders produced by mescaline, lysergic acid, and quinacrine, which are not characterized by either global cognitive impairment or by EEG slowing (3). This issue will be discussed later on. It is brought up at this point to underscore the probability that delirium as defined herein results from more than one pathophysiological process.

It is hypothesized that the various intracranial and systemic diseases which cause delirium do so by virtue of bringing about a diffuse or multifocal disturbance of cerebral metabolism. Many possible pathophysiological mechanisms may be involved. There may be deficiency of substrates for oxidative metabolism; impairment of the mechanisms for the liberation, conservation, or utilization of chemical energy stored in the fuels; disruption of synaptic transmission; disturbances in the normal ionic passage through excitable membranes; gross alterations in electrolyte concentration, water content, osmolality, and pH in the internal milieu; and impaired synthesis of macromolecules needed for renewal of the structural and functional elements of the neuron. In some cases there may be anatomical abnormalities in circuitry or disturbed equilibrium in functional relationships involving neural pathways necessary for integrative functions, or the presence of false neurotransmitters (6-9). It appears that at least one basic pathophysiological mechanism underlying delirium is a disturbance in the production or utilization of energy involving primarily cerebral cortex and/or subcortical structures whose integrated activity is necessary for the maintenance of wakeful awareness and organized cognitive processes.

Recent work that may have bearing on the pathogenesis of delirium will now be reviewed. Considering that a derangement of *cerebral metabolism* has been postulated to constitute a basic pathophysiological mechanism in delirium, current views on this subject will be discussed first. *Cerebral blood flow* is intimately related to the metabolism of the brain, and recent advances in measuring it have already been applied in the studies of delirium due to various causes (10-11). Both brain metabolism and blood flow are reflected in the *electroencephalogram*. EEG studies of delirium have so far provided the main direct information on the pathophysiology of the syndrome. Disturbances in *neurotransmission* have been proposed to underlie at least some cases of delirium and need to be examined in this context. The neural structures as well as the neurophysiological and biochemical mechanisms subserving and regulating the *sleep-wakefulness cycle* are highly relevant to delirium since the latter appears to be invariably accompanied by a disruption of the cycle and by fragmentation of the stages of sleep. Thus, the neurophysiology and biochemistry of arousal, wakefulness, and sleep need to be discussed. Particularly important are the studies on experimental delirium, one induced by drugs and other techniques. These studies have provided important information about the mechanisms underlying delirium and given support for a unitary conception of the syndrome. These studies will be referred to mostly in relation to the EEG findings and to the relevant hypotheses on the role of neurotransmission and the disturbances of the sleep-wakefulness cycle as they pertain to delirium.

CEREBRAL METABOLISM AND DELIRIUM

Studies of cerebral metabolism in delirium are lacking. It is generally assumed, however, that cerebral disorganization, which at the behavioral level is manifested by the syndrome of delirium, reflects a disturbance of brain metabolism. Indirect support for this contention is provided by studies of conditions such as hypoxia and hypoglycemia which can result in both delirium and coma. Siesjö et al. (8) have pointed out recently that many clinical disorders associated with psychological manifestations of transient cerebral dysfunction share a common feature, i.e. an abnormal alteration of brain metabolism. In addition to hypoglycemia, hypoxia, and ischemia, such factors as hyperthermia, acidosis, anxiety, and other clinically relevant variables may adversely affect cerebral metabolic rates and cognitive functioning. Normal state of the latter depends on intact brain function.

The brain constitutes only about 2 percent of body weight and yet its energy expenditure and oxygen consumption are disproportionately high for its size. The brain of a normal, conscious, young adult consumes about 20 percent of the total body basal oxygen (9). This high level of oxidative metabolism is used almost entirely for the oxidation of glucose and the production of energy. Adenosine triphosphate (ATP) serves as the immediate source of energy for the work of the neuronal cell. Because of its high energy requirements the brain is dependent on an uninterrupted supply of essential substrates, i.e. oxygen and glucose. Their stores in the brain are almost nil and hence these substrates must be continuously supplied by the cerebral circulation. Anaerobic glycolysis normally yields only about 5 percent of the ATP produced and cannot replace the aerobic oxidation of glucose as an adequate source of energy for the brain. Complete cessation of the cerebral blood flow in man results in loss of consciousness within about six seconds (9). Yet even if the cerebral blood flow continues at a normal or higher than normal rate, the supply of substrates may be insufficient if the arterial contents of oxygen or glucose fall below critical levels. A fall of arterial oxygen tension (PaO_2) to below 60 torr may already impair certain mental functions, such as short-term memory (8). The brain is relatively less vulnerable to glucose than to oxygen deprivation since its carbohydrate stores are relatively higher; also ketone bodies may be utilized instead of glucose, as occurs in starvation or diabetes. In these conditions glucose may constitute less than one-half of the oxidizable substrate and yet brain function remains normal (8). Despite this substitution, however, severe or prolonged hypoglycemia leads to irreversible neuronal damage.

Methods to measure cerebral metabolic rate (CMR) have depended largely on the measurement of cerebral blood flow (CBF) and the arteriovenous differences (AVD) in oxygen and glucose contents. Lately, however, important technical advances have occurred that permit simultaneous measurement of regional CBF as well as oxygen and glucose consumption in various areas of the brain and in different functional states. Techniques for the measurement of CBF will be described in the next section. Regional cerebral metabolic rate for oxygen ($rCMRO_2$) can now be measured in humans by using cyclotron-produced isotope oxygen-15. The isotope is injected into the subject's internal carotid artery, and a multidetector system, designed to measure up to thirteen regions of each cerebral hemisphere, monitors the time course of tracer movement through the injected hemisphere (12). Local cerebral glucose utilization can be measured by administering radioactive 2-deoxyglucose (13). The new method permits autoradiographic estimation of regional glucose consumption in the intact brain in animals. The autoradiographs reflect changes in local CMR resulting from changes in local neuronal activity. The latter has been shown to alter the former. Increased neuronal activity is accompained by increased oxygen consumption and energy utilization by brain cells. The latter require energy for two principal kinds of tasks: active transport and biosynthesis (8). The former involves mostly extrusion of sodium ions and accumulation of potassium ions in order to restore concentration gradients for these ions across the excitable membranes following depolarization. Furthermore, active transport includes axoplasmic transport from the body of the neuron to the periphery as well as the packaging of transmitters into synaptic vesicles and other sites. Biosynthetic work refers to resynthesis of the constantly degraded macromolecules, membranes, and cell organelles. Both biosynthesis and active transport require energy. The latter is provided by high energy phosphates, i.e. ATP or other nucleoside triphosphates such as phosphocreatine (8).

It has been found that the changes in local CMR, which reflect local functional activity of brain cells, are accompanied by changes in local CBF (14). There is thus a coupling of neuronal function, metabolic rate, and blood flow. Sokoloff (14) has proposed, on the basis of studies of local cerebral glucose utilization, that the changes in local metabolic rate may provide chemical mechanisms for the regulation and adjustment of the regional CBF. The nature of these mechanisms is still a matter of speculation. Products of increased metabolism, hydrogen ions, and adenosine have all been suggested as the coupling factors (15). Whatever the coupling mechanisms may prove to be, it has been established that increased neuronal activity is accompanied by elevated metabolic rate and increased blood flow. On the contrary, when the rate of neuronal firing decreases, both metabolic rate and blood flow decrease too. Thus, neuronal activity controls energy expenditure, but the latter does not control the former (16).

Lowry (16) has asserted that energy metabolism of the brain is controlled by neuronal activity. These two processes are closely coupled together. The consumption of glucose to produce ATP as the immediate source of energy is probably controlled at as many as ten steps. Brain metabolism can be reduced 40 to 50 percent by the administration of general anesthetics, for example, or increased by 500 percent for short periods by intense stimulation (16). When energy shortage is imminent, as in anoxia or hypoxia, neuronal activity is decreased, and energy reserves are thus conserved. Siesjö (15) has pointed out that CMR may be reduced to 25 percent normal by lowering body temperature to 22° or increased to 200 percent normal by immobilization stress without any disturbance of brain energy state, as assessed by tissue levels of ATP, ADP, and AMP.

Particularly important for the student of delirium is the relationship between mental activity, normal and abnormal, and cerebral metabolism. For a long time it has been assumed that brain metabolism is constant in different types of mental activity, with the possible exception of intense anxiety, and that a relatively strict correlation obtains between cerebral metabolic rate and the level of consciousness (9). Both these time-honored assumptions have been challenged in recent years (15). Cooper and Crow (17), for example, have found significant increases in cerebral oxygenation at localized areas of the brain during performance of mental tasks. During reading there were increases in oxygenation in the frontal regions, while mental arithmetic was accompanied by more widespread changes. These findings have been confirmed and greatly extended by measurements of regional CBF, to be discussed in the next section. The relationship between the level of consciousness and CMR was believed to be close. Sokoloff (9) summarized earlier work in this area and concluded that CMR and the level of consciousness showed "reasonably close correlation." Cerebral O_2 consumption in the normal alert state was found to be 3.5 ml/100g/min; in confusion —2.8 ml.; and in coma—2.0 ml. Thus, depressed levels of awareness were accompanied by parallel decrements in CMR. The generality of this finding has been questioned recently. Some drugs, such as ketamine or diazepam, may produce anesthesia or unconsciousness, or both, without a parallel decrease in oxygen consumption by the brain (15). Bachelard (6) asserts that coma is not simply due to energy failure but rather to sensitivity of specialized processes in the brain not necessarily involved in energy metabolism. Psychological symptoms and EEG changes tend to precede any detectable failure in energy metabolism and appear to be the result of biochemical changes other than reduced energy production.

Recent studies of hypoxia, hypoglycemia, and hepatic coma seem to support the above contention. With mild arterial *hypoxia* (6-7% oxygen) there is a marked increase in CBF and anaerobic glycolysis, as shown by increased arteriovenous difference in lactate, and without any change in rates of oxygen consumption by the brain. The increased glycolysis appears to involve activation of at least two enzymes: hexokinase and pyruvate kinase (6). Even moderately severe hypoxia affects other aspects of cerebral metabolism to a lesser extent than glycolysis. Changes in biologically active amino acids are relatively slight: there is only mild increase in the concentrations of ammonia and glutamate. Bachelard (6) points out, however, that changes in the metabolism of aromatic biogenic amines, i.e. dopamine, noradrenaline, and serotonin, do occur in hypoxia and may prove to be functionally important. These neurotransmitters may be especially sensitive to reduction in available oxygen, which is required for their synthesis via hydroxylation reactions. The latter are vulnerable to hypoxia. Furthermore, it appears that dopamine receptors may be even more sensitive to hypoxia than the hydroxylases. Behavioral disturbances induced in rats by mild hypoxia (8.65% oxygen) could be reversed by DOPA, in the presence of an inhibitor of peripheral DOPA decarboxylase (18).

Studies of *hypoglycemia* induced by insulin have shown that behavioral and EEG abnormalities could occur without any impairment of energy metabolism (6). Thus as in hypoxia, these abnormalities precede energy failure. How do they arise? Deoxyglucose-induced hypoglycemia provides some clues. Two-deoxyglucose is a glucose analogue that can inhibit the rate of glucose entry to the brain and thus leads to cellular hypoglycemia. Changes in behavior and EEG can result initially from deoxyglucose administration without any detectable effect on energy production. Thus, a mild reduction in available glucose can produce behavioral abnormalities which do not seem to result simply from reduced glucose utilization by the brain. These abnormalities have been hypothesized to be due to the sensitivity to hypoglycemia of glucoreceptors in the hypothalamic-pituitary system (6).

In *hepatic coma* there is reduced cerebral oxygen consumption and enhanced glycolysis before any demonstrable failure of energy metabolism (6). These changes are produced by the high ammonia concentrations in the brain. The latter removes ammonia by formation of glutamine, which accumulates in the brain in hepatic coma. The glutamine is partly converted to α-oxoglutaramate, which might yet prove to be the main toxic metabolite.

Hypoxia, hypoglycemia, hepatic encephalopathy, and other disorders leading to coma seem to share certain common features. An impairment of function, manifested in EEG and behavior, occurs *before* any demonstrable cell damage or failure of energy, as assessed from concentrations of ATP and creatine phosphate. Often the first metabolic change is enhanced glycolysis (6, 8). If a perturbation of energy state activates glycolysis, there follows an increase in glycolytic rate in relation to the rate of oxidation of pyruvate (8). It appears that in conditions such as hypoxia or hypoglycemia endogenous carbohydrate stores in the form of glycolytic and citric acid cycle intermediates are metabolized by the brain. Furthermore, substrate carbon is mobilized from amino acids by mechanisms involving transamination and deamination (8). Thus, oxidative metabolism may be upheld when the supply of substrates is reduced. The energy state is maintained, but there is derangement of intermediary metabolism.

Metabolic encephalopathies will be further discussed in Part II of this book. They have been cited in this chapter only to illustrate changing views on the mechanisms underlying the behavioral abnormalities in these clinically important pathological states. It appears now that it is incorrect to state that a failure in energy metabolism is a necessary condition for delirium to occur (6, 8). Disturbances in neurotransmission may yet prove to play a key role in the pathogenesis of the syndrome.

Certain conditions which increase or decrease functional

activity of the brain alter its energy demands correspondingly and are accompanied by parallel variations in energy production. These conditions are relevant to delirium. Amphetamine intoxication, anxiety, hyperthermia, and epileptic seizures increase cerebral functional activity, oxygen consumption, CBF, and CMR. *Anxiety* is particularly important in the present context. Betz (19) found an increase in CBF in human subjects in response to anxiety-provoking stimuli. Amount of bodily movement and the intensity of anxiety induced by the stimulation, as well as duration of the latter, appeared to be the main variables. Siesjö (8, 15) carried out animal experiments which showed that immobilization stress resulted in increases of up to 180 percent in cerebral oxygen consumption and in comparable elevation of CBF. Propranolol blocked these increases, and it was concluded that the effects of stress were mediated by catecholamines. These findings confirmed an earlier observation by King et al. (20) that intravenous infusion of adrenaline resulted in anxiety and a concomitant 20 percent increase in $CMRO_2$ and CBF. Siesjö (8) has suggested recently that anxiety and stress could increase cerebral energy consumption and that relief of anxiety by sedation was indicated in patients with abnormally compromised cerebral energy production, such as occurs in states of hypoglycemia, hypoxia, or ischemia.

Hyperthermia increases cerebral energy requirements. Animal studies have shown that $CMRO_2$ increases by about 5 percent for each 1°C increase in temperature (8). These findings may be relevant to the febrile delirium. Hyperthermia is known to induce delirium even in the absence of acute infection.

Also relevant to delirium are studies on cerebral metabolism in states of *wakefulness* and *sleep*. Creutzfeldt (21) has pointed out that changes in cerebral cortical activity and EEG patterns during metabolic reduction, such as obtains in hypoglycemia or hypoxia, are qualitatively similar to those during synchronized (slow-wave) sleep. Yet one cannot conclude from the similarity of EEG patterns that increased delta and theta activity necessarily implies decreased metabolism. In states of metabolic deficiency there is reduction in the activity of large groups of neurons. In synchronized sleep, however, some neurons are activated and others suppressed. Similarly, during arousal the majority of cortical neurons may show increased activity, but many cells show the opposite behavior. The difference in overall neuronal discharge rates between synchronized sleep and arousal is not dramatic. It appears that during cortical arousal the different temporal patterns of cortical neuronal activity are more important than the overall increase in the discharge rate. Actually, the latter may be predominantly decreased during desynchronization induced by electrical stimulation of the midbrain reticular formation (21). Only extreme states, such as seizure activity or coma, show significant increase or decrease, respectively, of discharge rates of cortical neurons.

Studies of CBF during *sleep* (22) have shown that REM sleep is accompanied by a marked increase in CBF, a moderate rise during transition from wakefulness to sleep, and a fall during awakening. These changes are thought to be secondary to the metabolic changes in the brain. A marked increase in CMR has been observed in REM sleep (22). Townsend et al. (23) have found an increase in CBF during REM sleep and a 10 percent decrease during slow-wave sleep. These changes are small but statistically significant. It is interesting in this regard that delirium has been often referred to as a waking dream, yet there appear to be important differences in the physiology of REM sleep and many cases of clinical delirium. In the latter, the EEG and CBF studies have pointed towards reduced or normal cerebral metabolism.

Engel and Romano (3) have asserted that advances in the knowledge of cerebral metabolism were essential for further progress in understanding the pathogenesis of delirium. They also predicted that a correlation between the degree of decrease in cerebral oxygen consumption and the mental status in delirium would be confirmed. Advances in the knowledge of brain metabolism in the twenty years since Engel and Romano wrote their paper have been spectacular but have thrown little light on the pathogenesis of delirium. It seems clear now that the syndrome is not a manifestation of a failure of cerebral energy metabolism and actually precedes it. It appears to be associated in many cases with a reduced cerebral metabolic rate but not a perturbation of the brain metabolic or energy state. Furthermore, normal or even increased cerebral metabolic rate may be associated with symptoms of delirium, as is the case in delirium tremens or ketamine administration. As a rule, however, reduction in the level of consciousness is associated with reduction of cerebral metabolic rate. The latter has been shown conclusively to be closely related to the functional activity in discrete structural and/or functional units of the central nervous system (13).

Schnaberth and Schubert (24) have studied the metabolism of the cerebrospinal fluid in patients with clouded consciousness. The latter showed significantly higher degrees of uncompensated metabolic (lactate) acidosis in the CSF than normally conscious control subjects. Thus, disturbances of cerebral function, due to various causes and manifested by reduction of consciousness, were found to correlate well with the pH, lactate, and HCO$_3$ levels in the CSF. These findings reflect reduced functional activity of cerebral neurons and derangement of cerebral metabolism in the direction of enhanced anerobic glycolysis. Increased CSF acidosis may in turn result in a disturbance of cerebral metabolism, and a vicious circle is created. The authors proposed that measuring lactate concentration in the CSF can have a prognostic value in patients displaying clouding of consciousness.

Sokoloff (19) observes that the correlation between the depression of consciousness and energy metabolism represents parallel but independent results of common underlying pathological processes. This viewpoint contrasts with the hypothesis that reduced brain metabolism *causes* disturbances of consciousness. Cerebral blood flow is a sensitive indicator of changes in cerebral activity associated with delirium and hence its studies are important for the understanding of the syndrome.

CEREBRAL BLOOD FLOW

Measurements of cerebral blood flow (CBF) have played an important role in attempts to correlate cerebral metabolic rate with levels of awareness and with various forms of mental activity in both normal and brain-damaged subjects (8-11, 15,

19, 22, 23, 25-31). Recent refinements in the techniques of measuring CBF have provided a powerful investigative tool which should throw new light on the pathogenesis of delirium. Engel and Romano (3) complained twenty years ago that the studies of CBF had been of limited value in elucidating the changes of cerebral metabolism in delirium, in part, because the techniques then available allowed only the measurement of the total oxygen uptake of the total brain and not of its functional parts. Sokoloff (31) has pointed out that patterns of behavior are likely to be more adequately reflected in the blood flow and metabolic rates in individual structural and functional units than in the brain as a whole. The development since 1961 of methods to measure regional cerebral blood flow (rCBF) has allowed a dramatic expansion of information about cerebral hemodynamics under various normal and morbid conditions (25, 27, 28).

Measurement of total CBF in man became possible with the introduction of the nitrous oxide technique by Kety and Schmidt (32) in 1945. The refinement of this technique by Lassen and Ingvar (33) in 1961 made it possible to measure rCBF in man. The new method at first involved injection into the common carotid artery of radioactive krypton-85, and later of xenon-133. These radioactive tracers have also been applied by inhalation. Xenon-133 is the most often used tracer at present (25).

Mean total CBF in a normal young adult is about 50 ml/min/ 100g of brain tissue. The value for children three to ten years old is higher, i.e. about 106 ml. (25). Unconsciousness occurs when CBF drops to 31 ml. Studies of rCBF, recently summarized by Ingvar (27), have shown that the distribution of blood flow in various parts of the brain of neurologically normal subjects changes with mental activity. In awake, resting subjects rCBF values are highest over premotor and frontal regions, suggesting a relatively high level of activity in these areas. During psychological testing which involved abstract thinking, memorizing, and problem solving, there was an increase of flow in the same areas, indicating increased activity in the association cortex of the dominant hemisphere. Ingvar concludes that man's conscious mental activity involves activation especially of precentral and frontal structures. These changes appear to involve two components: a regional one which involves areas of the brain necessary for the performance of specialized tasks, such as speech; and a general component reflecting an arousal reaction, and apparently related to the motivation and emotional state of the subject.

In Alzheimer's disease the total CBF is reduced roughly in proportion to the degree of intellectual deterioration (34). In the early stages of dementia, when only memory deficits were evident, the reduction of flow was particularly marked in the temporal regions. Patients showing global cognitive impairment had a reduction of temporal flow as well as lower mean hemispheric flow level. The demented subjects had a different rCBF pattern during performance of psychological tests from the normal individuals: the normally increased flow in pre-central and post-central regions was less pronounced or actually decreased. In chronic schizophrenics CBF level is normal, but rCBF distribution is not: the patients display a resting hypofrontal pattern, i.e. absence of normal high flow over premotor and frontal structures.

The above findings justify expectations that measurement of rCBF could advance our knowledge of cerebral metabolic rate in various brain structures during delirium caused by all kinds of factors. Only two studies of delirious patients have been published to date. Berglund et al. (10) studied rCBF in a case of bromide delirium using xenon inhalation technique. They found marked reduction of CBF as well as abnormal distribution pattern, in that the flow was low in frontal and parieto-occipital regions. This pattern resembled that found in presenile dementia.

The same authors studied rCBF in delirium tremens (11) and reported a decrease in CBF, but subsequently denied this (10). These very preliminary findings seem to support Engel and Romano's contention that the cerebral metabolic rate in delirium is reduced and correlates well with the degree of cognitive impairment. This rule does not seem to apply to delirium tremens despite the fact that it shares global cognitive impairment with delirium due to other causes. Furthermore, unchanged CBF levels in delirium tremens stand in contrast to increased CBF in REM sleep (23). This finding may reflect differences in regional metabolic activity, which has been shown to correlate with rCBF (29). CBF has also been shown to correlate with the frequency of the EEG (35). A decreased CBF is associated with a slow-wave EEG, and vice versa. There are exceptions to this rule, however. During slow-wave sleep the CBF is only slightly reduced in the presence of a large proportion of slow waves in the EEG. In children the cerebral oxygen uptake and CBF are high, and the EEG tends to be slow (35). Another exception is provided by cerebral anoxia, which induces lactacidosis in the brain and thus disrupts the normal metabolic regulation and the autoregulation of CBF (35). Following cerebral anoxic lesions one may find a high CBF despite the presence of a slow-wave EEG. Finally, reduced CBF in the presence of normal EEG has been reported (26).

CBF has long been thought to correlate well with the level of consciousness (9, 31). Reduction of the latter was found to be associated with modest decrease in CBF. More recently, however, this close correlation has been found to be lacking in some conditions. Carlsson et al. (36) report that diazepam caused only moderate reduction of CBF and did not lower cerebral oxygen uptake in rats. Yet in comatose patients the drug has been shown to cause a depression of both CBF and cerebral oxygen uptake (28). Ketamine, which has anesthetic properties, is also a potent cerebral vasodilator and stimulant, and it increases CMR and CBF (28).

In conclusion, functional neuronal activity and cerebral metabolism correlate well with blood supply to the brain. These variables also correlate, with notable exceptions, with the level of consciousness. When CBF is significantly reduced, the level of consciousness is correspondingly depressed and may range from delirium to coma. When arterial blood is deficient in oxygen and/or glucose, even normal or increased CBF will not prevent the onset of delirium. Reduced level of consciousness is usually, but not always, associated with reduction of CMR and CBF. CBF and supply of substrate may be adequate yet CMR may be reduced and the level of consciousness lowered. In this latter case there must be a reduction in neuronal activity and a corresponding drop in energy demand (31). Anesthesia with halothane, methoxyflurane, and nitrous oxide in a subject with a normal brain exemplifies this type of condition (28). Studies of rCBF in delirium have only begun. It appears that the syndrome may occur in conditions in which CBF is reduced, unchanged (delirium tremens), or even increased (hyperthermia). Application of the new methods for the simultaneous measurement of regional CBF as well as glucose and oxygen utilization in delirium should throw further light on the pathogenesis of delirium in the future. Yet it is well to keep in mind Sokoloff's (31) comment that it is very possible that "the mechanisms of behavior are far too subtle to be reflected in blood flow or metabolic rate, even if measured at the most minute level." Furthermore, discovery of meaningful correlations between psychopathological states or syndromes on the one hand, and cerebral activity, metabolic rate, and blood flow on the other, is hampered by problems of semantics and quantification of psychological variables. Psychopathological terms such as "depression of consciousness," "confusion," etc. are too vague to permit more than gross and imprecise correlations with neurophysiological and biochemical variables. Operational definitions and quantification of the various relevant psychopathological variables, such as attention, memory, cognitive impairment, delirium, etc., are necessary for the progress of our knowledge about relationships between cerebral events and their abnormal behavioral correlates.

ELECTROENCEPHALOGRAPHIC STUDIES

As stated earlier in this chapter, EEG studies of delirium due to various causes have offered most of the information we have on the pathophysiology of the syndrome and its clinical variants. EEG reflects, with exceptions noted in the preceding section, the functional and metabolic activity of the brain. Ingvar (35) asserts that the EEG may be viewed as a paraphenomenon of the metabolic activity underlying neuronal function. Neuronal activity determines $CMRO_2$, which in turn influences the CBF and the frequency of the background activity of the EEG. In general, reduced cerebral function, $CMRO_2$ and CBF are accompanied by a slowing of the EEG.

Pioneering studies of the EEG in delirium were carried out

by Engel, Romano, and their co-workers in the forties (37-43). Engel et al. (37) developed a quantitative method for the expression of frequency distribution in the EEG. They made a count of complete waves in 300 one-second intervals and expressed the distribution of frequencies per second as a percentage of the whole. This method yielded a spectrum of frequencies ranging from one to twelve per second, together with some low voltage activity. The distribution of waves per second, rather than that of individual wavelengths, was thus determined. Engel and co-workers found their method adequate to detect the magnitude of shifts in frequency under various conditions in which such shifts were diffuse rather than paroxysmal (37).

Romano and Engel (38) reported their major findings in 1944. They had studied fifty-three patients suffering from a broad range of cardiovascular, respiratory, cerebral, metabolic, infections, and toxic diseases. All their subjects displayed evidence of delirium characterized by an *increased fluctuation in the level of awareness,* loss of ability for abstract thinking, attentional deficits, and impairment of memory and calculation. All the patients showed EEG abnormalities that the investigators classified arbitrarily into five stages, enumerated in the order of increasing severity as follows:

Stage I: Appearance of a small amount of regular and irregular slow frequencies (5 to 7 c/sec);

Stage II: Further decrease in regularity of the tracing and an increase in both low voltage fast activity and regular and irregular theta waves;

Stage III: Low voltage fast activity and some regular and irregular slow frequencies (3 to 6 c/sec) predominate in the record;

Stage IV: Record irregular and disorganized, no recognizable alpha activity (8 to 12 c/sec), and predominance of slow frequency (2 to 7 c/sec) with small amounts of low voltage fast activity;

Stage V: Normal frequencies few or absent. Predominance of fairly regular, moderately high voltage slow activity (3 to 7 c/sec) (38).

The EEG abnormality reversed completely, or almost completely, to a normal pattern in most patients. The investigators concluded that delirium, as defined by them, was associated with an electrical disturbance of the brain, which was reversible to the extent that the manifestations of delirium were reversible. The EEG abnormalities included decrease in frequency, disorganization, and in the last stage, reorganization at a lower energy level. The researchers hypothesized that the decrease in frequency reflected reduced levels of, or responses to, cortical excitation, and the latter in turn was likely caused by reduced metabolic activity of the neurons or a decrease in the arousing effect of afferent impulses to the cortex. The abnormal electrical activity demonstrated by the EEG was postulated to arise from damaged or dying cells. The EEG abnormalities were considered to be nonspecific. They showed a direct correlation with the psychological deficits and abnormalities that define delirium as a clinical syndrome. The character of the EEG changes appeared to be independent of the specific underlying cerebral disorder but was related to the intensity, duration, and reversibility of the implicated noxious factors.

In subsequent papers, Engel, Romano, and their collaborators extended their original observations summarized above (39-43). They demonstrated that measures taken to correct a major physiological derangement underlying delirium in a given patient could lead to a reversal of the syndrome and its associated EEG abnormalities (39). For example, administration of 100 percent oxygen to delirious patients with congestive heart failure or pulmonary decompensation frequently resulted in an improvement of the EEG record.

Engel and his co-workers pioneered studies on experimentally induced delirium (40, 42). Engel and Rosenbaum (40) induced delirium by oral administration of alcohol to healthy volunteers and chronic alcoholics. The development of intoxication was accompanied by progressive slowing of the EEG background frequencies which correlated with changes in the level of awareness. *The degree of change in frequency* was found to be more significant than the appearance of any particular frequency. When the record taken prior to the experimental intoxication was fast or fast normal, the tracing obtained during gross intoxication had a frequency distribution within the normal range (8 to 12 c/sec). Experimental induction of delirium by means of exposure in the decompression chamber to simulated high altitudes, and thus anoxia, showed similar results to experimental acute alcoholic intoxication and hypoglycemia (42). By contrast, administration of quinacrine to healthy volunteers provoked a different psychological and EEG response (43). All of the subjects exhibited restlessness, tension, anxiety, irritability, and sleeplessness. Concurrently, their EEG records showed a sustained acceleration in frequency of the brain waves. The investigators concluded that quinacrine acts as a cerebral cortical stimulant and elicits a psychological reaction which is not delirium, but rather a syndrome characterized by heightened awareness.

Engel and Romano summarized their findings in two major review papers (3, 44). They interpreted their research results as demonstrating that the core psychological disturbance in delirium, namely an increased fluctuation in the level of awareness, is the result of derangement in cerebral cortical metabolism secondary to physical disease (44). In their most definitive statement to date, the investigators proposed that the metabolic derangement underlies all instances of delirium and that this is reflected psychologically in the disturbance in cognitive functions and physiologically in a relative generalized slowing of the EEG (3). Thus, these two abnormalities are a *sine qua non* of delirium. The EEG is to be viewed as the most sensitive and reliable indicator of cerebral insufficiency. The characteristic EEG changes coupled with the presence of increased fluctuation in the level of awareness, manifested by fluctuating impairment of cognitive functions, provide a basis for differentiation of delirium from other psychiatric disorders. Engel and Romano emphasize that a single normal EEG does not rule out delirium since the patient's predelirious record may have been faster. The slowing of the EEG in delirium is *relative* to the individual's premorbid tracing and may fall within the statistically normal range. Only serial recordings can settle the issue in some cases. Those delirious patients whose EEG shows no slow activity will be found to have either a fast normal or a faster than normal (more than 12 c/sec) record on recovery (4).

The generalizability of the findings and conclusions reported by Engel and Romano has been a subject of controversy. Their

critics, notably Victor and Adams (45), contend that it is erroneous to claim that delirium is always accompanied by an abnormal
EEG. They point out that in milder degrees of the syndrome
there is usually no EEG abnormality. It appears that this controversy reflects semantic, rather than empirical, issues. Victor
and Adams use a different terminology, and their definition of
delirium differs from that employed by Engel and Romano. For
the former writers, delirium represents a variant of acute confusional states, one characterized by gross disorientation, misperceptions, and psychomotor and autonomic nervous system
hyperactivity. This definition applies best to delirium tremens,
which Victor and Adams actually regard as a prototype of
delirium in general. This view is diametrically opposite to that
held by Engel and Romano (3), for whom delirium tremens
constitutes an atypical variant of delirium as a whole. Psychomotor hyperactivity is viewed by these authors as an associated
and inconstant rather than an essential feature of delirium.
They regard delirium tremens as a "more or less distinctive
syndrome noted in alcoholics," one which is closer to psychiatric
disorders produced by drugs such as mescaline, lysergic acid,
and quinacrine rather than to delirium.

It is necessary to be aware of the above semantic differences
if one is to evaluate properly the validity of statements made
by various writers concerning the relationship between delirium
and the EEG. The latter is usually either normal or shows
mixed slow and low voltage fast activity in delirium tremens
(3, 46, 47). Wikler (48) has found no specific changes in the
EEG (other than artifacts attributable to head movements,
blinking and scalp muscle activity) in this condition. He proposes that the EEG changes associated with delirium are related
to the etiological factors rather than to the overt behavioral
abnormalities.

Findings published during the last thirty years are generally
in agreement with those originally reported by Engel and
Romano, yet nobody has attempted to validate their results.
A major problem in this whole area of research is the use of
undefined or vague terms by the investigators and the generally
poor quality of the psychological assessment of the subjects.
Terms such as "delirium," "clouding of consciousness," "confu-

sional state," etc. are often used without any attempt to define them operationally, and this makes it difficult to interpret the EEG findings reported by the various authors. Flügel (49) has exhaustively reviewed the literature on the EEG findings in reversible organic psychoses caused by both intracranial and systemic diseases of various types: metabolic, traumatic, infectious, vascular, toxic, etc. He added the results of his own combined psychiatric and EEG study of 645 patients with reversible psychoses. His conclusions agree with those of Engel and Romano. He states that the characteristic EEG correlate of such psychoses consists of relative reduction in the frequency of the background activity in the milder cases and of the replacement of the alpha activity by abnormal slow waves in the more severe cases (49, p. 130). These EEG abnormalities are nonspecific with regard to the etiology of the reversible organic psychosis. Flügel observes that the nature and causes of the relationship between the latter and its concomitant EEG changes will be unclear as long as the neurophysiological basis of the EEG remains hypothetical.

Other authorities have expressed similar views (50, 51, 52). Kiloh et al. (51) state that conditions such as delirium, encephalopathy, and meningoencephalitis share both similar EEG abnormalities and the features of clouding of consciousness. In the absence of the latter the EEG is not as a rule significantly affected. The EEG abnormalities in these conditions are equivalent to those described by Engel and Romano. Yet, exceptions do exist. Cadilhac and Ribstein (50) have reviewed EEG findings in disorders of carbohydrate metabolism, hepatic and renal insufficiency, and electrolyte and acid-base disturbances. They point out that some very abnormal tracings may be found in the absence of manifestations of reduced consciousness and vice versa. Normal scalp EEG has been observed in patients in clinical coma due to pontomesencephalic hemorrhage. Seizure activity in structures such as the hippocampus and brain stem has been observed in the presence of normal scalp EEG despite clinical signs of clouding or loss of consciousness. A corticogram does not always reflect the pathology of the midbrain, brain stem or limbic structures despite the presence of reduced level of awareness (53, 54). In delirium tremens EEG is normal

(46) or shows transient, mild dysrhythmia (47). These exceptions are theoretically important and suggest that the syndrome of delirium may result from different pathogenic cerebral processes. For example, recent studies show that there is increased central noradrenergic activity in delirium tremens (55).

The finding of diffuse slowing of the basic frequencies in the EEG of patients with delirium raises the question of the behavioral correlates of such slowing. Changes in theta activity are most consistently related to the various components of attention (56). A review of studies of the relation between theta waves and various psychological variables indicates that theta activity accompanies the state of reduced alertness, that is to say receptivity to external stimuli (56). On the other hand, however, theta activity has been found to accompany active problem-solving and perceptual processing tasks (56). This discrepancy is not explicable at this time. Jenkins (57) studied the relation between diffuse EEG slowing and intellectual impairment. He found that tests involving perceptual organization of nonverbal stimuli were markedly affected in subjects displaying EEG slowing. Obrist et al. (58) found impaired intellectual performance in people sixty-years-old and older who had diffuse slow activity in the EEG. Such activity increased significantly after the age of seventy-five (59). In general, diffuse slowing of the background EEG activity in a waking person tends to correlate positively with reduced attention span and impaired cognitive functioning.

Delirium induced experimentally by various drugs has been studied electroencephalographically. These studies have yielded observations which throw some new light on the pathophysiology of delirium. Because of their importance and similar methodology, these studies will be reviewed now in a separate subsection.

Experimental Delirium and the EEG

In 1958 a group of Czech workers began to experiment with benactyzine, a strong anticholinergic agent (60). They observed that when this drug was administered in a dose of 15 to 70 mg. it would precipitate a delirium in healthy volunteers. The delirium lasted for three to five hours and was characterized by gross impairment of intellectual performance and memory;

disturbances of thinking, namely loss of directed thinking manifested by blocking and incoherence; visual hallucinations, with frequent appearance of zoopsia and micropsia; initially decreased, but in later stages increased, psychomotor activity; and neurologic symptoms, such as ataxia, dysarthria, and apraxia. The investigators found that the clinical features of the induced delirium resembled both delirium tremens and Korsakow's syndrome. The delirium could not be reversed by physostigmine. There was a drop in the excretion of 5-hydroxyindolacetic acid, which paralleled the development of delirious symptomatology. This finding led the researchers to hypothesize that the deliriogenic property of benactyzine depended on the drug's interference with both acetylcholine and serotonin metabolism. The EEG records taken during the induced delirium showed a breakdown of the background alpha activity and predominance of delta waves.

Also in 1958, Abood and Meduna (61) published their observations on deliriogenic properties of synthetic anticholinergic agents, namely various congeners of the piperidyl benzilates. One compound, designated JB-329, when administered to healthy volunteers in dosages of 5 to 10 mg. orally, elicited auditory and visual hallucinations, and delirium. JB-329, better known under its trade name Ditran®, was actually a mixture of two isomers: N-ethyl-2-pyrrolidyl-methyl-cyclopentylphenyl glycolate (70%) and N-ethyl-3 piperidyl cyclopentylphenyl glycolate (30%) (62). Gershon and Olariu (63) reported that Ditran could provoke in patients with a history of delirium tremens a delirium which was quite similar to the former. Deliriogenic effects of the drug could be counteracted by tetrahydroaminacrin, a compound with potent anticholinesterase activity. These early observations stimulated a considerable body of research on the behavioral and EEG effects of Ditran and have contributed to the understanding of the pathogenesis of delirium (62-73).

Itil (68-70) and Itil and Fink (71, 72) have reported on their extensive investigations of the behavioral and EEG changes induced by Ditran in man. Three main behavioral responses to the drug were observed (71). With a low dose (0.01-0.02 mg/kg) the changes consisted of slight fluctuation in attention and consciousness and were accompanied by occasional low voltage theta and delta activity. In higher doses (0.04-0.25 mg/kg) Ditran provoked in some subjects a stupor-like state. High doses of the drug (0.10-0.25 mg/kg) elicited reduction and fluctuation of awareness, perceptual distortions, thought disturbances, severe anxiety, and restlessness. These behavioral effects were accompanied by a reduction of alpha activity and the appearance of high voltage delta and theta waves with superimposed 20-40 c/sec fast beta activity. Both the behavioral and the EEG changes induced by Ditran were modified by administering various drugs during the experimental delirium. Intravenous chlorpromazine was found to interrupt the delirium and to induce coma and increased slowing of the EEG with decreased fast beta activity. Administration of tetrahydroaminacrin resulted in a reversal of the delirium in ten to twenty minutes and in decreased slow delta wave and fast beta activity. Intravenous LSD (0.001-0.002 mg/kg) produced increased alertness as well as psychomotor activity and restlessness. The investigators put forth a hypothesis that in delirium there are changes in central cholinergic and adrenergic mechanisms which affect the medial ascending reticular activating system and the medial thalamic diffuse projection systems. The former exercises mainly a cortical inhibitory function (expressed as the appearance of slow waves in the EEG), while the latter has a predominantly facilitatory influence on the cortex (expressed as fast activity in the EEG). Thus, a relative increase in either central inhibitory or stimulant function subserved by one or the other system, respectively, may determine the type of delirium, i.e. whether it is hyperactive or hypoactive. This hypothesis and the studies on which it was based provide a strong argument in favor of a unitary conception of delirium advanced by Engel and Romano.

Atropine® (0.04-0.30 mg/kg) induced more slow waves but less fast activity in the EEG than Ditran (72). The ratio of slow activity or fast activity was related to the clinical manifestations induced by either drug, especially to the degree of psychomotor activity and experience of hallucinations. An earlier study by Ostfeld et al. (74) had showed that atropine given to healthy volunteers in a dose of 10 mg. orally impaired recent memory and attention span, but did not induce illusions, hallucinations, delusions, or disorientation. The EEG showed a consistent shift towards lower amplitude and slow activity. Itil (69) observed that high doses of atropine and Ditran induced in some subjects a sleep-like state which differed significantly in both its clinical and EEG features from spontaneous sleep. He could not confirm the claims of earlier researchers that anticholinergic drugs elicited a dissociation of the EEG and behavior. In a later paper, Itil (70) reported on the digital computer analyzed EEG records during REM sleep, and following Ditran and LSD administration. He found that the EEG pattern characterized by both very slow and very fast activity occurred in REM sleep and in anticholinergic delirium. Itil hypothesized that both REM sleep and delirium depended on inhibition of the central cholinergic mechanism. Cartwright (67) noted that Ditran elicited EEG records markedly different from the experimental subjects' normal waking and sleep records. The EEG recorded during Ditran-induced delirium displayed features of both wakefulness and stages 1, 2, and 3 of sleep. REM's were found to be persistent and of very high amplitude. Mean total REM time on the night following Ditran administration was significantly reduced in comparison to the subject's pre-drug night. The content of dreams obtained from the experimental subjects on a night one to two weeks before or after the drug experience was quite similar to the content of Ditran-induced hallucinations. This led Cartwright to postulate that the fantasies produced under dreaming and drug conditions, respectively, were derived from the same substrate of ongoing mental life. She proposed that Ditran appeared to create a neurophysiological state different from and yet analogous to that of REM sleep and dreaming.

Behavioral and EEG effects of atropine, scopolamine, and Ditran are qualitatively similar (62). All three drugs induce delirium in normal volunteers when given in equivalent intramuscular doses. Subjects pass through an initial stage of drowsiness and "stupor," and then progress to what Ketchum et al. (62) have called a "pseudowakeful" state, characterized by disordered attention, impaired recent memory, defective abstract thinking and judgment, and disturbed time perception. Lucid periods are observed in even the most severely delirious subjects. Illusions and hallucinations, most often visual, are commonly present. Ditran delirium has been compared with and found similar to the acute alcoholic psychoses (64, 65) but different from LSD psychosis (73). It is associated with marked changes in cerebral potentials evoked by somatosensory and visual stimuli (66). The earlier portions of the evoked responses tend to be augmented or speeded up by Ditran, while the later portions are reduced or slowed by it. These changes could be interpreted as pointing to reduced activity of central data processing coupled with lowered inhibitory activity and thus increased responsiveness of the brain during Ditran delirium.

A number of other anticholinergic compounds have been used to induce experimental delirium (75-78). Scopolamine has been found to exert an increased deliriogenic effect after only one night of sleep deprivation (78). This drug is reported to decrease and postpone REM sleep. Physostigmine reverses the impairment of wakefulness caused by anticholinergic deliriants and by sleep loss (78).

Anticholinergic drugs have been the main group of substances used to induce delirium experimentally and observe its EEG correlates. Since the deliriogenic effects of these drugs have often been counteracted by *anticholinesterase compounds* such as physostigmine or tetrahydroaminacrine, it is important to know whether the anticholinesterases can provoke delirium in their own right. A few relevant experimental studies have been reported. Grob et al. (79) administered di-isopropyl fluorphosphate (DFP) to volunteers and observed increased electrical activity of the brain in seventeen of the twenty-three subjects. The EEG changes consisted of greater variations in potential, increased frequency, more irregularities in rhythm, and the intermittent appearance of high voltage slow waves. These changes appeared after two to seven days of daily intramuscular administration of 1 to 2 mg. of DFP. The onset and severity of these changes bore no relation to the plasma or red blood cell cholinesterase activity. The EEG changes could be inhibited in all subjects by the administration of 1.2 mg. of atropine intravenously. The authors interpreted their findings as suggesting that acetylcholine plays a role in central neural function. The behavioral symptoms induced by DFP included, in order of frequency: excessive dreaming, insomnia, tension, emotional lability, nightmares, drowsiness, mental confusion, and visual hallucinations. These symptoms were reduced but not abolished by atropine. It is not clear if one is justified to speak of delirium in this context.

Bowers et al. (80) administered an unspecified organophosphate anticholinesterase to young male volunteers and found behavioral changes which included difficulties in thinking, subjective sense of being slowed down, depression, irritability, and listlessness. The subjects performed serial sevens poorly or not at all, had defective retention and calculation, and minor difficulties with orientation. Hallucinations, illusions, and delusions were absent. Insight was preserved. The changes usually appeared only after whole blood cholinesterase had fallen to 40 percent of control or lower. The behavioral disturbance waxed and waned for about twenty-four hours. Disturbing dreams were often reported on the first postexperimental night. The syndrome elicited by the drug was thought to be similar to that described by Grob et al. (79). Its characteristic features consisted of difficulty in sustaining attention and a slowing of intellectual and psychomotor processes and thus represented a "state of altered awareness." Even though Bowers et al. invoke Engel and Romano and vaguely imply that the syndrome induced by the anticholinesterase agents is a delirium, this conclusion is open to question. There is little doubt that the behavioral effects elicited by the anticholinesterases are different from those induced by anticholinergic agents. Whether these effects represent delirium or a different organic mental disorder is far from clear. "Confusion" has been reported to be one of the common manifestations of organophosphorus insecticide poisoning in man (81, 82), but this term is so vague that its diagnostic value is almost nil. Decreased vigilance, slowing of information processing, psychomotor retardation, memory impairment, anxiety, and depression comprise the behavioral effects of organophosphate toxicity in man (81, 82). EEG abnormalities, especially frontocentral slowing, have been reported in men with histories of exposure to organophosphates (83, 84). Korsak and Sato (85) claim that chronic exposure to organophosphorus insecticides results in the EEG changes depending on whether the exposure to these agents was high or low. With the high exposure, the frontal regions show alpha rhythm as well as a tendency towards increased amounts of both theta (4 to 7 c/sec) and beta waves (22 to 25 c/sec). Some workers have claimed that chronic organophosphorus exposure may differentially affect only the left frontal region (85).

Physostigmine, another acetylcholinesterase inhibitor, has been administered intravenously in a dose of 3 mg. to healthy subjects. The drug induced a "physostigmine syndrome," characterized by decreased speech, slowed thoughts, mild sedation, and reduced motor activity. The capacity of short-term memory was significantly reduced (86). This description fits in well with that provided earlier by Bowers et al. (80). Physostigmine has also been reported to suppress manic symptoms and induce an anergic syndrome or depression (87, 88). Granacher (89) states that cognitive changes which he has observed with physostigmine are probably not a true delirium. Thus, it remains unclear whether anticholinesterase agents induce delirium.

In summary, experimental delirium induced by anticholinergic drugs supports a unitary conception of delirium, one in which global impairment of cognitive functions and attention which fluctuates over twenty-four hours is the main feature. The concomitant EEG changes correlate with the degree of reduced alertness elicited by the drug. If there is preponderance of diffuse slow EEG activity, sedation, drowsiness, memory impairment, and psychomotor underactivity dominate the clinical picture. If a considerable amount of fast EEG activity is superimposed upon a slow background activity, one finds clinically increased psychomotor activity, perceptual distortions, and delusional misinterpretation of internal and external information inputs. It appears that suppression of central cholinergic activity is one of the pathophysiological mechanisms that may underlie delirium.

Summary of the EEG Findings in Delirium

Bilateral, diffuse abnormality of the EEG background activity is an almost invariable feature of delirium. This abnormality typically consists of relative slowing, with or without superimposed fast activity. Relative preponderance of the latter is usually associated with the hyperactive variant of delirium.

Increased variability of the EEG frequencies and amplitudes tends to be accompanied by increased alertness, wakefulness, psychomotor activity, and perceptual distortions. These changes in the EEG tracings in delirium have been related to the activity of the reticular activating system and the medial thalamic diffuse projection system, respectively. Increased activity of one or the other of these systems appears to determine the type of delirium, i.e. whether it is hyperactive or hypoactive, as well as the degree of slowing and the amount of associated fast activity in the EEG. Slowing of the EEG found in delirium due to metabolic, infectious, and other factors correlates well with reduced alertness, awareness, and wakefulness on the one hand, and with diminished cerebral blood flow, oxygen consumption, and metabolic rate on the other. The EEG characteristics of the hyperactive variant of delirium may resemble those of REM sleep. In some cases of this variant, notably in delirium tremens, low voltage fast activity tends to predominate and return to normal as delirium subsides. In the hypoactive variant of the syndrome there is characteristically a predominance of relatively slow background activity that seems to correspond to that found in the period of transition from wakefulness to sleep. Roth (90) has called this transitional period "states of lowered vigilance" and ascribes its signs to the "insufficiency of the subcortical mechanisms of activation."

The EEG is a highly useful aid in the diagnosis of delirium, especially if serial recordings are made and show changes in background activity that parallel those in the level of alertness, wakefulness, and cognitive functioning (91). Like any other laboratory aid, the EEG must always be viewed in conjunction with pertinent clinical findings, psychological and other, and not as an isolated or pathognomonic finding. Furthermore, a single recording carried out during delirium may be read as normal and yet represent a relative abnormality if one uses the patient as his or her own standard for comparison. In such cases only serial recordings can disclose pathological changes. Furthermore, the EEG abnormalities may in some cases antedate or outlast delirium.

Recent advances in quantification of the EEG background

activity should help advance the knowledge of the EEG in delirium of different degrees of severity and due to various causes. Alterations in the amplitude and frequency of the EEG rhythms in states of diffuse cerebral pathology can be quantified and displayed graphically with the application of computer methods (92). Digital spectral analysis represents an important advance in recording and monitoring EEG background activity. Compression and graphic display of the EEG data is already being applied to monitor cerebral activity in medical and surgical settings. The somnogram and comagram are other useful additions to the techniques of monitoring electrophysiological changes in the brain during states of sleep and loss of consciousness (92). One may look forward to the development of an analogue to these new methods in the form of a "deliriogram" that could be used to record the EEG background activity and other relevant changes during delirium both during the daytime and at night. Another recent technical advance which appears to be highly relevant to delirium is neurometrics (93). This method applies computer technology for the quantification of diagnostically relevant features of the EEG as well as the detailed examination of average evoked responses. John et al. (93) claim that neurometrics provides a sensitive indicator of reception, encoding, processing, and evaluation of information. Neurometric methods are claimed to allow assessment of cerebral concomitants of cognitive functions without the use of verbal interaction or any other overt behavioral response. John et al. maintain that neurometrics is applicable to the study of cerebral dysfunction and the related cognitive impairment due to systemic diseases and drugs. One may expect that application of the above technological advances to the study of delirium will help clarify its relationship to the EEG changes.

The almost invariable presence of the EEG changes in delirium raises the question if this finding throws any light on the pathophysiology of the syndrome. The EEG reflects the activity of the cerebral cortex, modulated in varying degree by afferent impulses. Electrical potentials recorded from the scalp are summated synaptic potentials originating in the pyramidal cells of the cortex (51). Rhythmic discharges generated in the thalamic nuclei elicit responses in the cortical cells that are recorded as the electrical potentials. The frequencies of the latter as well as of the thalamic discharges are determined by the thalamic cells. Desynchronization of the cortical potentials during activation is brought about by impulses generated in the reticular formation that abolish the rhythmic discharges in the thalamic nuclei (51). The EEG changes that accompany delirium indicate an interference with the above mechanisms. Furthermore, these changes suggest a derangement of the processes subserving wakefulness and sleep. Acute cerebral disorders of any etiology tend to disorganize the twenty-four-hour sleep-wakefulness cycle (94). Such disorganization appears to be an invariable concomitant of delirium, which may thus be regarded as a disorder of wakefulness. The EEG changes in delirium seem to support this contention. They suggest an inquiry into the neurophysiological and biochemical mechanisms underlying wakefulness, sleep, and consciousness.

CEREBRAL SUBSTRATE OF SLEEP, WAKEFULNESS, AND ATTENTION IN RELATION TO DELIRIUM

It is generally acknowledged that a reticulothalamocortical system plays an important role in the regulation of the sleep-wakefulness cycle, and in attention (95). Moruzzi and Magoun (96) discovered the ascending reticular activating system (RAS), running the entire length of the brain stem. When stimulated it was shown to arouse sleeping animals and produce the fast pattern of arousal in the cortical EEG. The state of wakefulness in man depends at any time on continuous inflow of ascending impulses from the reticular formation which maintain the central tone of the forebrain (97). There is no universal agreement regarding which cerebral structures should be included in the RAS. The initial experiments by Moruzzi and Magoun involved the reticular formation of the lower brain stem. Later investigators included other structures, so that RAS is viewed now as stretching throughout the brain stem and extending to the diencephalon and the basal regions of the telencephalon (95). Some writers regard the hypothalamus as a direct extension of the brain stem RAS (95).

In both sleep and coma, the inflow of the tonic ascending impulses necessary for wakefulness is lacking. This releases the tendency of the thalamic nuclei to evoke a synchronized EEG. Stimulation of these thalamic regions at high frequencies elicits cortical activation similar to that induced by stimulation of the lower brain stem. The upper portion of thalamocortical projections has been termed the thalamic reticular system or the diffuse ("nonspecific") thalamic projection system (98). Low-frequency stimulation of the midline thalamic nuclei produces inattention, drowsiness, and sleep, and is accompanied by slow waves and spindle bursts in the EEG (95). These nuclei and their projections to the neocortex provide an extension of the RAS. The nonspecific nuclei bring about synchronization of widespread areas of cortex by virtue of their diffuse cortical projections. Descending afferents from the basal forebrain area and from the hypothalamus approach the nonspecific thalamic nuclei. These afferents are derived largely from the orbitofrontal cortex. The nuclei have other connections with the spinothalamic tract, hippocampal formation, and amygdaloid complex.

Some of the fibers of the reticular formation form the ascending reticular system, which plays a crucial role in activating the cortex and regulating the state of its activity (99). Other fibers of the formation form the descending reticular system. They run from the neocortex, the limbic system, caudate body, and thalamic nuclei to the reticular structures in the midbrain, hypothalamus, and brain stem. These descending pathways allow modification of the state of vigilance by the cortex. Thus, RAS influences the level of cortical excitability and of wakefulness and is, in turn, under cortical influence. This implies that the cortex may perform nonspecific activating functions (99). Activating influences on the RAS are derived primarily from the frontal cortex. Furthermore, the RAS appears to play the role of a modulator of the limbic system. Stimulation of the RAS in the rabbit elicits low voltage, fast electrical activity in the neocortex and concurrent theta activity in the cortex of the hippocampus. Luria (99) asserts that the medial zones of the hemispheres may be viewed as a system superimposed upon the RAS. Patients with lesions in those zones display disturbances of consciousness and memory which in some cases resemble those of delirium (99). Lesions of the upper part of the brain stem and the walls of the third ventricle may produce sleep or an oneiroid, drowsy state, accompanied by reduced cortical tone (99). RAS is responsible for alertness, i.e. general readiness to respond to external stimulation, and for wakefulness. Voluntary and selective attention, however, involve in addition the activity of the limbic and frontal cortex. Hence, in lesions involving the hippocampal structures there are attentional deficits, such as increased distractibility, inability to sustain attention, and frequent intrusion of irrelevant associations. Distinction between past and present, and between dream and reality, becomes confused; and organized, directed and selective mental activity is hampered. Frontal lobes can raise the level of alertness during performance of a task and thus take part in maintaining selective attention (99). Loss of the capacity for selective and sustained attention is one of the cardinal features of delirium. Another feature of it, namely defective memory, probably reflects the attentional deficits.

RAS, the medial regions of the cortex, and the diencephalon compose what Luria refers to as the functional unit for regulating cortical tone and the level of wakefulness and alertness. This unit works closely, that is, influences and is influenced by, the unit for reception, processing, and storing of information. In addition, RAS is intimately involved in the regulation of the sleep-wakefulness cycle. RAS exerts inhibitory control over the tonic activity of the preoptic hypnogenic region, the efferent impulses from which reciprocally inhibit the RAS (97). The other hypnogenic center is represented by the nucleus of the solitary tract in the medulla (97). Low-frequency stimulation of the bulbar or preoptic hypnogenic centers produces relaxed wakefulness as well as thalamocortical synchronization. According to Bremer (97), spontaneous sleep is the outcome of deactivation of RAS resulting from a sequence of disinhibitory and inhibitory processes. The serotonergic nuclei of the rostral pontine raphe seem to have a hypnotonic rather than a hypnogenic role (97). The serotonin-containing neurons, the raphe nuclei, are located in the lower midbrain and upper pons, and are included by some authorities within the reticular formation (95). Noradrenergic neurons are found throughout the brain stem RAS, but are most highly concentrated in the locus coeruleus of the pons (100). These two components of the RAS have been implicated in the regulation of the sleep-wakefulness cycle and the production of both the slow wave and REM sleep.

Attempts have been made to account for the alteration of the sleep-waking cycle by proposing a "monoamine theory" of the regulation of the states of vigilance (101). Serotonin-containing neurons have been postulated initially to be responsible for slow-wave sleep and for "priming" REM sleep. Ponto-mesencephalic noradrenergic neurons are, according to the theory, implicated in the "executive" mechanisms of REM sleep and in the maintenance of behavioral and EEG arousal. The brain stem is assigned a crucial role in the modulation of the sleep-wakefulness cycle, but it is conceded that structures in the hypothalamus and the basal forebrain area are also necessary for the regulation of the cycle. It has been proposed that activation of the serotonin-containing neurons may involve release from control by the ascending noradrenergic fibers from the rostral part of the locus coeruleus (101). Others have hypothesized that the latter inhibits the activity of the reticular cells except during REM sleep and that its inactivity allows initiation of REM sleep (101). The coerulo-cortical noradrenergic neuron system has been assigned an important role in regulating cortical arousal and the maintenance of wakefulness (101). There is a positive correlation between reduction of cortical arousal and the decrease of noradrenalin in the mesencephalon and the forebrain. It is suggested that the serotonin and catecholamine systems act antagonistically in slow-wave sleep and waking and agonistically in producing REM sleep. Increased activity in the locus coeruleus is accompanied by enhanced REM sleep. Morgane and Stern (101) conclude that evidence available to date indicates that serotonin and noradrenalin are implicated in the generation and maintenance of some aspects of the vigilance continuum but that the relevant chemical pathways and circuits cannot yet be identified as a sleep system. The role of each particular biogenic amine in the maintenance of a particular vigilance state is still controversial and open to question. The serotonergic and the noradrenergic systems appear to interact at different levels in the brain, and it is this interaction that is probably of crucial importance for the regulation of the sleep-wakefulness cycle and of its major components.

Cholinergic mechanism also appears to be involved in the regulation of the states of vigilance. Two major cholinergic systems in the brain have been identified: the ascending cholinergic reticular system and the cholinergic limbic system (95). The former consists of the dorsal and ventral tegmental pathways, respectively. High-frequency stimulation of the midbrain reticular formation desynchronizes the EEG and also produces increased output of acetylcholine from the cerebral cortex (95). Thus, the cholinergic system appears to be involved in electrocortical arousal. The cholinergic limbic system is intimately related to the hippocampal formation. Morgane and Stern (95) conclude that acetylcholine is involved in states of wakefulness, slow-wave sleep, and REM sleep. The most effective agent in inducing REM sleep is physostigmine. On the contrary, anticholinergic drugs, such as atropine, produce cortical synchronization and usually abolish REM sleep (95). Acetylcholine appears to act at different levels of the brain stem and, by interacting with the monoamine systems, to be involved in all three major states of vigilance. Cholinergic mechanisms in the brain stem and basal forebrain areas seem to enhance slow-wave and REM sleep. These mechanisms are particularly important for the student of delirium since the latter has been readily induced by administration of anticholinergic drugs and suppressed by anticholinesterases.

The knowledge that we possess at this time indicates that the transition to and the maintenance of the various states of vigilance involve integrated activity of a number of cortical and subcortical neuronal groups and their connecting pathways. Neurotransmitters discussed above, and possibly others as well, appear to play a key note in these processes. The latter become disrupted in delirium to a greater or lesser extent. Delirium involves impairment of information processing, reduced capacity for selective and sustained attention, and disruption of the sleep-wakefulness cycle. These abnormalities point towards involvement of both cortical and subcortical structures in the pathological process. It appears that in delirium the brain as a whole is involved rather than any single cerebral structure, such as the RAS or the limbic system. To state that delirium is a disorder of wakefulness implies that in this condition the normal alert waking state is disrupted by the intrusion of fragments of sleep stages and associated faulty awareness of self and environment. Many writers refer to such awareness as "consciousness." Subcortical structures subserving waking and alerting must be involved in this pathological state. At the same time, one may hypothesize that cortical functions are in part independently impaired as a result of a global metabolic derangement which underlies delirium.

The foregoing discussion is in accordance with current views on the physical basis of consciousness. Dimond (102), for example, points out that subcortical structures, and especially the brain stem, are essential for maintaining consciousness, since they regulate waking and alerting of the cortical centers that deal with the phenomena of subjective experience. He describes a circuit spanning the brain which runs from the parietal lobe at one side to that on the other and includes the splenium of the corpus callosum, the medial banks of the hemispheres, and the cingulate areas, and proposes that this circuit subserves consciousness. It is of interest in this regard that unilateral as well as bilateral medial temporo-occipital infarction may be accompanied by delirium (103). It has been suggested that release of the medial temporal region from other cortical areas or excitation of certain structures in the medial temporal lobe are the likely causes of delirium in these cases (103). A transient confusional state has also been reported after anterior cingulectomy (104). The patients reported a difficulty in distinguishing their images and dreams from perceptions. Some of them described the experience as "a sort of waking dream." Imagery and dreams were described as being unusually vivid after the operation. This "confusional state" appears to be either identical with or closely resembles delirium.

Delirium is viewed by many writers as a transitional state between alert wakefulness and coma. Plum and Posner (105) consider confusional states and deliria to be altered or clouded consciousness, that is, reduced wakefulness or awareness, progression of which leads to stupor and coma. These authors maintain that the presence of delirium indicates a generalized impairment of cerebral functions or at least bilateral lesions of limbic structures. If at least some cases of delirium represent a transition to coma, then the pathophysiology of and the EEG changes in the latter may be relevant to the former. Some authors maintain that EEG activity, level of consciousness, and degree of responsiveness are independent expressions of the same basic pathological process (106, p. 22). The degree of abnormality of each of these three parameters is said to vary according to the etiology and site of the responsible lesion. All types of EEG changes may be found at each degree of coma (106). Lesions in the pons or pontomesencephalic area may be accompanied by alpha activity in the EEG even in deep coma. EEG arousal may be found in about 20 percent of such cases (106). Global impairment of consciousness may accompany mesodiencephalic, deep hemispheric, and bilateral and diffuse hemispheric lesions. Brain stem lesions tend to produce coma or akinetic mutism rather than delirium. Extensive tumors of the brain stem may at times fail to impair consciousness, and coma may be produced without any apparent involvement of the mesencephalic reticular formation. Coma is positively correlated with the presence of diffuse slow background activity in the EEG, yet, all types of EEG abnormalities as well as alpha activity may at times be encountered (106). This is also the case in delirium. Diffuse slow background activity is an almost invariable concomitant of metabolic coma as well as delirium due to metabolic disorders. The level of unresponsiveness in metabolic coma is correlated with the degree of slowing of the EEG.

Of considerable interest are the EEG and behavioral studies of sleep in the states of coma (106). Twenty-four-hour polygraphic studies of comatose patients have been reported. EEG patterns of normal slow-wave sleep have been found in diurnal EEG's of some patients comatose after acute trauma. Polygraphic and behavioral evidence of slow-wave and REM sleep have been reported to occur in some subjects suffering from prolonged coma, mostly due to head trauma (106). It has been speculated that minute lesions of the upper midbrain and caudal diencephalon could produce loss of consciousness with preservation of slow-wave and REM sleep. These clinical and polygraphic findings underscore the complexity of the mechanisms and pathways subserving sleep-wakefulness cycle and awareness. These mechanisms may be disrupted in various patterns and thus result in different EEG records in the presence of behaviorally similar or even identical states. The same generalization appears to apply to delirium and the associated EEG abnormalities.

In summary, both direct and indirect evidence available today indicates that delirium, defined as a distinct psychopathological state, represents the final common path for a variety of pathophysiological processes and mechanisms. The latter appear to involve both cortical and subcortical structures whose integrated activity is necessary for the maintenance of the normal sleep-wakefulness cycle; alertness; and information reception, processing, and storage. Clinical delirium results from relative disintegration of these cerebral mechanisms. This disintegration is manifested behaviorally and electrophysiologically. The EEG shows a spectrum of abnormalities ranging from diffuse slowing of background activity, through mixed slow and very fast activity, to predominantly fast activity. It has been suggested that relative involvement of the medial reticular activating system and the medial thalamic projection system determines the degree of reduction of alertness and the corresponding degree of slowing or acceleration of the EEG background activity, respectively. This spectrum of alertness and the EEG background frequency appears to parallel the level of cerebral cortical excitability and arousal, analogous to slow-wave sleep and REM sleep, respectively. Delirium of alcohol and drug withdrawal states represents that end of the spectrum that is marked by increased arousal, alertness, and EEG frequency in the presence of impaired information processing and sustained and selective attention. Imbalance of normal noradrenergic, serotonergic, and cholinergic mechanisms appears to underlie delirium. The latter is thus viewed as a unitary behavioral syndrome brought about by several constellations of pathophysiological mechanisms involving both cortical and subcortical structures, their metabolism, and their neurotransmission.

REFERENCES

1. Susser, M.: *Causal Thinking in the Health Sciences.* New York, Oxford University Press, 1973.
2. Hart, B.: Delirious states. *Br Med J* 2:745-749, 1936.
3. Engel, G.L., and Romano, J.: Delirium, a syndrome of cerebral insufficiency. *J Chron Dis* 9:260-277, 1959.
4. Engel, G.L.: "Delirium," in *Comprehensive Textbook of Psychiatry,* Freedman, A.M. and Kaplan, H.S., Eds. Baltimore, Williams & Wilkins, 1967, pp. 711-716.
5. Jellinger, K.: Morphologische Grundlagen des organischen Psychosyndroms. *Wien Klin Wschr* 87:229-234, 1975.
6. Bachelard, H.S.: "Biochemistry of Coma," in Davison, A.N., Ed., *Biochemistry and Neurological Disease.* Oxford, Blackwell, 1976, pp. 228-277.
7. Fazekas, J.F., and Alman, R.W.: *Coma: Biochemistry, Physiology and Therapeutic Principles.* Springfield, Charles C Thomas, 1962.
8. Siesjö, B.K., Carlsson, C., Hagerdal, M., and Nordstrom, C.H.: Brain metabolism in the critically ill. *Crit Care Med* 4:283-294, 1976.
9. Sokoloff, L.: Neurophysiology and neurochemistry of coma. *Exp Biol Med* 4:15-33, 1971.
10. Berglund, M., Nielsen, S., and Risberg, J.: Regional cerebral blood flow in a case of bromide psychosis. *Arch Psychiatr Nervenkr* 223:197-201, 1977.
11. Berglund, M., and Risberg, J.: Regional cerebral blood flow during alcohol withdrawal related to consumption and clinical symptomatology. *Acta Neurol Scand, Suppl 64,* 56:480-481, 1977.
12. Raichle, M.: "Sensori-Motor Area Increase of Oxygen Uptake and Blood Flow in the Human Brain During Contralateral Hand Exercise: Preliminary Observations by the 0-15 Method," in Ingvar, D.H., and Lassen, N.A., Eds., *Brain Work.* Copenhagen, Munksgaard, 1975, pp. 372-376.
13. Sokoloff, L.: Relation between physiological function and energy metabolism in the central nervous system. *J Neurochem* 29:13-26, 1977.
14. Sokoloff, L.: "Influence of Functional Activity on Local Cerebral Glucose Utilization," in Ingvar, D.H., and Lassen, N.A., Eds., *Brain Work.* Copenhagen, Munksgaard, 1975, pp. 385-388.
15. Siesjö, B.K.: "Physiological Aspects of Brain Energy Metabolism," in Davison, A.N., Ed., *Biochemical Correlates of Brain Structure and Function.* London, Academic Press, 1977, pp. 175-213.
16. Lowry, O.H.: "Energy Metabolism in Brain and Its Control," in Ingvar, D.H., and Lassen, N.A., Eds., *Brain Work.* Copenhagen, Munksgaard, 1975, pp. 48-64.

17. Cooper, R., and Crow, H.J.: "Changes of Cerebral Oxygenation During Motor and Mental Tasks," in Ingvar, D.H. and Lassen, N.A., Eds., *Brain Work*. Copenhagen, Munksgaard, 1975, pp. 389-396.

18. Brown, R., Davis, J.N., and Carlsson, A.: DOPA reversal of hypoxia-induced disruption of the conditioned avoidance response. *J Pharm Pharmacol* 25:412-414, 1973.

19. Betz, E.: "CBF During Emotional Stimuli," in Ingvar, D.H., and Lassen, N.A., Eds., *Brain Work*. Copenhagen, Munksgaard, 1975, pp. 366-370.

20. King, B.D., Sokoloff, L. and Wechsler, R.L.: The effects of l-epinephrine and l-norepinephrine upon cerebral circulation and metabolism in man. *J Clin Invest* 31:273-279, 1952.

21. Creutzfeldt, O.D.: "Neurophysiological Correlates of Different Functional States of the Brain," in Ingvar, D.H., and Lassen, N.A., Eds., *Brain Work*. Copenhagen, Munksgaard, 1975, pp. 21-47.

22. Giuditta, A.: "The Biochemistry of Sleep," in Davison, A.N., Ed., *Biochemical Correlates of Brain Structure and Function*. London, Academic Press, 1977, pp. 293-337.

23. Townsend, R.E., Prinz, P.N., and Obrist, W.D.: Human cerebral blood flow during sleep and waking. *J Appl Physiol* 35:620-625, 1973.

24. Schnaberth, G., and Schubert, H.: Bewusstseinsstoerung und Liquormetabolismus. *Arch Psychiatr Nervenkr* 218:211-222, 1974.

25. Holman, B.L.: Concepts and clinical utility of the measurement of cerebral blood flow. *Semin Nucl Med* 6:233-251, 1976.

26. Siesjö, B.K.: *Brain Energy Metabolism*. London, Wiley, 1978.

27. Ingvar, D.H.: "Patterns of Brain Activity Revealed by Measurements of Regional Cerebral Blood Flow," in Ingvar, D.H., and Lassen, N.A., Eds., *Brain Work*. Copenhagen, Munksgaard, 1975, pp. 397-412.

28. Lassen, N.A., and Christensen, M.S.: Physiology of cerebral blood flow. *Br J Anaesth* 48:719-734, 1976.

29. Raichle, M.E., Grubb, R.L., Gado, M.H., Eichling, J.O., and Ter-Pogossian, M.M.: Correlation between regional cerebral blood flow and oxidative metabolism. *Arch Neurol* 33:523-526, 1976.

30. Cerebral Blood Flow. *Acta Neurol Scand*, Suppl. 64, Vol. 56, 1977.

31. Sokoloff, L.: "Cerebral Circulation and Behavior in Man: Strategy and Findings," in Mandell, A.J., and Mandell, M.P., Eds., *Psychochemical Research in Man*. New York, Academic Press, 1969, pp. 237-252.

32. Kety, S.S., and Schmidt, C.F.: The nitrous oxide method for the quantitative determination of cerebral blood flow in man: Theory, procedure, and normal values. *J Clin Invest* 27:476-483, 1948.

33. Lassen, N.A., and Ingvar, D.H.: The blood flow of the cerebral cortex determined by radioactive krypton-85. *Experientia 17*:42-43, 1961.
34. Ingvar, D.H.: "Brain Work in Presenile Dementia and in Chronic Schizophrenia," in Ingvar, D.H., and Lassen, N.A., Eds., *Brain Work*. Copenhagen, Munksgaard, 1975, pp. 478-497.
35. Ingvar, D.H.: Cerebral blood flow and metabolism related to EEG and cerebral functions. *Acta Anaesth Scand 45*:110-114, 1971.
36. Carlsson, C., Hagerdal, M., Kaasik, A.E., and Siesjö, B.K.: The effects of diazepam on cerebral blood flow and oxygen consumption in rats and its synergistic interaction with nitrous oxide. *Anesthesiology 45*:319-325, 1976.
37. Engel, C.L., Romano, J., Ferris, E.B., Webb, J.P., and Stevens, C.D.: A simple method of determining frequency spectrums in the electroencephalogram. *AMA Arch Neurol Psychiatr 51*:134-146, 1944.
38. Romano, J., and Engel, G.L.: Delirium. I. Electroencephalographic data. *AMA Arch Neurol Psychiatr 51*:356-377, 1944.
39. Engel, G.L., and Romano, J.: Delirium. II. Reversibility of the electroencephalogram with experimental procedures. *AMA Arch Neurol Psychiatr 51*:378-392, 1944.
40. Engel, G.L., and Rosenbaum, M.: Delirium. III. Electroencephalographic changes associated with acute alcoholic intoxication. *AMA Arch Neurol Psychiatr 53*:44-50, 1945.
41. Engel, G.L., Romano, J., and Goldman, L.: Delirium. IV. Quantitative electroencephalographic study of a case of acute arsenical encephalopathy. *AMA Arch Neurol Psychiatr 56*:659-664, 1946.
42. Engel, G.L., Webb, J.P., and Ferris, E.B.: Quantitative electroencephalographic studies of anoxia in humans; comparison with acute alcoholic intoxication and hypoglycemia. *J Clin Inves 24*:691-697, 1945.
43. Engel, G.L., Romano, J., and Ferris, E.B.: Effect of quinacrine (atabrine) on the central nervous system. *AMA Arch Neurol Psychiatr 58*:337-350, 1947.
44. Romano, J. and Engel, G.L.: Physiologic and psychologic considerations of delirium. *Med Clin N Am 28*:629-638, 1944.
45. Victor, M., and Adams, R.D.: "The Acute Confusional States," in Harrison, T.R., Adams, R.D., Bennett, I.L., Resnik, W.H., Thorn, G.W., and Wintrobe, M.M., Eds., *Principles of Internal Medicine*, 4th edition. McGraw-Hill, New York, 1962, pp. 354-362.
46. Allahyari, H., Deisenhammer, E., and Weiser, G.: EEG examination during delirium tremens. *Psychiatr Clin 9*:21-31, 1976.
47. Wikler, A., Pescor, F.T., Fraser, H.F., and Isbell, H.: Electroencephalographic changes associated with chronic alcoholic in-

toxication and the alcohol abstinence syndrome. *Am J Psychiatry* *113*:106-114, 1956.

48. Wikler, A.: Personal communication. October 5, 1977.
49. Flügel, K.A.: *Die Elektroenzephalographie der Funktionpsychosen.* Stuttgart, G. Thieme Verlag, 1974.
50. Cadilhac, J., and Ribstein, M.: The EEG in metabolic disorders. *World Neur* *2*:296-308, 1961.
51. Kiloh, L.G., McComas, A.J., and Osselton, J.W.: *Clinical Electroencephalography,* 3rd edition. New York, Appleton-Century-Crofts, 1972.
52. Pro, J.D., and Wells, C.E.: The use of the electroencephalogram in the diagnosis of delirium. *Dis Nerv Syst* *38*:804-808, 1977.
53. Hughes, J.R., Cayaffa, J., Leestma, J., and Mizuna, Y.: Alternating "waking" and "sleep" EEG patterns in a deeply comatose patient. *Clin Electroencephalogr* *2*:86-93, 1972.
54. Mirsky, A.F., and Pragay, E.B.: "The Relation of EEG and Performance in Altered States of Consciousness," in Kety, S.S., Evarts, E.V., and Williams, H.L., Eds., *Sleep and Altered States of Consciousness.* Baltimore, Williams & Wilkins, 1967, pp. 514-534.
55. Athen, D., Beckmann, H., Ackenheil, M., and Markianos, M.: Biochemical investigations into the alcoholic delirium: alterations of biogenic amines. *Arch Psychiatr Nervenkr* *224*:129-140, 1977.
56. Schacter, D.L.: EEG theta waves and psychological phenomena: A review and analysis. *Biol Psychol* *5*:47-82, 1977.
57. Jenkins, C.D.: The relation of EEG slowing to selected indices of intellective impairment. *J Nerve Ment Dis* *135*:162-170, 1962.
58. Obrist, W.D., Busse, E.W., Eisdorfer, C., and Kleemeier, R.W.: Relation of the electroencephalogram to intellectual function in senescence. *J Geront* *17*:197-206, 1962.
59. Busse, E.W., and Wang, H.S.: The value of electroencephalography in geriatrics. *Geriatrics* *20*:906-924, 1965.
60. Vojtechovsky, M., Vitek, V., and Rysanek, K.: Experimentelle Psychose nach Verabreichung von Benactyzin. *Arzneim-Forsch* *16*: 240-242, 1966.
61. Abood, L.G., and Meduna, L.J.: Some effects of a new psychotogen in depressive states. *J Nerv Ment Dis* *127*:546-550, 1958.
62. Ketchum, J.S., Sidell, F.R., Crowell, E.B., Aghajanian, G.K., and Hayes, A.H.: Atropine, scopolamine, and Ditran: Comparative pharmacology and antagonists in man. *Psychopharmacologia* (*Berl*) *28*:121-145, 1973.
63. Gershon, S., and Olariu, J.: JB 329—A new psychotomimetic: Its antagonism by tetrahydroaminacrin and its comparison with LSD, mescaline and sernyl. *J Neuropsychiatry* *1*:283-292, 1960.

64. Alpert, M., Angrist, B., Diamond, F., and Gershon, S.: "Comparison of Ditran Intoxication and Acute Alcohol Psychoses," in Keup, W., Ed., *Origins and Mechanisms of Hallucinations*. New York, Plenum Press, 1970, pp. 245-259.
65. Angrist, B., Urcuyo, L., and Gershon, S.: Response to incremental doses of Ditran in abstinent alcoholics and drug users. *Compr Psychiatry 15*:201-204, 1974.
66. Brown, J.C.N., Shagass, C., and Schwartz, M.: Cerebral evoked potential changes associated with the Ditran delirium and its reversal in man. *Rec Adv Biol Psychiatr 7*:223-234, 1965.
67. Cartwright, R.D.: Dream and drug-induced fantasy behavior. *Arch Gen Psychiatry 15*:7-15, 1966.
68. Itil, T.M.: Quantitative EEG changes induced by anticholinergic drugs and their behavioral correlates in man. *Rec Adv Biol Psychiatry 8*:151-173, 1966.
69. Itil, T.M.: Anticholinergic drug-induced sleep-like EEG pattern in man. *Psychopharmacologia (Berl.) 14*:383-393, 1969.
70. Itil, T.M.: "Changes in Digital Computer Analyzed EEG During 'Dreams' and Experimentally Induced Hallucinations," in Keup, W., Ed., *Origins and Mechanisms of Hallucinations*. New York, Plenum Press, 1970, p. 71-91.
71. Itil, T., and Fink, M.: Anticholinergic drug-induced delirium: Experimental modification, quantitative EEG and behavioral correlations. *J Nerv Ment Dis 142*:492-507, 1966.
72. Itil, T., and Fink, M.: EEG and behavioral aspects of the interaction of anticholinergic hallucinogens with centrally active compounds. *Prog Brain Res 28*:149-168, 1968.
73. Wilson, R.E., and Shagass, C.: Comparison of two drugs with psychotomimetic effects (LSD and Ditran). *J Nerv Ment Dis 138*:277-286, 1964.
74. Ostfeld, A.M., Machne, X., and Unna, K.R.: The effects of atropine on the electroencephalogram and behavior in man. *J Pharmacol Exper Ther 128*:265-272, 1960.
75. Arnold, O.H., and Kryspin-Exner, K.: Das experimentelle Delir. *Wien Z Nervenheilk 22*:73-93, 1965.
76. Bente, D., Stoerger, R., and Tautz, N.A.: Weitere klinische-experimentelle Untersuchungen zur Frage der durch zentrale Anticholinergica erzeugten Verwirrtheitszustände. *Arzneim-Forsch 16*:231-233, 1966.
77. Bauer, A.: Verlaufsanalyse der durch zentral anticholinergisch wirkenden Substanzen erzeugten Psychosen an Hand von 70 Fällen. *Arzneim-Forsch 16*:233-234, 1966.
78. Safer, D.J., and Allen, R.P.: The central effects of scopolamine in man. *Biol Psychiatry 3*:347-355, 1971.
79. Grob, D., Harvey, A.M., Langworthy, O.R., and Lilienthal, J.L.:

The administration of di-isopropyl fluorophosphate (DFP) to man. *Bull Johns Hopkins Hosp 31*:257-266, 1947.

80. Bowers, M.B., Goodman, E., and Sim, V.M.: Some behavioral changes in man following anticholinesterase administration. *J Nerv Ment Dis 138*:383-389, 1964.

81. Levin, H.S., and Rodnitzky, R.L.: Behavioral effects of organophosphate pesticides in man. *Clin Toxicol 9*:391-405, 1976.

82. Namba, T., Nolte, C.T., Jackrel, J., and Grob, D.: Poisoning due to organophosphate insecticides. *Am J Med 50*:475-492, 1971.

83. Dille, J.R., and Smith, P.W.: Central nervous system effects of chronic exposure to organophosphate insecticides. *Aerospace Med 35*:475-480, 1964.

84. Metcalf, D.R., and Holmes, H.H.: EEG, psychological, and neurological alterations in humans with organophosphorus exposure. *Ann NY Acad Sci 160*:357-365, 1969.

85. Korsak, R.J., and Sato, M.M.: Effects of chronic organophosphate pesticide exposure on the central nervous system. *Clin Toxicol 11*:83-95, 1977.

86. Davis, K.L., Hollister, L.E., Overall, J., Johnson, A., and Train, K.: Physostigmine: Effects on cognition and affect in normal subjects. *Psychopharmacology 51*:23-27, 1976.

87. Davis, K.L., Berger, P.A., Hollister, L.E., and Defraites, E.: Physostigmine in mania. *Arch Gen Psychiatry 35*:119-122, 1978.

88. Janowsky, D.S., El-Yousef, M.K., Davis, J.M., and Sekerke, H.J.: Parasympathetic suppression of manic symptoms by physostigmine. *Arch Gen Psychiatry 28*:542-547, 1973.

89. Granacher, R.P.: Personal communication. October 19, 1977.

90. Roth, B.: The clinical and theoretical importance of EEG rhythms corresponding to states of lowered vigilance. *Electroencephalogr Clin Neurophysiol 13*:395-399, 1961.

91. Fenton, G.: The straightforward EEG in psychiatric practice. *Proc Roy Soc Med 67*:911-919, 1974.

92. Bickford, R.: "Computer Analysis of Background Activity," in Remond, A., Ed., *EEG Informatics*. Amsterdam, Elsevier/North-Holland, 1977, pp. 215-242.

93. John, E.R., Karmel, B.Z., Corning, W.C., et al. Neurometrics. *Science 196*:1393-1410, 1977.

94. Remond, A., Ed.: *Handbook of Electroencephalography and Clinical Neurophysiology*. Vol. 7, Part 1, Amsterdam, Elsevier, 1975, p. 71.

95. Morgane, P.J., and Stern, W.C.: "Chemical Anatomy of Brain Circuits in Relation to Sleep and Wakefulness," in Weitzman, E., Ed., *Advances in Sleep Research*, Vol. 1. New York, Spectrum Publications, Inc., 1974, pp. 1-131.

96. Moruzzi, G., and Magoun, H.W.: Brain stem reticular formation and activation of the EEG. *Electroencephalogr Clin Neurophysiol* 1:455-473, 1949.
97. Bremer, F.: Cerebral hypnogenic centers. *Ann Neur* 2:1-6, 1977.
98. Brazier, M.A.B.: *Electrical Activity of the Nervous System*. 4th edition, Baltimore, Williams & Wilkins, 1977, pp. 186-208.
99. Luria, A.R.: *The Working Brain*. London, Penguin Books, 1973.
100. Amaral, D.G., and Sinnamon, H.M.: The locus coeruleus: Neurobiology of a central adrenergic nucleus. *Prog Neurobiol* 9:147-196, 1977.
101. Morgane, P.J., and Stern, W.C.: "The Role of Serotonin and Norepinephrine in Sleep-Waking Activity," in Bernard, B., Ed., *Aminergic Hypotheses of Behavior: Reality or Cliche?* Washington, D.C., National Institute on Drug Abuse Research, 1975, pp. 37-61.
102. Dimond, S.J.: Brain circuits for consciousness. *Brain Behav Evol* 13:376-395, 1976.
103. Medina, J.L., Chokroverty, S., and Rubino, F.A.: Syndrome of agitated delirium and visual impairment: A manifestation of medial temporo-occipital infarction. *J Neurol Neurosurg Psychiatry* 40:861-864, 1977.
104. Whitty, C.W.M., and Lewin, W.: Vivid day-dreaming; an unusual form of confusion following anterior cingulectomy. *Brain* 80:72-76, 1957.
105. Plum, F., and Posner, J.B.: *The Diagnosis of Stupor and Coma*. 2nd edition, Philadelphia, F.A. Davis Co., 1972.
106. Remond, A.: *Handbook of Electroencephalography and Clinical Neurophysiology*. Vol. 12. Amsterdam, Elsevier, 1975, pp. 5-77.

Additional References

Baldessarini, R.J., and Fischer, J.E. Substitute and alternative neurotransmitters in neuropsychiatric illness. *Arch Gen Psychiatry* 34:958-964, 1977.
Ballenger, J.C., and Post, R.M. Kindling as a model for alcohol withdrawal syndromes. *Br J Psychiat* 133:1-14, 1978.
Barchas, J.D., Akil, H., Elliott, G.R., et al. Behavioral neurochemistry: Neuroregulators and behavioral states. *Science* 200:964-973, 1978.
Creutzfeldt, O. "Physiological Conditions of Consciousness." In Proceedings of the 11th World Congress of Neurology, Amsterdam, Sept. 11-16, 1977. Amsterdam, Excerpta Medica, 1978, pp. 194-208.
Gibson, G.E., and Blass, J.P. Impaired synthesis of acetylcholine in brain accompanying mild hypoxia and hypoglycemia. *J Neurochem* 27:37-42, 1976.

Guilleminault, C., and Dement, W.C. 235 cases of excessive daytime sleepiness. *J Neurol Sci 31*:13-27, 1977.

Hagberg, B. Defects of immediate memory related to the cerebral blood flow distribution. *Brain and Language 5*:366-377, 1978.

Heiss, W.D. Regional cerebral blood flow measurement with scintillation camera. *Int J Neurol 11*:144-161, 1977.

Jacobs , B.L. Dreams and hallucinations: A common neurochemical mechanism mediating their phenomenological similarities. *Neurosci Biobehav Rev 2*:59-69, 1978.

Lenzi, G.L., Jones, T., McKenzie, C.G., et al. Study of regional cerebral metabolism and blood flow relationships in man using the method of continuously inhaling oxygen-15 and oxygen-15 labelled carbon dioxide. *J Neurol Neurosurg Psychiatry 41*:1-10, 1978.

Meyer, J.S.: Improved method for noninvasive measurement of regional cerebral blood flow by 133-Xenon inhalation. Part II: Measurements in health and disease. *Stroke 9*:205-210, 1978.

Mountcastle, V.B. Brain mechanisms for directed attention. *J Roy Soc Med 71*:14-28, 1978.

Nemoto, E.M. Pathogenesis of cerebral ischemia-anoxia. *Crit Care Med 6*:203-214, 1978.

Obrecht, R., Okhomina, F.O.A., and Scott, D.F. Value of EEG in acute confusional states. *J Neurol Neurosurg Psychiatry 42*:75-77, 1979.

Serafetinides, E.A., Walter, R.D., and Cherlow, D.G. "Amnestic Confusional Phenomena, Hippocampal Stimulation, and Laterality Factors." In *The Hippocampus*, Vol. 2, Isaacson, R.L. and Pribram, K.H., Eds. New York, Plenum Publishing Co., 1975, pp. 363-375.

Steriade, M. Cortical long-axoned cells and putative interneurons during the sleep-waking cycle. *Behav Brain Sci 3*:465-514, 1978.

Van Praag, H.M., and Bruinvels, J. *Neurotransmission & Disturbed Behavior.* Jamaica, New York, J.P. Medical & Scientific Books, 1978.

CHAPTER 7

DIAGNOSIS OF DELIRIUM

Diagnosis of delirium involves two essential steps or phases: first, the syndrome itself has to be recognized on the basis of its characteristic clinical features; and second, the underlying etiological factor (or factors) must be identified with the aid of a physical examination and special laboratory procedures. These two phases will now be discussed in practical detail.

CLINICAL DIAGNOSIS

To diagnose delirium is relatively easy once the symptoms have reached a certain level of severity. Every effort should be made, however, to detect the syndrome while the patient exhibits prodromal or mild symptoms of it. Such an early detection may allow one to identify the underlying cerebral disorder, whether primary or secondary to systemic disease, at its inception and to start appropriate treatment before a severe mental disorder has had time to evolve. Furthermore, early detection of delirium may help avoid serious complications of a full-blown syndrome, such as an accident or some degree of irreversible intellectual deficit.

Early or prodromal symptoms of delirium may be brought to a doctor's attention by the patient or by another observer, such as a family member, personal physician, nurse, etc. In either case, the key complaint concerns a perceived *change* in the person's ability to comprehend his or her surroundings and situation, and relate ongoing events to his or her knowledge and past experience. A typical way in which deliruim is presented to a doctor is a complaint by the patient or a report by an outside observer, or both, that he or she is "confused." Confusion in this context may imply difficulty in grasping the situation one is in, in orienting oneself in time and place, in distinguishing imagery from perceptions and dreams, in thinking with accustomed clarity, and in focussing and maintaining attention at will. The patient may voice no complaints at all, but an observer may notice that he or she has suddenly started to behave in a strange fashion and to exhibit unusual hyperactivity, drowsiness, withdrawal, bewilderment, or lapses of memory and judgment. A relatively sudden appearance of such unaccustomed behavior in someone who is known to be physically ill, or one who has recently undergone major surgery, or is known or suspected to abuse alcohol or other substances, should lead to a systematic diagnostic inquiry to rule out delirium. A person aged sixty years or over is particularly likely to develop the syndrome as a result of an infection, intake of drugs, hypoxia of any origin, and so forth.

A physician wrote that delirium is a syndrome which "no doctor likes to miss" (1). Like it or not, he frequently does miss it, especially in its early stage and mild form. One of the reasons for failing to diagnose delirium is unfamiliarity with its prodromal symptoms. The latter include insomnia, vivid dreams or nightmares, restlessness, distractibility, hypersensitivity to light and sounds, and subjective sense of difficulty in marshalling one's thoughts. Fleeting illusions and hallucinations, especially visual ones, may occur at this stage and alarm the patient. He or she may react to these prodromal symptoms with growing anxiety, which is liable to exacerbate the disorder. If the patient is in the hospital, a ward nurse or physician should be able to elicit a history of the symptoms by asking daily routine questions about the patient's sense of well-being, sleep, and alertness. Having obtained a history suggestive of incipient deliruim the nurse or doctor should immediately proceed to examine the patient's mental status by asking questions about his or her recent memory, attention, thinking difficulties, and any unusual experiences, especially during the preceding night. Such examination should be done in an informal, gentle, and nonthreatening manner. The patient should be told that any physically ill person may experience some mental symptoms, such as forgetfulness or difficulty concentrating, and that it is important for the doctor to be aware of this so that he can take proper therapeutic measures to avoid progression of the psychological difficulties.

It is often useful to ask the patient if he or she ever experienced delirium in the past, for example, in the course of a childhood ailment or after an operation. Once the patient is reassured that he or she is not going insane and that the doctor does not regard him or her as being "crazy"—a common fear—he or she is liable to be willing to report symptoms and cooperate in the mental status examination.

All too often, in the writer's experience, the ward staff fail to pay attention to changes in patients' behavior and to prodromal symptoms of delirium, with the result that the patient's mental disorder progresses and becomes noticed only when its manifestations create an emergency on the ward. Psychiatric consultants are frequently called to see a patient who attempted to leave the ward in the middle of the night, struck a nurse or another patient, or broke a window in an attempt to escape threatening hallucinations. Such crises are as a rule avoidable, since the patient seldom becomes severely disturbed without any premonitory signs and symptoms, which developed over a period of hours or a few days. Reading nurses' notes in the patient's chart usually reveals that his or her behavior had changed but nobody took proper notice of this fact until a dramatic event occurred and the patient became a focus of the staff's anxious and usually disapproving attention.

Delirium often becomes manifest for the first time during the night. The patient typically wakes up after a few hours of sleep and displays anxiety, bewilderment, and restlessness. He or she may report vivid dreams, or hallucinations, or both, and may be uncertain if his or her experiences represented dreams, perceptions of actual external events, or waking hallucinations. Such confusion is quite characteristic and should be inquired about since patients often do not report it spontaneously. The patient may be found to be trying to get out of bed, appear frightened and bewildered, fumble with the bedclothes, or wander aimlessly. A few questions asked at this point may suffice to elicit disorientation for time and place, misidentification of people, hallucinations, and general confusion. The appearance of such symptoms during the night in any physically ill person is highly suggestive, if not diagnostic, of delirium.

In general, the diagnosis of delirium is established when the following manifestations are elicited by history and direct observation:

1. Symptoms develop relatively rapidly, that is to say over less than one week;
2. There is evidence of impairment of directed thinking, recent memory, registration, and orientation (at least for time);
3. There is difficulty in mobilizing, focusing, maintaining, and shifting attention;
4. The patient is less than normally wakeful and alert, or on the contrary, displays heightened but indiscriminate alertness, that is, readiness to respond to external stimuli;
5. Sleep-wakefulness cycle is disturbed as manifested by excessive daytime drowsiness or insomnia, or reversal of the normal diurnal rhythm;
6. Attention and cognitive defects show a tendency to fluctuate unpredictably and irregularly during the day, and to become worse during a sleepless night;
7. Behavior is marked by increased or decreased psychomotor activity, or by changes from one extreme to the other;
8. Visual illusions and hallucinations commonly occur and may be accompanied by misperceptions in other sensory modalities, by fear, and by restlessness;
9. Fleeting, poorly systematized persecutory delusions may occur and intermingle with hallucinations;
10. The patient may at any time exhibit a more or less lucid period, marked by better contact with the environment, more sustained attention, and improved grasp of the situation.

The above set of diagnostic symptoms is usually elicited by history and a routine psychiatric interview. The presence of cognitive deficits and attention disturbances must be further confirmed by a systematic mental status examination and employment of appropriate psychological tests at the bedside. Questions aimed at eliciting cognitive impairment need to be pursued patiently and unobtrusively even in the face of the patient's maneuvers to evade them. Such maneuvers may take the form of circumlocution, sarcasm, perseveration, change of subject, silences, or outright and angry refusal to cooperate. The commonly used bedside tests will be discussed presently.

Delirium is diagnosed primarily on the basis of clinical observations. In the hospital such diagnostically important observations are usually made by the nurses, who see patients frequently both by day and by night. In the author's experience, nurses' notes in the patient's record provide the most useful diagnostic clues in cases of delirium. Notes made by the night nursing staff are particularly valuable. Phillips (2) gives an excellent account of what a night nurse is liable to observe: "Usually for three or four nights preceding the delirium the nurse will notice that the patient is restless and that when he awakens he is flighty, asking often, 'Where am I?' This confusion is momentary but each succeeding night it becomes more marked and lasts longer, extending into the day . . ." It is the duty of a night nurse to report and record her observations of such behavior in a patient before the delirium becomes florid or the patient slips into stupor.

It is important to keep in mind several common sources of error in diagnosing delirium, or rather errors which result in its being missed or misdiagnosed. First, a patient suffering from prodromal or mild symptoms of delirium is likely to look normal and behave appropriately. It is only during a conversation that the patient may voice diagnostically suggestive complaints or display cognitive and attentional defects. Second, many a delirious patient is quiet, listless, or just drowsy. It is erroneous to believe that delirium always, or even usually, features excited, loud, and restless behavior, frightening hallucinations, and persecutory delusions. A physician having such a skewed conception of delirium is liable to miss delirium in the quiet and generally inconspicuous patient. Third, the degree of psychological disturbance in terms of delusions, misinterpretations, hallucinations, and inappropriate behavior does not correlate with the degree of deficiency of attention and information processing and with the indices of cerebral dysfunction, such as the EEG abnormality. This implies that highly conspicuous and disturbing abnormal behavior does not necessarily reflect the severity of brain pathology. Fourth, the presence of psychiatric symptoms, such as schizophrenic thought disorders, various delusions, affective disturbance, and anxiety, neither increases nor decreases the probability that the patient is suffering from delirium. The latter is diagnosed on the basis of the criteria listed earlier which are independent of the symptoms under discussion here. And finally, delirium may be accompanied by either reduced or enhanced alertness, i.e. readiness to respond to external stimuli. In both instances, however, the patient's ability to respond to such stimuli selectively, voluntarily, and in a sustained manner is either abolished or obviously compromised.

Psychological Testing

Elaborate batteries of psychological tests that take an hour or longer to complete have no place in the diagnosis of delirium. A delirious patient is as a rule too ill, distractible, easily tired, and uncooperative to be able to sustain a prolonged psychological testing. The latter should be carried out at the bedside, be relatively simple, and take no more than twenty or thirty minutes. A number of such bedside test batteries have been proposed lately (3-8), and their validity and reliability have been documented to a varying degree. Some of these scales can be scored and thus provide a rough quantification of cognitive functioning for interindividual and intraindividual comparisons. The following tests and questions are included in most of the batteries and should be part of every mental status examination of a patient suspected of suffering from delirium:

1. Orientation: Date, day of the week, time of the day; ability to name the place, usually the hospital, the patient is in, and identification of the familiar persons in the environment by name, occupation, or both.

2. Recent memory: Ability to give a description of circumstances of, and reasons for, coming to the hospital, dates of major tests or operations since admission, length of hospitalization, dates of visits by relatives or

physicians, etc.;
Ability to recall three words and
three objects after five minutes;
Digit span.

3. Attention: Serial sevens or threes, depending
on the patient's level of education
and impairment;
Counting from twenty backwards.

4. Abstract thinking: Difference between a lake and a
river; Commonality between a
banana and an orange; Interpretation of one or two proverbs; Definition of a common word.

5. Speed and dynamics Word fluency test, i.e. asking the
of thought: patient to say as many single words
within one minute as he can, the
norm being about thirty words a
minute.

Some of the above tests have been scrutinized systematically
and their diagnostic value questioned (4, 8-10). Thus, subtraction of serial sevens from 100 down, strongly recommended
by Engel and Romano (11) is criticized by Smith (10), who
found that fewer than 50 percent of normals with above average
education were able to carry out the test without a single error.
Depression of mood significantly reduces patients' scores in the
serial sevens test, while increasing age is claimed to be associated
with greater accuracy of performance. Performance is related
to the ability to attend, concentrate, and understand (9). Subtraction of 3's from 100 or from 20 is, in this author's opinion,
more useful for the present purpose than the serial 7's. Despite
criticisms, however, the latter test continues to be widely used
and has been employed, along with orientation, to grade the
level of sensorium in patients with alcohol withdrawal syndrome
(12). Digit span test, part of Wechsler's intelligence scales, is
often used in the examination of the level of awareness even
though it has been shown to be of little value in discriminating
organic from functional cases (4). Despite these criticisms these
simple tests of memory, attention, calculation, abstract thinking,
and orientation have shown good correlation with the degree

of slowing of the EEG background activity and thus provide a reliable indicator of the severity of cerebral dysfunction (13). Recent scales that are brief and can be scored (3, 5) should be used consistently by clinicians and be correlated with the degree of EEG abnormality so that their value as a diagnostic screening aid could be definitely evaluated.

Of the more formal psychological tests the following have been used for the diagnosis of delirium by some investigators: Wechsler Memory Scale; Bender Visual Motor Gestalt; Graham-Kendall Memory-for-Designs; Benton Visual Retention; and Tien's Organic Integrity Test (6, 14). Lowy et al. (6) developed the Delirium Scale (D-Scale) designed to allow repeated quantitative evaluation of changes in cognitive functions, affect, and behavior in bedridden patients. The Scale is mainly suitable for research purposes. It consists of fifty-eight items in thirteen categories, necessitates the use of a simple recording apparatus for hand tapping, aiming, and tremor, and takes about forty minutes to administer. The D-Scale allows scoring and offers a comprehensive, quantified assessment of the patient's cognitive, psychomotor, and emotional functioning.

In summary, clinical and psychological diagnosis of delirium rests on the history of acute onset of characteristic symptoms reflecting disturbance of cognitive functions and attention, presence of disturbed sleep-wakefulness cycle, and at times illusions and hallucinations that are mostly visual in character. Clinical impression of impaired information processing and attention is confirmed by the use of bedside psychological testing aimed at eliciting cognitive and attentional deficits. These two sources of evidence allow the diagnosis of delirium as a clinical syndrome. Once such diagnosis has been arrived at, it should prompt an inquiry into the etiology of delirium in the given case.

ETIOLOGICAL DIAGNOSIS

Delirium is, by definition, a psychiatric disorder due to demonstrable cerebral disorder or dysfunction, primary intracranial or secondary to systemic disease. Many organic factors, listed in Chapter 5, can cause delirium by acting singly or in combination. Once the syndrome has been diagnosed on clinical grounds, it is imperative to treat the underlying illness rather than its symptom, viz. delirium. If the patient is known to have a physical illness that can give rise to delirium, for example pneumonia or hepatic failure, then the situation is clear, and extensive laboratory investigations are not usually needed. If, however, a person becomes delirious in the absence of a known organic condition that could be expected to cause it, an extensive search for the causal factors must be undertaken. This search may be rendered more focussed and deliberate if one attempts to answer the following questions; the answers may narrow the scope of the inquiry and thus its cost. It goes without saying that a thorough physical examination, including a neurological one, has been performed on every patient before laboratory investigations are planned and ordered. The following questions should aid a judicious planning of the search for the etiology of delirium:

1. What is the patient's age? The most common causes of delirium vary to some extent in each age group. Their listing may be helpful:

   A Childhood (three through sixteen years)

   Infection: measles, mumps, scarlet fever, rheumatic fever, influenza, meningitis, encephalitis

   Intoxication with drugs, poisonous plants, other poisonous substances

   Epilepsy

   Head trauma

   Acute glomerulonephritis

   Uremia

   Hypoglycemia

   Hyponatremia (water intoxication)

   Hypernatremia (dehydration)

   Migraine

   B Adolescence and young adulthood (17 through 40 years)

   Intoxication with deliriogenic substances, especially anticholinergic drugs, glue, etc. Withdrawal syndrome from alcohol, barbiturates, and other addictive sedatives and hypnotics

   Head injury

Infection: hepatitis, meningitis, encephalitis, infectious mononucleosis, pneumonia, influenza, typhoid
Postoperative delirium
Hypoglycemia
Epilepsy
Brain tumor
Uremia
Systemic lupus erythematosus
Multiple sclerosis
Severe burns
Intoxication with industrial poisons
Metabolic encephalopathy secondary to neoplasm, liver disease

C Middle age (41 through 65 years)
Withdrawal syndrome from alcohol and/or sedatives
Intoxication by drugs, alcohol, industrial poisons
Head injury
Epilepsy
Metabolic encephalopathy—renal, hepatic, pulmonary, pancreatic, secondary to neoplasm
Endocrinopathy—excessive or deficient secretion of adrenals, thyroid, etc.
Hypoxia secondary to cerebrovascular or cardiovascular disease, including myocardial infarction and cardiac arrhythmias
Hypoglycemia
Deficiency of thiamine, nicotinic acid, cyanocobalamin
Hypertensive encephalopathy
Infection: pneumonia, influenza, viral hepatitis, typhoid
Heat stroke
Autoimmune disease
Neurosyphilis
Presenile dementia with delirious episodes

D Old age (66 years and over)
Cerebrovascular disease or accident
Drug intoxication or withdrawal
Myocardial infarction, congestive heart failure, cardiac arrhythmia

Encephalopathy due to renal, hepatic, or pulmonary disease
Head injury
Vitamin deficiency
Infection of any type
Hypertensive encephalopathy
Brain tumor, primary or secondary
Endocrinopathy, especially hypothyroidism
Alzheimer-senile dementia
Subdural hematoma
Neurosyphilis

2. Is the patient known to suffer from a chronic disease, cerebral, renal, cardiac, hepatic, pulmonary, etc., which could predispose him or her to delirium?

3. Is the patient taking any potentially deliriogenic medications?

4. Is the patient known or suspected to abuse alcohol and/or other substances?

5. Is there a history of recent injury, especially trauma to the head and thus possibility of subdural hematoma?

6. Is there a history of recent intellectual decline, personality change, loss of consciousness, stroke, episodes of inappropriate or confused behavior? A positive answer would direct the inquiry to rule out the more *insidious* intracranial, metabolic, neoplastic, nutritional, vascular, and toxic diseases affecting brain function and thus capable of triggering delirious episodes.

7. What is the patient's occupation? Is he or she likely to be exposed to industrial poisons?

8. Is there a possibility of foul play in the form of poisoning by means of such agents as arsenic, insulin, etc.?

9. Is there any likelihood of surreptitious self-medication with potentially deliriogenic drugs, such as meperidine, insulin, digitalis, anticonvulsants?

10. Does the patient suffer from a chronic depressive or

schizophrenic psychosis with secondary malnutrition and vitamin deficiency?

11. Has the patient been recently exposed to intense heat, cold, sunlight, electrical injury? Any of these physical agents could result in delirium.

12. Is the patient known to suffer from allergy to specific drugs or foods? If so, this could point to an allergic encephalopathy or autoimmune disease.

13. Is the patient likely to suffer from a metabolic defect, such as porphyria?

14. Has the patient travelled recently to areas where certain infections and infestations are known to be endemic, say malaria, typhoid, rickettsial infections, yellow fever, etc.?

Answers to the above questions should be sought systematically in any patient who develops delirium in the absence of an obvious physical cause. The following list of laboratory investigations may serve as a general guide to be used discriminately and on the basis of a sound clinical judgment.

Laboratory Investigations:

1. Blood chemistries:

    A Serum levels of sodium, potassium, chloride, bicarbonate, calcium, phosphate, magnesium, BUN, liver enzymes, arterial blood oxygen tension, B_{12} and folate

    B Blood screen for the more common drugs, poisons

    C Levels of cortisol, thyroxin

2. Hemogram

3. Urinalysis

4. Electrocardiogram

5. Serum protein electrophoresis

6. L E cell preparation and ANA levels

7. X-rays of chest and skull

8. Serum serological tests for syphilis

9. CSF examination, including serology, culture, protein electrophoresis, glutamine

10. Electroencephalogram

11. Brain scan

12. CAT scan

It must be emphasized that in most cases only some of these tests are needed and that only occasionally will one encounter a patient whose delirium will not be readily accounted for unless extensive investigations outlined above are carried out. There is no justification, for example, to order an expensive test, such as the computerized axial tomography (CAT scan) unless more routine and cheaper tests, such as the EEG, brain scan, skull x-ray, or CSF examination have raised the suspicion of intra-cranial pathology.

The Electroencephalogram

The role of the EEG in the diagnosis of delirium is discussed in Chapter 6 and need not be repeated. Romano and Engel (13) have stated clearly that from a clinical viewpoint there is usually "no need to utilize the electroencephalogram in the diagnosis of delirium." The diagnosis is made primarily on clinical grounds, discussed earlier. The EEG is a useful aid in the diagnosis of delirium only if there is suspicion of primary intracranial, especially focal, pathology, or if doubt exists that the patient suffers from delirium rather than from one of the functional psychoses, a dissociative disorder, or an organic mental disorder caused by cerebral stimulants or nondeliriogenic hallucinogens. Acute schizophrenic, schizophreniform, or atypical psychosis is particularly likely to give rise to diagnostic difficulties and the EEG, especially serial recordings, may help solve the diagnostic dilemma (15). Slowing, with or without super-imposed fast waves, of the background activity is the single most significant EEG abnormality indicative of delirium. Like any other laboratory test, however, the EEG must always be viewed in conjunction with pertinent clinical findings, psychological and other.

The more common causes of delirium will be discussed in Part II of this book. Their discussion should help the physician in arriving at an etiological diagnosis of delirium. Differential diagnosis of the syndrome from other mental disorders is discussed in Chapter 8.

REFERENCES

1. Stead, E.A.: Reversible madness. *Med Times* 94:1403-1406, 1966.
2. Phillips, J.: Delirium. *Cleve Med J* 8:331-342, 1909.
3. Folstein, M.F., Folstein, S.E., and McHugh, P.R.: "Mini-mental state." *J Psychiatr Res* 12:189-198, 1975.
4. Hinton, J., and Withers, E.: The usefulness of the clinical tests of the sensorium. *Br J Psychiatry* 119:9-18, 1971.
5. Jacob, J.W., Bernhad, M.R., Delgado, A., et al.: Screening for organic mental syndromes in the medically ill. *Ann Internal Med* 86:40-46, 1977.
6. Lowy, F.H., Engelsmann, F., and Lipowski, Z.J.: Study of cognitive functioning in a medical population. *Compr Psychiatry* 14:331-338, 1973.
7. Pfeiffer, E.: A short portable mental status questionnaire for the assessment of organic brain deficit in elderly patients. *J Am Ger Soc* 23:433-441, 1975.
8. Withers, E., and Hinton, J.: Three forms of the clinical tests of the sensorium and their reliability. *Br J Psychiatry* 119:1-18, 1971.
9. Milstein, V., Small, J.G., and Small, I.F.: The subtraction of serial sevens test in psychiatric patients. *Arch Gen Psychiatry* 26:439-441, 1972.
10. Smith, A.: The serial sevens subtraction test. *Arch Neurol* 17:78-80, 1967.
11. Engel, G.L. and Romano, J.: Delirium, a syndrome of cerebral insufficiency. *J Chron Dis* 9:260-277, 1959.
12. Gross, M.M., Rosenblatt, S.M., Lewis, E., Chartoff, S., and Malenowski, B.: Acute alcoholic psychoses and related syndromes: Psychosocial and clinical characteristics and their implications. *Br J Addict* 67:15-31, 1972.
13. Romano, J., and Engel, G.L.: Delirium. 1. Electroencephalographic data. *Arch Neurol Psychiatry* 51:356-377, 1944.
14. Fjeld, S.P., Small, I.F., Small, J.G., and Hayden, M.P.: Clinical, electrical and psychological tests and the diagnosis of organic brain disorder. *J Nerv Ment Dis* 142:172-179, 1966.
15. Pro, J.D., and Wells, C.E.: The use of the electroencephalogram in the diagnosis of delirium. *Dis Nerv Syst* 38:804-808, 1977.

Additional References

Obrecht, R., Okhomina, F.O.A., and Scott, D.F. Value of EEG in acute confusional states. *J Neurol Neurosurg Psychiatry* 42:75-77, 1979.

Oxman, T.E. The use of computerized axial tomography in neuroradiologic diagnosis in psychiatry. *Compreh Psychiatry* 20:177-186, 1979.

Pincus, J., and Tucker, G.J. *Behavioral Neurology*. Oxford University Press, 1978.

CHAPTER 8

DIFFERENTIAL DIAGNOSIS

DELIRIUM NEEDS TO BE distinguished from other organic mental disorders (or organic brain syndromes) and from some of the so-called functional psychiatric disorders. In Chapter 7 the diagnosis of delirium was discussed in considerable detail. To recapitulate: several features of the syndrome help to distinguish it from other mental disorders:

1. *Mode of onset*: Delirium characteristically comes on rapidly, that is, in a matter of hours or several days and always under one week.
2. *Duration*: Delirium typically lasts several days or weeks, rarely a few months, and lifts completely. As a general rule, if symptoms have lasted longer than three months, then it is unlikely that one is dealing with delirium.
3. *Symptoms*: Delirium is characterized by global impairment of cognitive functions and disturbances of attention that tend to fluctuate in severity over the course of a day. There are thus rapid changes in alertness, attention, cognitive clarity, perceptual discrimination, memory and orientation, with relatively lucid intervals occurring unpredictably and for varying periods. Sleep-wakefulness cycle is disturbed. Illusions and hallucinations, especially in the visual sphere, are common. The patient is typically acutely ill, incapable of sustained purposeful activity, either excited or lethargic, or shifts between restless hyperactivity and apathy. He or she has difficulty in telling apart imagery, dreams, and true perceptions. If disorientation for place and person is present, the patient typically tends to mistake the unfamiliar for familiar surroundings and persons. The symptoms tend to be most conspicuous at night.

4. *EEG findings*: In delirium, the EEG is practically always abnormal and tends to correlate with the degree of cognitive impairment and attention disturbance, that is to say with the level of awareness. The EEG abnormality usually consists of a bilateral and diffuse slowing of the background activity, with or without intermixed fast activity. In some cases, notably in delirium of alcohol and drug withdrawal, fast activity tends to predominate. Serial tracings may be needed to demonstrate the EEG abnormality. The latter may antedate and outlast the symptoms of delirium.

If one keeps in mind the above characteristics of delirium, then the differential diagnosis of it should not usually pose major problems. We will now discuss the conditions from which delirium needs to be distinguished in clinical practice.

DIFFERENTIATION FROM OTHER ORGANIC BRAIN SYNDROMES

Dementia. The defining feature of dementia is an impairment of intellectual functioning, which is usually associated with personality change and reduced efficacy in performance in work and social situations (1). The syndrome may be reversible or not. The *onset* of dementia is, in contrast to delirium, often insidious, as in Alzheimer's senile dementia. The *duration* of dementia is invariably more prolonged than that of delirium. By the time the patient comes to a physician's attention, the symptoms have usually lasted for more than three months. Dementia is to be diagnosed when intellectual deficit is accompanied by radiological evidence of gross cerebral damage, or if it has lasted for at least three months without any signs of improvement, or both. The *symptoms* of dementia do not usually display diurnal fluctuations like those of delirium. Lucid periods in the course of a day are more characteristic of the latter. Rapid shifts in psychomotor activity are also a feature of delirium rather than dementia. Hallucinations, illusions, and confusion between imagery, dreams, and true perceptions are more commonly found in delirium. Disruption of the normal sleep-wakefulness cycle is more consistently a feature of the latter.

It should be emphasized that differential diagnosis between delirium and dementia on the basis of symptoms may be impossible to make in some cases. There is no sharp dividing line between the psychopathological manifestations of these two conditions. They shade over into each other and overlap. They may be viewed as a continuum of pathological states related to diffuse cerebral pathology, which may be completely, partly, or not at all reversible. Delirium may be the first manifestation of multi-infarct dementia, for example, or constitute a transitional phase between coma and dementia, as in some cases of severe head trauma. Furthermore, delirium may be superimposed upon dementia, as is often the case in degenerative cerebral diseases. So-called nocturnal confusion of the patient with senile dementia represents delirious episodes largely confined to the night.

To agonize if the label of delirium or dementia ought to be attached to a given case seems futile. If in doubt, one should assign the diagnosis of delirium, which carries the implication that the mental disorder is transient. If the clinical picture does not improve over a period of about three months, the diagnosis of dementia is to be assigned; it does not imply that the patient will not improve. As was stated earlier, the current tendency is to view dementia as a syndrome which need not be irreversible. If the EEG normalizes in a patient displaying global cognitive impairment, dementia is the diagnosis. The crucial point is that the diagnosis of both delirium and dementia should lead to an immediate search for the underlying cerebral disorder, its nature, and its etiology. If the latter is treated promptly and adequately, the mental disorder should clear up or at least improve unless widespread damage to the cerebral cortical neurons has occurred or the condition is at present untreatable.

Hallucinosis. This syndrome features continuous or recurrent hallucinations with or without delusional conviction that they represent true perceptions. Impairment of memory, orientation, attention, and directed thinking is absent or slight (1). Thus, the features of delirium are not present. This condition may be caused by various hallucinogenic drugs, such as LSD.

Amnestic syndrome. This is characterized by marked impairment of recent memory and retention, i.e. by retrograde and anterograde amnesia (1). Other cognitive deficits, such as disorientation and impaired concept formation, may be present, but it is the memory pathology that dominates the clinical picture. Occasionally, amnestic syndrome may coexist with delirium, as for example, in Wernicke's encephalopathy; the differential diagnosis should not otherwise present problems.

Organic affective syndrome. Here the clinical picture is that of depression or mania, and a coexistent cerebral disorder, or known exposure to a toxic substance, is believed to be of causal significance. Global impairment of cognitive functions is not a feature (1).

Organic delusional syndrome. This disorder resembles a paranoid psychosis or a schizophrenic disorder. Delusions, with or without hallucinations, are the main characteristic. A coexistent cerebral disorder, or known exposure to a toxic substance, is considered to be of etiological significance (1). Global impairment of cognitive functions is absent. This condition may be caused by drugs, such as amphetamines.

Organic personality disorder. Impaired capacity for the expression and control of emotions and impulses, disturbed ability for action planning, and impaired social judgment are the hallmarks of this disorder. It does not feature global cognitive impairment (1).

Intoxication and withdrawal. These disorders imply behavioral and autonomic disturbances associated with intake of certain toxic substances and with the sudden withholding of the substance to which the person is addicted, respectively (2). Global cognitive impairment is absent.

In summary, organic brain syndromes other than delirium lack the impairment of the level of awareness or consciousness. Dementia is characterized by relatively sustained rather than fluctuating global impairment of cognitive functions and lacks the marked disturbance of the sleep-wakefulness cycle. Hallucinosis and amnestic syndrome represent circumscribed, rather than global, cognitive abnormalities. Affective and delusional organic syndromes are similar to affective and schizophrenic disorders, respectively, and do not feature impairment of memory and orientation. These disorders may have a rapid onset like delirium, but they lack intellectual deficits and do not feature EEG slowing. The EEG in these conditions is either normal or accelerated or shows epileptiform potentials. When caused by drugs, these syndromes are often referred to as "toxic psychoses." It should be remembered that they are not coterminous with delirium. Psychoses caused by sympathomimetic amines, corticosteroids, methylphenidate, atabrine, LSD-25, mescaline, and other substances fall into this category. They are in most cases distinct from delirium in both symptoms and the EEG characteristics. Slowing of the EEG background activity is not a feature of these disorders.

DIFFERENTIATION FROM FUNCTIONAL PSYCHIATRIC DISORDERS

Schizophrenic Disorders

A disorder of cognition is the core psychopathology of both delirium and schizophrenic disorders. Yet, the characteristics of cognitive impairment are different in the typical cases of the two conditions (2). It is the atypical cases of schizophrenia, those characterized by disturbances of consciousness and attention, which may be difficult at times to distinguish from delirium.

Currently accepted operational criteria for the diagnosis of a schizophrenic disorder (2) make confusion with delirium unlikely to occur. A typical delirious patient does not exhibit characteristic delusions of being controlled, of thought broadcasting, or withdrawal. If delusions occur in delirium, they are characteristically fleeting, poorly organized, and highly influenced by the ongoing situation and events. Hallucinations differ: in delirium they are typically visual, in schizophrenic disorders—auditory. This distinction is relative since both these types of hallucinations may occur in either condition. Purely auditory hallucinations, especially of voices keeping up a running commentary on the patient's experiences and conduct, are unusual in delirium but are characteristic for schizophrenia. Formal thought disorder, accompanied by blunted or inappropriate affect, is not a feature of delirium. Thinking disorder in delirium is characterized by difficulty in controlling the train of thought, thus rendering it less effective as a tool for problem solving. It is less autistic or idiosyncratic and bizarre than in schizophrenia and more bound to ongoing information inputs. Schizophrenic patients do not as a rule show impairment of recent memory and retention or spatiotemporal disorientation. A schizophrenic may appear to be disoriented and claim to be on the planet Venus, for example. This, however, is an example of autistic thought or delusional disorientation (3). A delirious patient characteristically tends to mistake unfamiliar people and surroundings for familiar ones, and if there is confabulation to fill the gaps in memory and grasp, it is done with concrete, everyday details. Delirious patients typically show fluctuations in the severity of their symptoms in the course of a day and tend to display lucid intervals lasting minutes or hours; a schizophrenic does not display such striking oscillations of psychopathology. Catatonic symptoms may occur in both delirium and schizophrenia and cause diagnostic difficulties. A diagnostic sodium amytal interview may help in such a case: a delirious patient will display disorientation and other cognitive deficits which are absent in catatonic schizophrenia. Finally, an EEG may help settle the diagnosis if it shows diffuse slowing of the background activity, which is absent in uncomplicated schizophrenia.

Acute Schizophrenia and Related Atypical or Reactive Psychoses

Acute schizophrenia may at times cause diagnostic difficulties. Van Praag (4) states that when a schizophrenic disorder occurs as a response to marked psychological stress, the level of consciousness may be reduced during the first few days or weeks of the illness. Newmark et al. (5) observed disorientation to place, time, and person in 18 percent, 16 percent, and 7 percent, respectively, of a group of 112 schizophrenics. Vaillant (6) found "confusion" to be a favorable prognostic sign in schizophrenia and remarks that it contains features of "an organically determined delirium." A review of the autobiographical accounts of schizophrenic episodes has revealed subjective experience of memory deficits, impaired attention, and confusion (7). Scandinavian psychiatrists have separated from the class of schizophrenic disorders a group of similar conditions, but characterized by an acute onset in response to emotional trauma and by symptoms which often included confusion. Langfeldt (8) referred to them as "schizophreniform states;" Faergeman (9) called them "psychogenic psychoses;" McCabe and Strömgren (10) have adopted the label "reactive psychoses." More recently, McCabe and Cadoret (11) have used the term "atypical psychoses" for those which showed a similarity to both manic-depressive and schizophrenic disorders yet were identical with neither.

The nosological position of acute schizophrenia and related psychoses referred to above is in a state of flux. Current draft of the *Diagnostic and Statistical Manual of Mental Disorders, Third Edition,* (2) does not contain the category "acute schizophrenia." Instead, there are three new categories which seem to replace it, namely "schizophreniform disorder," "brief reactive psychosis," and "atypical psychosis." The features of the brief reactive psychosis include a recognizable stressor, sudden onset, and duration of less than one week. Its manifestations are declared to include "confusion with clouding of consciousness, disorientation and impairment of recent memory." The *Manual* states that this psychosis may only be distinguished from organic mental disorders on the basis of an absent history of a known organic etiological factor. If the psychosis lasts more than one week, the diagnosis of either schizophreniform or atypical psychosis would be made. Thus, it appears that the only reliable criterion for the differential diagnosis of these three psychoses from delirium would be the presence of a demonstrable organic causation or, in the case of a schizophreniform psychosis, relatively longer duration of the illness. These criteria would make a differentiation on descriptive grounds practically impossible at times.

This whole grey area of psychiatric classification has been poorly delineated and inadequately delineated from delirium for over a century. The disorders under discussion, those showing features of both a schizophrenic disorder and delirium (or "clouding of consciousness"), have received numerous designations in the past 150 years or so. Gomirato and Gamna (12) have listed many of them and tried to trace their tortuous and shifting course in the history of psychiatry. Nineteenth century English authors listed Bell's mania (13), acute delirium (14), typhomania (15), delirium of collapse (16), and acute confusional insanity (17), to mention just the most popular designations, for what seem to have been identical or at least overlapping disorders. Connolly's (17) description of what he called "acute confusional insanity" highlights the similarity of this condition to delirium. According to him, the confusional insanity has a sudden onset and lasts hours or days. Its manifestations include hallucinations, "a dreamy obscuration of the mind," disorientation for time and place, impairment of recent memory, "varied and disconnected delusions," emotional lability, and restlessness which may be followed by stupor. The disorder could arise from various causes, among which Connolly lists puerperium, postfebrile states, tuberculosis, nostalgia, abuse of alcohol, emotional shock, and sexual excess. Connolly viewed the disorder as distinct from mania, melancholia, and acute dementia, but one "intimately associated" with the latter condition.

Acute confusional insanity appears to be related to, if not identical with, amentia of Meynert (18), bouffées délirantes of the French authors (19), episodic confusions (20), oneirophrenia (21), acute exhaustive psychoses (22), etc. These psychoses are reportedly more frequent in the developing societies, or those going through political upheavals, and are probably of multiple etiology, including complex interplay of constitutional, infectious, nutritious, toxic, and psychosocial factors (19, 23, 24). Some writers invoke the role of stress of acculturation in the genesis of these psychoses in Africa (19, 23, 24). In the developed countries these syndromes are typically precipitated by a catastrophic event in the life of the person. Common clinical features include severe restlessness and excitement, vivid and often terrifying hallucinations, panic and confusion. Overactivity, insomnia, dehydration, and nutritional deficiencies that are commonly present may add a range of complicating factors and precipitate actual delirium (25, 26). Clinical diagnostic differentiation may then become impossible, and the overriding concern is to correct the complicating organic disorder and treat the excitement, overactivity, and insomnia.

A condition closely related to the foregoing syndromes is delirium acutum (acute lethal catatonia, acute pernicious psychosis) (25, 26). This syndrome has been described in association with organic diseases such as encephalitis, thyrotoxicosis, or epilepsy; schizophrenia; mania; depression. It combines features of delirium and a functional, often schizophrenic, psychosis. Its clinical features are malaise, irritability, anxiety, fatigue, and depersonalization lasting from several days to weeks and followed by a rapidly developing severe excitement, combativeness, incoherent speech, clouded consciousness, and hyperthermia. Once the latter develops, the patient may collapse and die (25, 26). For over 100 years now an inconclusive controversy has flared up periodically in Europe regarding the nosological position and etiology of this and related syndromes: Are they psychogenic or organic? They may occur in the absence of demonstrable organic disease. The etiology appears to be multifactorial.

Hart (27) in his thoughtful discussion of delirium and the syndromes under consideration here proposed that the latter may represent delirium brought about by chemical substances generated in states of excessive fatigue, emotional stress, or both. This is certainly a plausible hypothesis and one worth attempting to validate. Levin (28) has attempted to differentiate organic from "psychogenic" delirium on descriptive grounds. He proposed that in psychogenic delirium the patient shows no evidence of a coexistent organic disorder. He or she ignores or distorts elements of the environment in an attempt to fulfill a wish, but actually remains properly oriented, displays no fluctuations of awareness, and has no speech defect.

It appears clear from the preceding discussion that a heterogeneous group of transient psychoses may display some or all of the clinical manifestations of delirium, in the absence of a demonstrable cerebral disorder or recognizable organic cause. The nosological status of these psychoses and their relation to delirium will remain uncertain until systematic clinical and laboratory studies of them have been carried out. Differential diagnosis between these atypical psychoses and delirium should include the EEG and other laboratory tests aimed at demonstrating the presence of cerebral dysfunction and its presumptive organic cause or causes. If the EEG remains normal despite evidence of behavioral manifestations of delirium, the diagnosis of an atypical or schizophreniform psychosis becomes more likely. An interview using intravenous sodium amylobarbitone may be helpful in the differential diagnosis of these doubtful cases (29). Cognitive deficits caused by a cerebral disorder, and forming the nucleus of delirium, become accentuated by the drug. If such defects are concomitants of emotional turmoil in the absence of a cerebral disorder, they tend to clear up under the influence of the drug.

Affective Disorders

Both the manic and the major depressive disorders may occasionally cause difficulty in the differential diagnosis of delirium. Taylor and Abrams (30) report finding "confusion" in about 30 percent and visual hallucinations in about 26 percent of manic patients. "Confusion" in this context presumably implies spatiotemporal disorientation, but this is not clear. Distractibility is a common feature in both mania and delirium. Manic patients do not display global cognitive impairment which fluctuates during the day and tends to become worse at night. The EEG does not show slowing of the background activity in mania. Mentzos et al. (31) found confusional states resembling delirium in about 5 percent of 338 patients with manic-depressive disorders. These authors point out that on closer inspection it is possible to distinguish these states clinically from delirium. They claim that the patients appear to be disinterested or playful rather than truly disoriented. They tend to misidentify people in terms of important persons in their (that is, the patients') lives. They may display loss of awareness of personal identity—a very rare symptom in delirium. Furthermore, fluctuations in the degree of disorientation in the delirious patient, but not in the manic or depressed, follow those in the level of awareness and other cognitive functions or capacities. The differential diagnosis of these disorders from delirium requires obtaining a careful history and mental status examination. The EEG and sodium amytal interview may be resorted to in doubtful cases.

Factitious Disorder with Psychological Symptoms (Ganser Syndrome, Pseudodementia, Hysterical Twilight State, Hysterical Psychosis)

Whitlock (32), in a review of the Ganser syndrome, asserts that the basic disturbance is one of consciousness, which is clouded. He argues that the syndrome is a psychotic one, occurring either after acute head trauma or in the course of a psychosis. Ganser (33) himself referred to it as a hysterical twilight state, characterized by fluctuating level of consciousness, defects of memory, inability to answer correctly the simplest questions with a tendency to give only approximate answers, auditory and visual hallucinations, conversion symptoms, rather abrupt recovery and amnesia for the disorder following recovery. Tsoi (34) views it not as a psychosis but rather a disorder akin to malingering and hysteria. He could not, in contrast to Whitlock (32), distinguish Ganser syndrome from pseudodementia. There is controversy over the nosological position and clinical associations of Ganser syndrome. This rare condition may be difficult to differentiate from delirium. What distinguishes it from the latter is the inconsistency in the degree of cognitive impairment presented by the patient. He may be correctly oriented for time and place but have amnesia with loss of personal identity. His answers to simple questions are often inconsistent and tend to be grotesquely inaccurate, e.g. that two and two are five. EEG should be normal .

Dissociative Disorders

Psychogenic amnesia and fugue (2) bear a strong relation to Ganser syndrome. Both are characterized by sudden onset of a failure to recall important personal information and past history. In the fugue there is, in addition, a loss of awareness of personal identity, a tendency to travel, and assumption of a new identity. Delirium is readily distinguished from these disorders by a global rather than selective cognitive impairment, defect of registration (anterograde amnesia), and disorientation for time and place rather than for personal identity. In all dissociative states the normal EEG and the normal cognitive performance under sodium amytal interview may aid the diagnosis.

In summary, differential diagnosis of delirium from other mental disorders is likely to involve schizophrenic disorders, atypical and reactive psychoses, mania, dementia, and a factitious or dissociative disorder. In most cases delirium can be distinguished by finding its characteristic symptoms, by the associated abnormality of the EEG background activity, and, at times, by using a sodium amytal interview.

REFERENCES

1. Lipowski, Z.J.: Organic brain syndromes: A reformulation. *Compr Psychiatry 19*:309-322, 1978.
2. *Diagnostic and Statistical Manual of Mental Disorders.* 3rd edition, Draft. Washington, D.C., American Psychiatric Association, January 15, 1978.
3. Levin, M.: Varieties of disorientation. *J Ment Sci 102*:619-623, 1956.
4. van Praag, H.M.: About the impossible concept of schizophrenia. *Compr Psychiatry 17*:481-497, 1976.
5. Newmark, C.S., Raft, D., Toomey, T., Hunter, W., and Mazzaglia, J.: Diagnosis of schizophrenia: Pathognomonic signs or symptom clusters. *Compr Psychiatry 16*:155-163, 1975.
6. Vaillant, G.E.: Prospective prediction of schizophrenic remission. *Arch Gen Psychiatry 11*:509-518, 1964 .
7. Freedman, B.J.: The subjective experience of perceptual and cognitive disturbances in schizophrenia. *Arch Gen Psychiatry 30*:333-340, 1974.
8. Langfeldt, G.: *The Schizophreniform States: A Catamnestic Study Based on Individual Re-examinations.* Copenhagen, Munksgaard, 1939.
9. Faergeman, P.M.: *Psychogenic Psychoses.* London, Butterworths, 1963.
10. McCabe, M.S., and Stromgren, E.: Reactive psychoses. *Arch Gen Psychiatry 32*:447-454, 1975.
11. McCabe, M.S., and Cadoret, R.J.: Genetic investigations of atypical psychoses. 1. Morbidity in parents and siblings. *Compr Psychiatry 17*:347-352, 1976.
12. Gomirato, G., and Gamna, G.: *Die Verwirrtheitszustände.* Basel, Karger, 1957.

13. Bell, L.V.: On a form of disease resembling some advanced stages of mania and fever. *Am J Insanity* 6:97-127, 1849.

14. Editorial: Acute delirium in 1845 and 1860. *Am J Insanity* 21:181-200, 1864.

15. Williams, A.V.: Letter to the editor. *Am J Insanity* 8:146-149, 1851-2.

16. Weber, H.: On delirium or acute insanity. *Med–Chir Trans (Lond)* 30:135-159, 1865.

17. Connolly, N.: Acute confusional insanity. *Dubl J Med Sci* 89:506-518, 1890.

18. Pappenheim, E.: On Meynert's amentia. *Intern J Neurol* 9:311-326, 1975.

19. Collomb, H.: Bouffées délirantes en psychiatrie africaine. *Psychopathol Afric* 1:167-239, 1965.

20. Kasanin, J.: The syndrome of episodic confusions. *Am J Psychiatry* 93:625-638, 1936.

21. Meduna, L.J.: *Oneirophrenia: The Confused State.* Urbana, University of Illinois Press, 1950.

22. Adland, M.L.: Review, case studies, therapy, and interpretation of the acute exhaustive psychoses. *Psychiatr Q* 21:38-69, 1947.

23. German, G.A.: Aspects of clinical psychiatry in sub-Saharan Africa. *Br J Psychiatry* 121:461-479, 1972.

24. Jilek, W.G., and Jilek-Aall, L.: Transient psychoses in Africans. *Psychiatr Clin* 3:337-364, 1970.

25. Chrisstoffels, J., and Thiel, J.H.: Delirium acutum, a potentially fatal condition in the psychiatric hospital. *Psychiatr Neurol Neurochir* 73:177-187, 1970.

26. Tolsma, F.J.: The syndrome of acute pernicious psychosis. *Psychiatr Neurol Neurochir* 70:1-21, 1967.

27. Hart, B.: Delirious states. *Br Med J* 2:745-749, 1936.

28. Levin, H.L.: Organic and psychogenic delirium. *NY Med J* 99:631-633, 1914.

29. Ward, N.G., Rowlett, D.B., and Burke, P.: Sodium amylobarbitone in the differential diagnosis of confusion. *Am J Psychiatry* 135:75-78, 1978.

30. Taylor, M.A., and Abrams, R.: The phenomenology of mania. *Arch Gen Psychiatry* 29:520-522, 1973.

31. Mentzos, S., Lyrakos, A., and Tsiolis, A.: Akute Verwirrtheitszustände bei endogenen Psychosen. *Der Nervenarzt* 42:10-17, 1971.

32. Whitlock, F.A.: The Ganser syndrome. *Br J Psychiatry* 113:19-29, 1967.

33. Schorer, C.E.: The Ganser syndrome. *Br J Criminol* 41:120-131, 1965.

34. Tsoi, W.F.: The Ganser syndrome in Singapore: A report on ten cases. *Br J Psychiatry* 123:567-572, 1973.

Additional References

Akhtar, S., and Buckman, J. The differential diagnosis of mutism: A review and a report of three unusual cases. *Dis Nerv Syst* 38:558-563, 1977.

Cutting, J.C., Clare, A.W., and Mann, A.H. Cycloid psychosis: An investigation of the diagnostic concept. *Psychol Med* 8:637-648, 1978.

Heaton, R.K., Vogt, A.T., Hoehn, M.M., et al. Neuropsychological impairment with schizophrenia vs. acute and chronic cerebral lesions. *J Clin Psychol* 35:46-53, 1979.

Latcham, R., White A., and Sims, A. Ganser syndrome. *J Neurol Neurosurg Psychiatry* 41:851-854, 1978.

Manschreck, T.C., and Petri, M. The atypical psychoses. *Culture Med Psychiatry* 2:233-268, 1978.

Retterstöl, N. The Scandinavian concept of reactive psychosis, schizophreniform psychosis and schizophrenia. *Psychiatria Clin* 11:180-187, 1978.

Wells, C.E. Geriatric organic psychoses. *Psychiatric Annals* 8:57-73, 1978.

CHAPTER 9

MANAGEMENT OF DELIRIUM

Treatment of delirium has concerned physicians since antiquity. Specific therapeutic methods have varied, reflecting changes in the state of knowledge and the beliefs about the pathophysiology of the syndrome. Certain general principles of the management, however, have prevailed since antiquity and are still applicable today. Sedation of the restless and agitated delirious patient, securing rest and sleep, and providing a quiet environment and supportive nursing care have been the hallmarks of the treatment of this condition over the centuries. A brief historical account of the development of the therapeutic approaches to delirium follows.

HISTORICAL EVOLUTION OF TREATMENT

Some of the cardinal rules of the management of delirium were clearly spelled out at the beginning of the Christian era. Writers such as Aretaeus, Soranus, and Galen, active in the second century A.D., formulated therapeutic guidelines which in general are still valid. Aretaeus (1) taught that a phrenitic patient should be placed in a dark room if he was disturbed by the light, and in a bright one if he was afraid of the dark. Rest and sleep were to be aided by administering poppy boiled in oil. Soranus Ephesius (2) recommended that a delirious patient should be treated in a quiet and well-lit room, one devoid of pictures on the walls, since they might facilitate the occurrence of visual hallucinations. At times the patient had to be restrained physically and prevented from jumping out of the window. Venesection and cupping were indicated. Galen (3) taught that delirium was secondary to and symptomatic of many systemic diseases which affected the brain by "consensus" or "sympathetically." Thus, the treatment ought to be logically directed at the underlying condition. This was probably the first time in history that this crucial tenet of the treatment of delirium became acknowledged.

During the subsequent centuries medical writers modified and added details to the above general principles but basically did not change them until the nineteenth century when bloodletting, an important component of the treatment of delirium, gradually became abandoned. This mode of therapy was based on the prevailing misconceptions about the pathophysiology of delirium. Avicenna (3), for example, viewed the latter as a symptom of brain disease caused by black, yellow, or red bile; or by hot and burning blood perfusing the brain. It followed logically that the treatment should involve diversion of the disturbing humors from the brain and by removal or cooling of the overheated blood. Bleeding was done by means of phlebotomy or cupping glasses, and, later, by leeches. Gatinaria (2), a fifteenth century writer, recommended bleeding from the legs. Rivière (2), writing in the seventeenth century, urged that blood be removed from the veins of the head. He also advised that the whole body should be cooled but cautioned against the use of the cooling medicines. Among the latter were included oils of roses, violets, or water lilies.

Bloodletting continued to be a popular treatment for mental illness, including delirium, well into the nineteenth century. Esquirol (4), in his famous treatise on mental disorders published in 1835, deplored the abuse of this treatment and asserted that it should be confined to plethoric patients, "when the head is strongly congested" (4, p. 87). In such cases, leeches should be applied to the jugular vein and temporal arteries and cups to the base of the brain. Gallway (5) inveighed even more vehemently against bloodletting, especially when applied in the cases of delirium with "low or adynamic symptoms." He claimed that a physician who applied bloodletting to such cases, by means of "various instruments of professional torture to the head, in the shape of blisters, cupping-glasses, etc.," was liable to discover that he had "dealt his patient a knock-down blow, from which the chances are that he is effectually disabled from rising again." In 1813, Sutton (6) published his famous treatise on delirium tremens, a condition distinguished by him from other deliria on the basis of an adverse response to bloodletting but a good response to opium. By the 1890s bloodletting had gradually faded away from the treatment regimen (7). It had been replaced by such measures as application of evaporating lotions or the ice-bag to the head, cold baths, and other methods aimed at lowering fever and reducing the presumed hyperemia of the brain and raised intracranial pressure (8, 9). Yet as late as 1899 Hirsch (10) still found it necessary to condemn venesection as a treatment for delirium. He criticized the view that hyperemia of the brain was alone responsible for the syndrome and asserted that therapy should aim at stimulation and regulation of the circulation, rather than weaken the latter by venesection, purges, blisters, etc.

During the nineteenth century, three major aspects of the treatment of delirium became enriched and expanded: therapy of the underlying condition; sedation and inducing sleep; and general support. These three aspects will now be discussed.

An article in Rees's (11) authoritative encyclopedia, published in the early nineteenth century, states clearly that the remedies for delirium must be "varied according to its nature, and the concomitant symptoms." Salter (12), an eminent London surgeon, wrote in 1850 that it was essential to understand the underlying cause of delirium in a given patient if the latter was to be treated effectively. This principle is echoed by Verco (9): "In the treatment of delirium the best results will follow prescriptions according to causal indications." Hirsch (10) reaffirmed this teaching but also stressed the need for the symptomatic management of delirium regardless of its causation. Thus, by the beginning of the present century the key concept of the necessity to treat the pathological condition responsible for the delirium in an individual patient had been unequivocally spelled out. Progress in medical knowledge and therapy during the nineteenth century made it more feasible.

Sedation has been used for the treatment of delirium since antiquity. Opium remained by far the most popular drug for this purpose for centuries. In the nineteenth century, however, new sedatives enriched the physician's therapeutic armamentarium. Graves (13) announced in 1836 that he had scored a remarkable success treating delirium in the course of typhus with frequent doses of tartar emetic. He took pains to argue that the effectiveness of the drug in these cases was independent of its emetic action. During the following four decades other drugs came into use to ensure sedation and/or sleep in the delirious patient: bromides, chloral hydrate, and chloroform by inhalation (8, 9). By the end of the century, hypodermic injections of hyoscine, hyoscyamine, and ergotin had come into use (10). Morphine was being used by subcutaneous injection. Paraldehyde, introduced in 1882, and alcohol were favored by some. Barbiturates came into use in 1903. All these sedatives and hypnotics had been used for the symptomatic treatment of delirium until the introduction of the major and minor tranquilizers in the 1950s. As late as 1953 authors of a major review of delirium (14) recommended for its management paraldehyde, by the oral or parenteral route; chloral hydrate in doses of 1 to 2 gm. for sleep; intramuscular or intravenous amobarbital or secobarbital; and scopolamine. After the introduction of the modern psychotropic drugs the symptomatic treatment of delirium became dominated by them and a new therapeutic era began.

General supportive and nursing measures in delirium became quite sophisticated in the nineteenth century. Greiner (15) wrote a remarkable and fascinating book on delirium in 1817. The treatment that he recommended impresses one even today as advanced, sensitive, and humane. He argued that a delirious patient should be treated with respect. One must not speak in his presence as if he could not understand what was being said. Attention should be paid to his increased sensitivity to lights and sounds. Persons and objects that the patient dislikes should be kept away. A person whom he likes should stay with him, speak to him gently, and thus help to calm and orient him. The patient should not be left unattended since he might hurt himself as a result of frightening visions. Whatever the patient said or did in the course of delirium must never be used to judge his character, since he was not responsible for his words and actions. The latter tend to be expressions of fantasies and emotions that are beyond the control of the psyche. One could hardly improve on these precepts today.

Rees's (11) encyclopedia recommended these general supporting measures for the delirious patient: "Every source of irritation whatever, such as strong light, noises, conversation of visitors, motion or exertion of the body, etc., should be studiously avoided." Attention should be paid to the patient's state of nutrition, fluid intake, and bladder and bowels. Fothergill (8) advises that the patient should be kept in his own room and with a near relative in attendance, since unfamiliar surroundings and persons tend to provoke frightening fantasies and consequent attempts at escape. Attendants should try to restrain an agitated and fearful patient by appealing to "what is left of his reason," rather than by physical force. Phillips (16) stresses that the care of a delirious patient calls for careful nursing and close attention by the physician: "It requires tact, careful observation of details and infinite patience," he writes. Phillips warns that the patient may readily attempt to commit suicide or mutilate himself as a result of his mental condition. He recommends that windows should be barred, and the patient should not be left alone. Hawley (17) draws the attention of nurses to the exacerbation of delirium at night and describes symptoms which can help a nurse recognize the condition.

Thus, by the beginning of this century all the basic elements of the management of delirium had been clearly formulated. Indeed, therapeutic recommendations advanced by many early writers, especially during the last century, impress one by the high sensitivity to the plight and needs of the delirious patient. It is sobering to observe that we have added little of substance to the general management of delirium in the past fifty years and that its treatment in many hospitals falls far short of that taught by physicians a century ago and earlier. In the following outline of the contemporary treatment of the syndrome we will have to recapitulate precepts repeated by sensitive and observant physicians over the centuries.

GENERAL PRINCIPLES OF MODERN TREATMENT OF DELIRIUM

The management of delirium has two major aspects: first, elimination or correction of the underlying cause (or causes) by appropriate medical and/or surgical methods of therapy; and second, general symptomatic and supportive measures aimed at securing rest and sleep, nutrition, fluid intake, and essentially, optimal comfort for the patient. These two aspects of treatment, the causal and the symptomatic, obviously overlap, since malnutrition, dehydration, electrolyte imbalance, etc. may contribute to the onset, continuation, and severity of delirium. Causal treatment of the latter is in most cases beyond the scope of this book; it involves application of currently accepted medical therapeutic methods described in the appropriate textbooks. Only general guidelines will be discussed here, with special emphasis on the symptomatic and supportive measures (14, 18-23).

Identification and Adequate Treatment of the Underlying Pathology

As soon as delirium has been diagnosed on clinical grounds, a search begins for the etiological factor (or factors). In many cases more than one such factor is involved, and each of them has to be identified and either eliminated or corrected. A given patient may, for example, suffer from hypoxia, anemia, electrolyte imbalance, and toxic effects of one or more drugs. Unless all these etiological factors are identified and eliminated, the delirium is liable to continue.

One should obtain all available information about patient's recent and current intake of alcohol and any drugs. Drug intoxication as well as sudden withdrawal of alcohol, sedatives, and hypnotics are among the most common causes of delirium nowadays, and have largely replaced infections in this role. In the case of drug withdrawal syndromes, the sedative or hypnotic agent to which the patient has been addicted must be restored, or properly substituted, and withdrawn gradually. Virtually every known drug may cause delirium because of its overdosage, individual idiosyncrasy to it, interference with its detoxification and elimination related to hepatic or renal disease, etc. It follows that any medications which the patient has been receiving are potentially suspect and should be withheld or their dosage reduced, if at all possible.

Maintenance of Fluid and Electrolyte Balance and Nutrition

Correct any electrolyte imbalance that may be present and

maintain adequate fluid balance, nutrition, and vitamin supply. Many a delirious patient suffers from an exacerbation of a chronic disease or a life-threatening acute one, and shows evidence of malnutrition, dehydration, and subclinical vitamin deficiency. Following the onset of delirium such a patient is liable to neglect food and fluid intake. Furthermore, a restless and agitated delirious patient will readily exhaust his or her body stores of vitamins, especially of the B complex, and their deficiency may increase the severity of delirium. Thus, vitamin supplement should be given to every delirious patient.

Sedation and Sleep

Sedation is needed only if the patient is restless, excited, and fearful. Since insomnia and nocturnal exacerbation of symptoms are regular features of delirium, it is essential to ensure an adequate night's sleep. Medical writers since Hippocrates have observed that sound sleep usually indicates impending resolution of delirium and is thus a favorable prognostic sign.

The choice of sedative or tranquilizer presupposes that the cause of delirium has been determined. Otherwise, treatment with a particular psychotropic drug, or class of drugs, may be dangerous. For example, chlorpromazine could precipitate hepatic coma in a patient with advanced liver disease and delirium, or it could bring about a dangerous state of hypothermia in a delirious myxedematous subject (18). Furthermore, the sedative should be selected and its dose determined by taking into account the patient's age, weight, and any physical disorder he or she may have in addition to that which has been responsible for the delirium. For example, the presence of hypertension or coronary heart disease may not have contributed to the patient's delirium but would militate against the use of a psychotropic drug with a marked potential for inducing hypotension or cardiac arrhythmia. The selected drug and its dose should be effective in counteracting agitation and excitement and be relatively free of undesirable effects on cerebral functioning and on cardiovascular and respiratory functions. If delirium is believed to be due to an anticholinergic agent, one should obviously avoid using tranquilizers having anticholinergic properties. No single psychotropic drug available today is clearly superior and indicated for all cases of delirium. A particular physician's personal experience and thorough familiarity with the actions and side effects of a given drug will influence the choice in every case, as the following guidelines reflect (19-26). Drug treatment of delirium due to various specific causes will be further discussed in appropriate sections of Part II of this book.

The following groups of sedatives and tranquilizers have been recommended by various writers and require a critical discussion of their merits and disadvantages in the treatment of delirium:

Barbiturates: There is no place for this group of drugs in the treatment of delirium other than that due to drug withdrawal. They may make the delirious patient more obtunded or agitated, their cumulative effect could precipitate coma, and they have no remedial effect on delusions and hallucinations (19, 20).

Paraldehyde: This drug was often recommended for the management of delirium in the past. Its disadvantages include sterile abscesses with intramuscular injections, pulmonary edema after intravenous injection, and difficulty in adjusting the dosage with rectal administration (27). Newer drugs are preferable.

Benzodiazepines: Chlordiazepoxide and diazepam are the most popular drugs in this group. They are effective anxiolytic agents and have been recommended for the treatment of delirium, but their use in the latter condition needs to be reevaluated. They may at times bring about excessive sedation, intoxication, and occasionally, paradoxical excitement in the elderly (28). They are not effective against severe agitation, hallucinations, and delusions of the delirious patient (19). Chlordiazepoxide and diazepam have been widely used for the treatment of delirium tremens (27, 29-32). They are recommended for the treatment of hepatic encephalopathy, as they have less tendency to precipitate coma in this condition (33,34). In delirium due to other causes these drugs have been largely replaced by haloperidol.

Flurazepam hydrochloride, another diazepine, is an effective and relatively safe hypnotic (35). In doses of 15 to 30 mg. at bedtime it is recommended for relatively mildly delirious patients, especially those whose delirium is largely confined to a sleepless night, and whenever the use of a hypnotic is believed indicated.

Phenothiazines: Some authors recommend the use of one of the phenothiazine tranquilizers for the treatment of delirium (19, 20). An initial intramuscular injection of chlorpromazine 25 to 50 mg. may be repeated several times until sedation is achieved. Subsequently, an oral dose of 50 to 100 mg. every four to six hours should be effective in most patients (19). Perphenazine (10 to 15 mg. intramuscularly, or 8 to 16 mg. orally, either administered every four hours) has also been recommended for acutely disturbed patients (36).

It should be noted that chlorpromazine has serious disadvantages in the treatment of delirium. Adverse reactions have been reported in 12.2 percent of 556 medical patients treated with chlorpromazine (37): hypotension, tachycardia, cardiac arrest, drowsiness, coma, extrapyramidal symptoms, convulsions, hepatitis, and respiratory depression. In seven cases the drug reaction was life-threatening. Much higher frequency of adverse reactions —31.9 percent—has been reported in a similar study of psychiatric patients (38). Reactions were more frequent with higher daily doses and the intramuscular route. Jefferson (39) observed postural hypotension in 41 percent of patients receiving psychotropic drugs, mostly phenothiazines. Excessive sedation may occur with chlorpromazine. Phenothiazines may be hazardous in the geriatric, cardiac, hypertensive, and myxedematous patients, and those with hepatic disease. As Greenblatt et al. (24) caution, "Psychotropic drug treatment in medically ill patients should not be undertaken lightly." In this writer's opinion, if a delirious patient is sufficiently agitated, restless, fearful, and overactive either to directly endanger his or her health and life, or to make his or her medical management impossible, then an effective antipsychotic agent ought to be administered in an adequate dosage. The drug of choice for this purpose belongs not to the phenothiazines but to the next group of psychotropic drugs to be discussed.

Butyrophenones: The only member of this group of drugs commonly used in the United States is haloperidol. This drug is a very potent blocker of the central dopamine receptors compared to chlorpromazine (40). Since its introduction in 1958, haloperidol has been shown conclusively to have marked antipsychotic, anxiolytic, and antiemetic properties (41). The main advantages of this drug in the treatment of delirium are its effectiveness against the target symptoms of agitation, excitement, and fearfulness; its high potency; and its relatively low toxicity (41). For these reasons, haloperidol is currently the drug of choice for the management of the hyperactive delirious patient (21, 22, 25, 26, 41-46). It has been shown to be more effective than chlorpromazine in patients aged forty and over (44). It is preferred for the physically ill patient for the following reasons: it seldom causes marked hypotension; does not have known cardiotoxic effects; has relatively mild anticholinergic action; has no undesirable interaction with digitalis, diuretics, or other cardiovascular drugs; has a wide margin of safety; and seldom, if ever, causes delirium (21, 25, 26, 41, 45). Its most common side-effects are drowsiness, extrapyramidal reactions, especially acute dyskinesia and akathisia, mild hypotension, constipation, dry mouth, and blurring of vision due to anticholinergic effects (26, 41-46). Rarely, liver dysfunction with jaundice has been observed (47). Haloperidol is devoid of hypnotic effects but may indirectly promote sleep in the anxious and agitated patient. Sometimes the drug may delay sleep onset (41). Flurazepam hydrochloride may be administered at bedtime if the patient continues to suffer from insomnia despite adequate sedation.

The detoxification and inactivation of haloperidol occur largely in the liver and are accomplished by oxydative dealkylation (48). No psychoactive metabolites are produced and this helps define the relation of serum concentration of the drug to its antipsychotic effect (48). Traces of haloperidol can be found unmetabolized in the urine (48). Pharmacokinetic studies of the drug have shown that its therapeutic level in the serum could be 3 to 10 ng./ml. for many patients (49). The bioavailability of haloperidol is about 60 to 70 percent, which means that oral dose should be 1.4 to 1.7 times higher than the intramuscular one to result in equivalent serum concentration of the drug (49). Elderly patients may respond well to small doses of haloperidol (49). Barbiturates and diphenyl-hydantoin induce metabolism of haloperidol and thus depress its serum concentration (49). The serum half-lives of the drug range from ten to nineteen hours after intravenous, and twelve to thirty-eight hours after oral administration (50). Thus, administration twice daily should be sufficient in most cases. After oral administration there is a time-lag of almost 1.5 hours between ingestion and appearance of the drug in the serum. The serum concentration reaches maximum after four to six hours. After intravenous injection the peak of serum concentration and maximum sedative effect are reached within one hour. The extrapyramidal effects appear after twelve to sixteen hours (50).

Haloperidol can be administered orally in tablet form or as liquid concentrate, intramuscularly or intravenously. Ayd (51) states that intravenous administration of the drug affords rapid control of severe excitement in such conditions as delirium tremens, after a recent myocardial infarction, or in an acute postoperative psychosis. He states that this form of therapy is both safe and efficient. Dosage must be individualized and may range from 2 to 25 mg. Parenteral administration of haloperidol, even in relatively high doses, is less likely to induce extrapyramidal side effects than oral dosage (51). Dystonic reactions may be relieved rapidly by intramuscular or intravenous administration of 1 to 2 mg. benzotropine mesylate or 1 to 2 mg. biperiden (51). Subsequently, either of these drugs should be given in the same dosage every four to six hours for some four doses. The highest incidence of extrapyramidal effects has been observed in the elderly, in women, and with doses of 4 to 20 mg. daily (51). Prophylactic administration of anti-parkinsonian drugs is said to be ineffective (51).

A recent innovation in the management of the acute psychotic, including delirious, patients has been the regimen called "rapid tranquilization," which is somewhat analogous to digitalization (25, 26, 42, 45, 51-57). It involves giving intramuscular or intravenous doses of haloperidol 5 to 10 mg. every thirty to sixty minutes until tranquilization is achieved, usually after four to six injections. Subsequently, the drug is administered orally in doses one-half to two times higher than the parenteral. Moore (25) treated delirium in critically ill patients by administering haloperidol 5 to 10 mg. intramuscularly every hour until remission occurred. No patient required more than 30 mg. There were no limiting side effects. Ritter et al. (44) found haloperidol to be more effective than chlorpromazine in reducing "disordered sensorium." Similarly, Oldham (56) reports that rapid tranquilization with haloperidol was particularly effective in patients with confusional states. He asserts that cardiovascular disease, renal and hepatic insufficiency, blood dyscrasias, thyrotoxicosis, epilepsy, and acute infections constitute contraindications to high-dosage haloperidol treatment, but offers no evidence to substantiate this.

In the absence of controlled studies documenting the effects of haloperidol in the treatment of delirium due to various causes, no regimen may be regarded as clearly superior in effectiveness and safety. On the basis of the available literature and personal clinical experience the writer suggests the following guidelines.

For a severely agitated delirious adult, under sixty years, free of hepatic disease: 5 to 10 mg. intramuscularly every hour until tranquilization is achieved or severe side effects preclude further injections. One may expect that the effective total daily dose will be between 20 and 60 mg. As soon as desired tranquilization has been achieved, the patient should receive 10 to 20 mg. haloperidol orally twice a day. Intramuscular administration may have to be resorted to if the patient relapses or refuses oral medication. Intravenous route is not recommended for routine use because of the risk of severe cardiovascular complications (57). The oral dosage should be continued and gradually decreased depending on the individual patient's behavioral response. If the systolic blood pressure falls below 100 mm., treatment should stop.

An alternative treatment schedule would involve an initial dose of 5 to 10 mg. intramuscularly, followed by a repeated injection one hour later if the patient fails to respond. Otherwise, the injection is given twice or three times daily for a day or two; when adequate symptomatic control has been achieved, oral medication is started in equivalent or higher dosage. In either case, during the rapid tranquilization the patient should be recumbent and supervised.

For a mildly or moderately agitated, restless, and fearful delirious patient, lower doses are recommended. Haloperidol 5 to 15 mg. orally in the morning and at bedtime should be sufficient.

A patient sixty years old or older, or one frail and cachectic, should receive lower dosage under most circumstances. If the patient is severely restless, an initial dose of 3 to 5 mg. intramuscularly may be given and repeated after thirty minutes if no response has been observed. For milder delirium in the elderly one may use liquid concentrate in doses of 0.5 to 3 mg. twice daily (58). Extrapyramidal side effects are common in the elderly and may be controlled with benztropine mesylate 2 mg. orally at bedtime.

No absolute contraindications to haloperidol have been established. It is probably wise, however, to avoid using the drug in hepatic encephalopathy and in cases of anticholinergic delirium. It is effective in alcohol withdrawal syndrome (43) and as an adjunct in the management of barbiturate detoxification (59).

The above guidelines must be viewed as no more than that. No dogmatic or rigid dose schedule should be followed in the drug treatment of delirium, but rather a flexible regimen adjusted according to the individual patient's response. The nurse should be instructed to use her or his judgment when to administer the next dose, that is, to repeat it when the patient shows signs of renewed excitement and to delay it when the patient is asleep or appears stuporous. To avoid excessive or insufficient tranquilization, a p.r.n. order may be written to allow enough latitude in administration of the drug and while stating its maximum allowed dose over a twenty-four-hour period.

Provision of Optimal Sensory and Social Environment

Quality of the environment influences the onset, severity, and duration of delirium. Physicians since antiquity have been aware of this fact and formulated guidelines on how to modify environmental stimuli to minimize their potentially adverse effects on the delirious patient. Some of the relevant precepts were discussed earlier in this chapter, and they will now be recapitulated and expanded in the light of current knowledge and practice. One should stress that proper attention to the quality of the sensory and social environment of the physically ill is important not only for the adequate management of delirium but also for the *prevention* of its more harmful features, such as marked restlessness, agitation, panic, self-injury, attacks on others, hallucinations, and excessive autonomic arousal. Aspects of the environment that are believed to facilitate the occurrence of these undesirable features, and possibly of delirium itself, were discussed in Chapter 5. They include excessive and deficient sensory and information inputs for the patient, disruption of sleep, and stimuli provoking anxiety. We shall discuss measures to avoid these pathogenic factors.

One of the core characteristics of delirium is the patient's reduced ability to make sense of his or her environment and a related tendency to misinterpret it. This confusion is readily enhanced by surroundings that provide stimulation which is inadequate, excessive, unfamiliar, and/or ambiguous. Such sensory environment not only is more difficult for the patient to grasp but also facilitates the appearance of hallucinations and delusions, and thus increases the tendency for the patient to experience anxiety and to try to flee or fight the surroundings that he or she perceives as menacing. It is in such a setting that mishaps may occur. The following measures help prevent these undesirable developments.

The patient is best cared for in a quiet, well-lighted room with a dimmed light at night. A single room is preferable. Excessive noise and confusing sounds, such as the messages broadcast on the hospital intercom system, should be avoided. The patient should not be exposed to the bustle of a busy ward with all its unfamiliar, and thus confusing, sounds and sights. Patients tend to misinterpret these stimuli and to weave their fantasies, hallucinations, and delusions around them. On the other hand, a patient left alone for long periods, especially in a dark room, or one exposed to monotonous sounds of various apparatus, is liable to have inadequate sensory stimulation, and this may facilitate hallucinatory activity, impede spatiotemporal orientation, and promote irrational behavior. To counteract such sensory or perceptual deprivation the patient should be offered an adequate flow of orienting, reassuring, and unambiguous information. A radio or television set may help provide sensory stimulation but care should be taken that this is not counterproductive. For example, watching a noisy, violent television show is more likely to disturb the patient than calm him or her. Music has a soothing effect on many people and is a preferable source of stimulation for the agitated patient. On the other hand, a lethargic patient who has difficulty staying awake and attending to the environment may become more alert and in better contact when allowed to watch a reasonably quiet television show. Clearly, the staff have to use their judgment in adjusting the patient's environment according to his or her individual needs rather than following mechanically a set of iron rules.

Familiarity is another important aspect of the environment for a person with a compromised cerebral function. Fothergill (8) stressed one hundred years ago that a delirious patient should be treated in familiar surroundings if at all possible. Nowadays most such patients are hospitalized and thus find themselves in an unfamiliar environment. The disorganizing and threatening effects of the latter on the patient may be lessened by allowing a relative or friend whom the patient trusts to stay with him or her over and above routine visiting hours to provide a familiar social environment, help feed the patient, and administer oral medications. The relative should be told that the patient is delirious, that is, suffering from a temporary mental disturbance due to a physical illness. Such an explanation helps avoid fears that the patient has lost his or her mind, is "crazy" and will never recover. The family members should be asked to orient the patient, that is, state the date, and names of the hospital, doctors, and nurses in attendance, and also to talk about matters that interest him or her (60). Fothergill (8) quotes older authors who advised that attempts should be made "to rouse the patient's moral sentiments and affections, and to disperse his fugitive and chaotic ideas by recalling former associations and objects of affection or of ambition." Rynearson (60) rightly stresses the importance of involving the family in the care of the delirious patient to provide familiarity, enhance cognitive clarity, and counteract the sense of fear and isolation. It may also help to bring the patient a few photographs and other familiar objects and display them so that he or she can see them and be reassured by them.

Weisman and Hackett (61) have provided an excellent

example of applying the foregoing guidelines to the prevention and treatment of delirium after eye surgery. The cornerstone of their approach was a persistent attempt to provide the patients with perceptual cues to support reality testing, spatiotemporal orientation, and a sense of familiarity. Repeated explanations, encouragement, and description were employed to this end. These and other strategies discussed here are being increasingly employed in intensive care units, where the incidence of delirium tends to be relatively high. Turner (62) gives a detailed account of these measures in his book on the planning and operation of cardiovascular care units. His guidelines are relevant to other medical settings as well.

We have discussed the issues of sensory stimulation and familiarity of the environment. More needs to be said about the kind of information provided for the delirious patient. It is important to explain to him or her that he is delirious and what this implies. Since the word "delirium" is a familiar one to an average person, and is usually associated in people's minds with high fever and childhood ailments, it is not generally viewed as insanity and feared as such. The patient should be told that he or she may experience some difficulty in thinking, understanding, and remembering, and that the staff will help him or her to minimize this confusion. If hallucinations appear, they should be explained in a similar vein as transient symptoms of a physical illness and akin to waking dreams. Delusions are not to be directly challenged, but rather the patient should be offered alternative and more realistic explanations for his or her misinterpretations. For example, if the patient states that men intent on killing him are outside the room, it may help to let him get up and inspect what goes on there. It is then easier to point out that the people whom the patient sees are nurses, physicians, other patients, etc., who display no signs of hostility towards him or her. In addition to verbal information, one needs to provide other forms of it that help the patient maintain some cognitive control and thus a sense of security. A clock and a calendar should be placed in patient's sight to facilitate orientation. It is preferable to restrict the number of visitors and of staff interacting with the patient so as to avoid information overload, excitement, and fatigue. Finally, interruption of the patient's sleep should be reduced to a minimum.

Nursing Care

Nursing care of the delirious patient is most important (22, 63-68). Its cornerstones are careful observation, timely reporting, emotional support, and reorientation (64, 65). One nurse should preferably deal with the patient throughout each work shift and see the patient frequently and unhurriedly. A nurse is usually the first person to observe early symptoms of delirium and should alert the doctor in charge to this development. In this way prevention of severe disorganization and a psychiatric and medical emergency may be achieved by early diagnostic investigation, timely sedation, and close supervision of the patient. The nurses should tell the patient where he or she is, why, and what time it is. Physical restraint is best avoided since it tends to increase the patient's fear, excitement, and paranoid attitude. With close supervision and adequate and timely administration of antipsychotic drugs available nowadays, physical restraints should have no place in the management of delirium. If continuous nursing care cannot be provided and the patient is markedly disturbed, special attendants should be ordered to stay with him or her around the clock. This measure may help prevent accidents and undesirable medicolegal complications.

Gerdes (64) offers thoughtful guidelines for the nurses caring for delirious patients. She stresses that every such patient presents a different personality, educational background, intelligence, and severity of illness and of cognitive impairment. It follows that an evaluation of these factors needs to precede planning an approach to his or her general care and reorientation. Gerdes advises the nurses to focus conversations with the patient on topics that are most familiar to the latter. The nurse should try to speak clearly, in short and simple sentences, and mostly about concrete rather than abstract matters. These patients demand patience, forbearance, and understanding on the part of nursing staff. As Cohen and Klein (63) emphasize, "The nurse is a key figure in the care of the delirious patient." Her understanding of the patient's condition, calm acceptance of his or her often irrational talk and behavior, and attention to the patient's comfort and safety are key elements of good nursing care. The nurse can do a great deal to prevent and alleviate the most disturbing and hazardous aspects of delirium. The night nurse has special importance in this regard since delirium often first manifests itself and typically becomes worse during a sleepless night (17).

Psychiatric Consultation and Psychotherapy

The psychiatric consultant has a definite role to play in the management of delirium. The liaison psychiatrist is the physician most familiar with delirium, its causes, manifestations, and treatment. About 15 to 20 percent of patients referred for psychiatric consultation from medical and surgical wards and special units suffer from delirium. The role of the consultant in these cases falls into the following categories: diagnosis; advice on investigations; prescription and supervision of treatment with psychotropic drugs; counselling the staff regarding general management; and teaching how to recognize and treat delirium.

To be helpful, a psychiatric consultation should be requested as soon as delirium is suspected. Such a timely referral may enable the consultant to help prevent the development of florid symptoms and a psychiatric emergency. In the writer's experience as a liaison psychiatrist it happens all too often that an urgent consultation is requested because the patient is highly disturbed, disrupts the ward routine, threatens others, or has already managed to hurt himself or herself. Almost invariably, such an emergency had been preceded by mild delirious symptoms for hours or even days; but the staff, especially the physicians, failed to pay attention to them. Typically, a night nurse reports that the patient was awake and confused, and this information is duly recorded in the patient's chart, but no action is taken until a crisis arises.

Recognition of delirium is important not only because of its behavioral complications and the disturbance they may occasion, but also because of its medical significance. Appearance of delirium in a physically ill patient implies that cerebral function is disordered. This fact is important for several reasons:

first, it may indicate progression and/or complications of the disease; second, it may be a warning that the drugs that the patient is receiving are exerting a toxic effect; third, it may be a sign that the patient is becoming moribund; and fourth, it suggests that if the treatment is not instituted promptly, the patient may suffer irreversible brain damage. All these considerations are weighty enough to stress the importance of an early recognition and treatment of delirium and referral for psychiatric consultation to confirm the diagnosis and plan remedial measures.

The psychiatric consultant may elect to contribute directly to the patient's management as illustrated by Weisman and Hackett (61) in their paper quoted earlier. Their approach implies a form of supportive and directive psychotherapy carried out by the consultant. A different psychotherapeutic approach, called the confrontation problem-solving technique, has been employed by others (69, 70). This therapy involves presenting the patient with a statement dealing with a symptom or disturbed behavior exhibited by him or her. The statement is followed by a question: "What do you think or feel about what I told you?" This technique is claimed to enhance the patient's reality testing, capacity for reflection and self-examination, and adaptive behavior (70). The author has had no experience with this therapy, but it appears to be worth trying.

The psychiatrist may add an important dimension to the understanding and management of the delirious patient: an appraisal and appreciation of his or her personality, defenses, coping style, conflicts, fears, etc., as they are reflected in the patient's utterances and behavior. What the patient says and does in the course of delirium is not purely incidental but is rather imbued with personal meaning. To understand this meaning may help manage the patient. He or she can then be approached in a properly differentiated manner as an individual with particular concerns and ways of coping with them. The therapist's aim is to allay the patient's fear and reinforce rational control. Providing information, reorientation, and reassuring responses to the anxious and agitated delirious patient may go a long way towards calming him or her down and thus reducing the need for tranquilizing drugs. Paying careful attention to what the patient says, even if his or her talk is disjointed and incoherent, may provide useful clues to the choice of the psychological therapeutic approach. A patient expressing longing for a particular person, or the fears that his or her family have been harmed, or suspicion, or concern about death, or pregnancy or sexual fantasies offers hints regarding areas of special concern that need to be explored and their emotional charge reduced.

Finally, the liaison psychiatrist often plays the role of mediator and interpreter, or the liaison function proper, among patient, medical staff, and patient's family. This involves gathering information about the patient from all three sources, interpreting it and using it to clarify the situation for the patient, to explain his or her behavior to the staff and family, and to advise doctors, nurses, and family members how best to deal with the patient and why. Thus, the consultant may enable free flow of clarifying communications and foster understanding of the problems among all the persons involved in patient's care and the patient himself. Such a role is particularly important in the case of disturbed and disturbing delirious patients. It also has a place, however, in the mild cases and those lacking the disruptive, psychotic features. Skillful liaison may actually help prevent more florid symptoms and their complications.

Electroshock (ECT)

A number of reports published in the psychiatric literature over the past forty years have suggested that ECT may be a useful adjunct to the symptomatic treatment of delirium (71-74). Lieser (72) asserted that ECT could be life-saving in cases of delirium complicating general paralysis of the insane and the presenile dementias. Others reported the effectiveness of ECT in the management of delirium tremens and other deliria (71, 73, 74). This writer has occasionally resorted to ECT in cases where, regardless of the cause, the delirium was accompanied by severe overactivity which threatened patient's survival and failed to respond to large doses of tranquilizers. In such rare cases two or three ECT, given with all the anesthetic and medical precautions, have proved highly effective in controlling the patient's life-threatening restlessness and agitation. ECT cannot be viewed as part of routine treatment of delirium but may rarely be considered in severe and refractory cases.

In summary, the management of delirium has two major aspects: etiologic and symptomatic, respectively. Treatment of the underlying cause (or causes) is crucial and presupposes correct diagnosis of the etiology of delirium in the given patient. Symptomatic management follows these guidelines:

1. Close monitoring of the patient's mental state and behavior
2. Ensuring sleep; flurazepam hydrochloride 15 to 30 mg. at bedtime is a suitable hypnotic
3. Sedation of the restless, agitated, overactive, and/or fearful patient; haloperidol, orally or intramuscularly, is currently the drug of choice and its dosage must be adjusted for the individual patient
4. Environment should be structured so as to avoid sensory deprivation, overload, and monotony; reduce unfamiliarity; and provide adequate sensory stimulation and social support
5. Adequate nutrition, fluid intake, electrolyte balance, and vitamin supply need to be ensured
6. General nursing care, aimed at supporting the patient emotionally; provision of reorientation; and reporting symptoms are essential
7. Early psychiatric consultation is recommended
8. Electroshock may rarely be helpful

Management of delirium due to various specific conditions is discussed in Part II.

REFERENCES

1. *The Extant Works of Aretaeus, the Cappadocian.* F. Adams, Ed. London, Sydenham Society, 1861.
2. Diethelm, O.: *Medical Dissertations of Psychiatric Interest.* Basal, Karger, 1971.
3. Whitwell, J.R.: *Historical Notes on Psychiatry.* Philadelphia, Blakiston, 1937.
4. Esquirol, J.E.D.: *Mental Maladies.* New York, Hafner Publishing Co., 1965.

5. Gallway, M.B.: Nature and treatment of delirium. *Lond Med Gaz* 1:46-49, 1838.
6. Sutton, T.: *Tracts on Delirium Tremens, on Peritonitis and on Some Other Inflammatory Affections.* London, Underwood, 1813.
7. Tuke, D.H.: *A Dictionary of Psychological Medicine.* Philadelphia, Blakiston, 1892.
8. Fothergill, J.M.: The management of delirium. *The Practitioner 13*: 400-408, 1874.
9. Verco, A.: Delirium. *St Bart Hosp Rep (Lond)* 13:332-342, 1877.
10. Hirsch, W.: A study of delirium. *NY Med J* 70:109-115, 1899.
11. Rees, A.: *The Cyclopedia; or Universal Dictionary of Arts, Sciences, and Literature.* First American Edition. Vol. 12. Philadelphia, S.F. Bradford, 1818.
12. Salter, T.: Practical observations on delirium. *Prov Med Surg J* 1:677-684, 1850.
13. Graves, R.J.: Cases of violent delirium, occurring at an advanced stage of maculated or typhous fever, and treated successfully by doses of tartar emetic, frequently repeated. *Dubl J Med Sci* 9:449-466, 1836.
14. Cohen, S.: The toxic psychoses and allied states. *Am J Med* 15:813-828, 1953.
15. Greiner, F.C.: *Der Traum und das Fieberhafte Irreseyn.* Altenburg, F.A. Brockhaus, 1817.
16. Phillips, J.: Delirium. *Cleve Med J* 8:531-542, 1909.
17. Hawley, E.A.: Manifestations of delirium in the night-time. *Am J Nurs* 8:757-761, 1907/8.
18. Editorial: Organic psychosis. *Br Med J* 2:214-215, 1974.
19. Heller, S.S.: "The Organic Patient and Medical Problems," in Glick, R.A., Meyerson, A.T., Robbins, E., and Talbott, J.A., Eds., *Psychiatric Emergencies.* New York, Grune & Stratton, Inc., 1976, pp. 135-146.
20. Henry, W.D., and Mann, A.M.: Diagnosis and treatment of delirium. *Can Med Assoc J* 93:1156-1166, 1965.
21. Kiely, W.F.: Psychiatric syndromes in critically ill patients. *JAMA* 235:2759-2761, 1976.
22. Lipowski, Z.J.: "Delirium," in Conn, H.F., Ed., *Current Therapy.* 27th edition. Philadelphia, Saunders, 1975, pp. 804-806.
23. Lipowski, Z.J.: Delirium, clouding of consciousness and confusion. *J Nerv Ment Dis* 145:227-255, 1967.
24. Greenblatt, D.J., Shader, R.I., and Lofgren, S.: Rational psychopharmacology for patients with medical diseases. *Annu Rev Med* 27:407-420, 1976.
25. Moore, D.P.: Rapid treatment of delirium in critically ill patients. *Am J Psychiatry* 134:1431-1432, 1977.

26. Oldham, A.J., and Bott, M.: The management of excitement in a general hospital psychiatric ward by high dosage haloperidol. *Acta Psychiatr Scand* 47:369-376, 1971.

27. Thompson, W.L., Johnson, A.D., and Maddrey, W.L.: Diazepam and paraldehyde for treatment of severe delirium tremens. *Ann Intern Med* 82:175-180, 1975.

28. Baldessarini, R.J.: *Chemotherapy in Psychiatry.* Cambridge, Mass., Harvard University Press, 1977.

29. Brown, J.H., Moggey, D.E., and Shane, F.H.: Delirium tremens: a comparison of intravenous treatment with diazepam and chlordiazepoxide. *Scot Med J* 17:9-12, 1972.

30. Greenblatt, D.J., and Shader, R.I.: Benzodiazepines. *N Engl Med J* 291:1011-1015, 1974.

31. Sellers, E.M., and Kalant, H.: Alcohol intoxication and withdrawal. *N Engl Med J* 294:757-762, 1976.

32. Thompson, W.L.: Management of alcohol withdrawal syndromes. *Arch Intern Med* 138:278-283, 1978.

33. Editorial: Sedation in liver disease. *Br Med J* 1:1241-1242, 1977.

34. Murray-Lyon, I.M., Young, J., Parkes, J.D., Knill-Jones, R.P., and Williams, R.: Clinical and electroencephalographic assessment of diazepam in liver disease. *Br Med J* 2:265-266, 1971.

35. Greenblatt, D.J., Shader, R.I., and Koch-Weser, J.: Flurazepam hydrochloride, a benzodiazepine hypnotic. *Ann Intern Med* 83:237-241, 1975.

36. Fann, W.F., and Linton, P.H.: Use of perphenazine in psychiatric emergencies: the concept of chemical restraint. *Curr Ther Res* 14:478-482, 1972.

37. Swett, C.: Adverse reactions to chlorpromazine in medical patients. *Curr Ther Res* 18:199-206, 1975.

38. Swett, C.: Adverse reactions to chlorpromazine in psychiatric patients. *Dis Nerv Syst* 35:509-511, 1974.

39. Jefferson, J.W.: Hypotension from drugs. *Dis Nerv Syst* 35:66-71, 1974.

40. Tuck, J.R.: Effects of chlorpromazine, thioridazine and haloperidol on adrenergic transmitter mechanisms in man. *Eur J Clin Pharmarcol* 6:81-87, 1973.

41. Ayd, F.J.: Haloperidol: twenty years' clinical experience. *J Clin Psychiatry* 39:807-814, 1978.

42. Carter, R.G.: Use of oral haloperidol following rapid tranquilization of acutely disturbed patients. *West Va Med J* 74:55-56, 1978.

43. Palestine, M.L., and Alatorre, E.: Control of acute alcoholic withdrawal symptoms: a comparative study of haloperidol and chlordiazepoxide. *Curr Ther Res* 20:289-299, 1976.

44. Ritter, R.M., Davidson, D.E., and Robinson, T.A.: Comparison of

injectable haloperidol and chlorpromazine. *Am J Psychiatry 129*: 78-81, 1972.

45. Sangiovanni, F., Taylor, M.A., Abrams, R., and Gaztanaga, P.: Rapid control of psychotic excitement states with intramuscular haloperidol. *Am J Psychiatry 130*:1155-1156, 1973.

46. Stotsky, B.A.: Relative efficacy of parenteral haloperidol and thiothixene for the emergency treatment of acute excited and agitated patients. *Dis Nerv Syst 38*:967-970, 1977.

47. Fuller, C.M., Yassinger, S., Donlon, P., Imperato, T.J., and Ruebner, B.: Haloperidol-induced liver disease. *West J Med 127*:515-518, 1977.

48. Forsman, A., Folsch, G., Larsson, M., and Ohman, R.: On the metabolism of halopcridol in man. *Curr Ther Res 21*:606-617, 1977.

49. Forsman, A., and Ohman, R.: Applied pharmacokinetics of haloperidol in man. *Curr Ther Res 21*:396-411, 1977.

50. Forsman, A., and Ohman, R.: Pharmacokinetic studies on haloperidol in man. *Curr Ther Res 20*:319-336, 1976.

51. Ayd, F.J.: Haloperidol update: 1975. *Proc Roy Soc Med 69, Suppl 1*:14-22, 1976.

52. Anderson, W.H., and Kuehnle, J.C.: Strategies for the treatment of acute psychosis. *JAMA 229*:1884-1889, 1974.

53. Donlon, P.T., and Tupin, J.P.: Rapid "digitalization" of decompensated schizophrenic patients with antipsychotic agents. *Am J Psychiatry 131*:310-312, 1974.

54. Man, P.L. and Chen, C.H.: Rapid tranquilization of acutely psychotic patients with intramuscular haloperidol and chlorpromazine. *Psychosomatics 14*:59-63, 1973.

55. Reschke, R.W.: Parenteral haloperidol for rapid control of severe, disruptive symptoms of acute schizophrenia. *Dis Nerv Syst 35*: 112-115, 1974.

56. Oldham, A.J.P.: The rapid control of the acute patient by haloperidol. *Proc Roy Soc Med 69, Suppl 1*:23-25, 1976.

57. Garfinkel, P.E.: Efficient management of the acute psychotic patient: stabilization and maintenance with haloperidol. *Proc Roy Soc Med 69, Suppl 1*:26-31, 1976.

58. Godber, C.: The physician and the confused elderly patient. *J Roy Col Phys 10*:101-112, 1975.

59. Snyder, R.: Haloperidol in barbiturate detoxification. *Mil Med 142*: 885-886, 1977.

60. Rynearson, E.K.: The acute brain syndrome: a family affair. *Psychiatric Annals 7*:77-83, 1977.

61. Weisman, A.D., and Hackett, T.P.: Psychosis after eye surgery. *N Engl J Med 258*:1284-1289, 1958.

62. Turner, G.O.: *The Cardiovascular Care Unit*. New York, J. Wiley & Sons, 1978.
63. Cohen, S., and Klein, H.K.: The delirious patient. *Am J Nurs 58*:685-687, 1958.
64. Gerdes, L.: The confused or delirious patient. *Am J Nurs 68*:1228-1233, 1968.
65. McCown, P.P., and Wurm, E.: Orienting the disoriented. *Am J Nurs 65*:118-119, 1965.
66. Morris, M., and Rhodes, M.: Guidelines for the care of the confused patients. *Am J Nurs 72*:1630-1633, 1972.
67. Patrick, M.I.: Care of the confused elderly patient. *Am J Nurs 67*: 2536-2539, 1967.
68. Weymouth, L.T.: Nursing care of the so-called confused patient. *Nurs Clin North Am 3*:709-715, 1968.
69. Garner, H.: Confrontation technique applied to confusional and delirious states. *Ill Med J 137*:71-73, 1970.
70. Godbole, A., and Falk, M.: Confrontation-problem solving therapy in the treatment of confusional and delirious states. *Gerontologist 12*:151-154, 1972.
71. Dudley, W.H.C., and Williams, J.G.: Electroconvulsive therapy in delirium tremens. *Compr Psychiatry 13*:357-360, 1972.
72. Lieser, H.: Heilkrämpfe als leben-rettende Therapie. *Med Mschr 6*:350-358, 1957.
73. Roberts, A.H.: The value of ECT in delirium. *Br J Psychiatry 109*: 653-655, 1963.
74. Roth, M., and Rosie, J.M.: Use of electroplexy in mental disease with clouding of consciousness. *J Ment Sci 99*:103-110, 1953.

Additional References

Adams, M., Hanson, R., Norkool, D., et al. Psychological responses in the confused patient. *Am J Nurs 78*:1504-1512, 1978.

Anielanczyk, W. Delirious syndrome after haloperidol administration. *Psychiatria Polska (Gdansk)* 7:219-221, 1973.

Davidhizar, R., Ganden, E., and Wehlage, D. Recognizing and caring for the delirious patient. *J Psychiatr Nurs 16*:38-41, 1978.

Donlon, P.T., Hopkin, J., Schaffer, C.B., and Amsterdam, E. Cardiovascular safety of rapid treatment with intarmuscular haloperidol. *Am J Psychiatry 136*:233-234, 1979.

Donlon, P.T., Hopkin, J., and Tupin, J.P. Overview: Efficacy and safety of the rapid neuroleptization method with injectable haloperidol. *Am J Psychiatry 136*:273-278, 1979.

Forsman, A., and Öhman, R. On the objective evaluation of haloperidol effects in man: a pilot study. *Cur Ther Res 24*:179-192, 1978.

Fruensgaard, K. Parenteral treatment of acute psychotic patients with agitation: a review. *Curr Med Res Opin* 5:593-600, 1978.

Geller, B., and Greydanus, D.E. Haloperidol-induced comatose state with hyperthermia and rigidity in adolescence: Two case reports with a literature review. *J Clin Psychiatry* 40:87-88, 1979.

Greenblatt, D.J., Gross, P.L., Harris, J., et al. Fatal hyperthermia following haloperidol therapy of sedative-hypnotic withdrawal. *J Clin Psychiatry* 39:673-675, 1978.

Ketai, R., Matthews, J., and Mozdzen, J.J. Sudden death in a patient taking haloperidol. *Am J Psychiatry* 136:112-113, 1979.

McLay, W.D.S. Impaired consciousness: some grey areas of responsibility. *J Forens Sci Soc* 17:113-120, 1977.

Rosen, H.J. Double-blind comparison of haloperidol and thioridazine in geriatric outpatients. *J Clin Psychiatry* 40:17-20, 1979.

Scharbach, H. Complications psychiques des neuroleptiques. États confuso-oniriques. *Encéphale* 4:163-171, 1978.

Sellers, E.M. Clinical pharmacology and therapeutics of benzodiazepines. *Can Med Assoc J* 118:1533-1538, 1978.

Sinaniotis, C.A., Spyrides, P., Vlachos, P., and Papadatos, C. Acute haloperidol poisoning in children. *J Pediatr* 93:1038-1039, 1978.

PART II

ORGANIC CAUSES OF DELIRIUM

THE MORE COMMON organic causes of delirium are listed in Table 1, chapter 5. Their large number precludes a detailed discussion of all of them. Some of the listed factors only infrequently give rise to delirium and their clinical importance in this context is negligible. The purpose of this part is to draw attention to those substances and diseases whose association with delirium is more or less well established and which need to be considered in an attempt to determine the etiology of delirium in a given patient. Furthermore, the syndrome is common and thus practically important in certain clinical settings, such as surgical wards and recovery rooms or burn units, and in the practice of geriatrics. These special settings are dealt with separately to assist those health workers who are active in them. Emphasis is made throughout on distinct clinical features and pathophysiological mechanisms as well as on differences in the management of delirium associated with various organic factors. It is assumed that the reader is familiar with medical knowledge and terminology. This part is not intended to serve as a kind of minitextbook of medicine focused on delirium. Diagnosis, clinical features, and treatment of the various medical disorders that can give rise to this syndrome will not be dealt with here. Only information which is directly pertinent to delirium has been included. The writer has tried to keep the chapters brief and to bring out important data rather than to overwhelm the reader with a mass of details. It is a selective approach aimed at clarity in preference to completeness.

CHAPTER 10

INTOXICATION WITH MEDICAL DRUGS

A LARGE PROPORTION of the currently used drugs have been reported to give rise to delirium as one of their toxic side effects. The syndrome may be brought about by overdosage as well as by therapeutic dosage of various drugs. In the latter case one usually finds that allergy or individual sensitivity, or idiosyncrasy, to the offending agent is present, or that delirium has resulted from impairment of detoxification and/or elimination of the drug, or from synergistic action of therapeutic doses of two or more drugs on the CNS, or a combination of these factors. Inclusion of a given drug, or class of drugs, has been guided by the ease with which it can cause delirium and by its importance in medicine today.

ANTICHOLINERGIC DRUGS

Belladonna alkaloids and synthetic anticholinergics constitute the single most important group of deliriogenic substances. Their importance is related to the multiple therapeutic uses of drugs with anticholinergic properties in medicine, surgery, and psychiatry; the availability without prescription of various proprietary preparations containing anticholinergics; and the current tendency to abuse these drugs to induce altered states of consciousness, hallucinations, etc. This group of drugs constitutes one of the most common causes of delirium today. Anticholinergic delirium requires special treatment which differs from that recommended for delirium due to most other factors. Antipsychotic agents, such as phenothiazines and butyrophenones, have anticholinergic effects and are thus unsuitable for the treatment of delirium due to the drugs under discussion.

The propensity of belladonna alkaloids to cause delirium has been known since antiquity (1). Aretaeus of Cappadocia (2) listed poisoning by mandragora and hyoscyamus among the causes of phrenitis, a condition equivalent to delirium. Forbes (3) quotes Theophrastus, who described deliriogenic properties of belladonna alkaloids in the fourth century B.C.: "If you drink two drams, you will induce a greater madness; mind and eyes will see apparitions and startling fantasies. If you give three drams, he will labor under a madness from which he cannot free himself and ceaseless rages will ensue." The term "belladonna" was apparently introduced into scientific literature in the sixteenth century (3). Belladonna alkaloids were used for centuries for medicinal, religious, cosmetic, and homicidal purposes (1, 3, 4).

Belladonna alkaloids occur in plants of Solanaceae family. Deadly nightshade (*Atropa belladonna*), Jimson weed (*Datura stramonium*), devil's trumpet (*Datura metel*), dunal (*Datura metaloides*), angel's trumpet (*Datura suavolens*), and black henbane (*Hyoscyamus niger*) are the North American plants containing belladonna alkaloids and giving rise to poisoning (1, 5). These plants yield a mixture of the alkaloids atropine and scopolamine. Both these alkaloids and their methylated derivates have many uses in medicine. In addition, a large number of synthetic drugs endowed with anticholinergic properties are currently available (1). Antispasmodics, antihistamines, antiparkinsonian agents, phenothiazines, butyrophenones, and tricyclic antidepressants are the most common synthetic drugs having anticholinergic action. All of these drugs have been reported to cause delirium at times.

In Chapter 6 we discussed delirium induced experimentally with anticholinergic compounds, such as atropine, scopolamine, benactyzine, Ditran, amitriptyline, etc. With an adequate dose, delirium could be induced in all experimental subjects. Yet, the effects of anticholinergics on the central nervous system are to some extent variable and unpredictable (1). A combination of both CNS stimulation and depression is produced and characterizes a toxic state which some authors have termed the "CNS anticholinergic syndrome" (1). This designation should not be taken to imply that delirium due to anticholinergic agents has distinct psychopathological features from that caused by other factors. There is no evidence for the occurrence of drug-specific deliria with distinct identifying manifestations. Ketchum et al. (6) found that atropine, scopolamine, and Ditran produced qualitatively similar behavioral effects. The three compounds differed, however, in their potency, relative central affinity, and duration of their action. Scopolamine was found to have central potency eight to nine times that of atropine. All three drugs, given in large doses to normal volunteers, produced initial drowsiness, which progressed to stupor, and restlessness, which was at first superimposed upon reduced alertness and later tended to dominate the clinical picture. It is to be noted, however, that even therapeutic doses of scopolamine, and less often of atropine, may provoke delirium (1). Children and the elderly are particularly liable to develop delirium after small doses of anticholinergics (7). Even single doses of 1 percent scopolamine eyedrops have triggered delirium in some reported cases (8). Scopolamine ointment 0.35 percent may also have this effect (8). Atropine eyedrops are well known to bring about delirium in some patients (7). It is stated that fifteen drops of 1 percent atropine solution, containing 0.75 mg. of atropine per drop, may be sufficient to produce "mental confusion" (7).

Unusual sensitivity apart, relatively large doses of atropine and scopolamine are needed to provoke delirium. Ketchum et al. (6) found that intramuscular doses of 175 μg./kg. of atropine or 25 μg./kg. of scopolamine were adequate for this purpose. Safer and Allen (9) report that 10 μg./kg. of scopolamine administered intravenously produced delirium and that approximately four times that amount given orally would have this effect. Factors which enhance deliriogenic effect of scopolamine include: ambient temperatures higher than body temperature, sleep loss, pain, and bromides (9). Atropine doses higher than 5 to 10 mg. are usually needed to produce marked CNS effects. It is worth noting that in atropine toxicity therapy for schizophrenia doses of the drug of the order of up to 200 mg. intramuscularly have been used (10). Others used scopolamine, 5 to 50 mg. intramuscularly, for the same purpose. With these high doses, delirium was produced and followed by coma. Restlessness appeared within three-quarters of an hour after injection of the drug and was accompanied by excitement, uncoordination, confusion, and illusions and hallucinations. It is interesting to note that the restless patients could as a rule be calmed by kind reassurance (10). This underscores the importance of environmental support for reduction of anxiety and hyperactivity in delirium. Low-to-moderate (0.3-0.8 mg.) doses of scopolamine produce sedation; restlessness as a rule appears only with higher doses (9). However, paradoxical reactions in which relatively low dosage of the drug induces excitement and restlessness do occur (1).

Diagnosis of delirium due to anticholinergic agents is tentatively established when there is a history of recent intake of one or more of these drugs, and physical examination reveals presence of peripheral muscarinic blockade. The latter may suggest the etiology of delirium when history of drug exposure is absent or uncertain. The signs and symptoms of such blockade include: dilated and poorly reactive pupils, tachycardia, facial flushing, dryness of skin and mucous membranes, blurred vision, urinary urgency and difficulty in initiating micturition, rise in blood pressure, and constipation. In addition, clinical manifestations such as fever, ataxia, dysarthria, muscle twitching, hyperreflexia, convulsions, and overactivity are present in some cases (1, 6, 9-16). Granacher and Baldessarini (12, 13) advise that if the patient is an adult or adolescent, a test dose of physostigmine salicylate may help establish diagnosis. The drug is given by intramuscular or slow (to avoid convulsions) intravenous injection and in a dose of 1 to 2 mg. If no cholinergic signs appear and no change in the clinical picture appears within one-half hour, an additional 1 to 2 mg. of the drug may be injected. Pulse, mental state, and bowel motility change rapidly in response to physostigmine injection if anticholinergic intoxication is present (12). Ullman and Groh (17) found physostigmine helpful in diagnosing delirium due to over-the-counter sleeping pills. Physostigmine salicylate not only offers an effective treatment but also a diagnostic aid in anticholinergic delirium.

The following drugs, or groups of drugs, with anticholinergic properties may cause delirium:

Proprietary hypnotics. A large number of nonprescription hypnotics contain small quantities of scopolamine. Abuse of these

drugs for hallucinogenic and suicidal purposes has increased in
recent years and so has the incidence of delirium caused by them
(1, 12, 13, 14, 17, 18, 19). One recent list contains twenty-eight
different hypnotics, containing 0.125 to 0.5 mg. scopolamine per
tablet. Ten tablets of Sominex® or a similar preparation may
be enough to induce severe delirium.

Asthma powders. Belladonna alkaloids were used in the
past as treatment of asthma. Datura stramonium and Atropa
belladonna have been commonly used for this purpose (1, 11,
20, 21). Asthmador®, a nonprescription preparation, is still
popular in certain areas (11, 20). It is marketed as a powder
which is intended to be burned and its fumes to be inhaled
to provide relief from bronchospasm. Asthmador contains both
atropa and *datura* herbs, whose active principles are atropine
and scopolamine. Other asthma powders containing these
alkaloids are obtainable as cigarettes or pipe mixture. While
these preparations may occasionally produce delirium on inhalation, they have been abused by the young in recent years and
taken by mouth despite a label warning users of Asthmador
against oral intake. Gowdy (11) reviewed 212 reported cases
of intoxication with stramonium preparations taken for hallucinogenic purposes. From one to three teaspoonfuls of asthma
powder are usually dissolved in coke or beer, or swallowed
in capsules. Hallucinations were reported in nearly half of the
212 subjects; disorientation was found in about 20 percent.
Delirium induced by Asthmador is not different from that caused
by other anticholinergic preparations (20). It may last up to
twelve hours. Some persons may experience panic and paranoid
delusions during the peak of the intoxication and may exhibit
hyperactivity and combativeness.

Cycloplegics and mydriatics. Atropine, scopolamine, and
cyclopentolate have been used in eyedrops and been responsible
for a number of cases of delirium (1, 7, 8, 13, 22). As was
mentioned earilier, even a small number of drops may induce
delirium in the elderly, in children, and in subjects having
idiosyncrasy to these drugs (1, 8, 13). It is believed that delirium
due to eyedrops follows their being swallowed in tears and
absorbed from the gastrointestinal tract. It is claimed that fifteen

drops of 1 percent atropine solution may be sufficient to pre-cipitate delirium (7).

Antihistamines. Most of these agents have anticholinergic properties and may produce delirium. Orphenadrine (23), dimen-hydrinate (24, 25), diphenhydramine (26), and other anti-histamines (1, 27, 28) have been reported on occasion to cause it. Physostigmine (26) and tacrine (28) have been used to successfully reverse delirium due to some of these drugs.

Anti-parkinsonian agents. Belladonna alkaloids have been largely replaced by synthetic atropine-like drugs in the treatment of extrapyramidal motor disorders. These newer drugs, such as benztropine, trihexyphenidyl, and procyclidine, have all been reported to cause delirium in some patients (1, 29-33). Persons of all age-groups are susceptible to this complication and may develop it on therapeutic doses of the drugs (29). Individual susceptibility has been blamed for the occurrence of delirium in some cases (32). Benztropine mesylate is widely used for the control of extrapyramidal side effects of psychotropic drugs, and most cases of delirium have been reported in patients who were receiving both antipsychotic medications and benztropine (29, 32, 33). The incidence of benztropine delirium among psychiatric patients is reported to be low (29). The syndrome may come on within several hours of the first dose of benztropine and usually clears up within one week after withdrawal of the drug (29). As little as 2 mg. of the drug may produce delirium in some subjects (29). Physostigmine has been used success-fully for reversal of delirium and other toxic effects of these drugs (34).

Antispasmodics. Anticholinergic drugs are used as spasmo-lytics in a wide range of gastrointestinal disorders. Despite widespread use of these drugs singly and in combination with other agents, there are relatively few reports of delirium believed to be caused by them (1, 35, 36). Lomotil®, a spasmolytic preparation used for the symptomatic treatment of diarrhea, contains diphenoxylate hydrochloride 2.5 mg. and atropine sul-phate 0.025 mg. and may occasionally give rise to anticholinergic delirium in an abnormally sensitive person, usually a child (37).

Anticholinergic premedicants. Atropine and scopolamine

(hyoscine) have been widely used as part of premedication for the reduction of secretions, protection against vagal overactivity, sedation, and amnesia (38). Scopolamine has been used since 1902 to produce "twilight sleep," or rather amnesia, during labor (39). Common doses for premedication are 0.6 mg. of atropine and 0.4 mg. of scopolamine (hyoscine) (38). Kuhn and Savage (40) state that delirium occurs in about 20 percent of patients premedicated with scopolamine and can be reversed with physostigmine. They found that substitution of methscopolamine bromide for scopolamine hydrobromide sharply reduced the incidence of postoperative delirium. Scopolamine-induced delirium may occur in as many as 10 percent of women undergoing obstetrical anesthesia (1).

Antipsychotic drugs. Delirium induced by chlorpromazine and other phenothiazine derivatives used as antipsychotic agents has been reported by many authors since 1955 (41-48). Angst and Hicklin (41) claim that the incidence of delirium due to neuroleptics and antidepressants is 1 to 3 percent. Such incidence, however, is considerably higher with the latter drugs than with antipsychotic agents (48). Delirium with phenothiazine derivatives occurs most often in patients aged fifty years and over and those brain-damaged (41, 45). Helmchen (45) observed delirium in seventeen women treated with phenothiazines and other psychotropic drugs. These patients were more than fifty years old, and most of them displayed signs of cerebral disease. The delirium tended to follow rapid increases or decreases in dosage. Some of the women experienced prodromal symptoms of loss of energy and increased extrapyramidal motor activity.

Deliriogenic potential of an antipsychotic drug depends on two factors: central cholinergic activity and propensity for sedative-hypnotic effects (46). Chlorprothixene, thioridazine (12), and chlorpromazine are much more likely to cause delirium than fluphenazine, for example (46). High initial doses and combinations of drugs with anticholinergic activity are factors predisposing to delirium (41, 42). Some authors claim that psychological stress may be another predisposing factor (41). Physostigmine is effective in counteracting delirium due to phenothiazines (12, 13). Avoidance of polypharmacy, especially of combining several antipsychotic agents, or an antipsychotic drug with anti-parkinsonian, tricyclic antidepressant, and/or sedative drugs, should help prevent delirium. Furthermore, lower doses of these drugs are indicated in the treatment of the elderly and the brain-damaged.

Antidepressants. Tricyclic antidepressants have anticholinergic properties and have long been known to produce delirium (12, 13, 41, 45-52). Amitriptyline is particularly likely to give rise to this complication and has actually been used to induce delirium experimentally in subjects with alcoholic brain damage. Angst and Hicklin (41) state that incidence of delirium with antidepressants is between 1 and 3 percent. Helmchen and Hippius (46) report that delirium occurred in 7.9 percent of 152 patients treated with amitriptyline. The combination of relatively potent anticholinergic activity and sedative properties is probably responsible for the propensity of this drug to cause delirium. Davies et al. (47) have studied "confusional episodes" produced by antidepressants. They defined the episodes as a behavioral change "characterized by impaired orientation or memory or other evidence of acute intellectual impairment," with or without delusions or hallucinations. This definition indicates that the episodes represented delirium. They found the overall incidence of confusional episodes to be 13 percent, with the incidence of 35 percent in those aged forty and over. This is a much higher frequency of delirium than that reported by others (41, 46). The difference may reflect more permissive diagnostic criteria used by Davies et al. The confusional episode usually developed during the first two weeks following the administration of antidepressants and seemed to represent an idiosyncratic response to these drugs rather than one related to their dosage. The average episode lasted a week, but the duration could be as long as three weeks. The episodes had no tendency to recur even if medication was gradually reinstituted. Davies et al. found no evidence of dilated pupils or difficulty voiding in their confused patients; the majority also had a normal EEG. They do not mention the possibility that the episodes could represent anticholinergic delirium.

Tricyclic antidepressants may produce delirium which is

responsive to physostigmine, and yet may not show the striking peripheral parasympatholytic and pupillary signs seen with belladonna alkaloids (12, 13). Antimuscarinic potency of these drugs is much lower than that of scopolamine, atropine, trihexyphenidyl (Artane®), and benztropine (Cogentin®) (13). Nevertheless, tricyclic antidepressants seem capable of producing central anticholinergic toxicity even in ordinary doses, especially in the elderly (52). The prevalent current view is that delirium due to antidepressants represents central anticholinergic toxicity. In the past ten years a number of reports have documented the effectiveness of physostigmine in reversing delirium and other manifestations of intoxication with tricyclics (12, 13, 48-50).

Delirium due to antidepressant drugs may occur with average doses as well as with overdoses. In the latter cases it may usher in and/or follow coma or be the main behavioral manifestation of toxicity. Amitriptyline appears to be more potentially deliriogenic than imipramine and other tricyclics (46). Amitriptyline has the highest antimuscarinic potency of the tricyclic antidepressants (13).

Miscellaneous anticholinergic deliriants. Benzquinamide, an antiemetic agent, has recently been reported to produce delirium, which was successfully reversed with physostigmine (53). Various herbal medicines containing atropine and scopolamine have caused delirium (54).

Plants containing belladonna alkaloids are a common cause of anticholinergic delirium (1, 5, 12, 55-58). Although they are not medical drugs, these plants may be conveniently mentioned here, especially since poisoning caused by them needs to be considered in the differential diagnosis of anticholinergic delirium. Ingestion of Solanaceae plants may be accidental, especially in children, or deliberate for the purpose of inducing hallucinations. Jimson weed poisoning due to its deliberate ingestion appears to be on the increase, and delirium caused by it has been reported lately (55, 57). The EEG in Jimson weed delirium shows diffuse slowing of background activity, loss of alpha, and periodic bursts of slow activity. Delirium due to ingestion of Angel's trumpet has been reported to be increasing as a result of the growing popularity of this plant as a hallucinogen (58). The mushroom, **Amanita muscaria,** may at times produce a central anticholinergic syndrome (13). Delirium and other toxic effects of these plants and mushrooms are best treated with physostigmine (13, 55-58).

Treatment of Anticholinergic Delirium

For centuries the treatment of delirium due to belladonna alkaloids was purely symptomatic. Pedigo (59) wrote in 1888 that "opium, preferably in the form of hypodermic morphia, has held the highest place in the treatment of such cases." He noted that no specific antidote to belladonna existed and reported successful treatment of atropine poisoning with amyl nitrite. Pedigo was evidently unaware that twenty-four years earlier Kleinwächter (60) had treated atropine delirium with Calabar extract, which contains physostigmine, and had written that the favorable response of a severely intoxicated patient to Calabar was so prompt and distinct that one had to assume a cause and effect relationship. Kleinwächter declared that it would be necessary to carry out research to establish if Calabar extract would prove to be a potent antidote to atropine. This remarkable observation waited nearly 100 years to be appreciated and clinically applied. In 1949 Forrer (10) developed atropine toxicity therapy for schizophrenia, giving large doses of the drug intramuscularly. He found that physostigmine administered intravenously could reverse the central and peripheral effects of very high doses of atropine. Vojtechovsky et al. (61) tried but failed to reverse delirium experimentally induced by benactyzine with physostigmine. In 1967, Crowell and Ketchum (62) reported that physostigmine was effective in reversing delirium induced with scopolamine in healthy volunteers. In 1968, Duvoisin and Katz (63) reported excellent results with treating anticholinergic delirium with physostigmine and suggested that the latter could be used as an effective antidote against drugs possessing central anticholinergic properties. During the past ten years numerous reports have supported and extended this contention (1, 12, 13, 17, 25, 39, 48, 50, 53, 58, 62-64).

Granacher and Baldessarini (12, 13) recommend the following procedures for treatment with physostigmine:

1. Evaluation of the patient, with special attention to vital signs, pupillary size and responsiveness to light, bowel

sounds, urinary output, appearance of skin, and mental status;

2. Diagnostic dose, if etiology is unknown and anticholinergic delirium is suspected. Physostigmine salicylate (Antilirium) 1 mg. subcutaneously is given. If the person had taken anticholinergic drugs, the peripheral signs of muscarinic blockade will change only slightly or not at all; in the absence of such intake, cholinergic signs should appear in eleven to thirty minutes, and include lacrimination, miosis, sweating, salivation, and bradycardia;

3. Treatment begins with 1 or 2 mg. of physostigmine by intramuscular or slow intravenous injection. If no cholinergic signs and no clinical change appear in fifteen to thirty minutes, a second injection of 1 or 2 mg. should be given. If toxic signs persist or the patient relapses, further doses of physostigmine should be administered every thirty minutes to two hours. Treatment should be continued until clinical state improves or cholinergic toxicity develops;

4. Monitor changes in pulse, temperature, bowel motility, urine output, orientation, and recent memory;

5. Diazepam may be given in mild cases, or if physostigmine is not immediately available. An initial dose of 40 mg. orally, or 10 mg. intramuscularly, to be followed by 10 mg. every four hours;

6. Phenothiazines should not be used on account of their anticholinergic properties;

7. Atropine sulphate must be available to counteract physostigmine toxicity if such develops.

A striking response of delirium to the first injection of physostigmine may occur within one-half hour. In children and the elderly the dosage of physostigmine should be about 50 percent lower than in adults: 0.5 mg. initially, repeated, if necessary, every twenty minutes for a total of 2 mg. (13). Rumack (64) recommends 0.5 mg. by slow intravenous injection. If the child continues to show toxic effects and no clinical change occurs, the drug should be repeated at five-minute intervals until a maximum dose of 2 mg. has been reached.

Contraindications to physostigmine include asthma, diabetes, gangrene, coronary artery disease, heart block, peptic ulcer, ulcerative colitis, mechanical obstruction of bowel or bladder, glaucoma, pregnancy, hypothyroidism, and myotonia congenita and atrophica (13). Excessive or too rapid an administration of physostigmine may induce heart block, central and peripheral respiratory paralysis, bronchospasm, laryngospasm, and convulsions (13). Atropine sulphate, 0.5 mg., can be given by injection to counteract each milligram of physostigmine injected (13).

Physostigmine has been used to reverse delirium and coma due to drugs having anticholinergic effects and also to benzo-diazepines and barbiturates, which lack anticholinergic activity (65-67). The results with the latter two groups of agents have been variable (65), yet successful reversal of symptoms due to diazepam and lorazepam has been reported (66, 67). It appears that in these cases physostigmine acts as an analeptic. It causes an arousal response in the EEG and probably stimulates the reticular activating system (67). Physostigmine should not be viewed as a universal antideliriant drug, however. It has been proven ineffective in delirium tremens, for example (68).

Anticholinergic Delirium: Explanatory Hypotheses

The precise mechanism of anticholinergic delirium and of the action of physostigmine in its reversal are still obscure. There is striking individual variation in susceptibility to the deliriogenic effects of anticholinergic drugs. Some people become delirious after a dose of atropine or scopolamine of less than one milligram, while others may tolerate much higher doses without developing delirium. Itil and Fink (69) hypothesize that anticholinergic drugs, such as Ditran, change the balance of noradrenergic and cholinergic mechanisms in the medial ascending reticular activating system and the medial thalamic diffuse projection systems. As a result of the concurrent stimulation of these systems there is both cortical inhibition and excitation, a combination which causes delirium. Drachman (70) maintains that central cholinergic neurons are crucially involved in memory and learning. Cholinergic blockade results in memory impairment and cognitive deficits. Petersen (71) carried out experimental studies with scopolamine and found that the drug had its primary effect on the acquisition of new material and a minimal effect on the retrieval of already stored information. He raised and rejected the possibility that scopolamine might affect acquisition of new information as a result of impairment of attention. Petersen leans towards the hypothesis that scopolamine may interfere with the transfer of information from short to long-term memory. Since the hippocampal region is a cholinergic area that is probably involved in such a transfer, and scopolamine is an anticholinergic drug, it could conceivably bring about this type of memory pathology.

Drachman (70) raised the question whether scopolamine interferes with cognitive functions by reducing alertness or by direct interference with cholinergic neurons subserving memory and learning. He compared the effectiveness of physostigmine and d-amphetamine in reversing cognitive impairments induced by scopolamine in man and found that immediate memory was not impaired by the latter drug. Physostigmine produced no significant impairment on memory or cognitive tests. Physostigmine plus scopolamine largely reversed cognitive deficits induced by the latter drug alone. D-amphetamine plus scopolamine improved alertness but produced no significant improvement in cognitive functioning, and caused further deterioration in word storage. Drachman concludes that cholinergic neurons play a specific role in human memory and learning which appears to be independent of alertness and attention. This study does not, however, rule out the possibility that scopolamine, given in a dose sufficient to produce delirium, may affect both the cholinergic neurons in the hippocampal structures and the ascending cholinergic reticular system involved in cortical arousal, and thus impair concurrently acquisition and processing of information as well as alertness and wakefulness.

Physostigmine may exert dual action: it may counteract cholinergic blockade in the hippocampal structures and stimulate the reticular activating system. The latter activity is suggested by the ability of physostigmine to reverse sedation and coma due to agents as diverse as benzodiazepines and ketamine. At the same time, the drug is ineffective in delirium tremens, in which noradrenergic mechanisms seem to be predominantly involved, and sedation is absent. Physostigmine has been found to improve amnestic syndrome in a postencephalitic patient (72). This was interpreted as being due to central cholinergic potentiation in the limbic system. It was observed that the patient displayed improved selective attention and goal-directed behavior after physostigmine, an effect suggestive that the drug may enhance both vigilance and memory. Davis et al. (73) report that physostigmine infusion in normal subjects produced lethargy and impaired short-term memory, in contrast to *small doses* of anticholinergic agents. Ketchum et al. (6) state that after large doses of anticholinergic drugs the experimental subjects showed striking impairment of immediate and slightly delayed recall, and of attention span.

Anticholinergic delirium involves impairment of attention as well as memory and learning. Physostigmine appears to counteract both of these impairments by improving activation and, probably, memory storage and retrieval in the hippocampal structures. Elucidation of the role of the various brain areas and neurotransmitter mechanisms in anticholinergic delirium could throw new light on the pathophysiology of the syndrome as a whole. Meanwhile, this delirium appears to be increasing in frequency and poses a major health problem. Physostigmine provides the most effective antidote to it at present, but the effectiveness of other anticholinesterases, such as tetrahydro-aminocrin (tacrin), is worthy of further assessment.

SEDATIVES AND HYPNOTICS

Sedative-hypnotic drugs are the most often prescribed medications in the world today. One hundred twenty-eight million prescriptions for these drugs were filled in the United States in 1976 (74). Hypnotics alone accounted for 27 million prescriptions. Sedative-hypnotic drugs were involved in 35 percent of drug-related deaths in the United States in 1977 (74). Barbiturates alone accounted for 18 percent of these deaths and were thus second only to narcotics in this regard.

The incidence of delirium caused by these drugs is unknown. It appears, however, that intoxication rather than delirium is the most common psychiatric syndrome induced by them. Essig

(75) defines intoxication caused by sedatives and hypnotics as a syndrome consisting of drowsiness, impaired mentation, and motor incoordination. Isbell et al. (76) list confusion among the symptoms of chronic barbiturate intoxication and state that psychosis characterized by disorientation and unsystematized paranoid delusions occurs occasionally in the chronically intoxicated subject. "Impaired mentation" and "confusion" are terms indicative of some degree of impairment of cognitive functions, and their use in this context suggests that there is no sharp boundary between the syndromes of intoxication and delirium, respectively. In both of these conditions there is a disturbance of awareness and alertness, but delirium is a term reserved for a disorder in which global cognitive impairment sets in acutely, tends to fluctuate unpredictably over a twenty-four-hour period, and lasts no more than a few weeks. Hallucinations and unsystematized delusions are often present in delirium, but they are not a feature of simple intoxication. Delirium as defined in this book is a relatively uncommon complication of either acute or chronic poisoning with sedative-hypnotics. Bromides constitute the only exception to this general rule.

Kornetsky et al. (77) assert that the effects of drugs on cognitive performance are determined not only by the pharmacological activity of the given drug, but also by the specific reactivity of the person to it, and by the interaction of these two variables. Specific reactivity in this context includes idiosyncratic responses to the drug which may be manifested by paradoxical excitement or rage instead of sedation, or by delirium. The latter may thus result from an overdose of a sedative-hypnotic drug, or from an idiosyncratic response to a therapeutic dose of it. Furthermore, delirium is a common manifestation of the withdrawal syndrome from barbiturates and other hypnotic-sedative drugs, with the exception of bromides, which do not seem to lead to a withdrawal syndrome. These drugs will now be discussed as they pertain to delirium. Withdrawal syndromes are dealt with in Chapter 11.

Barbiturates. These drugs were introduced in 1903, and already in 1905 a report appeared, reporting delirium precipitated by barbital in a tuberculous woman (78, p. 61). Subsequent reports of both acute and chronic barbital intoxication showed that delirium was a relatively uncommon manifestation of such poisoning (78). Isbell et al. (76) state that a psychosis characterized by disorientation and paranoid delusions, presumably delirium, is seen only occasionally in patients with chronic barbiturate intoxication. These investigators studied the effects on humans of both large single doses and of chronic administration of barbiturates. In neither case did they observe delirium. None of their chronically intoxicated subjects displayed disorientation, hallucinations, or delusions. Acute poisoning by an overdose of barbiturates, or that due to hypersensitivity to these drugs, typically results in coma, but delirium not uncommonly precedes the onset of the latter and as a rule follows the emergence from unconsciousness. Acute poisoning most often results from ingestion for suicidal purposes, but it may also occur when a barbiturate drug is taken in combination with another CNS depressant, such as alcohol or an opiate, or with an anticholinergic agent. Such a combination appears to favor the occurrence of delirium, as exemplified by children who became delirious following administration of an antihistamine-barbiturate antiemetic medication (79) and by adults treated with both a barbiturate and diphenylhydantoin, chlordiazepoxide, lithium or an MAO inhibitor (80). Barbiturates may precipitate an attack of acute intermittent porphyria or hepatic encephalopathy and thus cause delirium indirectly. A similar effect may follow administration of barbiturates in patients with chronic pulmonary or renal insufficiency or hypothyroidism.

Delirium due to barbiturates is particularly likely to occur in the elderly. Gibson (81) points out that many a confused elderly person is receiving barbiturates, which may be responsible for the confusion. She describes one patient who became "excited and hallucinated throughout the night" following one dose of 200 mg. of amylobarbitone sodium. Robinson (82) asserts that a small dose of barbiturates may readily precipitate delirium in the older patients. This generally held opinion was challenged by McDonald et al. (83), who reported that amylobarbitone sodium given in a dose of 300 mg. at bedtime did not aggravate confusion in a group of elderly female psychogeriatric patients. Despite this finding we believe that barbiturates should not be given to geriatric patients because of the increased risk of inducing delirium even by therapeutic doses. *Chloral hydrate.* This hypnotic was introduced in 1869 and not long afterwards reports on its abuse appeared in the German psychiatric literature (78). Drowsiness with optic and auditory hallucinations are common features of chloral delirium. Lilliputian and haptic hallucinations are not uncommon. According to de Boor (78), Kraepelin studied psychiatric disorders due to chloral hydrate and found that they took the form of either delirium or hallucinosis. Visual hallucinations tended to resemble hypnagogic ones and often involved animals. The auditory hallucinations were found by Kraepelin to be mostly in the form of threatening and frightening voices. Margetts (84) reviewed exhaustively the reports of delirium due to chloral hydrate and described a case of his own, a woman who abused the drug. Margetts states that a number of famous men, such as Rossetti and Nietzsche, became addicted to chloral hydrate. The popularity of this drug has diminished in recent years and reports of delirium due to it have stopped.

Paraldehyde. Introduced in 1881, this drug is occasionally abused by alcoholics who became familiar with and dependent on it. The familiarity usually follows treatment of alcohol withdrawal syndrome with paraldehyde. Some persons prefer this drug to alcohol because they experience a faster and more satisfying response to it than they do to alcohol. Delirium due to paraldehyde intoxication has been described mostly in the German literature (78). The drug may be abused for a long time before delirium sets in. The latter does not seem to have any distinct characteristics.

Bromides. This group of sedatives was introduced into therapy in 1840 and achieved great popularity as well as notoriety, the latter due to the frequency of psychiatric complications following their use and abuse. A large literature on the mental disorders due to the intake of bromides has accumulated over the last 130 years and has continued into the 1970s despite decreased clinical use of this group of drugs. Recent reports stress that bromide abuse and intoxication constitute "a continuing problem" (85) and "a persistent peril" (86). There is little doubt, however, that bromism has become an uncommon condition in the United States (87). A recent survey of records at the Johns Hopkins Hospital over a period of twenty-three years reveals that only twenty-two patients were discharged with the diagnosis of bromide intoxication (87). The current source of the latter is mostly the continued use of proprietary compounds containing sodium, potassium, and/or ammonium bromides. Six such compounds were still on sale in the United States in 1976 (87). In addition, bromoureides, acyclic derivatives of urea containing bromide, are available on prescription and may cause bromism (88).

Levin (89) classifies psychiatric syndromes due to bromides as follows: 1. simple intoxication; 2. delirium; 3. transitory schizophrenia; and 4. hallucinosis. It appears that delirium is the most common of these four syndromes. Levin reports that of a group of seventy-four patients with bromide psychoses, 65 percent displayed delirium. The latter is usually seen in patients aged forty years and over. Bromide delirium occurs more often in women. It is typically preceded by simple intoxication for some days or weeks and usually lasts several days to weeks after discontinuation of the drug (89). Occasionally, bromide delirium may be followed by death or by a prolonged paranoid psychosis (90). The symptoms include disorientation; disorder of thinking; fear, depression, or emotional lability; hallucinations and illusions; transient delusions; and restlessness. Levin (91) describes a variety of visual symptoms in bromide delirium, such as photophobia; distortions of color, form, position, and size of perceived objects; delusions concerning the eyes; and frequent visual illusions and hallucinations. Pupils are often dilated and react sluggishly to light, and Argyll Robertson pupils may occur. Some observers stress that extreme excitement is a characteristic feature of bromide delirium (92). Confabulation may accompany memory impairment in the latter. In addition to the symptoms of delirium, the patients usually display neurological and dermatological signs. The former include slurred speech, ataxia, positive Romberg test, absent gag reflex, generalized muscular weakness, tremor, nystagmus, extensor plantar reflexes, deep reflex changes, dilated pupils, and ptosis (86, 87, 91-93). Cerebrospinal fluid may show increased pressure and protein concentration. The EEG shows diffuse slowing of background activity which may persist for weeks or even months after clinical recovery (86, 93). The skin is sometimes affected by an acneiform rash.

Diagnosis of bromide delirium may be difficult on clinical grounds alone. Laboratory tests are essential for correct diagnosis. The normal bromide content of the serum varies from 0.1 to 3.7 mg. per 100 ml. (88). There is disagreement about what serum bromide levels should be regarded as indicative of toxicity. It is reported that intoxication may occur with levels as low as 60 mg. per 100 ml. (86), but one usually finds higher serum bromide concentrations in a delirious patient. Levels of 150 mg. per 100 ml. and higher are more usual. There is no correlation between the severity of symptoms shown by the patient and the serum bromide level (86). Delirium may occur if relatively low levels have persisted for some weeks or months, as is the case in chronic intoxication. Wide variation in individual susceptibility to the effects of bromide ion exists. Cerebrovascular disease, renal insufficiency, and malnutrition tend to increase such susceptibility.

Trump and Hochberg (87) point out that an inappropriate elevation of the serum chloride may be the first clue to the diagnosis of bromism. The autoanalyzer method of measuring serum chloride concentration is the method that can show hyperchloremia in the cases of bromism. The Cotlove chloride titrator will not show excess chloride in the presence of bromide intoxication. It is claimed that a replacement of more than 40 percent of the chlorides by bromides in the blood is lethal, and that intoxication becomes manifest after at least 25 percent of the total halogens have been replaced by bromide (92). It follows that susceptibility to bromism is in part dependent on the amount of sodium chloride in the diet and increases when such intake is low. A saliva test for bromide has been recommended for identification of bromism, but serum bromide levels are still the usual diagnostic test (88).

Treatment of bromide delirium involves administration of ammonium chloride 6 g. per day and meralluride 2 cc. every day or every second day. Ethacrynic acid and mannitol have also been recommended. The objective is to achieve chloride loading and to speed up bromide excretion by diuresis (86, 87, 92). Haloperidol may be used to control excessive excitement. Hemodialysis may be necessary in severe cases and those with oliguria or an unstable cardiovascular system (87). Return to the premorbid state tends to lag behind the elimination of bromides from the system. Symptoms may persist for a few weeks after beginning of treatment or recur episodically apparently in response to rebound of serum bromide related to the movement of bromide ion from intracellular and extracellular compartments as a result of the concentration gradient brought about by diuresis (86). Prognosis with proper treatment is good. Even cases with extremely high serum bromide levels have been successfully treated (94).

Benzodiazepines. Diazepam, chlordiazepoxide, and oxazepam are among the most commonly prescribed drugs today. They have replaced barbiturates as anti-anxiety agents of choice. Flurazepam hydrochloride is the most commonly prescribed hypnotic among hospitalized medical patients (95). Intoxication with this group of drugs is usually manifested by drowsiness, tremor, and ataxia. "Confusion" is sometimes mentioned as a less common manifestation of the intoxication. This writer has not, however, found a single well-documented report of delirium due to intoxication with these drugs. Greenblatt et al. (96) quote a single report of "paradoxical delirium and confusion" ascribed to flurazepam. Shader et al. (97) review studies on the toxicity of benzodiazepines and mention "confusion-excitement-agitation" among the side effects of these drugs, but give no details regarding "confusion." Greenblatt et al. (95) report that flurazepam tends to cause "unwanted central nervous system depression" with higher doses and especially in the elderly. The commonest adverse reactions to benzodiazepines are drowsiness, confusion, and ataxia (98). Hall and Joffe (99) describe an "aberrant response" to diazepam consisting of tremulousness, apprehension, insomnia, depression, and suicidal ideation. Several patients were said to experience nocturnal confusion and memory deficit. It is not clear, although possible, that this aberrant response represented a mild delirium. Viscott (100) reported several cases of vivid hallucinations occurring after administration of chlordiazepoxide. The hallucinations were visual and occasionally auditory, came on just before or after awakening, and lasted several minutes. Some of the affected patients reacted to the visions as if they were real.

The anecdotal and sketchy reports quoted above suggest that delirium may be occasionally caused by benzodiazepines, but its occurrence, if any, appears to be rare. These drugs can cause physical dependence, and a withdrawal syndrome with delirium has occasionally been reported (see Chapter 11).

Miscellaneous sedative-hypnotics. Meprobamate, glutethimide, methyprylon, ethchlorvynol, ethinamate, and methaqualone can all cause both acute and chronic intoxication resembling that due to barbiturates. All of these drugs have addictive potential, and abstinence syndrome, sometimes manifested by delirium, may result from abrupt withdrawal of high doses of them. Intoxication with these drugs is characterized by drowsiness, impaired thinking, and ataxia. Disorientation, memory impairment, confusion, and dissociative or rage reactions have been observed in some intoxicated subjects (101). Gerald and Schwirian (102) report that adverse reactions to acute methaqualone intake include 'disorientation with respect to personal identity or location" and, very occasionally, impairment of memory. Delirium apparently due to glutethimide has been reported (103, 104). This drug has some anticholinergic activity, and patients intoxicated with it may show signs of peripheral muscarinic blockade (1). The presence of dilated pupils and other signs of the blockade in patients with glutethimide delirium should not lead to a diagnosis of an anticholinergic delirium.

The nonbarbiturate sedatives and hypnotics can cause intoxication whose manifestations may at times include delirium. The incidence of the latter is unknown but appears to be low. All these drugs can, if taken in excessive dosage and for a long time, result in physical dependence, and their rapid withdrawal can cause delirium. Such withdrawal delirium has been reported far more often than that due to intoxication.

NARCOTIC ANALGESICS

Opiates. In therapeutic amounts opiates can induce delirium, apparently on the basis of idiosyncrasy to these drugs (105, 106).

Morphine appears to cause delirium very rarely (78, 106). Miller and Jick (106) have found no cases of it among a large sample of hospitalized patients who had received the drug. *Meperidine*, on the other hand, was found to induce disorientation, bizarre feelings, hallucinations, or psychosis in 0.4 percent of over 3,000 hospitalized subjects who had received the drug parenterally. MacVicar (107) observed delirium after only two or three injections of meperidine administered for pain relief. The symptoms were dramatic: visual and auditory hallucinations, severe agitation, fear, and attempts to run out of the hospital. The delirium began with anxiety, was worse at night, and lasted up to three days. Chlorpromazine 50 to 100 mg. intramuscularly was reportedly effective in terminating it.

Pentazocine. The N- allyl derivative of the narcotic agent phenazocine, pentazocine was introduced in 1967 as a parenteral analgesic. In 1969 it became approved for oral usage. The drug has both narcotic agonist and antagonist properties and has become widely used for relief of acute and chronic pain. Shortly after its introduction, reports of hallucinations induced by it began to appear (108). In addition, confusion and disorientation were reported. The incidence of perceptual disturbances and other psychiatric side effects after therapeutic doses of the drug is variously reported as ranging from 1 to 10 percent (109, 110). Miller (110) found that hallucinations, disorientation, bizarre feelings, and vertigo were the most common adverse effects of pentazocine among about 1,400 patients hospitalized for various medical problems. Several of the hallucinating patients were reportedly "frankly psychotic" and displayed paranoid delusions. The psychotomimetic side effects were found to be dose related (111). Investigators at the Mayo Clinic observed confusion in four out of thirty patients who abused pentazocine and delirium in two who had also abused sedatives. Even though in most cases the reported psychotomimetic reactions (hallucinations, bizarre feelings, nightmares) were dose related, in some cases they were induced by only one dose of pentazocine 30 mg. intramuscularly (112). One must ask, of course, if the so-called psychotomimetic side effects of the drug represent delirium or some other organic brain syndrome.

Unfortunately, poor quality of the published reports makes it difficult to be certain in this regard. The various psychiatric adverse effects of the drug are said to include visual, tactile, and kinesthetic hallucinations, delusions, nightmares, euphoria, dysphoria, feelings of depersonalization, panic, and abnormal thoughts (113). All of these symptoms may occur in delirium but are not sufficient for its diagnosis. Description of some of the reported side effects suggests that in at least a proportion of the cases hallucinosis, rather than delirium, was present (108). Yet unequivocal cases of pentazocine-induced delirium have been reported (112, 114, 115). In one reported case the delirium induced by one injection of the drug persisted for a week (112). Kane and Pokorny (114) describe two patients who developed delirium apparently due to pentazocine. One experienced auditory hallucinations and had a vision of Christ reaching out his arms to her. The other patient, a parturient woman, had colored hallucinations of a baby with a deformed head. These psychotomimetic effects of the drug may be related to a rapid depletion of brain noradrenaline and dopamine caused by it (114).

There seems to be little doubt that pentazocine can induce delirium, but the occurrence of this complication appears to be quite low. Pentazocine abuse and withdrawal syndrome have been reported (111, 114). Withdrawal of the drug from a person who has abused it is not accompanied by delirium. When a patient complains of hallucinations, anxiety, nightmares, confusion, depersonalization, and bizarre thoughts following administration of pentazocine, one should view such symptoms as prodromata of delirium and switch to a different analgesic so as to avoid full development of the syndrome.

Psychotomimetic effects have been frequently observed following administration of narcotic antagonists such as *nalorphine* and *levallorphan* (110).

NONNARCOTIC ANALGESICS

Salicylic acid. Salicylic acid and its derivatives are among the most commonly used drugs. Each day 20 to 30 tons of aspirin are consumed in the United States (116). Salicylism accounts for about 25 percent of all poisonings. Intoxication with salicylates (salicylism) may be acute or chronic. Acute toxicity is either accidental or results from taking an overdose in a suicidal attempt. In addition, intolerance to salicylates may result in a severe reaction following therapeutic doses (116). Chronic intoxication may develop in the course of prescribed therapy with large doses of salicylates, or it can be a consequence of deliberate abuse of these drugs.

Delirium, even after one dose of the drug, has been reported (76). Following a single large oral dose of salicylate, especially of the acid or its methyl ester, the person may develop delirium with irritability, restlessness, and hallucinations. The delirium is usually followed by coma, which may end in death. Delirium may also be a manifestation of chronic salicylism (117-119). The incidence of delirium due to salicylates is unknown but appears to be low. A survey of acute toxicity of aspirin among over 2,000 hospitalized recipients of it mentions tinnitus and deafness, but not delirium, among the central nervous system effects (120). A recent review of aspirin intolerance also makes no mention of delirium (116). Greer et al. (117) found five cases of chronic salicylism admitted to the Mayo Clinic over a period of ten years. Confusion and hallucinations were among the symptoms shown by those patients. Other features of chronic salicylism included tinnitus, tremor, papilledema, and hyperventilation. Asterixis, paresthesia of the scalp, headache, convulsions, positive Babinski reflex, and absent tendon reflexes have been reported among the neurological symptoms and signs of salicylism (118, 119).

Delirium in salicylism appears to be related to metabolic changes, especially respiratory alkalosis that may be followed by a metabolic acidosis, which may exert adverse effects on cerebral function. A depression of the reticular activating system by the drug itself, or one secondary to its metabolic effects, has been postulated (119). Postmortem studies of subjects dying as a result of poisoning with salicylates have shown cerebral edema, congestion, hemorrhage, and injury to cerebral cortical cells (119). It was concluded that cerebral damage was due primarily to the selective toxic effects of the salicylates on the brain. Thalamus, hypothalamus, and other areas of the brain may be the seat of petechial hemorrhages (121). It appears that delirium in salicylate poisoning results from both direct toxic effects of the drug on the brain and, secondarily, as a result of hyperventilation and associated abnormalities in the acid-base balance. The EEG may be diffusely abnormal (119). Delirium due to salicylates may be facilitated by sedatives and by any disease, such as pulmonary insufficiency, accompanied by acidosis (118, 119).

It is not known at which serum levels of salicylates delirium is likely to appear. Tinnitus is usually the first symptom when serum levels exceed 20 mg./100 cc. Hyperventilation seldom occurs with levels below 35 mg./100 cc. Such levels may be exceeded in a person weighing 70 kg. by a single dose of 12 gm. of aspirin. One reported case developed psychosis at a serum salicylate level of 41.8 mg./100 ml., but that patient was acidotic to start with (118). Another reported case displayed mild confusion and a diffusely abnormal EEG with serum salicylate levels of 50 mg./100 ml. (119). It has been pointed out that the clinical state cannot be reliably correlated with serum salicylate level, since one patient with a level of about 90 mg./100 ml. may be comatose, while another may be awake and agitated (119). Treatment of salicylate delirium must be directed at elimination of the drug and correction of the acid-base imbalance.

Patients who abuse analgesics containing *phenacetin* may develop renal papillary necrosis and uremia and suffer delirium secondary to renal insufficiency (122). *Acetaminophen* (paracetamol) may cause liver damage and hepatic encephalopathy with delirium as its manifestation (123). An episode of delirium following administration of therapeutic doses of a mixture of acetaminophen and chlorzoxazone in a healthy young male has been reported (124).

Propoxyphene. This is a widely used non-narcotic analgesic. It is chemically related to methadone and can lead to dependence and withdrawal symptoms. The drug can be poisonous and fatal in overdoses, especially if it is combined with alcohol, tranquilizers, and sedative-hypnotics (125). Delirium due to propoxyphene has rarely been reported. Claghorn and Schoolar (126) report a woman who took about fourteen capsules daily for five months and developed delirium, which lasted for a month. Coma and convulsions can result from propoxyphene overdoses, but delirium appears to be rare. Generalized central nervous system depression develops rapidly with severe propoxyphene intoxication and thus rapid progression may perhaps prevent occurrence of delirium as a prelude to coma or seizures.

CARDIAC AND ANTIHYPERTENSIVE DRUGS

Digitalis. Delirium due to digitalis was first reported by Durozier in 1874 (1). Many cases of digitalis delirium have been reported in the literature since then, but some authors have questioned if digitalis as such ever causes the syndrome. Weiss (127), for example, argued that delirium thought to be caused by digitalis could actually be due to impaired cerebral circulation in patients suffering from congestive heart failure. A thorough recent review concludes that the existence of digitalis delirium remains a clinical impression, rather than an established fact (1). One cannot fault this cautious, if puristic, viewpoint, since no experimental studies have been carried out to settle the issue. Clinical opinions seem to endorse the view that digitalis may cause delirium independently of other factors. King (128) argues that it is unusual to see agitated delirium in a cardiac patient who is not receiving digitalis. He could reproduce delirium in a patient by administering digitalis in a smaller dose after an interval during which the patient was rational. Gillis et al. (129) have pointed out recently that digitalis is a neuroexcitatory drug whose extracardiac toxic effects, as well as the cardiac arrhythmias induced by it, are likely to be the result of the central nervous system activation. The neuropsychiatric side effects of digitalis occur with similar doses which precipitate cardiac arrhythmias. These side effects may precede, accompany, or follow the signs of cardiac toxicity, and they may occur without other evidence of digitalis intoxication (130).

The incidence of digitalis delirium is unknown. It is claimed that it occurs more readily in the elderly, in patients with cerebrovascular disease, and in those having aortic valve lesions (128, 130, 131). Psychiatric patients are said to be particularly vulnerable to digitalis toxicity if they receive lithium, have electrolyte imbalance of any origin, or have increased autonomic arousal (132). Digitalis has been used occasionally for self-poisoning (133). Any digitalis preparation can induce delirium. Both digoxin and digitoxin have been reported to do so. The former can pass the blood-brain barrier, although in minute amounts (1). Its therapeutic dose is close to the toxic one and digitalis intoxication is said to occur in about one in five patients treated with digitalis (1). About 25 to 50 percent of those intoxicated display neurological symptoms (130). The latter include many visual symptoms, weakness, drowsiness, dizziness, seizures, etc. (1). These side effects, as well as delirium, appear to be dose related. Determination of serum glycoside levels helps monitor digitalis treatment and avoid toxicity. Serum digoxin levels in excess of 2 mg./liter are liable to be toxic (1). Appearance of symptoms such as drowsiness, confusion, hyperactivity, restlessness, nightmares, insomnia, anxiety, and hallucinations in a patient receiving digoxin should always raise the question of delirium, either impending or actually present, and prompt determination of serum digoxin levels. If these levels are toxic, the drug should be reduced or discontinued. Continuation of the drug in toxic doses could result in full-blown delirium or lethal arrhythmia. Psychiatric symptoms may actually draw attention to the unrecognized fact that the patient has developed digitalis toxicity. If delirium does develop and is severe, haloperidol may be used for symptomatic treatment of excessive agitation (132). Factors which enhance digitalis toxicity, such as hypokalemia, need to be corrected. It is also important to keep in mind that delirium in a patient receiving digitalis often has multifactorial etiology and that the other potentially contributory factors need to be corrected in addition to discontinuation or reduction of the digitalis preparation.

Quinidine. Rarely has quinidine been reported to cause delirium (134, 135). Like other cinchona alkaloids, the drug may cause intoxication, cinchonism, whose manifestations occasionally include delirium (136). All antiarrhythmic drugs can produce adverse effects as a result of drug idiosyncrasy or allergy, of dose-related toxicity, or a combination of these factors (136).

Procainamide, lignocaine, diphenylhydantoin, and *mexiletine* have all been reported to cause confusion, hallucinations, or frank psychosis (136). Unfortunately, these terms are used so indiscriminately by the medical writers that one can only surmise that the symptoms to which they are referring may represent delirium.

Propranolol is one exception to the above statement. A case of delirium in a hyperthyroid and depressed woman who had received propranolol 60 mg. daily for a week has been reported (137). The delirium cleared up within two days following discontinuation of the drug. Propranolol may also induce visual and tactile hallucinations in the absence of disorientation and other symptoms of delirium (138). The latter syndrome may complicate the use of a combination of antiarrhythmic drugs (139). Propranolol readily crosses the blood-brain barrier and has sedative properties. Its reported neuropsychiatric effects include depression, vivid dreams, and insomnia (140). It induces changes in the EEG in that delta and fast activity increase while alpha waves decrease (141). Central nervous effects of propranolol have been invoked to account for its ability to counteract combativeness in patients who have sustained acute brain damage (142). Up to 320 mg. daily have been administered for this purpose without inducing delirium in the presumably brain-damaged subjects. This suggests that the deliriogenic potential of the drug is low.

Methyldopa. In doses used to control hypertension, methyldopa has been reported to have psychiatric side effects including depression, impairment of intellectual functions, and delirium (143-145). The latter featured marked paranoid delusions and visual hallucinations in one reported case (144). Delirium may apparently be precipitated in patients receiving methyldopa when haloperidol is administered concurrently (145). Both these drugs block central dopamine receptors and this synergistic activity may perhaps result in delirium in some persons. Methyldopa also depletes the brain of noradrenaline and serotonin. Nevertheless, delirium due to this drug alone appears to be rare.

Diuretics. Diuretics such as acetazolamide, chlorothiazide, ethacrynic acid, and furosemide may precipitate delirium, which is probably secondary to electrolyte imbalance. Patients with hepatic disease are particularly vulnerable. Hyponatremia may result from diuretic-reserpine combinations and become worse with the use of antidepressants as a result of increased fluid intake to counteract dryness of the mouth (146).

ANTICONVULSANTS

Mental symptoms may occur during therapy with all of the major anticonvulsant drugs (147-150). These adverse effects are said to occur in 15 to 20 percent of the patients (147). Confusional states, referred to by some authors as encephalopathy and by others as delirium or psychosis, have been reported with *diphenylhydantoin, phenobarbitone, primidone,* and *ethosuximide* (147-150). It appears from the published reports that simple intoxication, manifested by drowsiness, bradykinesia, and manifestations of cerebellar dysfunction, is the commonest form of anticonvulsant toxicity. Such intoxication merges imperceptibly with a reversible dementia, which implies the presence of definite intellectual impairment in addition to drowsiness and lethargy. Distinct delirious episodes appear to be uncommon.

The mental symptoms of acute and chronic anticonvulsant intoxication are related to the blood levels of the antiepileptic drugs rather than to their daily dosage (147, 150). Striking individual differences in the susceptibility to these effects have been observed. Some epileptic patients develop mental symptoms with blood levels of anticonvulsants which are regarded as therapeutic, i.e. 10 to 20 μg./ml., especially if therapy has been prolonged. These symptoms may occur in the absence of the usual signs of anticonvulsant toxicity, such as nystagmus and ataxia. Some authors claim that confusion appears when diphenylhydantoin levels exceed 40 μg./ml., but other writers point out that this is not always so (147, 150).

Trimble and Reynolds (150) hypothesize that the adverse mental effects of diphenylhydantoin, phenobarbitone, and primidone may result from the interference by these drugs with normal folate metabolism. Mental symptoms would be determined partly by genetic and other unspecific predisposing factors and partly by the duration and severity of the drug-induced folate deficiency. Whether such a postulated deficiency contributes to the occasional delirium is unknown, but seems plausible. Folate deficiency is known to cause delirium in nonepileptic subjects. It follows that when a patient receiving one or more anticonvulsants becomes delirious, blood levels of the drugs and serum folate and B_{12} values should be obtained.

ANTIBIOTIC, ANTIFUNGAL, ANTIMALARIAL, AND ANTITUBERCULOUS AGENTS

Antibiotics

Sulphonamides, penicillin, streptomycin, chloromycetin, gentamicin, cephalexin, and griseofulvin have all been reported to cause delirium occasionally.

Kline and Highsmith (151) were the first to report a toxic psychosis, a typical delirium with marked auditory hallucinations and persecutory delusions, in a girl who received *penicillin* intramuscularly and orally for ten days. Two days after the drug was discontinued she developed generalized urticaria, arthralgia, and fever. She apparently became delirious four days after developing what seemed to be serum sickness. The authors speculated that the delirium was due to penicillin sensitivity and related cerebral edema. Both her allergic and mental symptoms tended to subside after Pyribenzamine® was given. Yet, the etiology of that reported psychosis remains unclear.

In the last thirty years many papers have documented the occurrence of delirium in the course of penicillin treatment (152-155). Delirium has been linked with penicillin in two ways: as a manifestation of allergy to the drug and as a non-allergic reaction, possibly representing idiosyncrasy (153). The allergic reaction appears to be less common than the so-called pseudoanaphylactic reaction. According to Cohen (153), delirium associated with allergic manifestations may follow anaphylactic shock, clear up after a period of time, and leave in its wake apparently irreversible dementia. Allergic delirium is usually accompanied by fever, urticaria, angioneurotic edema, pulmonary edema, and arthralgia (153). Cerebral edema is believed to underlie this delirium.

The pseudoanaphylactic penicillin delirium follows immediately after intramuscular injection of aqueous procaine penicillin G (152, 153, 155). Its incidence is reported to be between 0.1 percent and 0.89 percent (152). Strictly speaking, the published reports do not use the term "delirium" for this disorder, but rather "acute psychotic reaction." It is the writer's impression that at least some of the reported cases do represent delirium. The symptoms include sudden anxiety and often a sense of impending death, violent behavior, perceptual disturbances, and paresthesiae. Auditory disturbances, such as ringing, noise, music, etc., reportedly occur in 60 to 70 percent of the cases. Visual disturbances, including lights, blurring, diplopia, and hallucinations were found in 30 to 50 percent of procaine penicillin reactions. Confusion and disorientation were reported in 20 percent of the cases (152). Blood pressure and pulse rate tend to be elevated, and signs of anaphylaxis are lacking (155). Convulsions may occur.

Several hypotheses have been advanced to account for the pseudoanaphylactic psychosis or delirium. Some believe that inadvertent injection of the drug into a vein may result in microembolism (152, 155). Since high concentration of penicillin in the brain is not believed to be likely to produce symptoms, concentration of free procaine has been blamed for the pseudoanaphylactic reaction. The latter resembles toxic reactions to local anesthetics in that it involves signs of cortical stimulation (155).

Conway et al. (154) report on penicillin encephalopathy, with confusion, drowsiness, convulsions and myoclonic twitching, following massive intravenous doses of penicillin. This appears to be a direct toxic effect of the drug on the brain. Such toxicity could be increased by any coexistent condition which increased permeability of the blood-brain barrier. This encephalopathy seems to involve cortical depression rather than activation and may represent a third mechanism for and variant of delirium due to penicillin therapy.

Chloramphenicol. When chloramphenicol is administered

orally it has been reported to induce delirium (156). Patients treated for typhoid tended to develop delirium when they were afebrile and the infection seemed to be under control (156). Similar effects have been observed in children. Hyperanabolic state, such as is encountered in the early stages of convalescence from infection or trauma, is said to predispose to chloramphenicol delirium (156). Mediation of this effect might be related to the drug's inhibitory effect on protein synthesis or to hepatic injury or to nutritional deficiency (156). Administration of large doses of vitamins has been recommended as a preventive measure against chloramphenicol toxicity.

Streptomycin (157), *gentamicin* (158), *cephalexin* (159), and *griseofulvin* (160) may all cause delirium in an occasional patient.

Antimalarial Drugs

Behavioral toxicity has been reported with quinacrine (atabrine) and chloroquine and its derivatives. Psychotic reactions are said to occur in 0.4 percent of patients treated with *quinacrine* (161). Over 300 cases of such reactions had been reported by 1966 (161). The nature of quinacrine psychosis remains unclear. Engel et al. (162) studied psychological and electroencephalographic effects of the drug on five normal adults. The investigators concluded that the drug acts as a cortical stimulant. The clinical symptoms included increased motor activity, restlessness, and insomnia. The EEG showed acceleration of the background activity. Engel et al. point out that the behavioral syndrome that they induced with quinacrine was not delirium. The subjects displayed heightened awareness and increased activity rather than global impairment of cognitive functions. The researchers emphasize, however, that if the intoxication is allowed to progress and excitement and anxiety mount, delirium may result. Thus, two types of toxic psychoses due to quinacrine may be seen: a paranoid psychosis similar to that observed with amphetamine (163) and delirium (161). In the latter, the patients are typically agitated, restless, hallucinated, and delusional. Convulsions may occur. The early symptoms include insomnia and increased dreaming, followed by an agitated paranoid psychosis with auditory and visual hallucinations. Delirium may develop from the paranoid state as Engel et al. have predicted.

Chloroquine. This drug was initially believed to be less toxic than quinacrine, yet reports of delirium associated with its administration have appeared in the past twenty years (161, 164). This complication is not very common: only about ten cases of "chloroquine psychosis" have been reported (164). This psychosis is very similar to that induced by quinacrine, is rapidly reversible after cessation of the drug, and may come on after several days to weeks following the institution of therapy. Seizures and death may follow intoxication. Delirium due to chloroquine may feature marked anxiety, depression with suicidal trends, and aggressiveness, symptoms that can mask cognitive impairment and lead to a false impression of a psychogenic psychosis. The effects of the drug on the EEG vary, but acceleration of the background activity appears to be a common change (164).

Antituberculous Drugs

Four drugs used for chemotherapy of tuberculosis may cause organic mental disorders: iproniazid, isoniazid, cycloserine, and ethionamide (1). As these drugs are usually administered in combination, it is not easy to identify the offending agent when psychosis develops.

Over 100 cases of *isoniazid* (INH) psychosis have been reported (1). Two types of psychosis due to the drug are observed: delirium and a schizophrenialike psychosis (1, 165). In the early stages of INH therapy some patients experience euphoria, enhanced activity, and at times, restlessness and agitation. The euphoria is believed to be due to relief of symptoms of tuberculosis (165). Acute INH poisoning as a result of overdosage can result in coma, generalized convulsions, and death (166). Delirium due to INH may feature marked paranoid delusions and be mistaken for a paranoid psychosis. Such delirium may at times persist for several weeks and even longer (1). INH delirium could result from pellagra induced by the drug. Administration of nicotinamide has reportedly alleviated the delirium in some cases (1). Intravenous administration of pyridoxine has been recommended (166) for acute poisoning with INH. The drug increases the excretion of pyridoxin, whose deficiency is believed to be responsible for peripheral neuropathy occurring in patients treated with large doses of INH.

Delirium due to *iproniazid* appears to be quite uncommon (1, 167). Behavioral adverse effects of *cycloserine* include symptoms such as nervousness, irritability, excitement, anxiety, depression, insomnia, drowsiness, nightmares, and difficulty in concentration (168). Delirium rarely develops and may be complicated by seizures. The EEG may show slowing or acceleration of the background activity (168, 169). Alcoholism and unstable personality are said to predispose to the development of psychiatric complications during cycloserine therapy (168). High doses of the drug were given to schizophrenic patients and provoked delirium in one of ten patients treated (169).

Ethionamide. Reportedly, ethionamide may induce psychosis, but the published reports are so inadequate in their description of psychopathology that it is impossible to judge if delirium does occur (1, 170).

CYTOTOXIC DRUGS

Several drugs used for the chemotherapy of cancer have various "neurotoxic" effects (171, 172). Description of the reported psychiatric side effects is generally so poor that it is impossible to know what proportion of the described reactions represent delirium.

Nitrogen mustard. Nitrogen mustard may rarely cause delirium (173). *Procarbazine* has been reported to induce "disorders of consciousness" such as depression, somnolence, confusion, hallucinations, agitation, and psychosis (172). It appears that at least some of these reactions represent delirium. In one series, drowsiness or disorientation were observed in about one-half of patients, but these symptoms occur in only about 10 percent of those treated with daily oral doses (172). Procarbazine inhibits brain monoamine oxidase and has a synergistic sedative effect with phenothiazines, barbiturates, and narcotics. Patients delirious due to this drug should not be treated with phenothiazines since both they and procarbazine may precipitate orthostatic hypotension (172).

L-asparaginase. L-asparaginase may induce delirium with slowing of the EEG. Five of nineteen adult patients in one series developed this complication (174). Delirium came on between the second and nineteenth day after the initial injection of the enzyme. The patients displayed slow mentation and varying level of consciousness. It has been suggested that delirium in these cases is due to the depletion of the brain of L-asparagine. Normal mentation returned in some cases with infusion of the latter. Delirium tends to be more common in adults than in children (174).

5-fluorouracil. Mental symptoms may be induced by 5-fluorouracil relatively infrequently (172). Two cases of delirium due to this drug have been reported (175). Both patients were elderly, received the drug intravenously for some weeks, and recovered within a month. The EEG was slowed in both.

Methotrexate. Methotrexate has been observed to induce "encephalopathy" (172). The drug does not cross the blood-brain barrier except when given after craniospinal radiotherapy. It can exert cerebral effects when given intrathecally (171, 172, 176, 177). Clinical symptoms of neurotoxicity are reported to occur in 5 to 55 percent of children receiving this form of therapy for meningeal leukemia (175). Delirium appears to be uncommon but has been observed (176). EEG shows diffuse slowing (176). It is important to bear in mind that not all the cases of intellectual or cognitive impairment due to methotrexate are progressive and irreversible (176, 177). Irreversible dementia may be a manifestation of leukoencephalopathy, which may follow methotrexate therapy (178). Computed tomography of the brain may help diagnose this condition and distinguish it from the clinically similar but transient delirium (178, 179). High concentration of methotrexate in the CSF, cranial radio-therapy, and altered brain metabolism have been suggested as likely determinants of the encephalopathy.

Vincristine and *vinblastine* have been reported to cause "mental changes" (171, 172). Whether delirium occurs is not clear.

HISTAMINE H₂-RECEPTOR ANTAGONISTS

A spate of letters to the editors of several journals have recently reported delirium as an adverse reaction to *cimetidine* (180-186). Of the eleven cases reported to date, six were in persons aged sixty-five and older, while five occurred in patients younger than sixty-five years. It is clear that the delirium is not confined to the elderly. This complication occurs with both average and high doses of cimetidine. Some of the patients are lethargic and drowsy; others are agitated, restless, and combative. Delirium clears up promptly after the drug is discontinued but may not respond to diazepam and haloperidol (183). Associated physical signs and symptoms may include slurred speech, dizziness, flushing, sweating, tachycardia, and dilated pupils. The underlying mechanism is unknown.

CORTICOSTEROIDS

Psychotic reactions to glucocorticoid drugs were frequently reported during the decade 1950 to 1960. Since then the number of reports has declined markedly. The difference in the frequency of reporting may reflect a lower incidence of psychosis with the currently used drugs, such as prednisone and prednisolone, as compared to cortisone and ACTH, which were the drugs used in the 1950s. Prednisone is the most commonly used glucocortical drug at present, and the incidence of psychosis ascribed to it is reported to be between one and 1.8 percent (187, 188). By contrast, the incidence of psychoses in the course of cortisone and ACTH treatment was about 4 percent (189). Thus, the current incidence of psychosis related to corticosteroid therapy is two to four times lower than it was in the 1950s. With doses of prednisone higher than 80 mg. per day, however, psychiatric reactions occur in 18.4 percent (188).

Nature of the steroid psychoses has been a subject of controversy: Are they mostly delirium, affective, or schizophreniform, or mixtures of all three? Glaser (190) in one of the early reports, described two types of psychosis: a primarily affective disorder and an organic reaction (toxic psychosis) with associated affective and/or paranoid-hallucinatory features. Clark et al.

(191) maintained that the steroid psychotic patients did not exhibit confusion, memory impairments, disorientation, and other manifestations of delirium, but rather featured schizophreniform and affective symptoms. More recently, French authors have asserted that the majority of the psychoses represent a confusional syndrome (delirium in our terminology) with superimposed manic, depressive, schizophreniform, or mixed clinical features (192). In their own series of fifteen patients these investigators found that ten had a confusional state, most often with superimposed manic symptoms. Thus, it appears that about two-thirds of steroid psychoses encountered nowadays represent delirium.

A number of predisposing and facilitating factors have been claimed to account for delirium in the course of steroid therapy. They include high dose of the steroid drug; rapid increase in the dose or abrupt discontinuation of the drug; presence of adrenal insufficiency, ulcerative colitis, or systemic lupus erythematosus; emotional instability of the patient; and coexistence of a cerebral damage or disorder of any etiology (187, 192). Even though delirium is more likely to occur with high doses, there is no consistent relationship between dosage and appearance of psychosis. Age and sex do not seem to have any influence. The type of steroid used is claimed by some to be important in that psychiatric complications are more common during therapy with cortisone and dexamethasone than with prednisone or prednisolone (187, 192).

The course of delirium induced by steroid drugs is highly variable and so are its manifestations. The onset is typically sudden, usually two to four weeks after initiation of therapy. Prodromal symptoms may precede the onset of delirium and include a combination of marked euphoria, anxiety, depression, insomnia, tension, and depersonalization (187). These symptoms are then added to those of delirium, usually with an admixture of affective, mostly manic, and/or schizophreniform features. The clinical picture tends to be quite heterogeneous, fluctuating, and confusing to the observer. Various constellations of psychiatric symptoms may be observed at different stages of the psychosis.

The EEG findings in steroid psychoses are also variable. Glaser (190) found no consistent pattern in his series of patients: about half of the records displayed some slowing of the background activity, but the EEG changes could also be found in the absence of manifest psychopathology. The most often observed EEG changes in steroid psychoses include decrease in amplitude and frequency of alpha activity, bursts of beta waves, and increased beta activity (192). Some authors state that, generally speaking, EEG changes do not occur frequently in steroid psychoses (187).

Much speculation has been devoted to the pathophysiology of steroid delirium (1, 187, 192, 193). Relevant hypotheses have focused on electrolyte imbalance, increased excitability of the brain, and changes in the balance of neurotransmitters. Hypokalemia is often found in patients receiving steroids, but it may be absent in those who develop psychosis (187). Increased excitability of the brain has been claimed to be a constant effect of glucocortocoids, but this claim remains controversial (192). These drugs may influence transport and turnover of noradrenaline in the brain and also cause a decrease in cerebral serotonin (1, 187, 192). Prednisone has been found to reduce total REM sleep, increase REM latency, and induce intermittent awakening (1). These effects on sleep have been ascribed to relative increase in noradrenaline and decrease of serotonin. Such sleep disturbances may conceivably facilitate the development of delirium in the presence of other causal factors. One has to conclude, however, that we do not yet understand the pathophysiology of steroid delirium. It has been proposed that steroids play no more than a facilitating role in the induction of delirium and that cerebral damage, metabolic disorder, or both, due to other factors, are usually present and perhaps constitute a necessary condition for delirium to develop (187). Quarton et al. (193) brilliantly reviewed the various explanatory hypotheses more than twenty years ago and concluded that "at the present time there is no completely satisfactory hypothesis." We have not progressed beyond that statement.

Treatment of steroid delirium involves gradual reduction of the dosage and either discontinuation of the drug or its substitution by a different steroid. If in the judgment of the physician continued therapy with the given steroid drug is indicated, then its dose should be reduced and the delirium treated with haloperidol. Electroshock may be effective in refractory cases (187). Patients who become delirious in the course of systemic lupus erythematosus treated with steroids present a difficult diagnostic and therapeutic dilemma at times. Computed tomography of the brain and the EEG may be of help in diagnosing cerebral lupus. If still in doubt, continue steroids and treat the excitement, agitation, and overactivity symptomatically. Haloperidol is an adequate drug for this purpose.

LITHIUM

Delirium is a recognized manifestation of neurotoxic effects of lithium (194-198). Agulnik et al. (194) report on three patients who became delirious with low blood lithium levels. One of the patients developed disorientation in all three fields, psychomotor slowing, distractibility, auditory and visual hallucinations, and incoherent thinking full of "archaic images." The authors comment that "Despite the similarity of this illness to delirium with occasional lucid intervals, the patient had no clouding of consciousness." This statement highlights the widespread confusion among psychiatrists and other physicians as to what constitutes delirium. The description quoted above is that of typical delirium, yet the diagnostic conclusion is just as typically muddled and erroneous.

Rifkin et al. (197) report on three more patients who developed delirium while receiving therapeutic doses of lithium and who showed no other signs of lithium toxicity. All three patients were thought to have concomitant cerebral impairment which might have accounted for their vulnerability to lithium neurotoxicity. All three recovered from delirium when lithium was discontinued.

Lithium neurotoxicity has been reported since its introduction to psychiatry in 1949 (196). Many cases of delirium have been observed (196, 198). Baldessarini and Lipinski (195) state that mild lithium neurotoxicity includes confusion, which with more severe intoxication may progress to stupor and coma.

Delirium may occur at both therapeutic and toxic blood lithium levels. The elderly are particularly vulnerable and may develop severe neurotoxicity only minutes after a single 100 mg. lithium dose (199). Severe intoxication more often develops after several days, unless an acute overdose has been ingested (195). There is increasing tremor, dizziness, weakness, ataxia, slurred speech, drowsiness, nystagmus, and deepening confusion. Severe intoxication usually develops at blood levels about 3 mEq/liter, but delirium can occur at levels as low as 1.15 mEq/liter (194). Convulsions, myoclonic movements, hyperreflexia, bilateral Babinski reflexes, opisthotonos, and other signs of neurotoxicity may be observed in severe cases (196, 198). EEG shows diffuse slowing.

Delirium ascribed to lithium has been reported by some writers to occur in about 10 percent of patients treated (196). This figure appears too high. A number of factors have been postulated to facilitate the occurrence of delirium and other signs of neurotoxicity in the patients treated with lithium:

Age. Delirium is said to occur particularly frequently in the elderly (199).

Organic brain disease. The evidence for its role as a predisposing factor is equivocal (196). Patients with dementia due to Huntington's chorea have been treated without evidence of neurotoxicity (196).

Sodium deficiency. Negative sodium balance leads to lithium retention and predisposes to neurotoxicity (196).

Concomitant physical illness. Renal insufficiency, febrile illness of any type, and congestive heart failure predispose to lithium toxicity, but the drug may be administered if proper precautions are taken (200).

Drug interaction. Concurrent administration of phenothiazines, haloperidol, diuretics, and methyldopa has been blamed for increasing the vulnerability to delirium (196, 198, 201-203). This matter is controversial. One study shows that a combination of lithium and haloperidol does not increase the probability of delirium (201). Not one of 425 patients treated concurrently with these two drugs showed "impairment of consciousness" (201).

Psychiatric diagnosis. Schizophrenic and schizoaffective patients have been reported to be more vulnerable to lithium-induced delirium than the manic-depressives (196).

Various mechanisms have been proposed to account for neuropsychiatric adverse effects of lithium. The ion has been assigned various actions on cerebral neurons, such as inhibition of the release of noradrenaline and dopamine, decrease of the synthesis and release of acetylcholine, and increase of metabolism of glucose (195). The relevance of these putative actions to lithium neurotoxicity is unclear. Lithium induces changes in the EEG which include slowing of the alpha activity (the most common change) and, in some subjects, generalized theta activity, focal theta waves, single delta or sharp waves, and paroxysmal changes (204). These changes in electrophysical activity of the brain suggest that lithium may have direct cerebrotoxic effect. Patients delirious in the course of lithium therapy show generalized and high voltage slowing of the background activity (204). Lithium tends to accentuate preexisting EEG abnormalities, whose presence has predictive value for the occurrence of neurotoxicity (196, 198). Lithium may also bring about delirium indirectly by inducing hypothyroidism (205).

Treatment of lithium delirium involves reduction of the dose or discontinuation of the drug, correction of fluid and electrolyte imbalance, and symptomatic therapy (195). There is no contraindication to the use of haloperidol for the control of agitation. Occurrence of delirium in the elderly patient may be partly prevented by a dose titration method (199). The drug is best avoided, or its dose should be kept low, in patients with evidence of cerebral disease, renal insufficiency, or congestive heart failure. Careful monitoring of symptoms, lithium blood levels, and the EEG are indicated in patients known to be predisposed to neurotoxicity.

ANTIPARKINSONIAN AGENTS

Drugs with anticholinergic activity which are used in parkinsonism are discussed in section A. L-Dopa has been reported to cause delirium in 4 to 13 percent of parkinsonian patients (1,

206). The true incidence of this complication is unknown, however, since the various reports use undefined terms such as organic brain syndrome, psychosis, delirium, or confusion. A typical statement asserts that the most common mental side effect of the drug is a set of symptoms that are similar to an organic brain syndrome, "with predominance of confusion and disorientation, sometimes progressing to frank delirium" (1). Celesia and Barr (206) found delirium in six out of forty-five patients treated with the drug. Five of the six patients had a mild chronic organic brain syndrome prior to the onset of therapy. Delirium developed as a rule about four months after initiation of treatment and was often associated with dyskinetic movements. Diminution or discontinuation of L-dopa was followed by lifting of delirium.

Several mechanisms for the deliriogenic effects of L-dopa have been suggested. The drug induces elevated dopamine levels in the brain and consequent excess of dopaminergic activity in limbic structures could account for the occurrence of delirium or at least for the presence of hallucinations. L-dopa might also act as a false neurotransmitter and alter cerebral metabolism. Brain serotonin levels are reduced during therapy with L-dopa, and this might provide another contributory mechanism (207). Administration of L-tryptophan relieved delirium in some patients receiving L-dopa (207).

Delirium has also been reported in parkinsonian patients receiving a combination of L-dopa and *carbidopa* (208). *Amantadine* may also induce delirium (209). The latter usually sets in shortly after the onset of therapy and may be preceded by urinary retention. Visual hallucinations and illusions precede the onset of delirium in some cases. Elderly patients appear to be particularly vulnerable.

DISULFIRAM

Disulfiram, used for the treatment of alcoholism, is reported to induce a "reversible toxic encephalopathy" (presumably delirium) in 2 to 20 percent patients treated with it (210). The reported higher incidence probably reflects use of larger doses of the drug. The incidence figures are quite unreliable in view of the inconsistent and undefined terminology used by the various authors. Disulfiram may induce three types of psychosis: delirium, delirium with affective or paranoid features, and a psychosis lacking organic features. Delirium accounts for 75 percent of the psychotic reactions to the drug (211).

The onset of delirium may follow initiation of therapy by days to months. There are often prodromal symptoms: concentration difficulties, forgetfulness, anxiety, depression, and drowsiness. Delirium follows and often features delusions, less often hallucinations (212, 213). Concurrent neurological symptoms may include ataxia, slurred speech, tremor, and Babinski reflexes (213). EEG shows diffuse slowing. Seizures may occur. The delirium lifts a few days to weeks after cessation of disulfiram therapy. Schizophrenic patients are said to be particularly prone to delirium while receiving the drug (213).

Several mechanisms have been proposed to account for disulfiram delirium: impaired consumption of oxygen, accumulation of carbon disulphide, and increase in cerebral dopamine concentration. Disulfiram inhibits β-hydroxylase and dopamine β-hydroxylase (212, 213).

Treatment consists of withdrawal of disulfiram and administration of haloperidol (213).

BISMUTH SALTS

Several recent reports have documented the occurrence and features of delirium in the course of encephalopathy caused by insoluble bismuth salts, especially *subnitrate* and *subgallate* (214-217). Supino-Viterbo et al. (217) have studied forty-five patients who developed encephalopathy while treated with bismuth subnitrate for a colonic disorder over periods ranging from one month to thirty years. All had bismuth blood levels about 150 μg./liter (normal less than 20 micrograms/liter). Patients experienced prodromal symptoms, such as depression, anxiety, irritability, and somnolence. Many suffered from prolonged insomnia and had visual hallucinations. Symptoms of increasing toxicity include disturbances of attention and memory and behavior suggestive of frontal lobe syndrome. Delirium set in rapidly against this more chronic background. It was typically accompanied by myoclonic jerks, dysarthria, tremor, and ataxia. Incontinence of urine and feces was common. The EEG showed generalized slowing of background activity, absence of alpha waves, and low voltage beta rhythm (217). Most patients displayed no responses to photic stimulation. The majority of the EEG records returned to normal over a period of weeks to three months. The patients usually recovered within three months after cessation of bismuth therapy.

All bismuth salts may induce the above features, including delirium. Bismuth may be absorbed from skin cream. It has been postulated that certain microorganisms in the gut can dissolve bismuth, which then crosses the blood-brain barrier (217). In the brain bismuth may inactivate thiol groups of enzymes and induce diminished utilization of oxygen and glucose and increased production of lactate. It is also possible that it may damage the blood-brain barrier and thus increase its permeability (216). Cerebral blood flow has been found to be reduced. An interesting feature in some cases of bismuth encephalopathy is a total insomnia (214). Patients experience vivid visual, auditory, and gustatory hallucinations, especially during the night. Imbalance of brain neurotransmitters, with increased levels of dopamine, may underlie the sleep disorders.

MISCELLANEOUS DRUGS

Practically every drug listed in the pharmacopeia may occasionally induce delirium in a susceptible individual. Many drugs may trigger delirium indirectly by virtue of their toxic effects on kidneys or liver and the consequent failure of these organs. Other examples of indirect mechanisms include dilutional hyponatremia (218), precipitation of heat stroke (219), and hypoglycemia (220). By means of these and other intermediate mechanisms a great many drugs lacking direct cerebrotoxic effects may bring about delirium. It is clear that to discuss all the drugs that have ever been reported to cause the syndrome would be pointless. Some drugs, however, not belonging unequivocally to those already discussed, may precipitate delirium and are of sufficient practical importance to justify their inclusion here.

Aminophylline (theophylline ethylenediamine) and *caffeine*. These drugs rarely give rise to delirium (221, 222). Aminophylline has caused severe poisoning, in some cases with delirium and seizures, in children (221). Caffeine also has recently been reported to have caused delirium in a man who had taken more than 1,000 mg. under conditions of severe physical effort, low temperatures, and sleep deprivation (222).

Bromocriptine. An ergot derivative used in the treatment of hyperprolactinemia and Parkinson's disease, bromocriptine, has reportedly caused "hallucinosis" in 1 to 16 percent of cases (223). It appears that delirium is the appropriate term for at least some of the cases of psychosis induced by this drug. It may be brought about by low daily dosage (2.5 to 5 mg. per day) and features violent behavior as well as "intense delusions" (223). These symptoms may persist for one to three weeks.

Camphor. Occasionally camphor is ingested by children and may lead to convulsions and delirium. De Boor (78) quotes Alexander and Purkinje, both of whom ingested camphor as self-experiments and experienced perceptual distortions and delirium. Monroe (224) writes that Vincent van Gogh used strong doses of camphor for insomnia and perhaps could have induced one of his psychotic episodes by this means.

Clozapine. A new neuroleptic agent, clozapine, has been reported to cause delirium (225). Patients suffering from the latter were found to have raised levels of 5-hydroxy-indoleacetic acid in the CSF and significantly reduced serotonin blood levels (225).

Cocaine. Usually cocaine induces euphoria, dysphoria, and a paranoid psychosis, but an overdose may result in delirium (226).

Colchicine. With colchicine, delirium or convulsions may be terminal events of severe acute poisoning (227). *Indomethacin* may cause delirium in a substantial proportion of users (228).

Ketamine (Ketalar). Ketamine is an anesthetic agent reported to cause emergence delirium more often than any other currently used anesthetic drug. Incidence of such reported emergence reaction has varied considerably from author to author. Knox et al. (229) found emergence delirium, defined as "confusion, with and without vocalization, excitement or irrational behavior" in about 40 percent of patients. On the other hand, these authors quote an earlier survey of over 12,000 unselected administrations, which revealed the incidence of delirium in 2.8 percent of patients. The delirium was unrelated to dose. Wantz (230) quotes an incidence of 13 percent. Other emergence phenomena observed after ketamine anesthesia include vivid dreams, visual hallucinations, sensation of floating, psychomotor disturbances, body image disturbances, and depersonalization (231, 232, 233). Such reactions are much less frequent in children, ranging from zero to 5 percent (234). A personal account of a "ketamine trip" reports some of the unpleasant sensory disturbances and body image distortions induced by the drug (235). Studies of attention, learning, and memory during ketamine emergence have shown impairment of short-term memory, good performance on backward digit span, and difficulty in organizing and comprehending environmental stimuli (236). Administration of the drug to experimental subjects has shown that reality testing and insight were relatively intact (237). These findings raise the question if ketamine induces delirium at all rather than a hallucinosis, with or without restlessness. Hefez and Lanyi (237) maintain that, in their experimental subjects, the drug did not impair orientation or recent memory. Ketamine is best described as a dissociative anesthetic which induces complete analgesia with only superficial sleep. Collier (231) has compared the emergence phenomena after ketamine anesthesia to those elicited by sensory deprivation experiments. Ketamine has been used for abreaction in 100 psychiatric patients and was found to be effective (238). Even though they reportedly exhibited disorientation in all three spheres, the patients had vivid recall of the drug state. French investigators have used ketamine as an initial sedative for the treatment of delirium tremens (239). Ketamine emergence phenomena have been prevented by premedication with lorazepam (240) and reduced by Innovar (230). Physostigmine has been reported to antagonize sensory disturbances induced by ketamine (241).

Phencyclidine. One of the most frequently used and dangerous drugs of abuse, phencyclidine is structurally related to ketamine and has been used as an anesthetic prior to the introduction of the latter. Its unsuitability as an anesthetic was due to severe emergence reactions such as agitation, excitement, disorientation, and hallucinations. For the past ten years or so it has become increasingly more abused and the cause of severe neuropsychiatric reactions (242-244). Known under a variety of names, such as PCP, angel dust, etc., it has been sold illegally as a "street drug" as a substitute for or ingredient of marijuana, tetrahydrocannabinol, mescaline, etc. Its effects include disturbances of body image, depersonalization, agitation, inability to speak, disorientation for time and place, anxiety, hallucinations, self-destructive behavior, catalepsy, and finally coma. This cluster of symptoms represents delirium, and it has been recommended that phencyclidine should be considered in the differential diagnosis of the syndrome (243). The drug has some anticholinergic activity. Autonomic effects include flushing, sweating, tachycardia, constricted pupils, and elevated systolic and diastolic blood pressure. Nystagmus, blurred vision, ataxia, tremors, slurred speech, and changes in deep tendon reflexes may all occur (242-244). Recovery from coma tends to be protracted and marked by delirium.

Management of phencyclidine delirium includes provision of a quiet environment to avoid exacerbation of symptoms and seizures and slow intravenous diazepam or haloperidol (242-244).

Nitrous oxide. Another anesthetic agent which has recently gained some popularity as a drug of abuse is nitrous oxide, which may give rise to delirium (245).

Metrizamide. A water-soluble contrast medium used for myelography and ventriculography, metrizamide may induce convulsions and delirium, the latter in about 2 percent of cases (246).

REFERENCES

1. Shader, R.I., Ed.: *Psychiatric Complications of Medical Drugs.* New York, Raven Publ., 1972.
2. *The Extant Work of Aretaeus, the Cappadocian.* F. Adams, Ed. London, Sydenham Society, 1861.
3. Forbes, T.R.: Why is it called "beautiful lady"? A note on belladonna. *Bull NY Acad Med* 59:403-406, 1977.
4. Johnson, C.B.: Mystical force of the Nightshade. *Int J Neuropsychiatry* 3:268-275, 1967.

5. Hardin, J.W., and Arena, J.M.: *Human Poisoning from Native and Cultivated Plants.* Duke Univ. Press, Durham, N.C., 1974.

6. Ketchum, J.S., Sidell, F.R., Crowell, E.B., Aghajanian, G.K., and Hayes, A.H.: Atropine, scopolamine, and Ditran: Comparative pharmacology and antagonists in man. *Psychopharmacol.* (Berl.) *28*:121-145, 1973.

7. Kounis, N.G.: Atropine eye-drops delirium. *Can Med Assoc J 119*: 759, 1974.

8. Freund, M., and Merin, S.: Toxic effects of scopolamine eye drops. *Am J Ophthalmol 70*:637-639, 1970.

9. Safer, D.J., and Allen, R.P.: The central effects of scopolamine in man. *Biol Psychiatry 3*:347-355, 1971.

10. Forrer, G.R.: Pharmacotoxic therapy with atropine sulfate. *J Nerv Ment Dis 117*:226-233, 1953.

11. Gowdy, J.M.: Stramonium intoxication. *JAMA 221*:585-587, 1972.

12. Granacher, R.P., and Baldessarini, R.J.: Physostigmine. *Arch Gen Psychiatry 32*:375-380, 1975.

13. Granacher, R.P., and Baldessarini, R.J.: "The Usefulness of Physostigmine in Neurology and Psychiatry," in *Clin Neuropharmacol,* Vol. 1, Klawans, H.L., Ed. New York, Raven Press, 1976, pp. 63-79.

14. Leff, R., and Bernstein, S.: Proprietary hallucinogens. *Dis Nerv Syst 29*:621-626, 1968.

15. Longo, V.G.: Behavioral and electroencephalographic effects of atropine and related compounds. *Pharmacol Rev 18*:965-996, 1966.

16. Parfitt, D.N.: An outbreak of atropine poisoning. *J Neurol Neurosurg Psychiatry 10*:85-88, 1947.

17. Ullman, K.C., and Groh, R.H.: Identification and treatment of acute psychotic states secondary to the usage of over-the-counter sleeping preparations. *Am J Psychiatry 128*:1244-1248, 1972.

18. Bernstein, S., and Leff, R.: Toxic psychosis from sleeping medicines containing scopolamine. *N Engl J Med 277*:638-639, 1967.

19. Thakkar, M.K., and Lasser, R.P.: Scopolamine intoxication from nonprescription sleeping pill. *NY St J Med 72*:725-726, 1972.

20. Jacobs, K.W.: Asthmador: A legal hallucinogen. *Int J Addict 9*:503-512, 1974.

21. DiGiacomo, J.N.: Toxic effect of stramonium simulating LSD trip. *JAMA 204*:173-174, 1968.

22. Ostler, H.B.: Cycloplegics and mydriatics. *Arch Ophthalmol 93*:432-433, 1975.

23. Bennett, N.B., and Kohn, J.: Case report: orphenadrine overdose. Cerebral manifestations treated with physostigmine. *Anesth Intensive Care 4*:157, 1976.

24. Jones, I.H., Stevenson, J., Jordan, A., et al.: Pheniramine as hallucinogen. *Med J Aust 1*:382--386, 1973.
25. Malcolm, R., and Miller, W.C.: Dimenhydrinate (dramamine) abuse: Hallucinogenic experiences wtih a proprietary antihistamine. *Am J Psychiatry 128*:1012-1013, 1972.
26. Lee, J.H., Turndorf, H., and Poppers, P.J.: Physostigmine reversal of antihistamine-induced excitement and depression. *Anesthesiology 43*:683-684, 1975.
27. Schipior, P.G.: An unusual case of antihistamine intoxication. *J Pediatr 71*:589-591, 1967.
28. Mendelson, G.: Pheniramine aminosalicylate overdosage. *Arch Neurol 34*:313, 1977.
29. Ananth, J.V., and Jain, R.C.: Benztropine psychosis. *Can Psychiatr Assoc J 18*:409-414, 1973.
30. Bolin, R.B.: Psychiatric manifestations of Artane toxicity. *J Nerv Ment Dis 131*:256-259, 1960.
31. Stephens, D.A.: Psychotoxic effects of benzhexol hydrochloride (Artane). *Br J Psychiatry 113*:213-218, 1967.
32. Warnes, H.: Toxic psychosis due to antiparkinsonian drugs. *Can Psychiatr Assoc J 12*:323-326, 1967.
33. Woody, G., and O'Brien, C.P.: Anticholinergic toxic psychosis in drug abusers treated with benztropine. *Compr Psychiatry 15*:439-442, 1974.
34. El-Yousef, M.K., Janowsky, D.S., Davis, J.M., and Sekerke, J.H.: Reversal of antiparkinsonian drug toxicity by physostigmine: a controlled study. *Am J Psychiatry 130*:141-145, 1973.
35. Greenblatt, D.J., and Shader, R.I.: Anticholinergics. *N Engl J Med 288*:1215-1219, 1973.
36. Asher, L.M., and Cohen, S.: The effect of banthine on the central nervous system. *Gastroenterology 17*:178-183, 1951.
37. Ginsburg, C.M., and Angle, C.R.: Diphenoxylate-atropine (Lomotil) poisoning. *Clin Toxicol 2*:377-382, 1969.
38. Mirakhur, R.K., Clarke, R.S.J., Dundee, J.W., and McDonald, J.R.: Anticholinergic drugs in anaesthesia. *Anaesthesia 33*:133-138, 1978.
39. Smiler, B.G., Bartholomew, E.G., Sivak, B.J., et al.: Physostigmine reversal of scopolamine delirium in obstetric patients. *Am J Obstet Gynecol 116*:326-349, 1973.
40. Kuhn, J.A., and Savage, G.J.: Belladonna alkaloid psychosis. *Delaware Med J 46*:239-242, 1974.
41. Angst, J., and Hicklin, A.: Deliröse Psychosen unter Neuroleptica und Antidepressiva. *Schweiz Med Wschr 97*:546-549, 1967.
42. Beszterczey, A., and Pecknold, J.C.: Toxic psychosis induced by high dosage of chlorpromazine therapy. *Can Med Assoc J 104*:884-889, 1971.

43. Chaffin, D.S.: Phenothiazine induced acute psychotic reaction: the psychotoxicity of a drug. *Am J Psychiatry 121*:26-32, 1964.

44. Greenberg, R.S., and Joseph, E.D.: A chlorpromazine organic psychotic reaction. *Mt Sinai J Med NY 29*:165-171, 1962.

45. Helmchen, H.: Delirante Abläufe unter psychiatrischer Pharmakotherapie. *Arch Psychiat Nervenkr 202*:395-411, 1961.

46. Helmchen, H., and Hippius, H.: Die unerwunschten psychischen Wirkungen der Psychopharmaka. *Der Internist 9*:336-344, 1967.

47. Davies, R.K., Tucker, G.J., Harrow, M., and Detre, T.P.: Confusional episodes and antidepressant medications. *Am J Psychiatry 128*:95-99, 1971.

48. Heiser, J.F., and Wilbert, D.E.: Reversal of delirium induced by tricyclic antidepressant drugs with physostigmine. *Am J Psychiatry 131*:1275-1277, 1974.

49. Johnson, P.B.: Physostigmine in tricyclic antidepressant overdose. *JACEP 5*:443-445, 1976.

50. Slovis, T.L., Ott, J.E., Teitelbaum, D.T., and Lipscomb, W.: Physostigmine therapy in acute tricyclic antidepressant poisoning. *Clin Toxicol 4*:451-459, 1971.

51. Tchen, P., Weatherhead, A.D., and Richards, N.G.: Acute intoxication with desipramine. *N Engl J Med 274*:1197, 1966.

52. Kramer, M.: Delirium as a complication of imipramine therapy. *Am J Psychiatry 120*:502-503, 1961.

53. Chapin, J.W., and Wingard, D.W.: Physostigmine reversal of benzquinamide-induced delirium. *Anesthesiology 46*:364-465, 1977.

54. Brown, J.K., and Malone, M.H.: "Legal highs"—constituents, activity, toxicology, and herbal folklore. *Clin Toxicol 12*:1-31, 1978.

55. Dew, J.M.: Toxic delirium induced by deliberate ingestion of Jimson weed. *J Kent Med Assoc 7*:434-436, 1977.

56. Mahler, D.A.: Anticholinergic poisoning from Jimson weed. *JACEP. 5*:440-442, 1976.

57. Mikolich, J.R., Paulson, G.W., Cross, C.J., and Calhoun, R.: Neurologic and EEG effects of Jimson weed intoxication. *Clin Electroencephalogr 7*:49-57, 1976.

58. Hall, R.C.W., Popkin, M.K., and McHenry, L.E.: Angel's trumpet psychosis. *Am J Psychiatry 134*:312-314, 1977.

59. Pedigo, L.G.: Case of atropia poisoning successfully treated with amyl nitrite, with remarks on treatment. *Va Med Mon 15*:81-87, 1888.

60. Kleinwachter, I.: Beobachtung uber die Wirkung des Calabar-Extracts gegen Atropin-vergiftung. *Berl Klin Wchshr 1*:369-371, 1864.

61. Vojtechovsky, M., Vitek, V., and Rysanek, K.: Experimentelle Psychose nach Verabreichung von Benactyzin. *Arzneim Forsch 16*:240-242, 1966.

62. Crowell, E.B., and Ketchum, J.S.: The treatment of scopolamine-induced delirium with physostigmine. *Clin Pharmacol Ther 8*: 409-414, 1967.

63. Duvoisin, R.C., and Katz, R.D.: Reversal of central anticholinergic syndrome in man by physostigmine. *JAMA 296*:1963-1965, 1968.

64. Rumack, B.: Anticholinergic poisoning: Treatment with physostigmine. *Pediatrics 52*:449, 451, 1973.

65. Walker, W.E., Levy, R.C., and Hanenson, B.: Physostigmine—its use and abuse. *JACEP 5*:436-439, 1976.

66. Larson, G.F., Hurlbert, B.J., and Wingard, D.W.: Physostigmine reversal of diazepam-induced depression. *Anesth Analg 56*:348-351, 1977.

67. Blitt, C.D., and Petty, W.C.: Reversal of lorazepam delirium by physostigmine. *Anesth Analg 54*:607-608, 1975.

68. Modestin, J.: Zur Pathogenese deliranter Zustände. *Confin Psychiatr 17*:42-52, 1974.

69. Itil, T., and Fink, M.: EEG and behavioral aspects of the interactions of anticholinergic hallucinogens with centrally active compounds. *Prog Brain Res 28*:149-168, 1968.

70. Drachman, D.: Memory and cognitive function in man: Does the cholinergic system have a specific role? *Neurology 27*:783-790, 1977.

71. Petersen, R.C.: Scopolamine-induced learning failures in man. *Psychopharmacology 52*:283-289, 1977.

72. Peters, B.H., and Levin, H.S.: Memory enhancement after physostigmine treatment in the amnesic syndrome. *Arch Neurol 34*:215-219, 1977.

73. Davis, K.L., Hollister, L.E., Overall, J., Johnson, A., and Train, K.: Physostigmine: Effects on cognition and affect in normal subjects. *Psychopharmacology 51*:23-27, 1976.

74. *FDA Drug Bulletin. 8*:5-6, 1978.

75. Essig, C.F.: Addiction to nonbarbiturate sedative and tranquilizing drugs. *Clin Pharmacol Ther 5*:334-343, 1964.

76. Isbell, H., Altschul, S., Kornetsky, C.H., et al.: Chronic barbiturate intoxication. *Arch Neurol Psychiatr 64*:1-28, 1950.

77. Kornetsky, C., Humphries, O., and Evarts, E.V.: Comparison of psychological effects of certain centrally acting drugs in man. *Arch Neurol Psychiatry 77*:318-324, 1957.

78. DeBoor, W.: *Pharmakopsychologie und Psychopathologie.* Berlin, Springer, 1956.

79. Schwartz, J.F., and Patterson, J.H.: Toxic encephalopathy related to antihistamine-barbiturate antiemetic medication. *Am J Dis Child 132*:37-39, 1978.

80. Kane, F.J., and Ewing, J.A.: Iatrogenic brain syndrome. *South Med J 58*:875-877, 1965.

81. Gibson, I.I.: Barbiturate delirium. *Practitioner* 197:345-347, 1966.
82. Robinson, G.W.: "The Toxic Delirious Reactions of Old Age," in *Mental Disorders in Later Life*. Kaplan, O.J., Ed. Stanford, Stanford Univ. Press, 1956, pp. 332-351.
83. McDonald, C., Mowbray, R.M., and Wilson, J.M.O.: A sequential trial of amylobarbitone sodium used as sedation for confused psychogeriatric patients. *Gerontol Clin* 12:335-338, 1970.
84. Margetts, E.L.: Chloral delirium. *Psychiatr Q* 24:278-299, 1950.
85. McDonald, C.E., Owens, D., and Bolman, W.M.: Bromide abuse: A continuing problem. *Am J Psychiatry* 131:913-915, 1974.
86. Blaylock, J.D.: Bromism: A persistent peril. *J Arkansas Med Soc* 70:130-135, 1973.
87. Trump, D.L., and Hochberg, M.C.: Bromide intoxication. *J Hopk Med J* 138:119-123, 1976.
88. Fried, F.E., and Malek-Ahmadi, P.: Bromism: Recent perspectives. *South Med J* 68:220-222, 1975.
89. Levin, M.: Transitory schizophrenias produced by bromide intoxication. *Am J Psychiatry* 103:229-237, 1946.
90. Levin, M.: Bromide delirium with unusual course. *Am J Psychiatry* 110:130-132, 1953.
91. Levin, M.: Eye disturbances in bromide intoxication. *Am J Ophthalmol* 50:478-483, 1960.
92. Serpe, S.J.: Bromide intoxication. *NY St J Med* 72:2086-2088, 1972.
93. Carney, M.W.P.: Five cases of bromism. *Lancet* 2:523-524, 1971.
94. Tillim, S.J.: Bromide intoxication and quantitative determination in serum. *Am J Psychiatry* 114:232-236, 1957.
95. Greenblatt, D.J., Allen, M.D., and Shader, R.I.: Toxicity of high-dose flurazepam in the elderly. *Clin Pharmacol Ther* 21:355-361, 1977.
96. Greenblatt, D.J., Shader, R.I., and Koch-Weser, J.: Flurazepam hydrochloride, a benzodiazepine hypnotic. *Ann Intern Med* 83: 237-241, 1975.
97. Shader, R.I., Greenblatt, D.J., Salzman, C., Kochansky, G.E., and Harmatz, J.S.: Benzodiazepines: Safety and toxicity. *Dis Nerv Syst* 36:23-26, 1975.
98. Greenblatt, D.J., and Shader, R.I.: *Benzodiazepines in Clinical Practice*. New York, Raven Press, 1974.
99. Hall, R.C.W., and Joffe, J.R.: Aberrant response to diazepam: A new syndrome. *Am J Psychiatry* 129:738-742, 1972.
100. Viscott, D.S.: Chlordiazepoxide and hallucinations. *Arch Gen Psychiatry* 19:370-376, 1968.
101. Essig, C.F.: Newer sedative drugs that can cause states of intoxication and dependence of barbiturate type. *JAMA* 196:714-717, 1966.

102. Gerald, M.C., and Schwirian, P.M.: Nonmedical use of methaqualone. *Arch Gen Psychiatry 28*:627-631, 1973.
103. Haas, D.C., and Marasigan, A.: Neurological effects of glutethimide. *J Neurol Neurosurg Psychiatry 31*:561-564, 1968.
104. Zvin, I., and Shalowitz, M.: Acute toxic reaction to prolonged glutethimide administration. *N Engl J Med 266*:496-498, 1962.
105. Cohen, S.: The toxic psychoses and allied states. *Am J Med 15*:813-828, 1953.
106. Miller, R.R., and Jick, H.: Clinical effects of meperidine in hospitalized medical patients. *J Clin Pharmacol 18*:180-189, 1978.
107. MacVicar, A.A.: Psychotic symptoms due to meperidine intoxication. *Can Med Assoc J 110*:1237, 1974.
108. DeNosaquo, N.: The hallucinatory effect of pentazocine (Talwin). *JAMA 210*:502, 1969.
109. Wood, A.J.J., Moir, D.C., Campbell, C., et al.: Medicines evaluation and monitoring group: Central nervous system effects of pentazocine. *Br Med J 1*:305-307, 1974.
110. Miller, R.R.: Clinical effects of pentazocine in hospitalized medical patients. *J Clin Pharmacol 15*:198-205, 1975.
111. Swanson, D.W., Weddige, R.L., and Morse, R.M.: Hospitalized pentazocine abusers. *Mayo Clin Proc 48*:85-93, 1973.
112. Byrd, G.J., and Kane, F.J.: Persistent psychotic phenomena following one dose of pentazocine. *Tex Med 72*:68-69, 1976.
113. Editorial: Mental side effects of pentazocine. *Br Med J 1*:297, 1974.
114. Kane, F.J., and Pokorny, A.: Mental and emotional disturbance with pentazocine (Talwin) use. *South Med J 68*:808-811, 1975.
115. Yost, M.A., and McKegney, F.P.: Acute organic psychosis due to Talwin (pentazocine). *Conn Med 34*:259-260, 1970.
116. Abrishami, M.A., and Thomas, J.: Aspirin intolerance—a review. *Ann Allergy 39*:28-37, 1977.
117. Greer, H.D., Ward, H.P., and Corbin, K.B.: Chronic salicylate intoxication in adults. *JAMA 193*:555-558, 1965.
118. Good, A.E., and Welch, M.H.: Hospital-acquired salicylate intoxication. Report of a case with psychosis, acidosis, and coma. *J Rheumatol 2*:52-60, 1975.
119. Brown, G.L., and Wilson, W.P.: Salicylate intoxication and the CNS. *Dis Nerv Syst 32*:135-140, 1971.
120. Miller, R.R., and Jick, H.: Acute toxicity of aspirin in hospitalized medical patients. *Am J Med Sci 274*:271-279, 1977.
121. Courville, C.B., and Myers, R.O.: Cerebral changes in salicylate poisoning. *Bull Los Angeles Neurol Soc 21*:124-136, 1956.
122. Murray, R.M.: Personality factors in analgesic nephropathy. *Psychol Med 4*:69-73, 1974.
123. Krenzelok, E.P., Best, L., and Manoguerra, A.S.: Acetaminophen toxicity. *Am J Hosp Pharm 34*:391-394, 1977.

124. Liederman, P.C., and Boldus, R.A.: Psychic side effects of a chlor-zoxazone and acetaminophen mixture. *JAMA* 202:64-66, 1967.
125. *FDA Drug Bulletin.* 8:14, 1978.
126. Claghorn, J.L., and Schoolar, J.C.: Propoxyphene hydrochloride, a drug of abuse. *JAMA* 196:1089-1091, 1966.
127. Weiss, S.: Effect of the digitalis bodies on the nervous system. *Med Clin N Am* 15:963-982, 1932.
128. King, J.T.: Digitalis delirium. *Ann Intern Med* 33:1360-1372, 1950.
129. Editorial: Digitalis: A neuroexcitatory drug. *Circulation* 52:739-742, 1975.
130. Sagel, J., and Matisonn, R.: Neuropsychiatric disturbance as the initial manifestation of digitalis toxicity. *S Afr Med J* 46:512-514, 1972.
131. Church, G., and Marriott, HJ.L.: Digitalis delirium. A report on three cases. *Circulation* 20:549-553, 1959.
132. Shear, M.K., and Sacks, M.H.: Digitalis delirium: Report of two cases. *Am J Psychiatry* 135:109-110, 1978.
133. Buchanan, J.: Self-poisoning with digitalis glycosides. *Br Med J* 3:661-662, 1967.
134. Gilbert, G.J.: Quinidine dementia. *JAMA* 237:2093-2094, 1977.
135. Quintanilla, J.: Psychosis due to quinidine intoxication. *Am J Psychiatry* 113:1031-1032, 1957.
136. Singh, B.N.: Side effects of antiarrhythmic drugs. *Pharmacol Ther C* 2:151-166, 1977.
137. Voltolina, E.J., Thompson, S.I., and Tisue, J.: Acute organic brain syndrome with propranolol. *Clin Toxicol* 4:357-359, 1971.
138. Shopsin, B., Hirsch, J., and Gershon, S.: Visual hallucinations and propranolol. *Br Psychiatry* 10:105-107, 1975.
139. Ilyas, M., Owens, D., and Kvasnicka, G.: Delirium induced by a combination of anti-arrhythmic drugs. *Lancet* 2:1368-1369, 1969.
140. Current status of propranolol hydrochloride (Inderal). *JAMA* 225:1380-1384, 1973.
141. Orzack, M.H., and Branconnier, R.: CNS effects of propranolol in man. *Psychopharmacol* (Berl.) 29:299-306, 1973.
142. Elliott, F.A.: Propranolol for the control of belligerent behavior following acute brain damage. *Ann Neurol* 1:489-491, 1976.
143. Adler, S.: Methyldopa-induced decrease in mental activity. *JAMA* 230:1428-1429, 1974.
144. Hawkins, D.J.: Acute organic brain syndrome psychosis with methyldopa therapy. *Mo Med* 73:476-481, 1976.
145. Thornton, W.E.: Dementia induced by methyldopa with haloperidol. *N Engl J Med* 294:1222, 1976.
146. Lewis, W.H.: Iatrogenic psychotic depressive reaction in hypertensive patients. *Am J Psychiatry* 127:1416-1417, 1971.

147. Leiber, L.: Psychological side effects of L-dopa and anticonvulsant medication. *NY St J Med* 77:1098-1102, 1977.
148. Plaa, G.L.: Acute toxicity of antiepileptic drugs. *Epilepsia* 16:183-191, 1975.
149. Roseman, E.: Dilantin toxicity. *Neurology* 11:912-921, 1961.
150. Trimble, M.R., and Reynolds, E.H.: Anticonvulsant drugs and mental symptoms: A review. *Psychol Med* 6:169-178, 1976.
151. Kline, C.L., and Highsmith, L.S.: Toxic psychosis resulting from penicillin. *Ann Intern Med* 28:1057-1058, 1948.
152. Bradberry, J.C., and Owens, J.: Acute psychotic reaction to procaine penicillin. *Am J Hosp Pharm* 32:411-413, 1975.
153. Cohen, S.B.: Brain damage due to penicillin. *JAMA* 186:899-902, 1963.
154. Conway, N., Beck, E., and Somerville, J.: Penicillin encephalopathy. *Postgrad Med J* 44:891-897, 1968.
155. Downham, T.F., and Ramos, D.P.: Non-allergic adverse reactions to aqueous procaine penicillin G. *Mich Med* 72:223-227, 1973.
156. Levine, P.H., Regelson, W., and Holland, J.F.: Chloramphenicol-associated encephalopathy. *Clin Pharmacol Ther* 11:194-199, 1970.
157. Porot, M., and Destaing, F.: Streptomycine et troubles mentaux. *Ann Med Psychol* 108:47-53, 1950.
158. Byrd, G.J.: Acute organic brain syndrome associated with gentamicin therapy. *JAMA* 238:53-54, 1977.
159. Saker, B.M., Musk, A.W., Haywood, E.F., and Hurst, P.E.: Reversible toxic psychosis after cephalexin. *Med J Aust* 1:497-498, 1973.
160. Lastnick, G.: Psychotic symptoms with griseofulvin. *JAMA* 229:1420-1421, 1974.
161. Good, M.I., and Shader, R.I.: Behavioral toxicity and equivocal suicide associated with chloroquine and its derivatives. *Am J Psychiatry* 134:798-801, 1977.
162. Engel, G.L., Romano, J., and Ferris, E.B.: Effect of quinacrine (atabrine) on the central nervous system. *Arch Neurol Psychiatry* 58:337-350, 1947.
163. Greiber, M.F.: Psychoses associated with the administration of atabrine. *Am J Psychiatry* 104:306-310, 1947.
164. Rockwell, D.A.: Psychiatric complications with chloroquine and quinacrine. *Am J Psychiatry* 124:1257-1260, 1968.
165. Pleasure, H.: Psychiatric and neurological side effects of isoniazid and iproniazid. *Arch Neurol Psychiatry* 72:313-320, 1954.
166. Brown, C.V.: Acute isoniazid poisoning. *Am Rev Resp Dis* 105:206-216, 1972.
167. Crane, G.E.: The psychiatric side effects of iproniazid. *Am J Psychiatry* 112:494-501, 1956.

168. Bankier, R.G.: Psychosis associated with cycloserine. *Can Med Assoc J 93*:35-37, 1965.
169. Simeon, J., Fink, M., Itil, T.M., and Ponce, D.: d-Cycloserine therapy of psychosis by symptom provocation. *Compr Psychiatry 11*:80-88, 1970.
170. Lansdown, F.S., Beran, M., and Litwak, T.: Psychotoxic reaction during ethionamide therapy. *Am Rev Resp Dis 95*:1053-1055, 1967.
171. Holland, J.: "Psychologic Aspects of Cancer," in *Cancer Medicine,* 2nd edition, Holland, J.F., and Frei, E., Eds. Philadelphia, Lea and Febiger, in press.
172. Weiss, H.D., Walker, M.D., and Wiernik, P.H.: Neurotoxicity of commonly used antineoplastic agents. *N Engl J Med 291*:75-81, 1974.
173. Roswit, B., and Pisetsky, J.E.: Toxic psychosis following nitrogen mustard therapy. *J Nerv Ment Dis 115*:356-359, 1952.
174. Holland, J., Fasaniello, S., and Ohnuma, T.: Psychiatric symptoms associated with L-asparaginase administration. *J Psychiatr Res 10*:105-113, 1974.
175. Greenwald, E.S.: Organic mental changes with fluorouracil therapy. *JAMA 235*:248-249, 1976.
176. Pizzo, P.A., Bleyer, W.A., Poplack, D.G., and Leventhal, B.G.: Reversible dementia temporally associated with intraventricular therapy with methotrexate in a child with acute myelogenous leukemia. *J Pediatr 88*:131-133, 1976.
177. Pochedly, C.: Neurotoxicity due to CNS therapy for leukemia. *Med Pediatr Oncol 3*:101-115, 1977.
178. Fusner, J.E., Poplack, D.G., Pizzo, P.A., and DiChiro, G.: Leuko-encephalopathy following chemotherapy for rhabdomyosarcoma: Reversibility of cerebral changes demonstrated by computed tomography. *J Pediatr 91*:77-79, 1977.
179. Bjorgen, J.E., and Gold, L.H.A.: Computed tomographic appearance of methotrexate-induced necrotizing leukoencephalopathy. *Radiology 122*:377-378, 1977.
180. Delaney, J.C., and Ravey, M.: Cimetidine and mental confusion. *Lancet 2*:512, 1977.
181. Grimson, T.A.: Reactions to cimetidine. *Lancet 1*:858, 1977.
182. Klotz, S.A., and Kay, B.F.: Cimetidine and agranulocytosis. *Ann Intern Med 88*:579-580, 1978.
183. Miller, A.A., Ambis, D., and Siegel, J.H.: Cimetidine and mental confusion. *N Engl J Med 298*:284-285, 1978.
184. Menzies-Gow, N.: Cimetidine and mental confusion. *Lancet 2*:928, 1977.
185. Nelson, P.G.: Cimetidine and mental confusion. *Lancet 2*:928, 1977.

186. Quap, C.W.: Confusion: An adverse reaction to cimetidine therapy. *Drug Intell Clin Pharm 12*:121, 1978.
187. Villareal, S.V., Escande, M., and Levet, C.: À propos des psychoses cortisoniques. *Ann Med Psychol 14*:523-530, 1974.
188. The Boston Collaborative Drug Surveillance Program: Acute adverse reactions to prednisone in relation to dosage. *Clin Pharmacol Ther 13*:694-698, 1972.
189. Ritchie, E.A.: Toxic psychosis under cortisone and corticotrophin. *J Ment Sci 102*:830-837, 1956.
190. Glaser, G.H.: Psychotic reactions induced by corticotrophin (ACTH) and cortisone. *Psychosom Med 15*:280-291, 1953.
191. Clark, L.D., Bauer, W., and Cobb, S.: Preliminary observations on mental disturbances occurring in patients under therapy with cortisone and ACTH. *N Engl J Med 246*:205-216, 1952.
192. Zerssen, D., von: "Mood and Behavioral Changes Under Corticosteroid Therapy," in *Psychotropic Action of Hormones*, Itil, T.M., Laudahn, G., and Herrmann, W.M., Eds. New York, Spectrum Publ., 1976, pp. 195-222.
193. Quarton, G.C., Clark, L.D., Cobb, S., and Bauer, W.: Mental disturbances associated with ACTH and cortisone: A review of explanatory hypotheses. *Medicine 34*:13-50, 1955.
194. Agulnik, P.L., Dimascio, A., and Moore, P.: Acute brain syndrome associated with lithium therapy. *Am J Psychiatry 129*:621-623, 1972.
195. Baldessarini, R.J., and Lipinski, J.F.: Lithium salts: 1970-1975. *Ann Intern Med 83*:527-533, 1975.
196. Johnson, G.F.S.: Lithium neurotoxicity. *Aust NZ J Psychiatry 10*:33-38, 1976.
197. Rifkin, A., Quitkin, F., and Klein, D.F.: Organic brain syndrome during lithium carbonate treatment. *Compr Psychiatry 14*:251-254, 1973.
198. Strayhorn, J.M., and Nash, J.L.: Severe neurotoxicity despite "therapeutic" serum lithium levels. *Dis Nerv Syst 38*:107-111, 1977.
199. Foster, J.R., Gershell, W.J., and Goldfarb, A.I.: Lithium treatment in the elderly. 1. Clinical usage. *J Gerontol 32*:299-302, 1977.
200. McKnelly, W.V., Tupin, J.P., and Dunn, M.: Lithium in hazardous circumstances with one case of lithium toxicity. *Compr Psychiatry 11*:279-286, 1970.
201. Baastrup, P.C., Hollnagel, P., Sorensen, R., Schou, M.: Adverse reactions in treatment with lithium carbonate and haloperidol. *JAMA 236*:2645-2646, 1976.
202. Cohen, W.J., and Cohen, N.H.: Lithium carbonate, haloperidol, and irreversible brain damage. *JAMA 230*:1283-1287, 1974.
203. Byrd, G.J.: Lithium carbonate and methyldopa: Apparent interaction in man. *Clin Toxicol 11*:1-4, 1977.

204. Zakowska-Dabrowska, T., and Rybakowski, J.: Lithium-induced EEG changes: relation to lithium levels in serum and red blood cells. Acta Psychiatr Scand 49:457-465, 1973.
205. Lindstedt, G., Nilsson, L., Walinder, J., Skott, A., and Ohman, R.: On the prevalence, diagnosis and management of lithium-induced hypothyroidism in psychiatric patients. Br J Psychiatry 130:452-458, 1977.
206. Celesia, G.G., and Barr, A.N.: Psychosis and other psychiatric manifestations of levodopa therapy. Arch Neurol 23:193-200, 1970.
207. Rabey, J.M., Vardi, J., Askenazi, J.J., and Streifler, M.: L-tryptophan administration in L-dopa-induced hallucinations in elderly Parkinsonian patients. Gerontology 23:438-444, 1977.
208. Lin, J.T.Y., and Ziegler, D.K.: Psychiatric symptoms with initiation of carbidopa-levodopa treatment. Neurol 26:699-700, 1976.
209. Postma, J.U., and Van Tilburg, W.: Visual hallucinations and delirium during treatment with amantadine (Symmetrel). J Am Ger Soc 23:212-215, 1975.
210. Knee, S.T., and Razani, J.: Acute organic brain syndrome: A complication of disulfiram therapy. Am J Psychiatry 131:1281-1282, 1974.
211. Liddon, S., and Satran, R.: Disulfiram (Antabuse) psychosis. Am J Psychiatry 123:1284-1289, 1967.
212. Heath, R.G., Nesselhof, W., Bishop, M.P., et al.: Behavioral and metabolic changes associated with administration of tetraethylthiuram disulfide (Antabuse). Dis Nerv Syst 29:99-105, 1965.
213. Hotson, J.R., and Langston, J.W.: Disulfiram-induced encephalopathy. Arch Neurol 33:141-142, 1976.
214. Billiard, M., Besset, A., Renaud, B., et al.: L'insomnie de l'encephalopathie bismuthique. Rev EEG Neurophysiol 7:147-152, 1977.
215. Burns, R., Thomas, D.W., and Barron, V.J.: Reversible encephalopathy possibly associated with bismuth subgallate ingestion. Br Med J 1:220-223, 1974.
216. Kruger, G., Thomas, D.J., Weinhardt, F., and Hoyer, S.: Disturbed oxidative metabolism in organic brain syndrome caused by bismuth in skin creams. Lancet 2:485-487, 1976.
217. Supino-Viterbo, V., Sicard, C., Risvegliato, M., Rancurel, G., and Buge, A.: Toxic encephalopathy due to ingestion of bismuth salts: clinical and EEG studies of 24 patients. J Neurol Neurosurg Psychiatry 40:748-752, 1977.
218. Moses, A.M., and Miller, M.: Drug-induced dilutional hyponatremia. N Engl J Med 291:1234-1239, 1974.
219. Shibolet, S., Lancaster, M.C., and Danon, Y.: Heat stroke: A review. Aviat Space Envir Med March, 1976, pp. 280-301.

220. Seltzer, H.S.: Drug-induced hypoglycemia. *Diabetes 21*:955-966, 1972.

221. Nolke, A.C.: Severe toxic effects from aminophylline and theophylline suppositories in children. *JAMA 161*:693-697, 1956.

222. Stillner, V., Popkin, M.K., and Pierce, C.M.: Caffeine-induced delirium during prolonged competitive stress. *Am J Psychiatry 135*:855-856, 1978.

223. Pearce, I., and Pearce, J.M.S.: Bromocriptine in Parkinsonism. *Br Med J 1*:1402-1404, 1978.

224. Monroe, R.R.: The episodic psychoses of Vincent van Gogh. *J Nerv Ment Dis 166*:480-488, 1978.

225. Banki, C.M., and Vojnik, M.: Comparative simultaneous measurement of cerebrospinal fluid 5-hydroxyindoleacetic acid and blood serotonin levels in delirium tremens and clorazapine-induced delirious reaction. *J Neurol Neurosurg Psychiatry 41*:420-424, 1978.

226. Post, R.M.: Cocaine psychoses: a continuum model. *Am J Psychiatry 132*:225-231, 1975.

227. Goodman, L.S., and Gilman, A., Eds.: *The Pharmacological Basis of Therapeutics*. 4th edition. London, Collier-MacMillan Ltd., 1970, p. 340.

228. Boardman, P.L., and Hart, F.D.: Side effects of indomethacin. *Ann Rheum Dis 26*:127-132, 1967.

229. Knox, J.W.D., Bovill, J.G., Clarke, R.S.J., and Dundee, J.W.: Clinical studies of induction agents. XXXVI: Ketamine. *Br J Anaesth 42*:875-888, 1970.

230. Wantz, G.P.: A method of preventing emergence reactions following ketamine anesthesia. *Anesth Rev*, July, 1977.

231. Collier, B.B.: Ketamine and the conscious mind. *Anaesthesia 27*:120-134, 1972.

232. Fine, J., and Finestone, S.C.: Sensory disturbances following ketamine anesthesia: recurrent hallucinations. *Anesth Analg 52*:428-430, 1973.

233. Hejja, P., and Galloon, S.: A consideration of ketamine dreams. *Can Anaesth Soc J 22*:100-105, 1975.

234. Meyers, E.F., and Charles, P.: Prolonged adverse reactions to ketamine in children. *Anesthesiology 49*:39-40, 1978.

235. Johnstone, R.E.: A ketamine trip. *Anesthesiology 39*:460-461, 1973.

236. Harris, J.A., Biersner, R.J., Edwards, D., and Bailey, L.W.: Attention, learning, and personality during ketamine emergence: a pilot study. *Anesth Analg 54*:169-172, 1975.

237. Hefez, A., and Lanyi, G.: Neuropsychiatric manifestations of ketamine hydrochloride. *Isr Ann Psychiatry 10*:180-187, 1972.

238. Khorramanzadeh, E., and Lotfy, A.O.: The use of ketamine in psychiatry. *Psychosomatics 14*:344-346, 1973.

239. Condi, M., Sallerin, T., and Devaux, C.: Utilisation de la ketamine dans le traitement du délirium tremens et des délires medicaux. *Anesth Analg 29*:377-394, 1972.
240. Lilburn, J.K., Dundee, J.W., Nair, S.G., et al.: Ketamine sequelae. *Anaesthesia 33*:307-311, 1978.
241. Balmer, H.G.R., and Wyte, S.R.: Antagonism of ketamine by physostigmine. *Br J Anaesth 49*:510, 1977.
242. Burns, R.S., Lerner, S.E., Corrado, R., et al.: Phencyclidine—states of acute intoxication and fatalities. *West J Med 123*:345-349, 1975.
243. Showalter, C.V., and Thornton, W.E.: Clinical pharmacology of phencyclidine toxicity. *Am J Psychiatry 134*:1234-1238, 1977.
244. Liden, C.B., Lovejoy, F.H., and Costello, C.E.: Phencyclidine. Nine cases of poisoning. *JAMA 234*:513-516, 1975.
245. Brodsky, L., and Zuniga, J.: Nitrous oxide: a psychotogenic agent. *Compr Psychiatry 16*:185-188, 1975.
246. Sortland, O., Lundervold, A., and Nesbakken, R.: Mental confusion and epileptic seizures following cervical myelography with metrizamide. *Acta Radiol, Suppl 355*:403-406, 1977.

Additional References

Abelson, H.T. Methotrexate and central nervous system toxicity. *Cancer Treatm Rep 62*:1999-2001, 1978.
Agarwal, S.K. Cimetidine and visual hallucinations. *JAMA 240*:214, 1978.
Allen, J.C. The effects of cancer therapy on the nervous system. *J Pediatr 93*:903-909, 1978.
Allen, J.C., and Rosen, G. Transient cerebral dysfunction following chemotherapy for osteogenic sarcoma. *Ann Neurol 3*:441-444, 1978.
Allen, R.M., and Flemenbaum, A. Delirium associated with combined fluphenazine-clonidine therapy. *J Clin Psychiatry 40*:236-237, 1979.
Allen, R.M., and Young, S.J. Phencyclidine-induced psychosis. *Am J Psychiatry 135*:1081-1084, 1978.
Anielańczyk, W. Delirious syndrome after haloperidol administration. *Psychiatria Polska (Gdansk) 7*:219-221, 1973.
Arena, F.P., Dugowson, C., and Saudek, C.D. Salicylate-induced hypoglycemia and ketoacidosis in a nondiabetic adult. *Arch Intern Med 138*:1153-1154, 1978.
Bartlett, J.D. Administration of and adverse reactions to cycloplegic agents. *Am J Optom Physiol Optics 55*:227-233, 1978.
Caroli, F., and Giuliano, G. Psychotropes et états confusionnels. *Rev Méd 20*:1173-1184, 1978.
Corbeil, R. Cimétidine et état confusionnel. *Vie Med Can 8*:15-16, 1979.
Daunderer, M. Akute Alkohol-intoxication: Physostigmin als Antidot gegen Äthanol. *Fortschr Med 96*:1311-1312, 1978.

Edmonds, M.E., Ashford, R.F.U., Brenner, M.K., and Saunders, A. Cimetidine: Does neurotoxicity occur? Report of three cases. *J Roy Soc Med* 72:172-175, 1979.

Flind, A.C., and Rowley-Jones, D. Mental confusion and cimetidine. *Lancet 1*:379, 1979.

Hall, R.C.W., Popkin, M.K., Stickney, S.K., and Gardner, E.R. Presentation of the "steroid psychoses." *J Nerv Ment Dis 167*:229-236, 1979.

Hollender, M.H., Jamieson, R.C., McKee, E.A., and Roback, H.B. Anticholinergic delirium in a case of Munchausen syndrome. *Am J Psychiatry 135*:1407-1409, 1978.

Hooper, R.G., Conner, C.S., and Rumack, B.H. Acute poisoning from over-the-counter sleep preparations. *JACEP 8*:98-100, 1979.

Ing, T.S., Daugindas, J.T., Klawans, H.L., et al. Toxic effects of amantadine in patients with renal failure. *Can Med Assoc J 120*:695-697, 1979.

Klawans, H.L. Levodopa-induced psychosis. *Psychiatric Annals 8*:447-451, 1978.

Kuhr, B.M. Prolonged delirium with propranolol. *J Clin Psychiatry 40*:198-199, 1979.

Kurland, M.L. Organic brain syndrome with propranolol. *N Engl J Med 300*:366, 1979.

Lieberman, A.N., Kupersmith, M., Gopinathan, G., et al. Bromocriptine in Parkinson disease: Further studies. *Neurology 29*:363-369, 1979.

McAllister, C.J., Scowden, E.B., and Stone, W.J. Toxic psychosis induced by phenothiazine administration in patients with chronic renal failure. *Clin Nephrol 10*:191-195, 1978.

McCrum, I.D., and Guidry, J.R. Procainamide-induced psychosis. *JAMA 240*:1265-1266, 1978.

Mogelnicki, S.R., Waller, J.L., and Finlayson, D.C. Physostigmine reversal of cimetidine-induced mental confusion. *JAMA 241*:826-827, 1979.

Palatucci, D.M. Paradoxical halide levels in bromide intoxication. *Neurology 28*:1189-1191, 1978.

Perry, P.J., Wilding, D.C., and Juhl, R.P. Anticholinergic psychosis. *Am J Hosp Pharm 35*:725-727, 1978.

Peterson, L.G., and Popkin, M.K. Psychiatric effects of cancer chemotherapeutic agents. Unpublished manuscript.

Pratt, T.H. Rifampin-induced organic brain syndrome. *JAMA 241*:2421-2422, 1979.

Raskind, M.A., Kitchell, M., and Alvarez, C. Bromide intoxication in the elderly. *J Am Geriatr Soc 26*:222-224, 1978.

Rubinstein, J.S. Abuse of antiparkinsonism drugs. *JAMA 239*:2365-2366, 1978.

Rumack, B.H., and Temple, A.R., Editors. *Management of the Poisoned Patient*. Princeton, Science Press, 1977.

Scharbach, H.   Complications psychiques des neuroleptiques. États confuso-oniriques. *Encéphale* 4:163-171, 1978.

Schentag, J.J., Calleri, G., Rose, J.Q., et al.   Pharmacokinetic and clinical studies in patients with cimetidine-associated mental confusion. *Lancet* 1:177-181, 1979.

Serby, M., Angrist, B., and Lieberman, A.   Mental disturbances during bromocriptine and lergotrile treatment of Parkinson's disease. *Am J Psychiatry* 135:1227-1229, 1978.

Sinianotis, C.A., Spyrides, P., Vlachos, P., and Papadatos, C.   Acute haloperidol poisoning in children. *J Pediatr* 93:1038-1039, 1978.

Sioris, L.J., and Krenzelok, E.P.   Phencyclidine intoxication: A literature review. *Am J Hosp Pharm* 35:1362-1367, 1978.

Skalpe, I.O.   Adverse effects of water-soluble contrast media in myelography, cisternography and ventriculography. *Acta Radiol (Suppl 355)*: 359-370, 1977.

Skullerud, K., and Halvorsen, K.   Encephalomyelopathy following intrathecal methotrexate treatment in a child with acute leukemia. *Cancer* 42:1211-1215, 1978.

Smith, R.C., Strong, J.R., and Samorajski, T.   Behavioral evidence for supersensitivity after chronic bromocriptine administration. *Psychopharmacol* 60:241-246, 1979.

Spring, G.K.   Neurotoxicity with combined use of lithium and thioridazine. *J Clin Psychiatry* 40:135-138, 1979.

Summers, W.K.   A clinical method of estimating risk of drug induced delirium. *Life Sci* 22:1511-1516, 1978.

Thompson, J., and Lilly, J.   Cimetidine-induced cerebral toxicity in children. *Lancet* 1:725, 1979.

Tindall, R.S.A., and Willerson, J.   Subacute phenytoin intoxication syndrome. *Arch Intern Med* 138:1168-1169, 1978.

Ulshen, M.H., Grand, R.J., Crain, J.D., and Gelfand, E.W.   Hepatotoxicity with encephalopathy associated with aspirin therapy in rheumatoid arthritis. *J Pediatr* 93:1034-1037, 1978.

Wesson, D.R., and Smith, D.E.   *Barbiturates: Their Use and Misuse.* New York, Human Science Press, 1976.

Wood, C.A., Isaacson, M.L., and Hibbs, M.S.   Cimetidine and mental confusion. *JAMA* 239:2550-2551, 1978.

CHAPTER 11

DELIRIUM DUE TO ALCOHOL AND DRUG WITHDRAWAL

ALCOHOL WITHDRAWAL DELIRIUM (DELIRIUM TREMENS)

PROBLEMS OF DEFINITION

T HERE IS A LACK OF general agreement on the definition and diagnostic criteria of delirium tremens. Gross et al. (1) state in their extensive review that the acute alcohol withdrawal syndrome is considered by many authorities to consist of three diagnostic groups: impending delirium tremens, acute alcoholic hallucinosis, and delirium tremens. These three groups of symptoms are differentiated according to three criteria: hallucinations, clouding of sensorium, and other signs of withdrawal, such as tremor. Delirium tremens is characterized by visual hallucinations, moderate to marked clouding of the sensorium, and moderate to marked signs and symptoms of withdrawal, i.e. tremulousness, insomnia, sweating, etc. Gross et al. point out, however, that 25 to 50 percent of the patients fail to meet these criteria. Auditory hallucinations, for example, are found in delirium tremens as often as the visual ones. The prevalence of hallucinations during the alcohol withdrawal syndrome is inversely related to age (1). Hallucinations and clouding of sensorium are positively correlated, but are to some extent independent features (1). There is overlap among the three traditionally recognized diagnostic groups within the alcohol withdrawal syndrome, and their separation in clinical practice is difficult.

Victor and Wolfe (2) confine the use of the term delirium tremens to a cluster of symptoms, which include profound confusion, hallucinations, increased speech and psychomotor activity, and overactivity of the autonomic nervous system, manifested by fever, tachycardia, sweats, and dilated pupils. These investigators distinguish between minor and major withdrawal syndrome, respectively. The former is manifested by tremor, mild sweating, hallucinations, seizures, and minimal disorientation. The major syndrome is equivalent to delirium tremens.

Diagnostic criteria for the alcohol withdrawal delirium in the current draft of the *Diagnostic and Statistical Manual of Mental Disorders, Third Edition* (3), include autonomic hyperactivity, disturbance of attention, disordered memory and orientation, reduced wakefulness or insomnia, perceptual disturbances, increased or decreased psychomotor activity, and a tendency for the symptoms to develop rapidly and to fluctuate in severity in the course of twenty-four hours. These criteria are the same as those used for the diagnosis of delirium generally, with only the added characteristic of autonomic hyperactivity.

Cutshall (4) traces back the definition of delirium tremens to Thomas Sutton, who was the first to use the term in 1813 and to distinguish the syndrome from other forms of phrenitis or delirium. Cutshall points out that the term has commonly been applied to the alcohol withdrawal state in general and proposes that the designation delirium tremens should not be applied until, and unless, the patient displays the following four manifestations: hallucinations or mental confusion, hyperkinesis, wakefulness, and tremor.

These four representative definitions overlap but are not equivalent. Since we are talking about a form of delirium, it should fit the descriptive definition adopted in this book. Some degree of global impairment of cognitive functions, i.e. memory, thinking, and perception, ought to be present for the term "delirium" to be applicable. The presence of hallucinations should not be considered necessary for the diagnosis of delirium in general, and of delirium tremens in particular. Gross et al. (5) found that patients suffering from an acute alcohol withdrawal syndrome displayed various constellations of symptoms, including hallucinations and clouding of sensorium. The latter was evaluated by these researchers and graded on the basis of orientation and performance of serial sevens. One-quarter of the patients with withdrawal symptoms lacked clouding of sensorium; 48 percent of them did not complain of hallucinations on admission. If one adopted the criteria for clouding of sensorium of Gross et al. (5), then the presence of disorientation should be regarded as a *sine qua non* for the diagnosis of withdrawal delirium.

It is clear that the term delirium tremens has been used inconsistently and thus statements by various authors regarding its incidence, pathophysiology, and treatment are difficult to interpret and compare. The best policy would be to adopt the term "alcohol withdrawal delirium" and grade it according to its severity. The term delirium tremens seems to be superfluous, but it is too entrenched to be dropped. It may be retained to designate the most severe degree of the alcohol withdrawal delirium, one featuring marked cognitive impairment, psychomotor and autonomic overactivity, hyperalertness, and hallucinations. Since most of the relevant literature since 1813 has used the term delirium tremens, it is impossible to review this literature without using it. It is hoped that once *DSM-III* is adopted, a more consistent terminology and diagnostic criteria will prevail.

CLINICAL FEATURES

The incidence of delirium tremens is unknown. Victor and Wolfe (2) state that if strict diagnostic criteria are used, the syndrome is relatively rare and occurs in about 5 percent of patients hospitalized for complications of alcoholism. On the other hand, Salum (6) found delirium tremens in about 44 percent of 1,026 male alcoholics hospitalized for acute mental and physical disturbances associated with drinking. Different diagnostic criteria are probably responsible for the wide discrepancy between these two reports. It is estimated that less than 1 percent of the alcoholics develop delirium tremens (1).

Age of patients varies from study to study and averages forty to fifty years (1). Men develop the syndrome four to five times as often as women. Delirium tremens occurs in alcoholics with a history of excessive drinking for at least several years, and the majority of patients give a history of more than ten years (1). Symptoms of abstinence or withdrawal come on as a rule some seven to twenty-four hours after cessation of drinking and consist mainly of tremor and hallucinations. This stage may be followed by convulsive seizures, whose peak incidence is at twenty-four hours. Delirium tremens, viewed as the most severe form or stage of alcohol withdrawal syndrome, develops seventy-two to ninety-six hours after cessation of drinking (2). This sequence of events is not invariable: seizures may not occur at all and delirium may not develop. If it does, it may emerge after three to four days of the tremulous-hallucinatory stage and without preceding seizures. If the latter do occur, however, they invariably come on before delirium (2). There is continuum of degree of severity of the withdrawal syndrome, with delirium tremens being its most severe stage, one that is reached, according to different reports, by 5 to 45 percent of alcoholics experiencing abstinence or withdrawal symptoms.

Clinical features of delirium tremens include gross global cognitive impairment or so-called clouding of sensorium, visual and auditory hallucinations, restlessness with hyperactivity, watchfulness with hyperalertness, insomnia, and signs of autonomic nervous system overactivity. The emotional tone varies and may range from pleasant or amused to panicky. A personal account of delirium by Root (7), published in 1844, speaks of the "horrors" that mark the experience of it. The large Swedish study reported by Salum (6) provides a wealth of information on the frequency of the various symptoms in patients with delirium tremens. Severe disorientation was noted in one-half of the patients; no patient was fully oriented, although about one in five displayed only a mild degree of disorientation. Visual hallucinations were observed in 97 percent, auditory in 79 percent, tactile in 39 percent, and gustatory or olfactory or both in 6 percent of the 552 cases of delirium. Delusions of persecution were present in 35 percent. Anxiety was noted in 65 percent, euphoria in 41 percent, depression in 13 percent, irritability in 48 percent, and aggressivity in 32 percent of the cases. Tremor was observed in 92 percent of patients on admission. General psychomotor hyperactivity was present in 92 percent, picking movements with fingers in 78 percent, attacks of clonic muscle jerks in 23 percent. One-third exhibited profuse sweating, one in five patients had vomiting or diarrhea or both. Fever was variable: none in 20 percent and in 57 percent the temperature was above 38°C at some time. Tachycardia with pulse rate of more than 90/min. was observed in 94 percent; in about one-third of the cases individual maximum values of over 120/min.

had been recorded. Both systolic and diastolic blood pressure were evaluated at some time in about two-thirds of the patients. The duration of delirium averaged three days; in only 5 percent did it last more than one week. Mortality was 3 percent and contrasts with the figure of 15 percent reported by Victor and Wolfe (2). Gross et al. (1) point out that in recent years the mortality rates have dropped to less than 1 percent.

Studies such as those of Gross et al. (1), Victor and Wolfe (2), Cutshall (4), Salum (6), and many others have helped clarify the clinical features and natural history of delirium tremens. These large-scale studies provide relatively little information, however, about the finer aspects of the patients' psychiatric symptoms and do not convey the quality of the subjective experience of delirium. More intensive clinical studies of individual patients have provided valuable data on these aspects of delirium.

DeBoor (8) has summarized the more important German studies in this area, especially those of Bonhoeffer, Kraepelin, and Naecke. Some of these authors pointed out that not all patients experience frightening illusions and hallucinations in the course of delirium tremens. Many hallucinations are marked by occupational and nonthreatening content. Hallucinations of animals were reported by only one-third of one series of patients, by 70 percent of another. The hallucinated animals may be small, but in the majority of cases, they are of natural size. Large, mythological animals occupy the visions of some patients. Not all patients hallucinate rats and mice as is popularly believed; in one study, quoted by DeBoor, not one patient reported such hallucinatory contents. Lilliputian hallucinations are not uncommon. There is a tendency for the patient to hallucinate many objects or animals simultaneously. Whole scenes, as well as inanimate objects, people, and plants may form the content of the visual hallucinations. The patients tend to accept them as real.

Auditory hallucinations, reported by some of the German writers, consisted mostly of threatening and abusive voices, but some patients hallucinated music or neutral sounds. Pressure on the eyeballs may elicit hallucinations. The patients display marked suggestibility and can be readily talked into hallucinating various objects or figures. Illusions are very common. Contents of dreams that the patient had experienced in the past may appear as hallucinations in delirium. Both hallucinations and delusions tend to reflect ongoing environmental and somatic stimuli, past experiences and dreams of the patient, and recent political events.

Saravay and Pardes (9) have studied auditory elementary hallucinations in delirium tremens. They found that 57 percent of their patients had experienced unstructured visual hallucinations such as shadows, spots, flashes of light, etc. Tinnitus was present in 40 percent. One-half of the patients reported simple phasic noises, such as clicks, reports, fluttering, and fading sounds. The authors hypothesize that these noises are not hallucinations in the usual sense of the word, but rather represent real noises produced by pathological contractions of the stapedius, tensor tympani, and tensor veli palatini muscles.

Gross et al. (10) have explored the relationship between sleep disturbances and hallucinations in alcohol withdrawal delirium. They describe a commonly observed sequence of events: an alcoholic patient suffers from insomnia which may actually precipitate a heavy drinking bout. Gradually nightmares develop and begin to interrupt sleep, but additional alcohol may initially secure return to it. The nightmares return and the patient becomes increasingly more uncertain if he is asleep and dreaming or awake and hallucinating. A predominantly sleepless state with hallucinations follows. The latter range from transient fragments to complex scenes. Initially, the hallucinations come on when the patient is alone, at night, and in the dark, and closes his eyes. This development may be arrested if the patient succeeds in obtaining sound sleep. Gross et al. hypothesize that an intimate relationship exists between dreams and waking hallucinations in these patients. This whole issue is discussed in Chapter 5.

In another study, Gross et al. (11) found a significant positive relation between hallucinations and clouding of sensorium. Gross (12) hypothesized that sensory superactivity, induced by a rebound from the cortical effects of alcohol, may in association with clouding of consciousness codetermine the appearance of hallucinations in delirium. This hypothesized rebound of sensory cortical activity is postulated to increase the proneness to hallucinate during wakefulness and increase REM activity during sleep.

Ditman and Whittlesey (13) compared subjective experience of delirium tremens with that of the state induced by LSD. Both similarities and differences beween these two experiential states could be discerned. The experience of delirium tremens was reported by people who had gone through it as marked by hallucinations accepted as real perceptions, and by anxiety, depression, and paranoid ideas. The LSD experience generally lacked these features. Both states were characterized by perceptual distortions, increased alertness, physical discomfort, and a sense of increased tempo of the train of thought. The authors were interested in the subjective experience of delirium tremens and LSD intoxication, respectively, and did not investigate other differences between the two states, such as the presence of disorientation and other cognitive deficits. The latter are present in delirium tremens but are absent in LSD intoxication. This difference is diagnostically important.

Ditman and Whittlesey found that a new experimental drug, J B 336, could induce a syndrome far closer in its characteristics to delirium tremens than the state provoked by LSD. The new drug was a centrally acting anticholinergic agent related to Ditran, which reproduced many features of delirium tremens when it was given to volunteers (14). The subjects passed through hallucinosis to delirium. Itil and Fink (15) induced delirium with Ditran and then administered LSD intravenously. What resulted was an increase in alertness, psychomotor activity, restlessness, perceptual distortion, and delusions. These behavioral changes were accompanied by a decrease in slow waves and an increase in fast activity in the EEG. A combination of Ditran and LSD reproduces the psychopathological and EEG features of delirium tremens more closely than either drug alone.

The above observations support the contention that delirium tremens defined as a psychiatric syndrome is not different from delirium due to causes other than alcohol withdrawal, an observation made on clinical grounds by Hoch (16) at the beginning of this century. He studied patients suffering from delirium due to drugs such as bromides and hyoscine and concluded that the drug-induced delirium shared a common psychopathological nucleus with delirium tremens. The alteration of consciousness and hallucinations were the same in both types of delirium. The differences consisted mostly in greater responsiveness, alertness, and wakefulness of the patients suffering from delirium tremens. Hayward (17), writing in 1822, stressed watchfulness as a characteristic feature of delirium tremens, which he proposed to rename "delirium vigilans." The hyperalertness of the delirium tremens patient contrasts with the drowsiness and reduced responsivity often seen in metabolic deliria (18), for example, and has given rise to the contention that the latter constituted a different class of mental disorders, one characterized by lowering of the level of consciousness. Yet already at the beginning of the last century it was recognized that delirium included two clinical variants "connected with two opposite conditions of the sensorium" (19). One variant was called acute or violent delirium (delirium ferox), the other was designated low delirium (delirium mite). The former was ascribed to increased flow of blood to the brain; the latter to "circulation through the brain too languid to support its functions" (19). These early conceptions seem to be partly confirmed by recent work which indicates that regional cerebral blood flow is reduced in bromide delirium but relatively unchanged in delirium tremens (20). This suggests a different pathophysiology of delirium tremens as compared to bromide delirium and, one might predict, other deliria which feature a reduction in alertness. Both types of delirium, however, share the same core, i.e. impairment of cognitive functions. They differ in the level of wakefulness and alertness. Such level is typically raised in delirium tremens and accounts for some of its characteristic clinical features. The latter do not justify, in this writer's opinion, the separation of delirium tremens from the class of deliria as a whole.

Gross et al. (1) point out that the clinical picture of delirium tremens helps in establishing the diagnosis. The patient is communicative and relates his experiences freely. He tends to be completely absorbed by his perceptual distortions and hallucinations and is unruffled by his actual circumstances and the glaring discrepancy between them and his inner experience. The quality of the latter tends to be rich and vivid, the content complex and variable. The visual hallucinations are distinguished by striking color, motion, multiplicity of objects, and often, by a touch of the fantastic, droll, and grotesque. One is reminded of the paintings of the Flemish master, Hieronymus Bosch, with his detailed and colorful depiction of both realistic and fantastic figures, objects, and scenes. Patients studied in the course of experimentally induced alcohol withdrawal delirium hallucinated being cut with knives or attacked by snakes or imaginary animals spitting acid; and they had visions of disembodied faces or heads, etc. (2). Auditory and kinesthetic hallucinations were also reported. Gross et al. (1) emphasize that hallucinations in delirium tremens are more frequent at night and intensified by closing the eyes. Both hallucinations and cognitive impairment (clouding of sensorium) tend to display striking fluctuations from moment to moment and are more marked at night.

ETIOLOGY AND PATHOGENESIS

From the time delirium tremens was first described at the turn of the nineteenth century a controversy has persisted regarding its cause and underlying pathophysiological mechanisms. Gross et al. (1) state that Lettsom, writing in 1787, held the view that delirium tremens was an alcohol withdrawal syndrome; while Pearson, in his observations on Brain Fever published in 1813, maintained that it was a direct effect of excessive drinking. This controversy has not been completely resolved, but important studies published in the past twenty-five years endorse the view that delirium tremens is indeed a result of abstinence or withdrawal of and not of intoxication by alcohol (1, 2, 21, 22). Gross et al. (1) observe that this hypothesis is generally accepted in America but not entirely accepted in Europe.

Alcohol is a central nervous system depressant whose prolonged and excessive intake results in the development of addiction, tolerance, and physical dependence (1). The latter becomes manifest when alcohol is withdrawn; delirium represents one of these manifestations. Alcohol intoxication produces behavioral symptoms that are not traditionally referred to as "delirium." This avoidance of the term in relation to acute alcohol intoxication is not shared by all observers, however. Engel and Rosenbaum (23), for example, assert that the administration of alcohol constitutes an easy way of inducing "an acute delirium which is rapidly reversible." They found that in experimental subjects

alcohol elicited changes in the level of consciousness that correlated with slowing of the EEG background activity. These
changes were the same as those induced by hypoglycemia or
hypoxia. The current custom, however, is to label the behavioral
effects of alcohol as "alcohol intoxication" or "alcohol idiosyncratic intoxication" and to distinguish these syndromes from
the alcohol withdrawal delirium (3).

Isbell et al. (21), in their classic experimental study, demonstrated that abrupt withdrawal of alcohol from chronically
intoxicated subjects induces an abstinence syndrome, which may
feature convulsions or delirium or both. Victor and Wolfe (2)
conclude on the basis of their own studies and those of others
that delirium tremens, and related disorders, are not the result
of alcohol intoxication, but of a reduction of blood alcohol levels
from a previously higher level. Furthermore, delirium tremens
requires a background of intense drinking for a period of many
weeks or months in a person who has, in most cases, abused
alcohol for five or more years (2, 4). Cutshall (4) reports that
the patients he studied had a mean daily consumption of one
liter of whiskey or two liters of wine. The mean duration of
excessive drinking in his series of subjects was 17.9 years. Isbell
et al. (21) found that the intensity of the withdrawal symptoms
correlated roughly with the quantity of alcohol intake and the
duration of intoxication.

Delirium tremens does not develop in all alcoholics—its incidence among them is estimated to be 1 to 15 percent (1)—and
this raises the question of individual predisposing factors to this
complication. Genetic, psychological, and nutritional predisposing factors have been proposed (1). Whitwell (24) found
supporting evidence for the hypothesis that more serious social
consequences of alcoholism and lower social class predispose an
alcoholic to the development of delirium tremens.

Postulated precipitating factors in delirium tremens involve
drinking pattern, dietary intake, gastrointestinal symptoms, infection, inflammation, trauma, and hepatic insufficiency (1, 2, 22).
Free choice drinking pattern, decreased food intake, gastritis,
acute infection, and trauma of accident or surgery are variables
observed to increase the probability of the occurrence and the
severity of delirium of alcohol withdrawal.

Several pathophysiological mechanisms have been described. They include metabolic disorders, disturbances of the sleep-wakefulness cycle, and alterations of biogenic amines. The underlying mechanisms responsible for the psychopathological manifestations of alcohol withdrawal delirium are still largely unknown (1, 22).

Metabolic derangements that have been postulated to underlie at least some of the symptoms of alcohol withdrawal include hypomagnesemia and respiratory alkalosis (1, 2, 22, 25, 26). Victor and Wolfe (2) found that hypomagnesemia during alcohol withdrawal correlated with vulnerability to seizures and photomyoclonus but not with delirium tremens, which in some patients developed only after return to normal of serum magnesium levels. Meyer and Urban (25) report that patients with withdrawal seizures have significantly lower CSF magnesium levels, which are not always accompanied by lower serum levels. Administration of magnesium sulfate decreases susceptibility to photomyoclonus, supporting the view that hypomagnesemia may be responsible for the latter (2). Stendig-Lindberg (26) found hypomagnesemia in eight out of eighteen patients with delirium tremens. He contends that a combination of hypomagnesemia with delirium tremens may be of etiological significance for the development of alcoholic encephalopathy, a term that includes alcoholic dementia and the Wernicke-Korsakoff's syndrome.

The early phase of alcohol withdrawal is said to be consistently associated with respiratory alkalosis (2). The reduction in pCO_2 and rise in arterial pH are greater in patients with seizures than in those with tremor and hallucinations. The alkalosis is most likely the result of hyperventilation (2). Lowered CO_2 tension may cause cerebral vasoconstriction, reduced cerebral blood flow, and thus hypoxia. Victor and Wolfe (2) hypothesize that hypomagnesemia and alkalosis account for photomyoclonus and spontaneous seizures of alcohol withdrawal. The relationship, if any, of these metabolic disturbances to the psychopathological manifestations of withdrawal are unclear (1).

Sleep disturbances in delirium tremens are discussed in Chapter 5, where references to the several relevant studies are also given. Mello and Mendelson (22) emphasize the fragmentation of sleep, rather than a decrease in total hours of sleep, as the predominant sleep pattern during withdrawal. Gross and Hastey (27) state that sleep onset REM, reduced time of REM onset, increased eye movement density, fragmentation of the individual REM periods, and reduction of slow wave sleep are manifestations of abstinence withdrawal. The relationship of these disturbances to the phenomenology of withdrawal delirium remains undetermined. Wolin and Mello (28) studied this problem and conclude that it is premature to assume a constant relationship between dream-hallucinatory episodes and REM activity. Hallucinations do not seem to represent a REM over-shoot or waking dreams. This whole issue is intriguing and calls for further research. Earlier hypotheses linking causally REM rebound during alcohol withdrawal with hallucinations of delirium tremens have failed to be confirmed (*see* Chapter 5 for further discussion).

A number of investigators have focused on the role of biogenic amines in the symptomatology of delirium tremens. Athen et al. (29) report evidence supporting the view that increased central noradrenergic activity takes place during the delirium. MHPG concentrations in the CSF of delirious patients were strikingly elevated: 13>percent in comparison to the control period at least fifteen days later. Urinary excretion of noradrenaline was also raised. These findings are important since they seem to reflect some of the key characteristics of delirium tremens such as psychomotor hyperactivity and hyperalertness. One may postulate that enhanced central noradrenergic activity, possibly coupled with reduced central cholinergic activity, constitutes a major biochemical derangement underlying psychopathological symptoms of delirium tremens. The EEG findings in this syndrome seem to fit in with this hypothesis. Isbell et al. (21) observed that during alcohol withdrawal the percentage of alpha activity declined and random spikes and paroxysmal bursts of slow high-voltage activity appeared, especially in frontal regions. Wikler et al. (30) in addition noticed low-voltage fast activity. These EEG changes differ from those of acute alcohol intoxication (23) and many other deliria in which reduction of wakefulness and alertness is accompanied by generalized slowing of the background activity. Clearly, different biochemical mechanisms must be involved in delirium tremens. Increased central noradrenergic activity seems to distinguish it from delirium due to various toxic and metabolic causes.

Explanatory hypotheses for the phenomena of the alcohol withdrawal syndrome and delirium have involved concepts of cellular adaptation to alcohol, denervation or disuse, super-sensitivity, and rebound (1, 22). Cells are believed to adapt to alcohol and thus homeostasis is achieved. When alcohol is withdrawn, counterregulatory mechanisms are activated and some functions that had been suppressed by it become transiently exaggerated. Rebound hyperexcitability of the nervous system results. More specifically, it has been proposed that alcohol may act primarily on the reticular activating system of the midbrain; during withdrawal, disuse supersensitivity of this structure is accompanied by increased cortical excitability. These hypotheses remain to be tested.

TREATMENT

A variety of therapeutic regimens have been claimed to be effective in the alcohol withdrawal syndrome (1, 2, 4, 31-39). No single approach to treatment has gained universal acceptance. Cutshall (4) asserts that the most effective therapy for delirium tremens is to try to prevent its onset. This distinction is important when one attempts to evaluate the various therapeutic regimens: did the reported patients represent cases of alcohol withdrawal short of or in the stage of delirium tremens? Cutshall (4) maintains that no drug will shorten delirium tremens to any marked extent. Victor and Wolfe (2) claim that available data fail to demonstrate the effectiveness of currently used drugs in preventing, shortening, or reducing the mortality from delirium tremens. These authors assert that the most important aspect of the management of this condition consists of administration of fluids and correction of electrolyte depletion, especially of sodium, potassium, and magnesium. Fisher and Abrams (32) echo this assertion and point out that failure to correct electrolyte and acid-base abnormalities in delirium tremens may permit the development of life-threatening ventricular tachycardia and fibrillation. A review of the large literature on the treatment of delirium tremens is beyond the scope of this book. Only the major aspects of it and the more commonly used drugs will be briefly reviewed.

Examination of the patient. When first seen, every patient should be carefully examined for evidence of injury or infection, especially head trauma, subdural hematoma, pneumonia, meningitis, and hepatic failure. X-rays of skull and chest, and lumbar puncture are indicated (2, 38). Serum electrolyte levels, including magnesium and other routine blood chemistries should be obtained.

General management. Any medical complications that may be present require immediate appropriate treatment. Constant observation and repeated examination of the patient are essential. Precautions against self-injury or injury to others by a severely agitated and delusional patient are mandatory. The patient may have to be restrained in a lateral or prone position. A special attendant or a member of the family should stay with the patient if circumstances allow it. A reassuring staff is claimed to obviate the need for psychoactive drugs (39).

Dehydration, electrolyte imbalance, and vitamin deficiency need to be corrected. Intravenous fluids should be administered, their quantity depending on the degree of fluid depletion. IV fluid intake of 4 to 10 liters in the first day may be needed (38). Hypomagnesemia and hypokalemia, which are common in delirium tremens, should be corrected. Magnesium sulfate IV, 2 gm. every six hours during the first day, has been recommended for patients with intact renal function (38). Others have suggested that diazepam or propranolol may be used instead (36). Thiamine, 100 mg., should be added to the IV fluid and supplemented by daily multivitamins.

Sedation. Benzodiazepines, haloperidol, paraldehyde, propranolol, hydroxyzine, and other drugs have their ardent advocates (1, 2, 32, 34-38). The drugs have been selected for the treatment of delirium tremens either because of their cross tolerance to alcohol or on account of their known sedative effects. Over 135 different drugs and drug combinations have been applied, using one or the other criterion or both, during the past twenty-five years (36). Phenothiazines, barbiturates, paraldehyde, and antihistamines are not recommended on account of their toxicity (36). Chlordiazepoxide, a drug cross-tolerant with alcohol, is effective in preventing the development of delirium tremens and convulsions (34). Diazepam, given intravenously or orally, is equally effective (38). These two drugs are as effective as other agents used for the treatment of alcohol withdrawal and, in addition, have welcome anticonvulsant activity and relatively low toxicity. Their drawbacks include the need to adjust the dosage to the individual variations in biotransformation, to the severity of the withdrawal symptoms, and to the presence of hepatic disease (37). Both drugs are absorbed erratically after intramuscular injection and should be administered orally or intravenously (32).

It has been stressed that the choice of the sedative drug is not as crucial as the adjustment of its dosage so as to calm the patient (38). Widely different doses of diazepam have been required for this purpose. It follows that no suggested dosage schedule should be followed rigidly. The objective is to keep the patient calm but not oversedated. In a patient with mild to moderate agitation and anxiety chlordiazepoxide 25-100 mg. or diazepam 5-20 mg. orally every six hours is usually effective. Initial dose may be repeated every two hours if agitation continues unabated. In the case of severe agitation, intravenous administration is more effective. Diazepam 5 mg. or chlordiazepoxide 25 mg. is given IV every five to fifteen minutes until the patient is calm. Subsequently, either drug should be given either orally or IV every two to six hours to maintain adequate sedation (36, 38).

Electroconvulsive therapy. A number of anecdotal reports have described the effectiveness of this form of treatment in delirium tremens. A retrospective study suggested that one ECT could arrest the delirium in some patients (31). The value of ECT for the treatment of delirium tremens remains uncertain.

SEDATIVE-HYPNOTIC WITHDRAWAL

Abrupt reduction in dosage or cessation of a habitual intake of almost every sedative-hypnotic drug in current use may result in a withdrawal syndrome, with delirium as one of its chief manifestations. These drug withdrawal deliria have clinical characteristics that resemble closely those of the alcohol with-

TABLE 11-I

DRUGS WHICH MAY CAUSE WITHDRAWAL DELIRIUM

Barbiturates
Chloral hydrate
Paraldehyde
Meprobamate
Glutethimide
Ethinamate
Ethchlorvynol
Methyprylon
Methaqualone
Chlormethiazole
Chlordiazepoxide
Diazepam
Oxazepam
Nitrazepam
Clorazepate
Morphine (rarely)
Propoxyphene
Amphetamine (unproven)
Thiothixene (rarely if at all)

drawal delirium. They typically feature the following symptoms: global cognitive impairment with disorientation, attention disturbance, restlessness, agitation, irritability, insomnia, visual and auditory hallucinations, delusions, and anxiety. In addition, somatic symptoms are regularly present and may include sweating, fever, tremor, tachycardia, orthostatic hypotension, raised blood pressure, weakness, anorexia, nausea, vomiting, and rapid weight loss (40-44). In general, delirium and/or generalized convulsions constitute the major clinical manifestation of barbiturate and related sedative withdrawal syndrome (45).

Table 11-I lists the drugs known or suspected to cause withdrawal delirium. Even though the general features of the drug withdrawal delirium are similar regardless of which particular sedative-hypnotic is involved, the frequency and thus clinical importance of the delirium due to specific drugs vary widely. For this reason they are discussed in separate sections. Since treatment is essentially the same for drug withdrawal deliria, it is discussed at the end of this section.

Barbiturates

Classic experimental studies by Isbell et al. (43) demonstrated that abrupt withdrawal of barbiturates in subjects chronically intoxicated by them produced an abstinence syndrome which included delirium. The latter occurs in 60 percent of the cases, while convulsions follow withdrawal in 75 percent of patients (21). Experimental subjects of Isbell et al. received secobarbital sodium, pentobarbital sodium, or amobarbital sodium in doses which were gradually increased to a maximum of 1.3 to 3 gm. daily. The total period of intoxication ranged from 92 to 144 days. After twelve to sixteen hours following abrupt withdrawal of the barbiturate the subjects began to complain of anxiety and weakness, and displayed anorexia, insomnia, and coarse tremor of hands and face. Twenty-four to thirty hours after the last dose these symptoms became worse and in addition the patients developed muscle twitching, vomiting, and increased startle responses. After thirty to sixty hours following withdrawal most subjects had convulsions. In four out of five patients delirium developed after a period of insomnia. Delirium came on thirty-six hours to thirteen days following the last dose. All patients recovered. The EEG during withdrawal showed paroxysmal bursts of high amplitude, slow waves (4-6 cycles per second). These changes preceded the grand mal seizures. Increased percentages of waves 6-7 c/sec persisted for about two weeks.

Wikler (44) has summarized the earlier studies on barbiturate withdrawal. He points out that delirium usually develops between the fourth and seventh day of abstinence and may or may not be preceded by convulsions. The symptoms are worse at night. Occasionally, delirium may be ushered in by a schizophrenia-like or amnestic-confabulatory syndrome. The delirium lasts a few days to about two weeks. Sudden recovery may follow prolonged spontaneous sleep. In other patients, however, the recovery progresses gradually. Administration of barbiturates does not abolish the delirium. Intake of as little as 1.0 g. of barbiturates daily for a month or more may be sufficient to result in delirium after rapid withdrawal. The EEG changes during the withdrawal syndrome include diffuse slowing of the background activity and high voltage, diffuse, bilaterally synchronous bursts of spikes, sharp waves, irregularly shaped delta waves, or two to four cycles per second "spike and dome" complexes. These changes generally subside by the fourth or fifth day, but mild slowing of the background activity may persist longer. EEG changes during the phase of delirium are difficult to assess because of muscle artifacts.

Considerable attention has been devoted to the role of sleep disturbances in the barbiturate withdrawal delirium. Evans and Lewis (46) advanced a hypothesis that REM sleep rebound is responsible for the occurrence of delirium during drug withdrawal. These researchers argued that barbiturates suppress REM sleep initially but then tolerance develops and REM levels return to the baseline levels. On rapid withdrawal of the drug there is an immediate overswing or rebound of REM sleep which persists for several weeks. Mental activity concomitant with REM sleep intrudes into wakefulness and constitutes delirium. Evans and Lewis conclude that there is a common mechanism underlying both REM sleep and the drug withdrawal delirium. This attractive hypothesis was called into question when more recent work failed to confirm that REM rebound occurs regularly after a period of barbiturate-induced REM suppression (47). Both barbiturates and benzodiazepines can suppress REM sleep, with relatively greater suppression of eye movement activity than of emergent stage 1 EEG. Both these classes of drugs also suppress stage 4 sleep. After withdrawal, eye movements rapidly return to baseline levels, but stage 4 sleep takes a longer time to do so; rebound, in the sense of overshoot, is usually lacking (47). Tachibana et al. (48) studied sleep patterns in patients suffering from delirium due to alcohol and meprobamate withdrawal, that is conditions believed to have the same underlying mechanisms as the barbiturate withdrawal delirium. These investigators did not find rebound increases in REM sleep reported by others. They did, however, find stage 1 REM with tonic EMG (stage 1–REM) in delirium tremens. This type of sleep occupied a large portion of the total sleep time of patients with meprobamate delirium. Tachibana et al. (48) postulate that delirium due to alcohol and meprobamate withdrawal could occur as a result of increased dissociation of the phasic features of REM sleep from its tonic features. They speculate that such dissociation might also occur during wakefulness and result in hallucinations. This interesting hypothesis needs to be tested in barbiturate and other drug withdrawal delirium. The reasons for the contradictory findings regarding REM rebound remain to be elucidated.

Wulff (49) studied a group of patients who exhibited symptoms of barbiturate withdrawal. Such symptoms occurred only in patients addicted to barbiturates which are rapidly excreted as determined by the blood levels. Gault (42) has reviewed major hypotheses trying to account for barbiturate addiction and withdrawal. He notes that two major types of such hypotheses have been put forth: chronic disuse hyperexcitability, and transmitter surfeit and supersensitivity of receptors, respectively. The former hypothesis asserts that chronic barbiturate intoxication suppresses the central nervous system in such a way that upon rapid withdrawal of the drug a hyperexcitability analogous to that which follows denervation or chronic disuse of tissue results. The same explanation has been proposed to account for the whole class of drugs that share the propensity to depress the CNS. These drugs display the phenomenon of cross-tolerance, that is, one of them can substitute for another in suppressing specific abstinence symptoms. The other type of explanatory hypothesis asserts that CNS depressants bring about accumulation of transmitter substance in the presynaptic terminals and in the axons of presynaptic neurons. After withdrawal of the depressant drug there is release of the excess transmitter, resulting in exaggerated response to stimuli. A related hypothesis proposes that the observed hyperexcitability in withdrawal states results from an increase in the number of receptors in the postsynaptic areas. These issues have not yet been resolved.

Nonbarbiturate Sedative-Hypnotics

Both the older drugs, such as chloral hydrate (50) and paraldehyde (51), and the newer ones, introduced since 1950, are capable of inducing intoxication, physical dependence, and withdrawal delirium practically indistinguishable from those due to barbiturates (40, 41, 52, 53). Meprobamate, glutethimide, methyprylon, ethchlorvynol, ethinamate, clomethiazole, and methaqualone share these features. Clinical features of withdrawal delirium due to these agents are the same as those listed in the section on barbiturates and need not be repeated. Brief comments on each of the newer drugs follow.

Meprobamate abuse may result in a withdrawal syndrome, with convulsions, delirium, or both, after an intake of 2.4 or more grams daily for about a month or longer, followed by rapid withdrawal (53). One reported patient died during the withdrawal (54). In one controlled study delirium developed in eight of forty-seven patients (55). As the popularity of meprobamate has waned, reports on withdrawal delirium due to it have stopped.

Glutethimide withdrawal delirium and convulsions have been reported following dosage close to that regarded as therapeutic, i.e. 2.5 g. daily for about three months (53, 56, 57).

Methyprylon withdrawal delirium has been reported following daily dosage of 4.5 g. for an unknown period (58).

Ethchlorvynol withdrawal delirium may occur after daily intake of 1 g. or more for a period of months or years (59-61).

Ethinamate withdrawal delirium has been reported following daily dosage of 13 g. for about two years (62).

Clomethiazole withdrawal delirium is mentioned by one author but no details are provided (41).

Methaqualone withdrawal symptoms with convulsions, but apparently without delirium, have been reported after 1,500 to 2,000 mg. daily for several months (63). Japanese workers claim that delirium occurs in about 10 percent of patients when methaqualone is withdrawn (64). Withdrawal delirium has also been observed in Britain (65).

Benzodiazepines

Chlordiazepoxide, diazepam, oxazepam, nitrazepam, lorazepam, and clorazepate appear to be able to give rise to addiction and withdrawal delirium (41, 52, 53). The incidence of the latter is low, much lower than after withdrawal of barbiturates or nonbarbiturate sedative hypnotics. It is reported that serious withdrawal symptoms may follow withdrawal of therapeutic doses of benzodiazepines (41, 52). More typically, however, prolonged heavy intake is involved, with daily dosage that is equivalent to 100 mg. or more of diazepam (66). Some authors state that withdrawal symptoms may follow prolonged daily intake of only 60 to 80 mg. (67). Maletzky and Klotter (68) have recently reviewed the whole problem of addiction to diazepam, but report no cases of withdrawal delirium. In fact, it appears that the occurrence of diazepam addiction is still a matter of controversy despite the publication of a number of reports supporting its existence. Fruensgaard (41) found ten patients who had been receiving benzodiazepines among thirty treated for "withdrawal psychosis." He observes that withdrawal delirium due to benzodiazepines tends to occur rather late, i.e. on about the seventh day. Some of his patients had been taking as little as 30 mg. of chlordiazepoxide or 20 to 30 mg. diazepam daily for several years. Barten (69) reported withdrawal delirium and convulsions in a woman who had taken about 60 mg. of diazepam daily for several months. Patients experienced auditory, visual, gustatory, and olfactory hallucinations, and displayed a marked recent memory impairment and confabulations. The delirium lasted about one week. Floyd and Murphy (70) describe five cases of diazepam withdrawal delirium following chronic use of the drug. Delirium due to withdrawal of other benzodiazepines has been rarely reported (41, 52). Considering the widespread use of these drugs, there is a distinctly low incidence of addiction and withdrawal delirium.

Miscellaneous Drugs

Several drugs have been claimed to bring about withdrawal delirium, but the evidence for it appears to be inconclusive. They are mentioned briefly for the record.

Opiates. Occurrence of delirium as part of opiate withdrawal is a matter of some controversy. Isbell (72), a brilliant student of drug withdrawal, states plainly that convulsions and delirium are not observed following withdrawal of analgesic drugs. Fruensgaard (41) asserts that withdrawal psychosis occurs in morphine addicts "very seldom." De Boor (8) reviews German literature up to about 1955 and states that even when morphine is withdrawn suddenly, delirium does not follow. He does quote one investigator, however, who claims to have observed delirium. Wikler (44) does not mention delirium in his description of the opiate withdrawal syndrome. One may conclude that if an opiate addict exhibits delirium during withdrawal, addiction to other drugs, such as barbiturates, or intoxication or some other cause of the delirium should be investigated.

Propoxyphene addiction and withdrawal have been reported. Withdrawal from even high doses has not resulted in delirium (73). Fruensgaard (41), however, describes a woman who took 520 mg. of d-propoxyphene daily for about eight years; when she tried to stop, she developed delirium.

Amphetamine withdrawal delirium has been occasionally reported (74, 75), but most authorities deny that it exists.

Thiothixene withdrawal delirium has been observed in one case (76). Such delirium has not been reported following withdrawal of other neuroleptics (77).

TREATMENT OF BARBITURATE AND RELATED DRUG WITHDRAWAL DELIRIUM

The patient should be hospitalized. Withdrawal from these drugs may be accompanied by convulsions, and occasionally, status epilepticus may develop. The usual method of treatment involves substitution of pentobarbital or phenobarbital, and subsequent gradual withdrawal of the drug. If the patient is already delirious, 100 mg. phenobarbital intravenously over ten minutes should be given, or alternatively 200 mg. intramuscularly. Subsequently, the drug should be administered orally in four divided doses for a total of about 500 to 600 mg. daily. If toxic signs, such as ataxia, nystagmus, or slurred speech, are present, the dose of phenobarbital is omitted. Otherwise, the dose is reduced by 30 mg. daily. If the patient is in the predelirious phase of withdrawal, the dose is calculated according to the amount of drug he or she reports to be using. Phenobarbital 30 mg. substitutes for each 100 mg. of the short-acting barbiturate. The patient is stabilized for two days and then withdrawal begins. If an intermediate-acting barbiturate is preferred, then pentobarbital may be used, 100 mg. being equivalent to 30 mg. phenobarbital. If the patient's usual dose is unknown, a test dose of 200 mg. pentobarbital is given, and the response is observed after one hour. The patient's requirement for the drug is estimated according to the clinical signs elicited. If the patient becomes sleepy and grossly ataxic, it indicates a habitual intake of about 400 mg. or less and no withdrawal regimen is needed. Mild ataxia and dysarthria indicate an intake of 500 to 600 mg. daily; nystagmus—700 to 800 mg.; if no toxic signs appear—the patient must have been taking more than 800 mg. daily. In the latter case, a second test dose of 300 mg. is given, and if it has no effect, the patient will need 1600 mg. of pentobarbital daily. The substitute dosage is divided into four daily doses. After one or two days of stabilization the dose is reduced by 100 mg. of pentobarbital daily. If the patient becomes tremulous, anxious, or cannot sleep, the withdrawal should be stopped for a day or two or until these symptoms clear up (53, 78, 79).

General care during the withdrawal is important. The patient should be carefully observed and his or her temperature, pulse, and blood pressure measured three times daily. Nutrition and hydration should be adequate. Haloperidol has been recommended as an aid in relieving symptoms of barbiturate withdrawal delirium (80). Withdrawal from benzodiazepines may be accomplished by gradually tapering the addicting agent.

REFERENCES

1. Gross, M.M., Lewis, E., and Hastey, J.: "Acute Alcohol Withdrawal Syndrome," in *The Biology of Alcoholism,* Vol. 3, Kissin, H., and Begleiter, H., Eds. New York, Plenum Press, 1973, pp. 191-263.
2. Victor, M., and Wolfe, S.M.: "Causation and Treatment of the Alcohol Withdrawal Syndrome," in *Alcoholism: Progress in Research and Treatment,* Bourne, P., and Fox, R., Eds. New York, Academic Press, 1973, pp. 137-169.
3. *Diagnostic and Statistical Manual of Mental Disorders.* 3rd edition. Washington, D.C., American Psychiatric Association, January 15, 1978.
4. Cutshall, B.J.: The Saunders-Sutton syndrome: An analysis of delirium tremens. *Q J Stud Alcohol 26*:423-448, 1965.
5. Gross, M.M., Rosenblatt, S.M., Lewis, E., et al.: Acute alcoholic psychoses and related syndromes: Psychosocial and clinical characteristics and their implications. *Br J Addict 67*:15-31, 1972.
6. Salum, I., Ed.: Delirium Tremens and Certain Other Acute Sequels of Alcohol Abuse. *Acta Psychiatr Scand, Suppl 235,* 1972.
7. Root, J.: *The Horrors of Delirium Tremens.* New York, J. Adams, 1844.
8. DeBoor, W.: *Pharmakopsychologie und Psychopathologie.* Berlin, Springer Verlag, 1956.
9. Saravay, S.M., and Pardes, H.: Auditory elementary hallucinations in alcohol withdrawal psychosis. *Arch Gen Psychiatry 16*:652-658, 1967.

10. Gross, M.M., Goodenough, D., Tobin, M., et al.: Sleep disturbances and hallucinations in the acute alcoholic psychoses. *J Nerv Ment Dis 142*:493-514, 1966.

11. Gross, M.M., Rosenblatt, S.M., Lewis, E., et al.: Hallucinations and clouding of sensorium in alcohol withdrawal. *Q J Stud Alcohol 32*:1061-1069, 1971.

12. Gross, M.M.: Sensory superactivity. *Adv Exper Med Biol 35*:321-330, 1973.

13. Ditman, K.S., and Whittlesey, J.R.B.: Comparison of the LSD-25 experience and delirium tremens. *Arch Gen Psychiatry 1*:47-57, 1959.

14. Alpert, M., Angrist, B., Diamond, F., and Gershon, S.: "Comparison of Ditran Intoxication and Acute Alcohol Psychoses," in *Origins and Mechanisms of Hallucinations*, Keup, W., Ed. New York, Plenum Press, 1970, pp. 245-259.

15. Itil, T., and Fink, M.: Anticholinergic drug-induced delirium: experimental modification, quantitative EEG and behavioral correlations. *J Nerv Ment Dis 143*:492-507, 1966.

16. Hoch, A.: A study of some cases of delirium produced by drugs. *Studies in Psychiatry 1*:75-93, 1912.

17. Hayward, G.: Some remarks on delirium vigilans; commonly called "delirium tremens," "mania a potu," or "mania a tremulentia." *N Engl J Med Surg 11*:235-243, 1822.

18. Davidson, E.A., and Solomon, P.: The differentiation of delirium tremens from impending hepatic coma. *J Ment Sci 104*:326-333, 1958.

19. "Delirium," in *The Cyclopaedia; or Universal Dictionary of Arts, Sciences, and Literature*, 1st American edition, Vol. 12, Rees, A., Ed. Philadelphia, S.F. Bradford, 1818.

20. Berglund, M.: Personal communication, February 27, 1978.

21. Isbell, H., Fraser, H.F., Wikler, A., et al.: An experimental study of the etiology of "rum fits" and delirium tremens. *Q J Stud Alcohol 16*:1-33, 1955.

22. Mello, N.K., and Mendelson, J.H.: "Alterations in States of Consciousness Associated with Chronic Ingestion of Alcohol," in *Neurobiological Aspects of Psychopathology*, Zubin, J., and Shagass, C., Eds. New York, Grune & Stratton, Inc., 1969, pp. 183-218.

23. Engel, G.L., and Rosenbaum, M.: Delirium. III. Electroencephalographic changes associated with acute alcoholic intoxication. *Arch Neurol Psychiatry 53*:44-50, 1945.

24. Whitwell, F.D.: A study into the etiology of delirium tremens. *Br J Addict 70*:156-161, 1975.

25. Meyer, J.G., and Urban, K.: Electrolyte changes and acid base balance after alcohol withdrawal. *J Neurol 215*:135-140, 1977.

26. Stendig-Lindberg, G.: Hypomagnesemia in alcohol encephalopathies. *Acta Psychiatr Scand 50*:465-480, 1974.
27. Gross, M.M., and Hastey, J.M.: "Sleep Disturbances in Alcoholism," in *Alcoholism: Interdisciplinary Approaches To An Enduring Problem,* Tarter, R.E., and Sugarman, A.A., Eds. Reading, Mass., Addison-Wesley Publ. Co., 1976.
28. Wolin, S.J., and Wello, N.K.: The effect of alcohol on dreams and hallucinations in alcohol addicts. *Ann NY Acad Sci 215*:266-302, 1973.
29. Athen, D., Beckmann, H., Ackenheil, M., and Markianos, M.: Biochemical investigations into the alcoholic delirium: Alterations of biogenic amines. *Arch Psychiatr Nervenkr 224*:129-140, 1977.
30. Wikler, A., Pescor, F.T., Fraser, H.F., and Isbell, H.: Electroencephalographic changes associated with chronic alcoholic intoxication and the alcohol abstinence syndrome. *Am J Psychiatry 113*:106-114, 1956.
31. Dudley, W.H.C., and Williams, J.G.: Electroconvulsive therapy in delirium tremens. *Compr Psychiatry 13*:257-260, 1972.
32. Fisher, J., and Abrams, J.: Life-threatening ventricular tachyarrhythmias in delirium tremens. *Arch Intern Med 137*:1238-1241, 1977.
33. Funderburk, F.R., Allen, R.P., and Wagman, A.M.I.: Residual effects of ethanol and chlordiazepoxide treatments for alcohol withdrawal. *J Nerv Ment Dis 166*:195-203, 1978.
34. Kaim, S.C., and Klett, C.J.: Treatment of delirium tremens. *Q J Stud Alcohol 33*:1065-1072, 1972.
35. Knott, D.H., and Beard, J.D.: Diagnosis and therapy of acute withdrawal from alcohol. *Curr Psychiatr Ther 10*:145-152, 1970.
36. Sellers, E.M., and Kalant, H.: Alcohol intoxication and withdrawal. *N Engl J Med 294*:757-762, 1976.
37. Sellers, E.M., Zilm, D.H., and Degani, N.C.: Comparative efficacy of propranolol and chlordiazepoxide in alcohol withdrawal. *Q J Stud Alcohol 38*:209-218, 1977.
38. Thompson, W.L.: Management of alcohol withdrawal syndromes. *Arch Intern Med 138*:278-283, 1978.
39. Whitfield, C.L., Thompson, G., Lamb, A., et al.: Detoxification of 1,024 alcoholic patients without psychoactive drugs. *JAMA 239*: 1409-1410, 1978.
40. Essig, C.F.: Addiction to nonbarbiturate sedative and tranquilizing drugs. *Clin Pharmacol Ther 5*:334-343, 1964.
41. Fruensgaard, K.: Withdrawal psychosis: A study of 30 consecutive cases. *Acta Psychiatr Scand 53*:105-118, 1976.
42. Gault, F.P.: A review of recent literature on barbiturate addiction and withdrawal. *Bol Estud Med Biol 29*:75-83, 1976.

43. Isbell, H., Altschul, S., Kornetsky, C.H., et al.: Chronic barbiturate intoxication. *Arch Neurol Psychiatry 64*:1-28, 1950.
44. Wikler, A.: Neurophysiological aspects of the opiate and barbiturate abstinence syndromes. *Proc Assoc Res Nerv Ment Dis 32*:269-286, 1953.
45. Essig, C.F.: Clinical and experimental aspects of barbiturate withdrawal convulsions. *Epilepsia 8*:21-30, 1967.
46. Evans, J.I., and Lewis, S.A.: Drug withdrawal state. *Arch Gen Psychiatry 19*:631-634, 1968.
47. Feinberg, I., Hibi, S., Caveness, C., and March, J.: Absence of REM rebound after barbiturate withdrawal. *Science 185*:534-535, 1974.
48. Tachibana, M., Tanaka, K., Hishikawa, Y., and Kaneko, Z.: A sleep study of acute psychotic states due to alcohol and meprobamate addiction. *Adv Sleep Res 2*:177-205, 1975.
49. Wulff, M.H.: *The Barbiturate Withdrawal Syndrome.* Copenhagen, Munksgaard, 1959.
50. Margetts, E.L.: Chloral delirium. *Psychiatr Q 24*:278-299, 1950.
51. Kehrer, F.: Uber Abstinenzpsychosen bei chronischen Vergiftungen. *Z Neur 3*:485-502, 1910.
52. Allgulander, C.: Dependence on sedative and hypnotic drugs. *Acta Psychiatr Scand Suppl 270*, 1978.
53. Essig, C.F.: Newer sedative drugs that can cause states of intoxication and dependence of barbiturate type. *JAMA 196*:714-717, 1966.
54. Swanson, L.A., and Okada, T.: Death after withdrawal of meprobamate. *JAMA 184*:780-781, 1963.
55. Haizlip, T.M., and Ewing, J.A.: Meprobamate habituation: A controlled clinical study. *N Eng J Med 258*:1181-1186, 1961.
56. Johnson, F.A., and VanBuren, H.C.: Abstinence syndrome following glutethimide intoxication. *JAMA 180*:1024-1027, 1962.
57. Lloyd, E.A., and Clark, L.D.: Convulsions and delirium incident to glutethimide (Doriden) withdrawal. *Dis Nerv Syst 20*:524-526, 1959.
58. Jensen, G.R.: Addiction to Noludar: A report of two cases. *NZ Med J 59*:431-432, 1960.
59. Flemenbaum, A., and Gunby, B.: Ethchlorvynol (Placidyl) abuse and withdrawal. *Dis Nerv Syst 32*:188-192, 1971.
60. Garza-Perez, J., Lal, S., and Lopez, E.: Addiction to ethchlorvynol. A report of two cases. *Med Serv J Can 23*:775-778, 1967.
61. Wood, H.P., and Flippin, H.F.: Delirium tremens following withdrawal of ethchlorvynol. *Am J Psychiatry 121*:1127-1129, 1965.
62. Ellinwood, E.H., Ewing, J.A., and Hoaken, P.C.S.: Habituation to ethinamate. *N Eng J Med 266*:185-186, 1962.
63. Swartzburg, M., Lieb, J., and Schwartz, A.H.: Methaqualone withdrawal. *Arch Gen Psychiatry 29*:46-47, 1973.

64. Kato, M.: An epidemiological analysis of drug dependence in Japan. *Int J Addict 4*:591-621, 1969.
65. Ewart, R.B.L., and Priest, R.G.: Methaqualone addiction and delirium tremens. *Br Med J 3*:92-93, 1967.
66. Preskorn, S.H., and Denner, L.J.: Benzodiazepines and withdrawal psychosis. *JAMA 237*:36-38, 1977.
67. Peters, U.H., and Boeters, U.: Valium-Sucht. *Pharmakopsychiat Neuro-Psychopharm 3*:339-348, 1970.
68. Maletzky, B.M., and Klotter, J.: Addiction to diazepam. *Int J Addict 11*:95-115, 1976.
69. Barten, H.H.: Toxic psychosis with transient dysmnestic syndrome following withdrawal from Valium. *Am J Psychiatry 121*:1210-1211, 1965.
70. Floyd, J.B., and Murphy, C.M.: Hallucinations following withdrawal of Valium. *J Kent Med Assoc 74*:549-550, 1976.
71. Adriani, J.: "Drug Dependence in Hospitalized Patients," in *Acute Drug Abuse Emergencies*, Bourne, P.G., Ed. New York, Academic Press, 1976, pp. 231-250.
72. Isbell, H.: Medical aspects of opiate addiction. *Bull NY Acad Med 31*:886-901, 1955.
73. Miller, R.R., Feingold, A., and Paxinos, J.: Propoxyphene hydrochloride. A critical review. *JAMA 213*:996-1006, 1970.
74. Askevold, F.: The occurrence of paranoid incidents and abstinence delirium in abusers of amphetamine. *Acta Psychiatr Neur Scand 34*:145-164, 1959.
75. Streltzer, J., and Leigh, H.: Amphetamine abstinence psychosis—does it exist? *Psychiatr Opinion 13*:47-51, 1977.
76. Ferholt, J.B., and Stone, W.N.: Severe delirium after abrupt withdrawal of thiothixene in a chronic schizophrenic patient. *J Nerv Ment Dis 150*:400-403, 1970.
77. Lacoursiere, R.B., Spohn, H.E., and Thompson, K.: Medical effects of abrupt neuroleptic withdrawal. *Compr Psychiatry 17*:285-294, 1976.
78. Bourne, P.G., Ed.: *Acute Drug Abuse Emergencies*. New York, Academic Press, 1976.
79. Wikler, A.: Diagnosis and treatment of drug dependence of the barbiturate type. *Am J Psychiatry 125*:758-765, 1968.
80. Snyder, R.: Haloperidol in barbiturate detoxification. *Milit Med 142*: 885-886, 1977.

Additional References

Agrawal, P. Diazepam addiction. A case report. *Can Psychiatr Assoc J 23*:35-37, 1978.

Allgulander, C., and Borg, S. Case report: A delirious abstinence syndrome associated with clorazepate (Tranxilen). *Br J Addict* 73:175-177, 1978.

Ballenger, J.C., and Post, R.M. Kindling as a model for alcohol withdrawal syndromes. *Br J Psychiatry* 133:1-14, 1978.

Cutting, J. A reappraisal of alcohol psychoses. *Psychol Med* 8:285-295, 1978.

Daunderer, M. Akute Alcohol-intoxication: Physostigmin als Antidot gegen Äthanol. *Fortschr Med* 96:1311-1312, 1978.

DeBard, M.L. Diazepam withdrawal syndrome: A case with psychosis, seizure, and coma. *Am J Psychiatry* 136:104-105, 1979.

Deiker, T., and Chambers, H.E. Structure and content of hallucinations in alcohol withdrawal and functional psychosis. *Q J Stud Alcohol* 39:1831-1840, 1978.

Dencker, S.J., Wilhelmson, G., and Carlsson, E. Piracetam and chlormethiazole in acute alcohol withdrawal: A controlled clinical trial. *J Intern Med Res* 6:395-400, 1978.

Editorial: Benzodiazipine withdrawal. *Lancet* 1:196, 1979.

Eisenberg, S. Cerebral blood flow and metabolism in patients with delirium tremens. *Clin Res* 16:71, 1968.

Greenblatt, D.J., Gross, P.L., Harris, J., Shader, R.I., and Ciraulo, D.A. Fatal hyperthermia following haloperidol therapy of sedative-hypnotic withdrawal. *J Clin Psychiatry* 39:673-675, 1978.

Heiss, W.D. Regional cerebral blood flow measurement with scintillation camera. *Intern J Neurol* 11:144-161, 1977.

Hession, M.A., Verma, S., and Bhakta, K.G.M. Dependence on chlormethiazole and effects of its withdrawal. *Lancet* 1:953-954, 1979.

Holzbach, E., and Bühler, K.E. Die Behandlung des Delirium tremens mit Haldol. *Nervenarzt* 49:405-409, 1978.

Kramp, P., and Rafaelsen, O.J. Delirium tremens: A double-blind comparison of diazepam and barbital treatment. *Acta Psychiatr Scand* 58:174-190, 1978.

May, P.R.A., and Ebaugh, F.G. Pathological intoxication, alcoholic hallucinosis, and other reactions to alcohol. *Q J Stud Alcohol* 14:200-227, 1953.

Pevnick, J.S., Masinski, D.R., and Haertzen, C.A. Abrupt withdrawal from therapeutically administered diazepam. *Arch Gen Psychiatry* 35:995-998, 1978.

Smith, D.E., and Wesson, D.R. *Diagnosis and Treatment of Adverse Reactions to Sedative-Hypnotics.* Rockville, Md., National Institute on Drug Abuse, 1974.

CHAPTER 12

DELIRIUM DUE TO METABOLIC DISORDERS

In a general sense, all delirium is a manifestation of a diffuse disturbance of cerebral metabolism. From the clinical and practical point of view, however, it is convenient to distinguish a class of etiological factors in delirium which may be regarded as systemic disorders of metabolism having secondary effects on the brain. These cerebral effects are sometimes referred to as metabolic encephalopathies and delirium is often one of their behavioral or psychiatric manifestations. Metabolic disorders are among the most common and thus most important causes of the syndrome in clinical practice today, sharing this distinction with intoxication by drugs. Hypoxia, hypoglycemia, electrolyte imbalance, and renal, hepatic, and respiratory insufficiency constitute prominent causes of delirium and deserve separate, if brief, discussion. All of these conditions may also cause stupor and coma (1).

HYPOXIA

Hypoxia refers to a reduction in the oxygen concentration or tension in the body. The importance of adequate oxygen supply for cerebral function and some of the consequences of hypoxia for the latter are discussed in Chapter 6. The normal brain in a conscious human accounts for about 20 percent of the total body basal oxygen consumption. The level of awareness shows fairly close correlation with the cerebral metabolic rate. Siesjö (2) points out that the metabolic basis of consciousness or awareness is twofold. First, appropriate transmembrane ion gradients must be maintained in order that communication between cells be safeguarded. Second, to enable such communication, appropriate transmitters need to be synthesized, released, and inactivated;

and, in addition, the postsynaptic membranes must be in an excitable state. For the monoamines to be synthesized an adequate oxygen tension and precursor availability are needed. Synthesis of acetylcholine requires normal production of pyruvate. In conditions of lack of oxygen, or substrate, or both, cerebral function fails before there is evidence of depletion of brain energy reserves. Psychological symptoms and EEG changes tend to precede any detectable failure in energy metabolism and seem to reflect changes in the metabolism of aromatic biogenic amines, i.e. dopamine, noradrenaline, and serotonin. Hydroxylation reactions and dopamine receptors appear to be particularly sensitive to hypoxia (3). Thus, as Siesjö (2) asserts, pathways subserving communication between cells are especially vulnerable to metabolic failure and hence to hypoxia.

The supply of oxygen to the brain depends on the cerebral blood flow (CBF) and the oxygen content of the blood. CBF depends on the cerebral perfusion pressure, i.e. the difference between the mean systemic arterial pressure and the cerebral venous blood pressure. The level of the mean systemic arterial blood pressure at which brain damage is produced in man is about 50 mm. Hg. (4). The lower limit of the oxygen saturation of the arterial blood for normal mental function is 85 percent. The limit for consciousness is 55 to 60 percent saturation (5). Oxygen deprivation for one or two minutes, especially in a person with cerebrovascular disease, is liable to be followed by delirium and stupor. Hypoxic damage to the brain may occur in a variety of clinical conditions characterized by inadequate supply of oxygen or glucose to the neurons. Areas of the brain that are selectively vulnerable to hypoxia include the arterial boundary zones, the Ammon's horns, the thalamus, and the cerebellum (4).

Graham (4) distinguishes six categories of cerebral hypoxia: 1. stagnant, which may be ischemic and due to local or generalized arrest of blood supply, or oligemic, which is due to local or generalized reduction in blood supply; 2. anoxic and hypoxic —in the former there is an absence of oxygen in the lungs, and in the latter—reduced oxygen tension in the lungs; 3. anemic, which results from abnormally low hemoglobin concentration or from unavailability of hemoglobin for oxygen transport, as in carbon monoxide poisoning; 4. histotoxic, which is due to poisoning of respiratory enzymes in the neurons; 5. hypoglycemic; and 6. febrile convulsions and status epilepticus.

Plum and Posner (1) distinguish three types of anoxia, i.e. anoxic, anemic, and ischemic. These authors subdivide the clinical categories of ischemic and hypoxic cerebral damage into acute, chronic, and multifocal. This classification is useful for the student of delirium since it allows grouping of the clinical conditions in which hypoxia and ischemia are instrumental in bringing about delirium. Acute diffuse ischemia or hypoxia is due to such causes as cardiac arrest, syncope, inhalation of carbon monoxide, or acute pulmonary embolism. Subacute or chronic diffuse hypoxia may be due to myocardial infarction, severe anemia, congestive heart failure, and pulmonary disease. Multifocal cerebral ischemia or anoxia occurs in such disorders as hypertensive encephalopathy, polycythemia, multiple small emboli originating in the heart, fat embolism, cerebral malaria, disseminated lupus erythematosus, polyarteritis nodosa, and multi-infarct cerebral disease (dementia). Some of these conditions will now be discussed.

Myocardial infarction. Delirium may follow myocardial infarction. Data on the incidence and prevalence of this complication are scarce. Trubnikov and Zorina (6) have observed delirium in 6.6 percent of 1,058 patients suffering from acute myocardial infarction. Delirium was more common among the aged, an observation consonant with that of others. Libow (7) asserts that myocardial infarction presents with confusion in 13 percent of elderly patients. The Russian investigators found that delirium usually came on in the third or fourth day after infarction and lasted two to five days (6). Significantly, 37 percent of the delirious patients died. This finding suggests that delirium following acute infarction may represent an adverse prognostic sign. Nearly one-half of the patients studied by Trubnikov and Zorina had been chronically intoxicated with alcohol, and this factor was believed to have contributed to the delirium. Observations from coronary care units give discrepant figures on the frequency of delirium. Hackett et al. (8) found it in 10 percent of patients; Cay et al. (9) observed it in about 3.5 percent, and Parker and Hodge (10) in only 11 among

500 patients treated in the coronary care unit. Various factors have been proposed to account for the CCU delirium; they are discussed at length in Chapter 5. Cerebral hypoxia in these patients could result from cardiac arrhythmias, congestive heart failure, or an episode of severe hypotension. Moderate anemia in conjunction with cerebrovascular disease predisposes elderly patients to delirium after myocardial infarction even when the reduction in cardiac output is not marked (1).

Cardiac arrhythmia. Sudden and temporary interference with normal heart function due to various types of cardiac arrhythmia, whether associated with myocardial infarction or caused by other conditions, may result in diffuse cerebral ischemia and delirium (11-16). Diminished cardiac output, subsequent decreased carotid blood flow, and reduced cerebral perfusion may all be the consequences of a cardiac dysrhythmia (16). Clark (11) has emphasized that mental confusion and related abnormal behavior are a rather common mode of presentation of paroxysmal cardiac arrhythmias in the elderly. It is essential to diagnose the arrhythmia correctly and treat it promptly to avoid permanent brain damage and intellectual deficit or dementia. Prolonged electrocardiographic monitoring (such as with the Holter system) is recommended for patients who suffer from delirious episodes and in whom transient cerebral dysfunction due to a cardiac dysrhythmia is suspected (16). Paroxysmal tachyarrhythmias, intermittent complete heart block, bundle branch block, and severe bradycardia all seem to be possible causes of episodes of delirium, especially in the elderly (11-18). Dizziness, seizures, and/or syncope seem to be the more common manifestations of these arrhythmias than delirium. Patients suffering from an abnormally slow heart rate due to acquired complete heart block may show improvement in mental functioning after implantation of an artificial pacemaker (14, 15, 19). Patients with *chronic cardiovascular disease* may show signs of cognitive dysfunction. Diminished cerebral blood flow and cerebral embolization have been blamed for the intellectual deficits (20, 21). Such patients may be expected to be vulnerable to delirium in response to sudden further reduction in cerebral perfusion or other factors compromising brain function. Michael (22) found delirium in about 1 percent in a large sample of patients with *cardiac decom-*

pensation. This complication was five times more common in women. Eisenberg et al. (23) studied patients with severe congestive heart failure who showed "mental aberrations" or "mental confusion." Six of these patients had alternating states of mental confusion and alertness, and thus appear to have suffered from episodes of delirium. As a group, the confused subjects showed a profound reduction in cerebral perfusion and a decrease in cerebral oxygen consumption. The mean cerebral blood flow was 26 ml. per minute per 100 g.; cerebral oxygen consumption was 2.71 ml. per minute per 100 g. The six patients with episodes of mental confusion were studied both when they were confused and lucid. While confused, they showed a significant decrease in cerebral blood flow, increase in cerebral vascular resistance, and decrease in cerebral oxygen consumption and arterial carbon dioxide content. Eisenberg et al. observe that the onset of mental confusion in patients with advanced congestive heart failure has grave prognostic implications in that it often heralds deterioration of the physical condition followed by death.

Hypertensive encephalopathy. Multifocal cerebral hypoxia is exemplified by hypertensive encephalopathy. There is a sudden elevation of arterial pressure, and symptoms such as severe headache, generalized or focal seizures, delirium, stupor, and coma (1, 24). The symptoms may last minutes, hours, or days and leave without sequelae. They may complicate acute glomerulonephritis, essential hypertension, toxemia of pregnancy, etc. Cerebral blood flow is decreased and cerebral arterioles constricted. Multiple small thrombi form in the brain and cerebral edema supervenes.

Pulmonary embolism. Pulmonary embolism may result in decrease in cardiac output and decreased cerebral blood flow and thus ischemia. Mental changes are said to occur in about 60 percent of patients (1). They usually come on after recovery of consciousness whose loss may be the initial acute event and one associated with seizures. The patient is delirious, tachypneic, and often anxious. He or she usually complains of dyspnea, either at rest or on exertion. Pulmonary embolism should be considered in any patient who suddenly faints or becomes delirious, or both, without any obvious reason, and displays tachypnea. Determination of the blood gases and lung scan are needed to establish the diagnosis. There is decreased arterial PO_2 (less than 80 mm. Hg.) and a reduced $P CO_2$ (1).

Endocarditis. The result of endocarditis may be embolic ischemia of the brain and delirium (1, 25, 26). In infective endocarditis the mental symptoms may range from mild confusion to a full-blown delirium with hallucinations and delusions. Delirium may occur in as many as 50 percent of patients and is especially common among the elderly, in whom it may be the most prominent manifestation of the disease (26). Bademosi et al. (25) found neuropsychiatric complications in 38 percent of patients with infective endocarditis; in two of them psychiatric symptoms were the cause for admission.

Fat embolism. Trauma, pancreatitis, and other conditions may be complicated by fat embolism and result in cerebral hypoxia and delirium (1).

Decompression sickness. Liberation of gases into body fluids and tissues during or after decompression at too fast a rate causes decompression sickness. Cerebral ischemia and raised intracranial pressure are some of the consequences, and delirium may be one of their clinical manifestations (27).

Nitrogen narcosis. Divers using compressed air may suffer from nitrogen narcosis (28). Various factors, such as rapid compression, anxiety, exertion, fatigue, and increased oxygen partial pressure, tend to increase the narcotic effect. The mental symptoms consist of initial mild impairment of cognitive functions and euphoria, followed by confusion and hallucinations. These latter more severe effects tend to appear at more than 10 ATA (atmospheric absolute) (28).

Air embolism. The passage of gas into the pulmonary veins and systemic circulation results in air embolism. Cerebrovascular occlusion may be one of the consequences of air embolism from mediastinal emphysema or pneumothorax and result in delirium, loss of consciousness, or both (29).

High altitude sickness. This is a condition in which low oxygen supply results in cerebral hypoxia and delirium. The mental effects of acute exposure to altitude are related to the degree of oxygen unsaturation of the arterial blood (5). There is still no general agreement regarding the degree of acute hypoxia necessary to cause the earliest signs of decrement in mental performance. Crow and Kelman (30) assessed performance on a free-recall memory test and a scanning task in subjects acutely exposed to simulated altitudes of 12,000 feet and found no evidence of impairment. Pugh (5) asserts that memory and intelligence begin to show disturbance at between 12,000 and 18,000 feet, depending on the rapidity of ascent, duration of exposure, and individual susceptibility. He states that the accepted limit for normal mental function is 85 percent oxygen saturation of the arterial blood, which corresponds to an altitude of 10,000 feet for people breathing air and 33,000 feet for those breathing oxygen. The limit for consciousness, Pugh asserts, is 55 to 60 percent saturation. The level at which delirium may occur is unknown. Sarnoff and Haberer (31) studied disturbances of consciousness at altitudes using simulated chamber flights. They found that from 10,000 to 18,000 feet all subjects showed some slight degree of EEG slowing. Above 18,000 feet, high voltage slow-wave activity occurs intermittently for increasing periods of time. The first signs of the EEG slowing preceded the disturbance of consciousness by sixty seconds when the subjects were tested at 26,000 feet. Consciousness is lost with sudden exposure to oxygen lack in five to seven minutes at 25,000 feet (5). Prolonged exposure to altitude may result in mountain sickness. The symptoms of the latter have been documented in mountaineers and others. Hillary spent 10 minutes on the summit of Mt. Everest, i.e. at about 27,700 feet. After that interval he began to notice confusion and had to put himself back on oxygen (5). The mental effects of high altitudes in climbers are the result not only of low oxygen supply but also cold, fatigue, etc., which can be expected to increase susceptibility to delirium. Impairment of judgment and retardation of thought and action are common mental manifestations of mountain sickness (5).

Anemia. Delirium will not be caused by anemia unless the oxygen-carrying capacity of the blood is reduced by more than half (1).

Thrombotic thrombocytopenic purpura. Delirium may be the first manifestation of thrombotic thrombocytopenic purpura in about one-third of the patients (32). The syndrome is probably related to the occlusion of small vessels, small infarcts, and petechial hemorrhages occurring diffusely in the gray matter. About 27 percent of the patients presenting with an organic brain syndrome improve (32).

Multifocal cerebral ischemia and delirium may also result from *polycythemia vera* (33), *macroglobulinemia* (1), *disseminated intravascular coagulation* (1), and *cerebral malaria* (1, 34-37). In the latter, there is believed to be plugging of cerebral vessels by clumped erythrocytes infected with Plasmodium falciparum and by pigments (34). Others explain cerebral hypoxia in this condition by endothelial proliferation, anemia, decreased oxygen-carrying capacity of the infected erythrocytes, etc. Incidence of cerebral malaria in those infected with P. falciparum is about 2 percent (34). Stupor, convulsions, and coma may follow. Wintrob (37) reports on four cases of what appeared to be delirium observed in Liberia. The patients showed vivid hallucinations, paranoid delusions, and agitation.

Carbon monoxide (CO) poisoning. An important cause of acute cerebral hypoxia and related encephalopathy is carbon monoxide poisoning (38-42). It is a rather common means of suicide, especially with the use of automobile exhaust fumes. Accidental intoxication with household gas, leaking gas mains, black smoke inhalation during fire, etc., may occur. About 1,500 deaths from accidental or deliberate exposure to carbon monoxide occur in this country annually. Estimated mortality is 30 percent. Housewives, garage workers, and motor vehicle operators are the major groups at risk. CO poisoning should always be suspected in patients sustaining burns from fires in enclosed spaces. The carboxyhemoglobin which results from a combination of carbon monoxide with hemoglobin is a relatively stable compound which interferes with the oxygen-carrying capacity of the blood. Cerebral hypoxia follows.

The incidence of delirium in CO poisoning was found in one well-documented series of patients to be between 17 and 25 percent (39). It appears that delirium may be the main mode of presentation of CO poisoning or can come on after the patient has emerged from coma. It may last hours to up to four weeks (40). Furthermore, the syndrome may be a manifestation of delayed postanoxic encephalopathy (1). The latter comes on hours to as long as three weeks after the initial hypoxia and is typically preceded by a lucid and seemingly normal interval. Suddenly, delirium and/or other manifestations of cerebral dysfunction appear, and the patient may develop coma and die. A few patients recover fully; other survivors display signs of cerebral damage in the form of dementia, amnestic syndrome, organic personality syndrome, or a combination of these organic mental disorders (40). The latter may develop without the intervention of delayed encephalopathy in which there is damage to the white matter of the cerebral hemispheres with sparing of the nerve cells (1). The cause of this leukoencephalopathy is unknown, but cerebral edema or damage to regional vasculature have been suggested to play a causative role. The encephalopathy has been described most often in association with CO poisoning, but it may also occur in other settings, such as cardiac arrest, drug overdose, or hypoglycemia.

Adequate treatment of acute CO poisoning is essential if lasting neuropsychiatric sequelae are to be prevented. Ginsburg and Romano (38) recommend the following guidelines: 1. determination of carboxyhemoglobin level on admission after acute exposure; 2. blood and urine screen for drugs depressing the central nervous system which the patient may have taken; 3. determination of arterial blood gases and correction of acidosis; 4. ECG should be recorded and arrhythmia, if any, treated; 5. adequate oxygenation, if possible with hyperbaric therapy; 6. avoidance of tranquilizers that decrease REM sleep; 7. treatment of cerebral edema with steroids or mannitol; and 8. bedrest for two to four weeks to help avoid delayed leukoencephalopathy.

HYPOGLYCEMIA

The importance of glucose as the main substrate of cerebral metabolism is discussed in Chapter 6. Studies of hypoglycemia induced by insulin have shown that behavioral and EEG abnormalities can occur without any impairment of energy production. It has been proposed that these abnormalities may reflect sensitivity to hypoglycemia of glucoreceptors in the hypothalamic-pituitary system (3). There is little, if any, reduction in the cerebral rate of oxygen utilization even if the level of blood glucose is reduced to that at which coma supervenes. This finding indicates that oxidative metabolism is maintained at the expense of endogenous substrates, namely glycolytic metabolites, citric acid cycle intermediates, amino acids, and phospholipids (*see* Chapter 6).

In healthy men subjected to a twenty-four-hour fast, plasma glucose levels do not fall below 60 mg. per deciliter, but in healthy premenopausal women such levels are generally lower and may decrease to 58 mg. per deciliter (43). The arterial blood glucose concentration at which neuropsychiatric symptoms appear varies widely, but is seldom above 40 mg. per deciliter. Lower blood glucose levels, even as low as 20 mg. per deciliter or less, have been recorded in symptom-free subjects. In most cases of spontaneous hypoglycemia giving rise to symptoms, the glucose concentration is 30 mg. per deciliter or less (44).

Plum and Posner (1) state that acute hypoglycemic encephalopathy may present in one of four forms: delirium, coma, a stroke-like form, and an epileptic attack with single or multiple general convulsions. Marks and Rose (44) distinguish between acute and chronic neuroglycopenia. The former starts with malaise, anxiety, feelings of unreality, restlessness, hunger, palpitations, profuse sweating, facial flushing, and tremulousness. These symptoms may progress to delirium and coma. Chronic neuroglycopenia is characterized by insidious personality changes, impairment of memory, episodes of delirium often with paranoid or schizophreniform features, and gradual progression to dementia. Recurrent severe hypoglycemic episodes as well as a single prolonged coma may result in irreversible intellectual deficit. A study of 850 cases of islet-cell tumors showed that the incidence of psychiatric disorders was 12 percent (45). About one-half of these patients failed to show improvement in mental status after surgery. This poor prognosis underscores the importance of an early diagnosis and management of hypoglycemia.

Fasting hypoglycemia is caused by a variety of disorders. Fajans and Floyd (43) have classified the latter into four major groupings: 1. organic hypoglycemia, in which a recognizable anatomic lesion exists, e.g. hyperinsulinism due to disease of pancreatic islet beta-cell disease, nonpancreatic tumors, and pituitary and adrenocortical hypofunction; 2. deficiency of specific hepatic enzyme (in infancy and childhood); 3. functional hypoglycemia, in which there is no demonstrable anatomic lesion, e.g. severe inanition; and 4. hypoglycemia caused by exogenous agents, such as alcohol, insulin, and oral hypoglycemic and other drugs (46-48). Postprandial or reactive hypoglycemia, such as that after gastrectomy, may occasionally result in delirium (49). Laboratory diagnosis of hypoglycemia due to the various conditions cannot be discussed here (43).

The most common cause of fasting hypoglycemia is a functioning islet-cell tumor (45,50-54). Insulinoma is a rare tumor, occurring more often in women and in older people (53). Hypoglycemic symptoms may occur for several or more years before diagnosis is made. They come on irregularly and vary in duration. They occur typically in the late afternoon or in the early morning before breakfast. Confusion or abnormal behavior were reported in 80 percent of hypoglycemic episodes in one series of patients (53). In that series, spontaneous symptoms or those induced by provocative tests occurred in fifty-six out of sixty patients. In another reported series, mental confusion was observed in about 30 percent of patients (51). In most cases hypoglycemic episodes occur spasmodically at first and are separated by symptom-free intervals of weeks or months. The frequency of the episodes may be less than six per year (51). Gradually, the frequency, duration, and severity of hypoglycemia increase. Delirium may be misdiagnosed as a functional psychiatric illness, and the patient's underlying organic disease may remain unrecognized for years.

Hypoglycemic symptoms are the same regardless of the underlying cause. Neuroglycopenia and delirium depend for their development on the rate and degree of decrease in blood glucose concentration as well as on individual susceptibility, which is variable. Most reports on organic psychiatric symptoms due to hypoglycemia to be found in the literature are related to islet-cell tumors and to iatrogenic hyperinsulinism. The symptoms are relieved by intravenous administration of glucose. In one reported case delirium was stopped by intramuscular phenothiazines (50). The symptoms of hypoglycemia, or rather neuroglycopenia, may include outbursts of anger, violence, paranoid delusions, catalepsy, dysarthria, ataxia, diplopia, vertigo, hemiparesis, perceptual disturbances such as macropsia, micropsia, chromatopsia, and visual hallucinations, etc. (45). Hypoglycemic symptoms have been misdiagnosed as hysteria, schizophrenia, mania, and endogenous depression. In one series of ninety-one patients with hyperinsulinism a psychiatric diagnosis was initially made in sixteen (55). Delirium may last minutes or hours and is usually followed by amnesia. Nonrecognition of this syndrome is likely the reason for the misdiagnosis of some patients as cases of functional psychosis or behavioral disorder.

The EEG in hypoglycemia shows diffuse slowing, epileptiform activity, or foci of slow activity (45). Engel et al. (56) induced mild hypoglycemia experimentally and found that when blood glucose levels were reduced to 35 to 49 mg. per deciliter, a distinct shift to lower frequencies occurred.

HEPATIC ENCEPHALOPATHY

Hepatic encephalopathy has been defined as a disturbance of cerebral function in which consciousness is particularly affected and which can complicate all forms of liver disease (57). Neuropsychiatric symptoms complicating liver disease have been recognized since antiquity. Excellent clinical accounts of psychiatric disorders, especially of delirium, occurring in the course of liver disease were published in the nineteenth century (57).

There is some evidence that clinical manifestations of hepatic encephalopathy are due to complex metabolic derangement involving both cerebral cortex and the centrencephalic system (57). The rate of cerebral oxidation is decreased even though there appears to be no failure of glucose and oxygen supply to the brain. The reduced oxygen uptake and utilization have been ascribed to various toxic factors, such as ammonia. The latter interferes with the energy metabolism of brain tissue. It is not established, however, if the reduction in energy metabolism is responsible for the symptoms of hepatic encephalopathy.

Three clinical types of hepatic encephalopathy have been distinguished: chronic portasystemic encephalopathy, cirrhosis with a precipitant, and acute liver failure (57). Cirrhosis with a precipitant is the most commonly seen form. Psychiatrically, mental disorders due to liver disease include delirium, dementia, and organic personality syndrome. Delirium can occur in all three clinical types of encephalopathy. Episodes of delirium complicate the late stages of all forms of cirrhosis. It may be precipitated by overbrisk diuresis, gastrointestinal hemorrhage, infection, alcohol ingestion, surgery, and drugs such as opiates, barbiturates, tranquilizers, and antihistamines.

Acute liver failure is usually due to viral hepatitis, acetaminophen self-poisoning, alcoholic hepatitis, drugs such as halothane and methyldopa, and poisoning with carbon tetrachloride. Delirium may be preceded by euphoria or depression, posturing, antisocial behavior, nightmares, headache, dizziness, etc. It is typically of the hyperactive type, with psychomotor overactivity, noisy and belligerent behavior, and seizures. Drowsiness is common. The delirium may progress to or follow stupor and coma. Jaundice may be absent and make diagnosis difficult at first. Prognosis is poor (57, 58). Chronic portasystemic encephalopathy may feature intermittent episodes of delirium related to such factors as increased dietary intake of protein or infection (57).

Clinical features of delirium due to chronic liver disease are variable. Degree of cognitive impairment may vary from slight to profound. Somnolence during the day and insomnia at night are common initial features. The patient tends to be slow in speech and movement, and apathetic. He or she may show memory impairment, inability to concentrate, constructional apraxia, spatial disorientation, tendency to aimless wandering, unformed visual hallucinations, macropsia, etc. These manifold symptoms tend to fluctuate from day to day and precede the onset of delirium, stupor, and/or coma by days or weeks. Psychometric tests have documented intellectual and attentional deficits and abnormalities in these patients (59-62). Delirium itself may be difficult to distinguish sharply from the more chronic cognitive and attentional deficits which accompany chronic hepatic encephalopathy, and these two mental disorders merge into each other. Delirium is typically hypoactive with intermittent agitation and restlessness. The patient tends to be apathetic, depressed, or euphoric; his or her speech is slurred and monotonous and may feature perseveration and dysphasia. Visual hallucinations are common and usually simple, i.e. colored stars (often green or red) or flashing lights. Catatonic posturing has been reported. In an alcoholic patient, symptoms of hepatic encephalopathy may be mixed with those of delirium tremens. Flapping tremor (asterixis) and exaggerated tendon reflexes accompany delirium in encephalopathy (57, 63, 64). The patient may at any time slip into stupor and coma and display delirium again after emerging from the latter.

The EEG in hepatic encephalopathy shows changes during both wakefulness and sleep (57, 65, 66). The mean frequency of the background activity slows down to the delta range. Initially, there is an increase in amplitude and a slight slowing. As the patient develops stupor, further slowing and increase in amplitude of the waves appear. Triphasic waves occur in hepatic coma and carry a poor prognosis. The degree of slowing correlates well with the clinical state, although the EEG changes may be initially more severe than the mental state of the patient would suggest, and they may persist after the patient's mental disorder has lifted. Sleep is profoundly disturbed in hepatic encephalopathy (66). There is reduction in slow-wave sleep, with absence of stage-four sleep, increase in the percentage of REM sleep, and gradual breakdown of the sleep function as the encephalopathy worsens. Correlations were established between the clinical and EEG severity and the arterial ammonia level on the one hand and the EEG features, duration, and organization of sleep on the other.

Diagnosis of delirium as a manifestation of hepatic encephalopathy depends on history, clinical features, and laboratory tests. History of chronic liver disease, with or without signs of chronic hepatic encephalopathy, or portacaval shunt, or both, is suggestive, but not conclusive, evidence that the delirium is due to hepatic failure. The patient may actually be delirious due to alcohol or drug withdrawal, intoxication with drugs, or other factors. History of liver disease may be lacking in some patients. Clinical features are helpful: disorders of sleep, with somnolence preceding the delirium and drowsiness during it; slow and slurred speech, and monotonous voice; mask-like face; general psychomotor hypoactivity; perseveration; flapping tremor; and increased muscle tone with exaggerated deep tendon reflexes are all suggestive of hepatic encephalopathy. Laboratory tests include the EEG, examination of cerebrospinal fluid (CSF), and blood chemistries. The EEG changes have been described. They are a sensitive indicator of the level of awareness but are nonspecific with regard to the cause of the reduced level of awareness. The CSF is usually clear and colorless. Ammonia level tends to be more raised than in the blood. There is no characteristic change in cells, protein, glucose, or electrolytes. One fairly consistent change is an elevated level of glutamine which does not regularly reflect the degree of the encephalopathy. Blood (especially arterial) ammonia concentration is usually, but not invariably, elevated; it does not correlate with the level of awareness. Hepatic encephalopathy is virtually always present when the blood ammonia concentration exceeds 3 mg. per ml., but about 10 percent of patients with severe encephalopathy have ammonia levels within the normal range. Hypoglycemia, hypokalemia, and alkalosis are common in liver failure and may aggravate encephalopathy (57).

Pathogenesis of hepatic encephalopathy has been the subject of considerable speculation. The proposed mechanisms have included the following: 1. *ammonia toxicity;* serum ammonia levels are raised in most patients with hepatic encephalopathy. Hyperammonemia induced experimentally in human volunteers is accompanied by lower alertness, decreased interaction with people, and tremor (67). On the other hand, arterial and CSF ammonia levels in hepatic encephalopathy do not correlate with the level of awareness. The brain stem and subcortical centers are particularly involved in the encephalopathy, yet ammonia toxicity does not affect them; 2. *false neurotransmitters;* bacterial action on the colonic contents may result in the formation of false neurotransmitters, such as octopamine, which replaces noradrenaline and dopamine. Disturbances in consciousness might be due to displacement of these normal neurotransmitters from widely spread CNS neurons (68). This hypothesis has some experimental support; 3. *tryptophan and serotonin;* tryptophan levels in the CSF are increased in hepatic encephalopathy. Brain tryptophan concentration is a chief determinant of the synthesis and turnover of serotonin, which are increased in hepatic encephalopathy. Both serotonin and tryptophan have been implicated in the pathogenesis of hepatic encephalopathy, but the issue remains controversial (68, 69); 4. *short-chain fatty acids.* Patients with hepatic encephalopathy have high levels of these acids in blood and CSF. The role of the acids in production of mental symptoms in liver failure is open to question (68).

Treatment of delirium due to hepatic disease involves therapy for the underlying condition and, at times, sedation. Medical treatment aims at reduction of blood ammonia levels with lactulose, sterilization of the gut with neomycin, and correction of hypokalemia. Prednisone and prednisolone have been advocated for severe alcoholic hepatitis. Levodopa has been used successfully to counteract delirium and coma in liver failure. Details of these treatments cannot be discussed here (57, 59, 70, 71). Sedation is best avoided if at all possible since all sedatives are liable to precipitate coma (57, 72). On occasion, however, a delirious patient may be severely agitated and belligerent, and sedation may be necessary. Phenothiazines are contraindicated. Chlorpromazine may cause stupor, which is apparently related to increased sensitivity to the drug (72). Diazepam is the drug of choice. It is best given by slow intravenous injection and in small doses. Special care should be taken in patients with previous history of encephalopathy. Repeated doses are best avoided since the drug is liable to accumulate. Oral doses of 5 to 10 mg. may be given to induce sleep at night (72, 73).

UREMIC ENCEPHALOPATHY

Encephalopathy may complicate both acute and chronic renal failure; it may be acute or chronic (74-78). Furthermore, encephalopathy may also complicate treatment of renal failure (79-84). As early as 1868, Addison (85) wrote "On the Disorders of the Brain Connected With Diseased Kidneys" and noted "psychotic manifestations." Baker and Knutson (86) described six psychiatric syndromes complicating uremia: 1. asthenic form, characterized by malaise, fatigue, poor memory and concentration, lassitude, and gradual progression to lethargy, coma, and death; 2. acute delirium, by far the most common syndrome;

3. schizophrenic form, featuring catatonic symptoms; 4. depressed form; 5. manic form; and 6. paranoid form. It appears that some "asthenic" cases represent what we call dementia. Baker and Knutson actually observe that uremia may lead to irreversible brain damage.

Stenbäck and Haapanen (77) studied delirium in patients with acute renal failure as well as those suffering from chronic kidney disease. The criterion for inclusion into the study was "azotemia," defined as blood urea value of 50 mg. per 100 ml. or higher. The patients were divided into two groups: those with serum urea concentration of 50 to 199 mg. per 100 ml. and over ("low urea" group); and those with 250 mg. per 100 ml. and over ("high urea" group). Delirium was observed in about 35 percent of patients with acute renal failure and in about 45 percent of those with chronic renal failure. Delirium was more likely to accompany serum urea concentrations higher than 250 mg. per 100 ml.; about 80 percent of all cases of delirium belonged to this "high urea" group. Convulsions often accompanied delirium in chronic uremia. Multiple metabolic disturbances accompany acute renal failure and are likely to contribute to the onset of delirium. Increased blood urea nitrogen levels, hyponatremia, hypochloremia, hypokalemia, hyperkalemia, hypocalcemia, hypermagnesemia, and metabolic acidosis may all occur. Autopsy findings in patients dying from uremia have shown neuronal degeneration, mostly in the cerebral cortex, reticular formation, and the sensory nuclei of the brain stem (77).

Acute renal encephalopathy may complicate acute renal failure or supervene in the course of chronic kidney disease with chronic encephalopathy. The latter may be reversible or not. Chronic encephalopathy features cognitive deficits, such as impaired ability to select and process information. Poor performance on tests of choice-reaction time, auditory short-term memory, serial sevens, number recall, mental arithmetic, and time perception has been reported (76, 87, 88). In a stable phase of chronic encephalopathy the patients are oriented but show the above deficits of memory and intellectual performance. The patient is typically tired and apathetic and may be depressed. Evidence of cognitive deficits is usually present when blood urea is only moderately raised (less than 200 mg. per

100 ml.), but may not be apparent on the bedside clinical testing unless the levels of 200 mg. are exceeded (76). Chronic salt depletion, hypertension, anemia, impaired drug tolerance, and nutritional deficiencies may contribute to the chronic encephalopathy (76). The neuropsychiatric disorders in uremia do not show regular correlation with either blood urea nitrogen or the multiple metabolic and biochemical disturbances. A patient may have delirium with BUN levels of 50 mg. per 100 ml. or less, while other patients are free of signs of encephalopathy with BUN values over 200 mg. per 100 ml. On the whole, however, delirium does occur more often when blood urea exceeds 250 mg. per 100 ml., especially when such a change develops rapidly (75, 77). Delirium may come on whenever a rapid progression of the underlying kidney disease takes place and/or a sudden change in electrolyte concentration occurs.

An episode of acute encephalopathy with delirium may develop in the setting of chronic renal failure as a result of a number of possible precipitating factors. The latter include salt depletion, water intoxication, hypertensive encephalopathy, systemic and urinary infection, congestive heart failure, intravascular coagulation, and neurological complications, such as Wernicke's encephalopathy (75, 76). Rapid changes in electrolytes may precipitate delirium (78). Clinical features of the latter have been referred to as the "hyperexcitable syndrome," characterized by irritability, hallucinations, aggressive behavior, and central nervous system and muscle hyperexcitability (76). The patient may display some degree of disorientation for time, such as failure to state accurately the time of day, as the earliest symptom of a developing delirium (75). As delirium progresses, the patient is likely to appear anxious, restless, and bewildered. Psychomotor activity is liable to shift from lethargy to excitement and back. Baker and Knutson (86) describe it well: "The entire course of the illness may shift rapidly from states of overactivity with aggressiveness, crying, laughing, singing, dancing, and swearing to states of lethargy with incoherent muttering, self-condemnatory delusions, mutism, or even catatonia." Hallucinations are common, fleeting, and usually frightening. They are usually both auditory and visual. The emotional state of the patient is variable and may feature anxiety, depression, or euphoria. Delusions may be present and are usually persecutory in character. Speech may be slurred or incoherent, with the patient mumbling or muttering to himself. Lucid intervals may occur at any point. An occasional patient may display schizophrenia-like features, such as catatonic posturing and mutism, negativism, waxy flexibility, etc. (86, 89).

Various neurological symptoms accompany delirium of renal failure. Involuntary movements, such as tremor and asterixis, akinesia, rigidity, choreoathetosis, trismus, myoclonus, and oculogyria may occur (75). Asterixis (flapping tremor) is usually most marked when delirium is present. Convulsions may occur. Dysfunction of practically every cranial nerve may be encountered in uremia (76).

The EEG in uremic encephalopathy is abnormal both during wakefulness and sleep (76, 90, 91). There is usually slowing of background activity with frequencies of 5 to 7 cycles/second. Bursts of paroxysmal slow waves and spike discharges may occur. Arousal responses may be abnormal in that various stimuli may induce bursts of slow waves. When serum creatinine concentration was used to express the degree of kidney failure, it was found that increasing percentages of slower EEG frequencies correlated with increasingly severe degrees of renal failure (90). The sleep EEG in uremia features reduced slow-wave (stages 3 and 4) and REM stages and an increased number of awakenings. The changes are similar to those of hepatic encephalopathy. The sleep cycles become better organized after hemodialysis. Awakenings are decreased and slow-wave sleep is increased. A correlation has been found between increased blood urea levels and the disturbance of sleep (91).

Pathogenesis of uremic encephalopathy is unknown and subject to speculation. Several hypotheses have been put forth to account for the encephalopathy. First, presence of a neurotoxin in blood has been postulated, but no such substance has yet been identified. Urea is not a neurotoxin (75). Phenolic acids have been implicated but their role in this context remains debatable (76). Second, brain permeability changes have been demonstrated in nephrectomized rats. Thus, as a result of increased permeability of the blood-brain barrier and/or altera-tions in the choroid plexus, various potentially neurotoxic sub-stances may have access to the brain. Such substances are believed to decrease cerebral oxygen consumption and exert stimulatory or inhibitory effects on various cerebral structures (75, 76). Third, cerebral oxygen utilization is reduced in uremic subjects. There is no correlation, however, between oxygen utilization and the mental state, the serum urea and electrolyte values, and the acid-base state of the uremic patients (75). Fourth, electrolyte and acid-base abnormalities have been sus-pected of being responsible for the mental disorders in uremia, but no single abnormality has been shown to consistently produce adverse mental changes. Systemic metabolic acidosis will not produce the latter as long as the pH of the CSF is not markedly altered. Severe hyponatremia has been blamed for the so-called dialysis disequilibrium syndrome. The most consistent finding has been the onset of delirium following rapid change of serum urea and electrolyte levels (75). Arieff et al. (74) studied uremic encephalopathy induced by bilateral ureteral ligation in dogs. These researchers found that acute uremia is associated with an increase in brain calcium content, due to the secondary hyper-parathyroidism in uremia. These changes in brain calcium may underlie some of the mental symptoms. Following rapid hemo-dialysis CSF pressure in the uremic dogs rose from 4 to 28 cm H_2O, and the EEG showed a further slowing of the background activity. Brain osmolality was significantly greater than that of plasma. As a result of the osmotic gradient between brain and plasma, movement of water into brain took place. After rapid dialysis, in addition to the increases in the CSF pressure, and brain osmolality and water content, there was also a fall in the pH of CSF. Cerebral edema results after rapid hemodialysis and may be responsible for the dialysis disequilibrium syndrome to be discussed presently. Fifth, an abnormality of neurotrans-mitter metabolism has been proposed to account for the involun-tary movements in uremia (75). It may be concluded that the pathogenesis of the mental disorders, neurological disturbances, and EEG abnormalities in renal failure is still largely unknown (74).

Encephalopathy with delirium may complicate not only

acute and chronic renal failure but also treatment of these conditions (75, 76, 78-84). A variety of causative factors may operate in delirium occurring in the course of dialysis and/or after renal transplantation: hypotension, cerebral edema, thiamine deficiency, intracranial bleeding, central nervous system infection, brain neoplasm, drugs (corticosteroids, methyldopa, diazepam, flurazepam, phenothiazines), seizures, and secondary hyperparathyroidism with hypercalcemia. It must be emphasized that, as a rule, hemodialysis results in an improvement of uremic encephalopathy and associated organic mental disorders. Yet some factors more or less inherent to dialysis may precipitate delirium. Dialysis disequilibrium syndrome is the best known example of acute encephalopathy directly related to hemodialysis. The syndrome may appear during or up to twenty-four hours after hemodialysis; it features headache, nausea, vomiting, twitching, tremor, cardiac arrhythmias, delirium, and convulsions. This syndrome is particularly liable to complicate rapid hemodialysis and has become less frequent since the introduction of modern techniques (75, 76). Experimental work aimed at elucidation of the pathogenesis of the syndrome has already been mentioned. The current opinion seems to be that osmotically active intracellular acids bring about entry of water into the brain and cerebral edema. This development follows rapid hemodialysis and may underlie the disequilibrium syndrome. The latter may be prevented by the use of glycerol in the dialysate (74, 75, 76).

Other factors which may bring about delirium in a hemodialyzed patient include subdural hematoma, seizures, viral encephalitis, Wernicke's encephalopathy, hypotension, subarachnoid hemorrhage, and drugs. Flurazepam and diazepam have been implicated in delirium during maintenance hemodialysis (82). In some cases of delirium the etiology cannot be identified (92, 93). Contribution of psychological stress occasioned by dialysis to the onset of delirium during it has been emphasized by some authors but remains an untested hypothesis (79, 92, 93).

A study of renal homograft recipients revealed significant psychopathology in 32 percent of 292 patients studied (83). Thirty-eight percent of these patients had had psychiatric symptoms prior to transplantation. Preoperative organic brain syndromes were usually relieved by successful transplantation. About 10 percent of postoperative patients developed an organic brain syndrome related to the administration of steroids, defective renal function, hypertension, and sepsis. Depression was a common finding in those who developed delirium as well as in other patients. The main causes of severe depressive reactions were threatened rejection of the transplanted organ, infection, and drugs. Seven patients attempted suicide (83). Following renal transplantation old infections may become reactivated and new ones may develop as a result of increased susceptibility to them in patients treated with immunosuppressive drugs. An incidence of CNS infections of 10 percent has been reported in renal transplant recipients (76). Bacterial and fungal infection of the meninges, brain abscess, toxoplasmosis, and viral encephalitis have all been observed in these patients and may cause delirium (76). Malignant neoplasms, especially of the brain, have been reported in renal transplant recipients (75, 76). Progressive multifocal leukoencephalopathy is a rare complication after renal transplantation and results in dementia. The latter may be initially mistaken for delirium and viewed as a transient disorder. Prednisone may give rise to delirium in the transplant patient. Patients suffering from systemic lupus erythematosus with renal failure may develop delirium at any phase of treatment of the renal complications (75, 76). Psychological studies of transplant patients show that about 50 percent of them show cognitive deficits suggestive of irreversible dementia (84). Such patients are likely to have a history of medical complications in the course of dialysis. This implies that permanent brain damage may occur during uremic encephalopathy and/or its treatment by dialysis and cannot be reversed by renal transplantation. Kiley et al. (94) report that the EEG tends to return to the normal range following immediately successful renal transplantation and that this provides convincing evidence of chronic uremic encephalopathy in most cases. Yet it is well known that the EEG may revert to the normal range while cognitive deficits may remain permanent following an acute or subacute cerebral disorder.

An important clinical problem is to distinguish delirium and reversible dementia from the progressive dialytic encephalopathy (dementia dialytica) complicating renal hemodialysis (76, 80, 95-100). Dementia dialytica (98) is distinct from the acute encephalopathies occurring in the course of dialysis. It is a rare and lethal complication of the latter, one featuring dementia, dysphasia, dyspraxia, facial grimacing, multifocal seizures, myoclonus, and a relentlessly progressive course leading to death in three to fifteen months (86, 97, 98). The earliest changes observed in one group of patients included disorientation for time and place and impaired judgment (98). Other patients may attract attention on account of stuttering, dysphasia, dysgraphia, hallucinations, delusions, delirium, and "bizarre" behavior (96, 97, 98). These symptoms develop suddenly or insidiously after many months or a few years on dialysis. The EEG changes in dialysis dementia consist of diffuse high amplitude slow waves with bifrontal predominance. Occasionally bifrontal negative spikes or triphasic waves may be seen. The changes are bilaterally symmetrical, and there is usually no evidence of focal brain discharges. The EEG abnormalities suggest involvement of both the reticular formation of the brain stem and the cerebral cortex (80). These changes are nonspecific and not diagnostic of dialysis dementia. Radionuclide studies have revealed alteration in CSF dynamics (80). Psychological studies have confirmed the presence of dementia in these patients (100). The latter showed deterioration of intellectual processes, disturbances in visual-motor integration, and general decline of cognitive functioning (100).

Many pathogenic mechanisms have been suggested for dialysis dementia. Recurrent hypoglycemia, vitamin deficiency, accumulation of heavy metals and aluminum, phosphate depletion, seizure disorder, hypercalcemia, diazepam toxicity, and slow virus infection of the central nervous system have been implicated (80, 95, 99). Aluminum intoxication hypothesis has found support from the finding that aluminum concentrations are higher in patients dying with dialysis encephalopathy than in dialyzed controls and uremic patients who were not dialyzed (95, 99). It has been proposed that these high aluminum levels are due to dialysis with fluid containing water with high aluminum concentrations (99). Dialysis with deionised water does not seem to contribute to the brain aluminum levels.

Differential diagnosis between acute dialytic encephalopathy with delirium, a subacute or chronic encephalopathy with reversible dementia, and dialysis dementia is difficult, yet prognosis in these three disorders is vastly different. Several observers point out that delirium may occur in the course of dialysis dementia (96, 97). Others claim that the symptoms of the latter may fluctuate during the disease and thus suggest a reversible cerebral disorder (100). Buchanan et al. (79) urge caution in diagnosing dialysis dementia, which carries a hopeless prognosis. Similarity of the clinical picture and the EEG findings between reversible and progressive dialysis encephalopathy, respectively, makes such diagnostic errors difficult to avoid. Combination of delirium, progressive dementia, speech and language disorders, and severe EEG slowing, developing in a patient who had been on hemodialysis for more than one year, point to the diagnosis of dialysis dementia. Yet caution is advised. A patient showing such symptoms has recently been reported to have recovered after transplantation (101). Other similar cases have reportedly recovered after parathyroidectomy (102), diazepam treatment (103), and withdrawal of treatment with benzodiazepines (82). RISA cisternography may help in the differential diagnosis (80). Every effort should be made to rule out treatable causes of dementia listed earlier before concluding that the patient has irreversible and progressive cerebral and mental disease.

Management of delirium occurring in patients with renal disease involves, as always, identification and treatment of the underlying cause (or more often multiple causes). General measures are the same as for any delirious patient. Agitation and excitement are probably best managed with haloperidol, starting with lower doses such as 2 or 3 mg. intramuscularly.

ENCEPHALOPATHY OF RESPIRATORY FAILURE

Respiratory failure may be caused by pulmonary as well as many extrapulmonary diseases, such as obstruction of the upper airways, trauma to the chest or head, myasthenia gravis, etc. Respiratory failure has been defined as inadequate or impaired gas exchange, that is to say hypoxemia with or without hyper-carbia (104). The encephalopathy of respiratory failure is a consequence of cerebral hypoxia or hypercarbia, or both. Acute respiratory failure is diagnosed by examination of arterial blood gases and finding of hypoxemia with or without hypercarbia. The former finding reflects inadequate lung function and implies the presence of subnormal partial pressure of oxygen (PaO_2) in the arterial blood. Hypercarbia refers to elevated arterial blood carbon dioxide tension (PCO_2). Delirium may be brought about by hypoxemia, hypercarbia, or both (104).

Most of the few studies of mental disorders due to respiratory failure have involved patients with chronic obstructive pulmonary disease (chronic pulmonary insufficiency, pulmonary encephalopathy) (105-108). Acute pulmonary decompensation in such patients is commonly associated with delirium. Respiratory failure may also develop in a subject with normal lungs due to a decrease in total ventilation (104). In either case, mental symptoms, including delirium, result from hypoxia with or without hypercarbia. Hypoxia was discussed earlier in this chapter. Its effects differ depending on the rate of its development. If the oxygen saturation of arterial blood falls abruptly to about 60 percent, a disturbance of awareness is liable to become manifest. On the other hand, chronic hypoxia with oxygen saturation as low as 60 percent may be tolerated (106). The same appears to be true of hypercapnia. Experimentally induced acute hypercapnia produces mental confusion when the arterial PCO_2 reaches about 70 mm. Hg. Patients with chronic pulmonary disease, however, may be mentally clear with levels of 60 to 70 mm. and are said to tolerate PCO_2 levels up to 90 mm. Hg. (107). In one reported series of patients with chronic lung disease obvious mental changes were noted at PCO_2 levels ranging from 48 to 148 mm. Hg. (107). Carbon dioxide behaves as an anesthetic drug. Moderate hypercapnia (PCO_2 of 50 to 60 mm. Hg.) in man approximately doubles the cerebral blood flow and at the same time produces a reduction in glucose utilization (109). Thus, hypercapnia appears to resemble barbiturate anesthesia and hypoglycemia in that the brain becomes partially depleted of carbohydrate substrate and has to oxidize endogenous substrate to sustain production of energy (109). It is believed that most of the metabolic effects of hypercapnia are due to the fall in cell pH. A good correlation has been found between the severity of neuropsychiatric symptoms in patients with pulmonary insufficiency and the intensity of acidosis in the CSF (1).

Patients with chronic pulmonary insufficiency may develop delirium as well as neurological symptoms and signs which may include flapping tremor (asterixis), headache, multifocal myoclonus, papilledema, twitching of the extremities, and convulsions (1, 106, 107). The patient tends to be forgetful, inattentive, drowsy, and irritable. Falling asleep at work or during conversation may attract attention to the patient (106). The presenting picture may be that of episodic delirium or stupor (105, 106). Delirium develops as a result of acute exacerbation of respiratory failure in patients suffering from chronic pulmonary obstructive disease. Such development is most often precipitated by respiratory infection or excessive sedation. In addition, extrapulmonary conditions, such as congestive heart failure, hypotension, or electrolyte abnormalities, may contribute to or be responsible for the development of delirium in these patients (107). The highest incidence of delirium seems to occur in patients showing PCO_2 levels above 75 mm. Hg. (107). Yet no consistent correlation between the degree of mental abnormality and the degree of deviation from normal of concentration of any examined chemical in the blood could be found in one series (107). The patients usually show both hypoxia and hypercapnia. The latter may be absent, but if present may give rise to CO_2 narcosis, which features delirium as well as drowsiness, headache, hypertension, tachycardia, sweating, and asterixis (104). Coma and death may follow. Hallucinations, delusions, and "mania" have been observed in 14 percent of fifty patients suffering from acute pulmonary decompensation (107).

The EEG in patients with pulmonary insufficiency encephalopathy shows slowing of the background activity, appearance of theta and delta waves, and increased voltage (106). Night sleep in this disorder is similar to that in renal and hepatic insufficiency, featuring reduced slow-wave sleep and prolonged awakenings (110).

Patients with chronic obstructive pulmonary disease and both hypoxemia and hypercapnia may develop delirium, stupor, or coma after administration of oxygen. The latter removes the stimulus of hypoxia needed to maintain respiration in the presence of hypercapnia. As a result, the latter increases and consciousness becomes more reduced (1). Oxygen should be administered in low doses (1, 104). Continuous oxygen therapy has resulted in improved cognitive functioning in patients with chronic obstructive pulmonary disease (108).

Management of delirium in patients with respiratory failure involves, first of all, treatment of the underlying hypoxemia, hypercapnia, electrolyte imbalance, etc. Sedation should be avoided as far as possible so as not to compromise the respiration further. Benzoctamine has recently been recommended as a safe sedative for patients with respiratory failure (111). The author has used haloperidol without any complications.

Delirium has recently been reported in a patient with obstruction of the airway after irradiation of carcinoma of the nasopharynx (112). The patient developed paroxysmal hypersomnia with periodic respiration and brief episodes of delirium with visual and auditory hallucinations between sleep and waking. He showed PCO_2 of 50 mm. Hg. and normal oxygen saturation.

PANCREATIC ENCEPHALOPATHY

Delirium may complicate pancreatic disease, especially acute pancreatitis (113-118). Benos (115) claims that at least 168 cases of such delirium have been reported in the medical literature. The incidence of delirium in pancreatic disease is variously given as ranging from 4 to 53 percent (114). Delirium comes on forty-eight to seventy-two hours after onset of acute pancreatitis and lasts several days (113). It is often mistakenly regarded as delirium tremens and shows marked similarity to the latter (115, 117). Schuster and Iber (117) studied thirty patients with pancreatitis and compared them with thirty alcoholic patients admitted with the diagnosis of pneumonia. An "impressive alcoholic background" was judged to be present in all but two of the patients with pancreatitis. Sixteen (53%) of the latter suffered "acute hallucinatory psychosis" during an attack of pancreatitis. Hallucinations were visual, auditory, or both. In the comparison group of alcoholics with pneumonia 13 percent developed delirium. The authors conclude that pancreatitis is more likely to induce delirium in alcoholic patients than pneumonia. Alcohol withdrawal did not seem to be the cause of the observed delirium.

The term "pancreatic encephalopathy" has been given to delirium and various neurological symptoms arising in the course of acute pancreatitis (116). Various putative causes have been postulated, among them cerebral and pulmonary fat embolism, hypoxia, hyperglycemic-hyperosmolality syndrome, disseminated intravascular coagulation, toxic effects of the enzymes on the brain, and hypoglycemia (114, 116, 118). Diagnosis is based on the evidence of acute pancreatitis, delirium, multifocal neurological signs, and diffuse slowing of the EEG. The pathological picture is mostly that of widespread demyelinization and diffuse petechial hemorrhages in the brain (118). Treatment with anti-enzymes is said to improve prognosis (118).

VITAMIN DEFICIENCY

Deficiency of several vitamins can result in delirium. Conditions most often associated with vitamin deficiencies in the United States include old age; depression; dementia; alcoholism; iatrogenic deficiency occurring in renal hemodialysis, or drug-induced, or due to intravenous hyperalimentation; and gastrointestinal disease. Delirium due to vitamin deficiencies in the elderly is not uncommon even in the affluent countries (119). Persons aged sixty years or over are particularly vulnerable to such deficiencies as a result of chronic debilitating illness, poor appetite, depression, dementia, and poverty. A number of surveys have documented inadequate nutrition and subnormal blood levels of various vitamins in older persons in the United States (120). Deficiencies of thiamine, niacin, cyanocobalamine (vitamin B12), and folic acid are reasonably well established as potential causes of delirium. The status of vitamin C, riboflavin, and pyridoxine deficiencies is unclear in this respect.

Thiamine deficiency. Malnutrition of any cause may result in thiamine deficiency. It is most often encountered in association with chronic alcoholism but by no means confined to the alcoholic population. Severe thiamine deficiency has been reported with gastrointestinal disease and hyperemesis gravidarum, in patients on renal hemodialysis, in starvation, and in those treated with intravenous fluids or hyperalimentation (121-128). Wernicke's encephalopathy is a syndrome caused by thiamine deficiency. It features delirium, ophthalmoplegia, nystagmus, ataxia, and a severe memory deficit with or without confabulation. In one large study, 56 percent of patients displayed a "global confusional state" (delirium in our terminology) on admission (128). This delirium is typically quiet or hypoactive and features apathy, inattention, severe disorientation, and marked memory impairment. Hallucinations are not common unless delirium tremens coexists. The delirium persists for up to two months after institution of treatment; the symptoms usually begin to subside within several days (128). As the delirium clears up, the impairment of memory—an amnestic syndrome—emerges more clearly (128). Prompt treatment is essential to minimize permanent memory deficits. Thiamine is administered parenterally.

Nicotinic acid (niacin) deficiency. This deficiency is manifested by pellagra and the nicotinic acid deficiency encephalopathy, which features delirium, cog-wheel rigidity, and grasping and sucking reflexes (129, 130, 131). Delirium may occur in the absence of physical signs of pellagra (129). Gregory (129) states that three psychiatric disorders occur in pellagra: depression, delirium, and dementia. Endemic pellagra was eliminated in the United States over thirty years ago, but sporadic cases of it still occur, most often in association with alcoholism (131). "Dementia" was reported in 50 percent of a recent small series of patients (131). It is not clear what type of mental disorder these patients suffered from, but about half of them had disorientation and memory impairment. Dermatitis is commonly present in pellagra; neuropathy, glossitis, and diarrhea less consistently so. Confirmation of the diagnosis of pellagra involves either a therapeutic trial with niacin or determination of urinary excretion of 2-pyridone (131). Plasma tryptophan values are reduced.

Vitamin B12 deficiency. This vitamin deficiency is well known to lead to organic mental disorders. The precise nature of the latter is not clear since some writers refer to delirium while others speak of dementia or psychosis in this context (132-135). Eilenberg (132) studied seventeen patients wtih pernicious anemia and diagnosed "organic states" in seven of them: one acute confusional state, five dementias, and one alcoholic hallucinosis. One of Eilenberg's patients had presented with acute confusional state (presumably delirium). Holmes (134) states that mental symptoms in vitamin B12 deficiency are varied and may include disorders of mood, mainly depression; memory defects; confusion; paranoid delusions; auditory and visual hallucinations; incontinence of urine and feces; and violent maniacal behavior. In his own series of fourteen patients Holmes found "confusion and memory defect" in all of them. Four of the patients had developed psychological symptoms before the onset of anemia or neurological signs. This observation has been confirmed by others (136). Psychiatric manifestations of vitamin B12 deficiency may precede any abnormality of the peripheral blood and marrow, and any signs of subacute combined degeneration of the cord (136). Samson et al. (135) studied fourteen patients with pernicious anemia and found delirium in thirteen. Diagnostic criteria for the latter included disturbance in level of awareness and shift towards slower frequency ranges in the EEG. Eleven of the thirteen patients had abnormally slow records. Ten of the thirteen patients cleared completely in response to treatment with vitamin B12. Semantic problems account for the uncertainty regarding the nature of psychiatric manifestations of vitamin B12 deficiency. It appears that the majority of the patients exhibiting mental symptoms due to such deficiency suffer from a reversible dementia, i.e. a protracted impairment of intellectual functions and alertness of insidious onset. Subacute delirium would be another suitable term for these abnormalities. An occasional patient with vitamin B12 deficiency presents with typical acute delirium. If the organic mental disorder is not treated properly, i.e. with adequate doses of vitamin B12, an irreversible dementia of some degree of severity is liable to develop (134, 135).

The EEG in patients with vitamin B12 deficiency and organic mental disorders shows diffuse slowing of the background activity (132, 135). This abnormality correlates with the clinical findings. Improvement in both the EEG and mental state follows administration of vitamin B12 and occurs at about the same time as the maximum reticulocyte response (135). Cerebral blood flow is increased and cerebral metabolic rate decreased in patients with pernicious anemia (135).

Vitamin B12 deficiency occurs most often in pernicious anemia; other causes include gastrectomy, intestinal malabsorption, nutritional deficiency, and administration of drugs, especially anticonvulsants (137, 138). It is important to consider vitamin B12 deficiency in the differential diagnosis of every patient presenting with unexplained delirium, dementia, or both.

Folic acid deficiency. It has been claimed that folic acid deficiency causes reversible dementia (137, 139-142), but this effect is still open to question (140). Insufficient intake, malabsorption, and metabolic defect due to certain drugs, such as methotrexate, or to vitamin B12 deficiency are the usual types of folate deficiency encountered clinically (140). Several cases of reversible dementia believed to be due to folate deficiency have been reported (141, 142). It is not clear if the latter ever gives rise to delirium.

HYPERVITAMINOSIS

Excessive intake of vitamin A occasionally results in an organic mental disorder (143, 144). Acute vitamin A intoxication may feature delirium with increased alertness and hypersensitivity to auditory stimuli. The patients had taken high doses, at least 150,000 units daily, of vitamin A for prolonged periods.

DISORDERS OF FLUID AND ELECTROLYTE METABOLISM

Brain function may be affected by disturbance of the electrolyte concentration of two major sources: first, there may be a disorder of blood or whole-body electrolytes affecting the brain secondarily; and second, a disorder of the brain may result in disturbance of the salt and water balance which in turn affects cerebral function. The blood-brain barrier is freely permeable to water and thus changes in the osmolality of the blood plasma are readily transmitted to the CSF and the extracellular fluid of the brain. Penetration of inorganic cations and anions from blood into brain is, on the contrary, slow. Disturbances of the concentrations of potassium, calcium, and magnesium in the blood do not have a marked effect on the function of the CNS thanks to the mechanisms which tend to keep ionic composition of the CSF and the extracellular fluid of the brain stable (145). On the contrary, the brain is highly vulnerable to variations in plasma osmolality. An increase in the latter will cause shrinkage of the brain cells, while a decrease leads to their swelling. Delirium is the main psychiatric manifestation of acute electrolyte and fluid disorders (146, 147). Many clinical conditions bring about delirium, because they give rise to these disorders. Burns, major surgery, renal failure, and infections are important examples of conditions that are often associated with delirium and mediated in part by fluid and electrolyte imbalance. Deficiency and excess of fluid and of the more important ions and cations will now be discussed from the point of view of their capacity to cause delirium.

Hypernatremia. Hypernatremia is usually associated with a high osmolality of body fluids, and its manifestations reflect hyperosmolality. Its common causes include vomiting, diarrhea, excessive administration of salt, increased loss of water due to fever or hyperventilation, treatment with salt-retaining steroids, hypothalamic lesions and diabetes insipidus, and severe burns (146, 148). There is thus deficient water intake, or water is lost in excess of salt, or salt is retained in excess of water. Thirst normally protects a conscious adult from insidious development of hypernatremia and dehydration. When thirst is suppressed by hypothalamic damage due to a tumor, such as craniopharyngioma, pinealoma, glioma, or metastasis, or to sarcoidosis, for example, the patient is liable to become severely dehydrated and hypernatremic.

The development of hypernatremia may be rapid or insidious, and this influences its effects on mental function. Gradual onset may allow awareness to remain undisturbed despite serum sodium level of 170 or more mEq. per liter. Depression of sensorium ranging from lethargy to coma may occur. The EEG shows slowing of the background activity but may be normal (149). The earliest manifestations of hypernatremic encephalopathy are usually drowsiness, delirium, and seizures. Coma may occur but is less common than delirium. Hyperreflexia, tremor, and muscular weakness and rigidity are the usual neurological findings (148). Permanent brain damage may result, especially in children.

Hyponatremia. Dilution and/or depletion of body sodium stores results in hyponatremia. The syndrome of water intoxication, resulting from dilutional hyponatremia, may be due to compulsive water drinking or psychogenic polydipsia in an occasional schizophrenic, alcoholic, or neurotic patient (150-159). Dilutional hyponatremia caused by water retention usually results from failure of the kidneys to excrete a water load and produce a dilute urine. Interference by tumor or infection with the control of secretion of the antidiuretic hormone (A.D.H.) or abnormal secretion of that hormone by bronchogenic carcinoma, for example, may result in the syndrome of inappropriate secretion of A.D.H. (160). Hyponatremia results from such secretion. The syndrome has been reportedly triggered by drugs such as haloperidol, thioridazine, and amitriptyline (161). Delirium is a common manifestation of the syndrome (162, 163). Demeclocycline and lithium may be used to correct the hyponatremia (160). Other causes of the latter include administration of diuretics, adrenal insufficiency, hemodialysis, and loss of salt-containing body fluids followed by attempts at their replacement with water. Various drugs may induce dilutional hyponatremia (164).

Mental symptoms are related to the level of serum sodium, the rapidity of its fall, and the etiology. Insidious development of hyponatremia may be tolerated until serum sodium falls to about 100 mEq. per liter. Delirium develops in subjects deprived of sodium and having serum sodium levels of below 115 m. moles per liter (149). Delirium due to acute water intoxication usually is not observed until sodium has fallen below 125 m. moles per liter (149). In addition to delirium, patients may suffer from dizziness, lethargy, drowsiness, headache, restlessness, weakness, muscular twitches and tremors, cramps, ataxia, and seizures. Coma, irreversible brain damage, and death may follow. Patients treated with diuretics and tricyclic antidepressants for concomitant depression and hypertension are liable to develop delirium as a result of combined sodium loss and excessive water intake due to dry mouth and thirst (165). Low sodium syndrome with delirium is a known clinical association (166). Treatment depends on the etiology of hyponatremia (160).

Hyperkalemia. Delirium may be caused indirectly by hyperkalemia as a result of cardiac arrhythmias induced by elevated serum potassium levels. Severe hyperkalemia affects neuromuscular excitability and may cause paralysis, paresthesias, dysphonia, and irritability.

Hypokalemia. Delirium may be caused by hypokalemia, but this development is uncommon. Profound hypokalemia may occur in familial periodic paralysis without any mental symptoms (167). Hypokalemia may result from vomiting, diarrhea, diuretics, diabetic acidosis, renal tubular acidosis, aldosteronism, Cushing's syndrome, laxative addiction, excessive ingestion of licorice, etc. (167). The common symptoms include muscular weakness, muscle cramps and pains, lethargy, apathy, drowsiness, and irritability. Delirium may occur, as may coma. The EEG is rarely abnormal with potassium depletion.

Hypercalcemia. Delirium may be caused by hypercalcemia, and it may be the chief presenting complaint of the hypercalcemic patient (168). Other neuropsychiatric symptoms include lassitude, drowsiness, anxiety, depression, incontinence, muscle weakness, stupor, and coma. The more common causes include hyperparathyroidism, nephrolithiasis, neoplastic disease (carcinoma of the breast, lung, and kidney, multiple myeloma, lymphomas), hypervitaminosis D, sarcoidosis, milk-alkali syndrome, hyperthyroidism, hypothyroidism, adrenal insufficiency, and immobilization (169, 170, 171). Hypercalcemia may be acute, subacute, or chronic, and presents a life-threatening emergency (169, 171). It is, therefore, important to keep in mind that delirium may be a major manifestation of acute or subacute hypercalcemia.

Neuropsychiatric symptoms may develop when calcium levels are only 12 mg. per 100 ml., yet they may be lacking with levels as high as 16 mg. per 100 ml. Anorexia, nausea, vomiting, headache, and difficulty walking are among common early symptoms. There is nothing characteristic about the delirium. The EEG shows diffuse slowing of background activity interrupted by high-voltage bursts of delta waves (172). These abnormalities subside within two months of instituting therapy. Hypercalcemia as such is claimed not to cause EEG changes unless additional complicating factors are present and the blood-brain barrier to calcium is altered (173).

Treatment of acute hypercalcemia involves administration of mithramycin, calcitonin, furosemide, adequate hydration, indomethacin, etc. (169, 171).

Hypocalcemia. Delirium, seizures, irritability, fatigue, weakness, and depression may be caused by hypocalcemia. It usually results from hypoparathyroidism, acute and chronic renal insufficiency, vitamin D deficiency, osteoblastic metastases, calcitonin secreting tumors, acute pancreatitis, pseudohypoparathyroidism, and renal tubular acidosis.

Some patients develop symptoms when serum calcium levels fall rapidly below 8.5 mg. per 100 ml.; others, with chronic hypocalcemia, may remain free of symptoms with calcium levels as low as 5 to 6 mg. per 100 ml. Delirium is liable to come on when hypocalcemia develops acutely. Muscle cramps, paresthesias, tetany, seizures, choreiform movements, etc. may precede or accompany delirium. The EEG shows progressive slowing of background activity with falling calcium levels, low voltage fast activity, and sharp waves and spikes. The latter tend to appear only when calcium values are under 6.5 mg. per 100 ml. They are an expression of neuronal excitability and convulsive potential (174).

Emergency treatment of hypocalcemia involves slow intravenous injection of 10 to 20 ml. of calcium gluconate. Patients are particularly vulnerable to dystonic reactions to phenothiazines (148).

Hypermagnesemia. Hypermagnesemia occurs infrequently. Its most common causes are renal failure and treatment with magnesium salts. The symptoms include narcosis (175). It is not clear if delirium occurs.

Hypomagnesemia. Delirium as well as weakness, tremors, muscle fasciculations, irritability, tetany, and convulsions may be caused by hypomagnesemia (175-177). Hypomagnesemia may be a result of starvation, malabsorption syndrome, severe diarrhea, diuretics, primary aldosteronism, nonketotic diabetes, hyperparathyroidism, hypoparathyroidism, cancer, delirium tremens, etc. (175).

Hypomagnesemia usually occurs in association with other electrolyte abnormalities, such as hypocalcemia and hypokalemia, and so it is difficult to tease apart its specific clinical effects (148). Levels of about 1 mEq. per liter may lead at times to delirium and seizures, while levels as low as 0.3 mEq. per liter may produce no symptoms. Treatment consists of giving magnesium sulphate parenterally.

Nonketotic hyperglycemia. Serum hyperosmolality leading to a metabolic encephalopathy is produced by nonketotic hyperglycemia. It commonly occurs in elderly diabetics and features blood glucose levels of over 600 mg. per 100 ml. and plasma osmolality of at least 350 mOsm./Kg. without ketoacidosis (178). Depression of sensorium in this condition correlates highly with the plasma osmolality (178). Clinical manifestations of nonketotic hyperglycemia may include reduction or loss of consciousness, visual hallucinations, seizures, focal neurological signs, vestibular dysfunction, etc. (179). The EEG shows slowing of the background activity, disappearance of the alpha rhythm, and paroxysmal focal spike and wave discharges (179).

The patient with ketotic hyperglycemia shows gradual reduction in the level of awareness, progressing from lethargy to stupor and coma. It appears that delirium, with or without hallucinations, may precede stupor (179). Hyperosmolality, which seems to be responsible for the mental abnormalities, results from a combination of dehydration, loss of electrolytes, and hyperglycemia. Treatment consists of administering insulin and hypotonic sodium chloride infusion.

SYSTEMIC ACID-BASE DISORDERS

Acidosis. Deviation of the arterial pH below 7.40 is implied by acidosis. There may be a primary respiratory acidosis with increased PCO_2 or primary metabolic acidosis with a compensatory hyperventilation and decreased PCO_2. A patient with metabolic alkalosis may hyperventilate and have compensatory respiratory acidosis with increased PCO_2 (normal value 40 mm.

Hg.). Respiratory acidosis may be acute or chronic. It was discussed under the heading of respiratory failure.

Metabolic acidosis occurs in diabetic ketoacidosis; renal failure; lactic acidosis; methanol, ammonium chloride, and salicylate intoxication; diarrhea; renal tubular acidosis; etc. (104). In pure metabolic acidosis patients initially tend to have a normal pH in the CSF and be alert despite marked reduction of the serum pH. Posner and Plum (180) state that systemic acidosis as such does not lead to encephalopathy unless CSF acidosis supervenes. Delirium and coma are manifestations of the latter. They develop more readily in patients with respiratory failure, probably as a result of CSF acidosis. A patient with diabetic ketoacidosis may display delirium during the progression to and after recovery from coma (181).

Alkalosis. In contrast to acidosis, alkalosis is associated with delirium rather than coma (1). Respiratory alkalosis occurs when CO_2 removal by the lungs exceeds its production in the body with resulting hypocapnia. It is due to hyperventilation, mechanical overventilation, pneumonia, hepatic failure, etc.

Metabolic alkalosis is defined by a blood pH above that predicted for the prevailing PCO_2. It may result from loss of acid through vomiting, chloride depletion, or following hypercapnia; excessive intake of alkalis; excessive secretion of mineralocorticoids; etc.

Alkalosis gives rise to a mild encephalopathy (1). In acute respiratory alkalosis there is constriction of cerebral arterioles and consequent reduction of cerebral blood flow. Mild confusion and EEG slowing follow. These changes occur more readily in the younger subjects probably due to greater cerebral vascular reactivity in those under thirty-five years of age. Excessive hyperventilation results in a reduction of cerebral cellular oxygenation. Voluntary hyperventilation for about three minutes induces symptoms such as lightheadedness, faintness, feelings of unreality, blurring of vision, paresthesias, and sometimes loss of consciousness (182). Occasionally hallucinations may occur (183). The EEG shows generalized slowing. These effects amount to a mild delirium. Severe metabolic alkalosis may also give rise to delirium (1).

ERRORS OF METABOLISM

Several errors of metabolism may give rise to neuropsychiatric syndromes. Hepatolenticular degeneration (Wilson's disease), porphyria, and carcinoid syndrome are the most important members of this group of conditions.

Wilson's disease. This disease may present with a psychiatric disorder and thus give rise to diagnostic error (184). Delirium is not usually considered a complication of Wilson's disease unless hepatic disease and related encephalopathy develop. This writer has seen a patient with unrecognized Wilson's disease and associated hepatic disease, who developed agitated delirium as a manifestation of the latter. An internist diagnosed the acute behavior disorder as "hysteria" and administered chlorpromazine, 25 mg. intravenously. The patient slipped into coma and had to be hospitalized for it. When she came to some twelve hours later, the author was called in consultation and was asked to transfer the patient to psychiatry for treatment of her "hysterical stupor." Having noticed yellow sclerae and flapping tremor as well as signs of delirium, the writer suggested that hepatic encephalopathy was the cause of the patient's mental disorder. History of a chronic tremor of the hands emerged in the meantime and pointed to Wilson's disease as the underlying condition.

Porphyria. In its acute intermittent form, porphyria is notorious for the frequency and diversity of its neuropsychiatric manifestations. Delirium is the most common mental disorder complicating acute porphyria. Its frequency in three of the largest published series of patients ranged from 18 to 52 percent (185). Roth (186) quotes several investigators who have found that the most common psychiatric disturbance in porphyria is delirium. The latter may vary in severity from mild to severe and, on occasion, progress to coma. The typical course of an acute attack involves exposure to an inciting agent or event, such as barbiturates, sulfonamides, alcohol excess, menstruation, or infection, which is followed by severe abdominal pain, pains and paresthesias in the extremities, delirium, nausea, vomiting and constipation (187). Some patients develop seizures, flaccid quadriparesis, respiratory paralysis, vesical symptoms, hypertension, tachycardia, sensory loss, transient blindness, diplopia, fever, etc. (185, 187, 188). During the attack dark urine is passed by about 75 percent of patients (187). Some authors have stressed the high frequency of hysterical personality traits in porphyrics; they have claimed that these traits are responsible for some of the clinical features of an acute attack and that they become overshadowed by the symptoms of an organic brain syndrome (186). Central nervous system involvement has been reported in 40 to 80 percent of patients. The EEG shows diffuse slowing in about 80 percent of cases (187). Some patients display schizophrenia-like features during an acute attack of porphyria, and these symptoms may lead to an erroneous diagnosis of a functional psychosis (185, 188).

Pathogenesis of acute intermittent porphyria is still obscure. Two major pathogenic mechanisms have been postulated: a deficit of heme-synthesis in the nervous system and neurotoxic effect from the excessive production of porphobilinogen and/or delta-aminolevulinic acid, respectively. Decreased activity of uroporphyrinogen-I-synthetase has been demonstrated in various tissues and been postulated to occur in the neurons (188). The resulting decreased hemesynthesis could prevent the neurons from obtaining sufficient quantity of essential heme-containing proteins. The neurotoxic hypothesis has been challenged on various grounds, including the observation that there is no correlation between the severity of the acute attack and the amounts of delta-aminolevulinic acid and porphobilinogen excreted in the urine. Neither compound is harmful when given to normal humans. More recent work, however, indicates that either or both of these substances might be responsible for the neuropsychiatric symptoms of porphyria, by virtue of modifying synaptic transmission in the central nervous system (188). If the neurotoxic hypothesis is correct, then suppression of the enzyme, delta-aminolevulinic acid synthetase, necessary for the synthesis of the acid should have beneficial therapeutic effect, since the production of the acid and porphobilinogen would be blocked. Hematin suppresses the enzyme and has been shown to be of value (188). Propranolol is also beneficial in acute porphyria, and this effect is explained in part by the drug's putative repression of the delta-aminolevulinic acid synthetase induction (188).

The carcinoid syndrome. This syndrome is of considerable

interest for the student of delirium because of its association with disorders of indole metabolism. Major et al. (189) found "episodes of confusion" in 35 percent of twenty-two patients with carcinoid tumor. The confusional episodes (presumably delirium) were said to overlap with depressive and anxiety syndromes. The investigators hypothesized that decreased levels of serotonin in the brain were responsible for confusion and depression in the patients. Lehmann (190) quotes other observers who found that "confusion" was the most common mental abnormality in patients with carcinoid syndrome and occurred in about 25 percent of the cases. He reports on his own patient who displayed florid delirium followed by catatonic stupor. Administration of L-tryptophan seemed to have a beneficial effect on the delirium. Slowing of the EEG accompanies the delirium (190). Main clinical features of the carcinoid syndrome include attacks of erythematous flushing of the head and neck, tachycardia, bronchospasm, diarrhea, cardiac valvular lesions, and hypotension. The attacks of flushing may be provoked by eating, alcohol, or excitement. The syndrome is usually due to carcinoid tumors, especially in the ileum, but on occasion hyperserotonemia may be found without a neoplasm (191). Serotonin does not penetrate the blood-brain barrier and thus a functional deficiency of brain serotonin may exist despite high blood levels. Production of serotonin by a carcinoid tumor accounts for about 60 percent of dietary tryptophan and insufficient quantity of the latter is available for serotonin synthesis in the brain. Lehmann (192) claims that mental symptoms occur in several conditions, such as carcinoidosis, pellagra, and some drug-induced diseases (p-chlorophenylalanine, levodopa, and alphamethyldopa), which are all characterized by tryptophan and serotonin deficiency.

Delirium has been reported in patients with some of the above conditions. A patient with hyperserotonemia, without coresponding 5-hydroxyindoluria, suffered from episodes of flushing, paroxysmal hypertension and loss of consciousness, followed by delirium and amnesia for the episode (191). Patients with carcinoidosis who were treated with p-chlorophenylalanine (PCPA) developed delirium in a proportion of cases (193, 194).

Gruner (194) has reviewed the literature on this subject and reported on a patient of his own. The latter developed delirium on 1 g. of PCPA daily. The syndrome came on suddenly at night, with marked psychomotor hyperactivity, aggressive behavior, and paranoid delusions. The patient had striking hypersensitivity to auditory stimuli, tactile and visual hallucinations, severe insomnia, and illusions. The delirium lasted two weeks. The author draws attention to the schizophrenialike features of this patient's delirium. The EEG at the height of the latter showed marked slowing of the background activity. PCPA given to normal subjects has not been reported to cause delirium. Not all carcinoid patients treated with the drug become delirious. It appears quite unlikely that serotonin deficiency alone gives rise to delirium, but it is more probable that this condition has to be combined with other metabolic factors or neurotransmitter changes in order to bring about cerebral decompensation.

ENDOCRINE DISORDERS

Several of these disorders have already been discussed in relation to the abnormalities of glucose and electrolyte metabolism. These and other endocrinopathies are dealt with here only insofar as they give rise to delirium. Several recent reviews of psychiatric disturbances complicating endocrine disease contain some relevant information (195, 196, 197). In many instances it has been necessary to read the original case reports to reach an opinion as to what type of psychiatric syndrome the patient actually displayed.

Beaumont (195) quotes Manfred Bleuler, who stated that mental disorders associated with endocrine dysfunction can be classified into acute organic brain syndrome, the chronic organic or amnestic syndrome, and the endocrine psychosyndrome. The latter does not feature abnormalities of cognitive organization and performance but rather those of mood, drives, and personality. Our focus here is on the acute organic brain syndrome or delirium.

Panhypopituitarism. Commonly associated with psychiatric disorders, especially with Bleuler's endocrine psychosyndrome, is panhypopituitarism. Delirium occurs not infrequently (195). Smith et al. (196) quote Escamilla and Lisser, who reported on 100 verified cases of hypopituitarism and found that 64 percent of them had presented with psychiatric symptoms. The incidence of delirium in this disorder is unknown. Court and Diaz (198) state that patients with disturbances of consciousness, ranging in severity from mild confusion to coma, can be observed in patients with Sheehan's syndrome. Hypoglycemia, electrolyte imbalance, hypothermia, and hypotension may be responsible for the delirium and coma. It appears that delirium may precede or follow coma, or be the only disorder of awareness in patients with hypopituitarism (199, 200). One notes that the organic mental disorders associated with this endocrinopathy are reported to have rather slow onset and last at times as long as two years (200). It is possible that these disorders represent dementia rather than delirium, or a combination of both these syndromes.

Hypothyroidism. There is a large number of clinical reports on the mental disorders associated with hypothyroidism. Beaumont (195) asserts that mental symptoms are "almost always present" in hypothyroidism and are often among the presenting features. Browning et al. (201) assert that the psychosis of myxedema is delirium, presumably due to a disturbance of cerebral metabolism as suggested by the concomitant slowing and lowering of the voltage of the EEG background activity. One notes, however, that in five of the seven patients studied by Browning et al. the "sensorial impairment" could only be detected by formal testing and seemed to be quite stable and prolonged. Thus, the term dementia appears to be more appropriate than delirium to diagnose these patients. A review of the literature leads one to the following conclusions:

Memory impairment, mental slowness, some degree of intellectual deterioration, and irritability are very common manifestations of hypothyroidism. They are of slow onset and usually long duration and thus comprise dementia of some degree of severity and varying extent of reversibility by thyroid therapy (197, 201-203). It is claimed that hypothyroid patients with a mental illness of more than two years' duration are not likely to recover fully (203). Those who show disturbance of consciousness tend to have better prognosis (203). Psychoses, mostly paranoid and/or depressive, without concurrent signs of significant cognitive impairment, but often with visual or auditory hallucinations, may occur but seem to be uncommon. Easson (204) was able to find only nineteen such patients among admissions to the Mayo Clinic between 1947 and 1958. He postulates that psychosis in these patients is related to the stress occasioned by internal and external bodily changes. Easson quotes Kraepelin as stating that, in myxedematous patients, "In rare cases there may appear conditions of confusion with hallucinations and delusions." An extensive review of the literature supports this contention. Delirium is distinctly uncommon in hypothyroidism and is most likely to occur in thyroidectomized patients and in those who have undergone rapid change in thyroid status as a result of medication (205-208). Royce (209) in his review of severe impairment of consciousness in myxedema notes that about 100 such cases were reported between 1953 and 1963. He points out that hypoxia, hypercarbia, hyponatremia, and hypopituitarism are the main factors directly responsible for the depression of consciousness in patients with myxedema. Hypothermia may be another causative factor. Drugs, such as barbiturates and phenothiazines, may also depress consciousness in these patients. It is conceivable that the same factors might precipitate delirium in the hypothyroid patient.

The EEG in hypothyroidism is abnormal in most patients and usually consists of mild slowing of alpha rhythm and poor or absent response to eye opening and closure (210). About 25 percent of patients have low voltage, diffusely slowed records. These changes improve in parallel with clinical improvement. In addition, a decrease in stages 3 and 4 of sleep have been found in hypothyroidism (210). Cerebral blood flow and metabolic rate are reduced. All these factors may contribute to the delirium occasionally seen in this disorder.

Hyperthyroidism. Hyperthyroidism rarely gives rise to delirium nowadays. Its incidence is of the order of 3 to 4 percent (211). The frequency of delirium was apparently higher in the past when thyroid crisis was a relatively common occurrence (212). Occasionally, a patient may present with apathy or lethargy and delirium (213). Such presentation occurs most often in the elderly and in patients with absent palpable goiter and marked cardiovascular symptoms. These apathetic patients may progress through delirium to stupor and coma. The much more common clinical picture of thyrotoxicosis features hyperactivity, nervousness, anxiety, and tremor.

The EEG is often abnormal. Patients with more severe hyperthyroidism tend to show slow background activity. In one study, 41 percent of patients had activity below 7 cycles per second (214). A considerable proportion of patients show slow activity following antithyroid therapy; some display an increase in paroxysmal and fast activity. Cerebral blood flow and oxygen uptake are usually increased (1).

Hypoparathyroidism. Hypoparathyroidism may lead to delirium, dementia, and seizures. Delirium is the most common form of psychosis in hypoparathyroidism, one not necessarily associated with tetany and convulsions but improving with return to normal of calcium levels (215). Greene and Swanson (216) found five cases of delirium in a series of eighteen patients. Anxiety, depression, and a sense of impending catastrophe were common. Delirium tends to arise within three to four months following the onset of hypoparathyroidism. The latter may represent a complication of thyroidectomy (217). Delirium in hypocalcemia is discussed in the section on the latter. Patients operated for parathyroid adenoma may develop acute anxiety, followed by delirium, ten to fourteen days after operation (218).

Hyperparathyroidism. This disease may present with psychiatric symptoms (219). Delirium appears to be uncommon nowadays since the disease is diagnosed earlier and at less severe stages. In a recent series of sixteen patients only one displayed delirium (220). "Mental disturbances" are reported in about 20 to 30 percent of patients with primary hyperparathyroidism but they usually consist of such symptoms as decreased recent memory, mild depression, irritability, drowsiness, lethargy, and fatigue (220). Delirium is usual with plasma calcium levels above 16 mg. per 100 ml. but may occur with lower concentrations (221). It tends to occur abruptly and may lead to prompt surgery (196). Stupor and coma may follow delirium (222). The latter may also occur shortly after removal of a parathyroid adenoma.

Hypercalcemia and magnesium deficiency have been blamed for mental symptoms in hyperparathyroidism (221). Both are discussed in earlier sections.

Hypoadrenalism (Addison's disease). In about 65 percent of the cases this disease is associated with mental abnormalities (196). The reported disturbances have included irritability, depression, apathy, paranoid psychosis, and delirium. The incidence of the latter is unknown (223). It is probably most likely to come on prior to impending adrenal crisis. Some writers assert that "a large percentage" of untreated and inadequately treated patients with Addison's disease are mildly delirious (1). The pathogenesis of delirium in this disease probably involves factors such as hypoglycemia, hyponatremia, and, perhaps, hyperkalemia.

Hyperadrenalism (Cushing's disease). This disease is accompanied by mental abnormalities in about 25 percent of cases (196). Of course, terms like "mental abnormalities" have no precise meaning and convey minimum useful information, but they are widely used in the generally inadequate descriptive literature on the psychopathology of endocrine disorders. Regestein et al. (224) found four patients with delirium among seven with Cushing's syndrome. Other writers have reported single cases of delirium in this context (225, 226). Paranoid and depressive features may figure prominently in delirious patients with Cushing's syndrome and result in erroneous diagnosis of a functional pychosis. On the other hand, depressive and/or paranoid psychoses, lacking cognitive impairment, may also occur. Delirium due to exogenous steroids is discussed in Chapter 10. The EEG in Cushing's syndrome is usually either normal or consists of mild slowing of background activity, excessive fast activity, and minor paroxysmal changes (227).

REMOTE EFFECTS OF NEOPLASM

Delirium may be one of the manifestations of the remote effects of a malignant and, less often, benign neoplasm on the brain. "Remote" in this context implies that the encephalopathy occurs in the absence of involvement of the cranial contents by

the tumor. The whole subject of organic mental disorders complicating neoplasm and its treatment has been neglected by
researchers (228). Data on their incidence are also nonexistent.
Davies et al. (229) reported intellectual impairment in 28
percent of terminal cancer patients. Holland and Glass (230)
found delirium in fifteen of nineteen patients hospitalized for
preterminal stages of advanced cancer. Levine et al. (228) diagnosed an organic brain syndrome in 40 of 100 consecutive
patients with cancer referred for psychiatric consultation.

Delirium may arise in a cancer patient as a result of many
possible mechanisms: metastases to the brain; infiltration of the
meninges, the brain, or both; infection; destruction of organs
such as liver or kidney; metabolic effects on brain function;
limbic encephalitis; malnutrition; and complications of therapy.
Cerebral metastases comprise about 20 percent of brain neoplasms.
The latter give rise to delirium, dementia, or both in about
70 percent of cases (231). The faster the tumor grows and the
earlier it gives rise to increased intracranial pressure, the more
likely is delirium to become manifest. Nonmetastatic encephalopathies seem to be at least as common a cause of delirium as
cerebral metastases. For example, carcinoma of the lung is said
to metastasize to brain in about 37 percent of patients. Schmid-
Wermser et al. (232) investigated the records of 142 patients
who had died of bronchogenic carcinoma. Brain metastases had
been diagnosed clinically in 44 percent of the cases but histo-
logically proven in only 20 percent. Delirium ("disturbances of
consciousness") was present in about 80 percent of all patients
suspected of having brain metastases and was almost equally
distributed among those who proved to have a brain tumor
and those who did not. It follows that at least as many patients
without cerebral metastases displayed delirium. The most
important causes of the latter included cardiovascular insufficiency, respiratory failure, and hypercalcemia.

There are basically four groups of remote effects of neoplasm
on the brain, most of which can, theoretically at least, give rise
to delirium (233-237).

    A. Viral and/or degenerative disorders
        1. Multifocal leukoencephalopathy
        2. Diffuse polioencephalopathy

3. Subacute limbic encephalitis

B. Disordered metabolic or endocrine function
   1. Hyperadrenalism
   2. Hypercalcemia
   3. Hypoglycemia
   4. Hyponatremia or water intoxication
   5. Hyperserotonemia
   6. Hyperthyroidism
   7. Hyperviscosity and increased coagulability of the blood

C. Nutritional and hematapoietic disorders
   1. Undernutrition
   2. Anemia
   3. Erythrocytemia
   4. Thrombocytopenia

D. Encephalopathy secondary to therapy
   (*see* Chapter 10)

Progressive multifocal leukoencephalopathy. Widespread subcortical demyelination is involved. The disease may complicate especially Hodgkin's disease and leukemia (238). Periods of delirium, irritability, drowsiness, and fluctuating levels of awareness with periods of alertness and orientation interspersed with confusion are common early features. The EEG is diffusely slow (1). Dementia gradually sets in and the disease progresses to coma and death. Various focal neurological signs are prominent.

Diffuse polioencephalopathy. This disease may present with delirium, dementia, and/or depression (233). The EEG is diffusely abnormal. The brain shows patchy degeneration of the ganglion cells of the gray matter.

Limbic encephalitis. This is an uncommon complication of cancer, particularly of oat cell carcinoma of the lung. Charatan and Brierly (239) have reported on a "toxic confusional psychosis running a fluctuating course" in patients with primary lung carcinoma. These episodes of delirium are gradually superseded by progressive dementia.

Hyperadrenalism. Hyperadrenalism has been reported in association with tumors of the bronchus, pancreas, kidney, etc.

These neoplasms are believed to secrete ACTH and severe hypercorticolism results. The incidence of related psychiatric disorders is reportedly high (235). *Hypercalcemia* may be associated with malignant neoplasms of the lung, kidney, ovary, pancreas, and the reticuloendothelial system (170). *Hypoglycemia* may result from secretion of insulin or related hormones by mesenchymal tumors, such as fibroma or fibrosarcoma. Primary hepatic carcinoma may also cause hypoglycemia. *Water intoxication* and hyponatremia may result from the inappropriate secretion of the antidiuretic hormone by bronchial carcinoma. Brain tumors may stimulate such secretion by direct effects on hypothalamic-pituitary action (160). *Serotonemia* is a feature of carcinoid tumors discussed earlier. *Hyperthyroidism* may occur rarely with a hydatidiform mole secreting thyrotropin. *Hyperviscosity* is usually associated with dysproteinemias, such as excessive macroglobulinemia in multiple myeloma. The patient typically presents with delirium, lethargy, somnolence, and disorientation (240). The EEG is diffusely slowed. The delirium is believed to be at least partly caused by concurrent hypercalcemia. *Disseminated intravascular coagulation* is an uncommon complication of many diseases, including carcinoma (240). Thromboembolic disease may be the main clinical effect of the coagulation defect. Nonbacterial thrombotic endocarditis is one of the manifestations of the chronic form of the latter, that also seems to be most common in patients with malignant tumors, especially carcinoma of the pancreas. Clinical features may be those of cerebral embolism or widespread vascular occlusions with micro-infarcts. Delirium may be one of the manifestations of this disorder (241). *Thrombocytopenia* associated with cancer may give rise to delirium as a result of bleeding into the brain. *Undernutrition* is common in advanced cancer, especially that involving the gastrointestinal tract. Avitaminosis may follow inadequate nutrition and cause delirium. *Anemia*, whether nutritional, due to depression of bone marrow, blood loss, chronic infection, radiotherapy, or chemotherapy is common and while unlikely to cause delirium directly, is likely to predispose to it and facilitate its onset. *Hypoxia* may result from tumor-related respiratory or cardiovascular failure, or other causes, and lead to delirium.

There are other potential metabolic and vascular mechanisms whereby a neoplasm may give rise to insufficient supply of substrate for cerebral energy production, to disturbed fluid and electrolyte equilibrium, to disordered acid-base balance, to cerebral ischemia, and other pathological states which may be manifested by delirium. It follows that if this syndrome develops in a patient known to have a neoplasm, the various treatable and potentially reversible factors, which may cause delirium in the cancer patient, ought to be looked for. On the other hand, delirium may be the presenting manifestation in a patient not known to suffer from a malignancy. Possible presence of the latter should always be considered in a patient forty years or older who develops delirium without a readily explicable cause.

DISORDERED TEMPERATURE REGULATION

Hypothermia. Hypothermia may give rise to delirium, stupor, and coma (242). Accidental exposure, myxedema, hypopituitarism, hypothalamic disorder, etc. may be the causative factors involved. Reduction of body temperature below 32.2°C is likely to be associated with some degree of clouding of sensorium. This effect is likely a reflection of reduction of cerebral metabolic rate, which decreases by about 5 percent for each degree of drop in body temperature below the normal levels.

Heatstroke. Commonly heatstroke features hyperactive delirium among its manifold clinical manifestations (243). It is prevalent in hot climates, during heat waves in urban areas, and in hot industrial environments, and may be caused by drugs such as atropine, chloropromazine, tricyclic antidepressants, glutethimide, etc. Heatstroke may be preceded by a short period of general weakness or delirium or both. The onset is usually sudden. Loss of consciousness and high body temperatures are prominent from the start. Delirium with vivid hallucinations may occur instead at temperatures above 40°C. Cessation of sweating (anhydrosis) is a very frequent feature. Seizures, extreme hyperirritability, rigidity, muscle cramps, coarse tremor, dystonic movements, ataxia, dysarthria, etc. may occur. After regaining consciousness, most patients report vivid and frightening dreams (243). Delirium may come on after recovery from coma and last several days. Brain damage may occur. Tachycardia, hyperventilation, nausea, vomiting, and diarrhea are common symptoms. Hyperthermia causes increased cerebral blood flow and metabolic rate. At or just above 42°C brain energy failure develops (109). Edema or congestion of the brain are usually present in heatstroke.

Electrical injury. Severe, accidental electric shock may occasionally cause delirium, sometimes with mutism (244).

REFERENCES

1. Plum, F., and Posner, J.B.: *Diagnosis of Stupor and Coma.* 2nd edition. Philadelphia, F.A. Davis Co., 1972.
2. Siesjö, B.K.: "Metabolic Basis of Consciousness," in 11th World Congress of Neurology. Amsterdam, Excerpta Medica, 1977, p. 671.
3. Bachelard, H.S.: *Biochemistry and Neurological Disease.* Oxford, Blackwell, 1976, p. 228-277.
4. Graham, D.I.: Pathology of hypoxic brain damage in man. *J Clin Pathol 30 Suppl (Roy Coll Path) 11*:170-180, 1978.
5. Pugh, L.G.C.E.: "The Effect of Acute and Chronic Exposure to Low-Oxygen Supply on Consciousness," in Schaefer, K.E., Ed., *Environmental Effects on Consciousness.* New York, MacMillan, 1962, pp. 106-116.
6. Trubnikov, G.V., and Zorina, Z.N.: Acute psychoses in myocardial infarction. *Kardiologia 13*:76-81, 1973.
7. Libow, L.S.: Pseudo-senility: acute and reversible organic brain syndromes. *J Am Geriatr Soc 21*:112-120, 1973.
8. Hackett, T.P., Cassem, N.H., and Wishnie, H.A.: The coronary-care unit. *N Engl J Med 279*:1365-1370, 1968.
9. Cay, E.L., Vetter, N., Philip, A.E., and Dugard, P.: Psychological reactions to a coronary care unit. *J Psychosom Res 16*:437-447, 1972.
10. Parker, D.L., and Hodge, J.R.: Delirium in a coronary care unit. *JAMA 201*:702-703, 1967.
11. Clark, A.N.G.: Ectopic tachycardias in the elderly. *Geront Clin 12*:203-212, 1970.
12. Cole, S.L., and Sugerman, J.N.: Cerebral manifestations of acute myocardial infarction. *Am J Med Sci 223*:35-40, 1952.
13. Ferrer, M.I.: Mistaken psychiatric referral of occult serious cardiovascular disease. *Arch Gen Psychiatry 18*:112-113, 1968.
14. Lagergren, K.: Effect of exogenous changes in heart rate upon mental performance in patients treated with artificial pacemakers for complete heart block. *Br Heart J 36*:1126-1132, 1974.

15. Lavy, S., and Stern, S.: Transient neurological manifestations in cardiac arrhythmias. *J Neurol Sci* 9:97-102, 1969.

16. Sand, B.J., Rose, H.B., and Barker, W.F.: Effect of cardiac dysrhythmia on cerebral perfusion. *Arch Surg* 111:787-791, 1976.

17. Scheinman, M., Weiss, A., and Kunkel, F: His bundle recordings in patients with bundle branch block and transient neurologic symptoms. *Circulation* 48:322-330, 1973.

18. VanDurme, J.P.: Tachyarrhythmias and transient cerebral ischemic attacks. *Am Heart J* 89:538-540, 1975.

19. Dalessio, D.J., Benchimol, A., and Dimond, E.G.: Chronic encephalopathy related to heart block. *Neurology* 15:499-503, 1965.

20. Kezdi, P., Zaks, M.S., Costello, H.J., and Boshes, B.: The impact of chronic circulatory impairment on functioning of central nervous system. *Ann Intern Med* 62:67-79, 1965.

21. McDaniel, J.W.: Cognitive dysfunction with cardiovascular disease. *Psychon Sci* 20:280-281, 1970.

22. Michael, J.C.: Psychosis with cardiac decompensation. *Am J Psychiatry* 93:1353-1362, 1937.

23. Eisenberg, S., Madison, L., and Sensebach, W.: Cerebral hemodynamic and metabolic studies in patients with congestive heart failure. 11. Observations in confused subjects. *Circulation* 21: 704-709, 1960.

24. Finnerty, F.A.: Hypertensive encephalopathy. *Am J Med* 52:672-678, 1972.

25. Bademosi, O., Falase, A.O., Jaiyesimi, F., and Bademosi, A.: Neuropsychiatric manifestations of infective endocarditis: a study of 95 patients at Ibadan, Nigeria. *J Neurol Neurosurg Psychiatr* 39:325-329, 1976.

26. Greenlee, J.E., and Mandell, G.L.: Neurological manifestations of infective endocarditis: a review. *Stroke* 4:958-963, 1973.

27. Edmonds, C., and Thomas, R.L.: Medical aspects of diving—part 4. *Med J Aust* 2:1367-1369, 1972.

28. Edmonds, C., and Thomas, R.L.: Medical aspects of diving—part 5. *Med J Aust* 2:1416-1419, 1972.

29. Edmonds, C., and Thomas, R.L.: Medical aspects of diving—part 3. *Med J Aust* 2:1300-1304, 1972.

30. Crow, T.J., and Kelman, G.R.: Psychological effects of mild acute hypoxia. *Br J Anaesth* 45:335-337, 1973.

31. Sarnoff, C.A., and Haberer, C.E.: The technique of studying disturbances of consciousness at altitude. *J Aviat Med* 30:231-240, 1959.

32. Silverstein, A.: Thrombotic thrombocytopenic purpura. *Arch Neurol* 18:358-362, 1968.

33. Ekiert, H., Gogol, Z., Jarzebowska, E., et al.: Psychic disturbances

and EEG patterns in polycythemia vera. *Polish Med J* 6:1041-1046, 1967.

34. Daroff, R.B., Deller, J.J., Kastl, A.J., and Blocker, W.W.: Cerebral malaria. *JAMA* 202:679-682, 1967.

35. Kastl, A.J., Daroff, R.B., and Blocker, W.W.: Psychological testing of cerebral malaria patients. *J Nerv Ment Dis* 147:553-561, 1968.

36. Koranyi, E.K.: Two cases of malaria presenting with psychiatric symptoms. *Biol Psychiatry* 11:445-449, 1976.

37. Wintrob, R.M.: Malaria and the acute psychotic episode. *J Nerv Ment Dis* 156:306-317, 1973.

38. Ginsburg, R., and Romano, J.: Carbon monoxide encephalopathy: need for appropriate treatment. *Am J Psychiatry* 133:317-320, 1976.

39. Smith, J.S., and Brandon, S.: Acute carbon monoxide poisoning—3 years of experience in a defined population. *Postgrad Med J* 46:65-70, 1970.

40. Smith, J.S., and Brandon, S.: Morbidity from carbon monoxide poisoning at three-year follow-up. *Br Med J* 1:318-321, 1973.

41. Bow, H., and Ledingham, I.McA.: *Carbon Monoxide Poisoning.* Amsterdam, Elsevier, 1967.

42. Rose, E.F., and Rose, M.: Carbon monoxide: a challenge to the physician. *Clin Med* 78:12-21, 1971.

43. Fajans, S.S., and Floyd, J.C.: Fasting hypoglycemia in adults. *N Engl J Med* 294:766-772, 1976.

44. Marks, V., and Rose, C.F.: *Hypoglycemia.* Philadelphia, F.A. Davis, 1965.

45. Laurent, J., Debry, G., and Floquet, J.: *Hypoglycemic Tumors.* Amsterdam, Excerpta Medica, 1971.

46. Turkington, R.W.: Encephalopathy induced by oral hypoglycemic drugs. *Arch Intern Med* 137:1082-1083, 1977.

47. Scarlett, J.A., Mako, M.E., Rubenstein, A.H., et al.: Factitious hypoglycemia. *N Engl J Med* 297:1029-1032, 1977.

48. Seltzer, H.S.: Drug-induced hypoglycemia. *Diabetes* 21:955-966, 1972.

49. Hafken, L., Leichter, S., and Reich, T.: Organic brain dysfunction as a possible consequence of postgastrectomy hypoglycemia. *Am J Psychiatry* 132:1321-1324, 1975.

50. Boyd, I.H., and Cleveland, S.E.: Psychiatric symptoms masking an insulinoma. *Dis Nerv Syst* 28:457-458, 1967.

51. Frerichs, H., and Creutzfeldt, W.: Hypoglycemia. 1. Insulin secreting tumors. *Clin Endocrin Metab* 5:747-767, 1976.

52. Leichty, R.D., Alsever, R.N., and Burrington, J.: Islet cell hyper-insulinism in adults and children. *JAMA* 230:1538-1543, 1974.

53. Service, J.F., Dale, A.J.D., Elveback, L.R., and Jiang, N.S.: Insulinoma. Clinical and diagnostic features of 60 consecutive cases. *Mayo Clin Proc* 51:417-429, 1976.

54. Todd, J., Collins, A.D., Martin, F.R.R., and Dewhurst, K.E.: Mental symptoms due to insulinomata. *Br Med J* 2:828-831, 1962.
55. Breidahl, H.D., Priestley, J.T., and Rynearson, E.H.: Clinical aspects of hyperinsulinism. *JAMA 160*:198-201, 1956.
56. Engel, G.L., Webb, J.P., and Ferris, E.B.: Quantitative electro-encephalographic studies of anoxia in humans; comparison with acute alcoholic intoxication and hypoglycemia. *J Clin Invest* 24:691-697, 1945.
57. Sherlock, S.: *Diseases of the Liver and Biliary System*. Fifth edition. Oxford, Blackwell Scientific, 1975.
58. Zacharski, L.R., Litin, E.M., Mulder, D.W., and Cain, J.C.: Acute, fatal hepatic failure presenting with psychiatric symptoms. *Am J Psychiatry 127*:382-386, 1970.
59. Steigman, F., and Clowdus, B.F.: *Hepatic Encephalopathy*. Springfield, Ill., Charles C Thomas, 1971.
60. Elsass, P., Lund, Y., and Ranek, L.: Encephalopathy in patients with cirrhosis of the liver. A neurophysiological study. *Scand J Gastroent 13*:241-247, 1978.
61. Rehnstrom, S., Simert, G., Hansson, J.A., et al.: Chronic hepatic encephalopathy. A psychometrical study. *Scand J Gastroent 12*:305-311, 1977.
62. Zeegen, R., Drinkwater, J.E., and Dawson, A.M.: Method for measuring cerebral dysfunction in patients with liver disease. *Br Med J* 2:633-636, 1970.
63. Davidson, E.A., and Solomon, P.: The differentiation of delirium tremens from impending hepatic coma. *J Ment Sci 104*:326-333, 1958.
64. Jaffe, N.: Catatonia and hepatic dysfunction. *Dis Nerv Syst 28*:606-608, 1967.
65. Hawkes, C.H., and Brunt, P.W.: The current status of the EEG in liver disease. *Digest Dis 19*:75-80, 1974.
66. Kurtz, D., Zenglein, J.P., Girardel, M., et al.: Étude du sommeil nocturne au cours de l'encephalopathie porto-cave. *Electro-encephalogr Clin Neurophysiol 33*:167-178, 1972.
67. Eichler, M.: Psychological changes associated with induced hyper-ammonemia. *Science 144*:886-888, 1964.
68. Fischer, J.E.: Hepatic coma in cirrhosis, portal hypertension, and following portacaval shunt. *Arch Surg 108*:325-336, 1974.
69. Ono, J., Hutson, D.G., Dombro, R.S., et al.: Tryptophan and hepatic coma. *Gastroenterology 74*:196-200, 1978.
70. Fischer, J.E., Funovics, J.M., Falcao, H.A., and Wesdorp, R.I.C.: L-dopa in hepatic coma. *Ann Surg 183*:386-391, 1976.
71. Lesesne, H.R., Bozymski, E.M., and Fallon, H.J.: Treatment of alcoholic hepatitis with encephalopathy. *Gastroenterology 74*: 169-173, 1978.
72. Editorial: Sedation in liver disease. *Br Med J* 1:1241-1242, 1977.

73. Murray-Lyon, I.M., Young, J., Parkes, J.D., et al.: Clinical and electroencephalographic assessment of diazepam in liver disease. *Br Med J* 2:265-266, 1971.

74. Arieff, A.I., Guisado, R., and Massry, S.G.: Uremic encephalopathy: studies on biochemical alterations in the brain. *Kidney Int* (*Suppl 2*) 7:194-200, 1975.

75. Neary, D.: Neuropsychiatric sequelae of renal failure. *Br J Hosp Med* 15:122-130, 1976.

76. Nissenson, A.R., Levin, M.L., Klawans, H.L., and Nausieda, P.L.: Neurological sequelae of end stage renal disease (ESRD). *J Chron Dis* 30:705-733, 1977.

77. Stenbäck, A., and Haapanen, E.: Azotemia and psychosis. *Acta Psychiatr Scand* 43 (Suppl. 197), 1977.

78. Tyler, H.R.: Neurologic disorders seen in the uremic patient. *Arch Intern Med* 126:781-786, 1970.

79. Buchanan, D.C., Abram, H.S., Wells, C., and Teschan, P.: Psychosis and pseudo dementia associated with hemodialysis. *Int J Psychiatr Med* 8:85-97, 1977-78.

80. Mahurkar, S.D., Meyers, L., Cohen, J. et al.: Electroencephalographic and radionuclide studies in dialysis dementia. *Kidney Int* 13:306-315, 1978.

81. Ockner, S.A., McDonald, F.D., and Merrill, J.P.: Toxic psychosis following nondialytic therapy of chronic renal failure. *JAMA* 217:74-76, 1971.

82. Taclob, L., and Needle, M.: Drug-induced encephalopathy in patients on maintenance hemodialysis. *Lancet* 2:704-705, 1976.

83. Penn, I., Bunch, D., Olenik, D., and Abouna, G.: "Psychiatric Experience with Patients Receiving Renal and Hepatic Transplants," in Castelnuovo Tedesco, P., Ed., *Psychiatric Aspects of Organ Transplantation.* New York, Grune & Stratton, 1971.

84. Waniek, W., Pach, J., Hartmann, H.G., and Beersiek, F.: Hirnleistungsstörungen bei Patienten eines Dialyse-Transplantations-Programms. *Schweiz med Wschr* 107:832-835, 1977.

85. Addison, T.: "On the Disorders of the Brain Connected with Diseased Kidneys," in *A Collection of the Collected Works of Thomas Addison.* London, New Sydenham Society, 1868.

86. Baker, A.B., and Knutson, J.: Psychiatric aspects of uremia. *Am J Psychiatry* 102:683-687, 1946.

87. McDaniel, J.W.: Metabolic and CNS correlates of cognitive dysfunction with renal failure. *Psychophysiology* 8:704-713, 1971.

88. Ginn, H.E.: Neurobehavioral dysfunction in uremia. *Kidney Int* (*Suppl. 2*) 7:217-221, 1975.

89. Reimer, D.R., and Nagaswami, S.: Catatonic schizophrenia associated with cerebral arterial malformations and with membranous glomerulonephritis. *Psychosomatics* 15:39-40, 1974.

90. Teschan, P.E.: Electroencephalographic and other neurophysiological abnormalities in uremia. *Kidney Int (Suppl 2)* 7:210-216, 1975.
91. Passouant, P., Cadilhac, J., Baldy-Moulinier, M., and Mion, C.: Étude du sommeil nocturne chez des urémiques chroniques soumis à une épuration extrarenale. *Electroencephalogr Clin Neurophysiol* 29:441-449, 1970.
92. Glick, I.D., Goldfield, M.D., and Kovnat, P.J.: Recognition and management of psychosis associated with hemodialysis. *Calif Med 119*:56-59, 1973.
93. Merrill, R.H., and Collins, J.L.: Acute psychosis in chronic renal failure: case reports. *Milit Med 139*:622-624, 1974.
94. Kiley, J.E., Woodruff, M.W., and Pratt, K.L.: Evaluation of encephalopathy by EEG frequency analysis in chronic dialysis patients. *Clin Nephrol* 5:245-250, 1976.
95. Alfrey, A.C., LeGendre, G.R., and Kaehny, W.D.: The dialysis encephalopathy syndrome. *N Engl J Med* 294:184-188, 1976.
96. Burks, J.S., Alfrey, A.C., Huddlestone, J., et al.: A fatal encephalopathy in chronic hemodialysis patients. *Lancet 1*:764-768, 1976.
97. Chokroverty, S., Bruetman, M.E., Berger, V., and Reyes, M.G.: Progressive dialytic encephalopathy. *J Neurol Neurosurg Psychiatry* 39:411-419, 1976.
98. Editorial: Dementia dialytica. *JAMA* 226:190, 1973.
99. McDermott, J.R., Smith, A.I., Ward, M.K., et al.: Brain-aluminium concentration in dialysis encephalopathy. *Lancet 1*:901-904, 1978.
100. Madison, D.P., Baehr, E.T., Bazell, M., et al.: Communicative and cognitive deterioration in dialysis dementia: two case studies. *J Speech Hear Dis* 42:238-246, 1977.
101. Sullivan, P.A., Murnaghan, D.J., and Callaghan, N.: Dialysis dementia: recovery after transplantation. *Br Med J 2*:740-741, 1977.
102. Ball, J.H., Butkus, D.E., and Madison, D.S.: Effect of subtotal parathyroidectomy on dialysis dementia. *Nephron 18*:151-155, 1977.
103. Nadel, A.M., and Wilson, W.P.: Dialysis encephalopathy: a possible seizure disorder. *Neurology 26*:1130-1134, 1976.
104. Rogers, R.M., ed.: *Respiratory Intensive Care.* Springfield, Ill., Charles C Thomas, 1977.
105. Arieff, A.J., and Buckingham, W.B.: Fluctuating "acute dementia" due to emphysema with pulmonary insufficiency. *Trans Am Neurol Assoc* 95:203-205, 1970.
106. Austen, F.K., Carmichael, M.W., and Adams, R.D.: Neurologic manifestations of chronic pulmonary insufficiency. *N Engl J Med* 257:579-590, 1957.
107. Dulfano, M.J., and Ishikawa, S.: Hypercapnia: mental changes and extrapulmonary complications. *Ann Intern Med* 63:829-841, 1965.

108. Krop, H.D., Block, A.J., and Cohen, E.: Neuropsychologic effects of continuous oxygen therapy in chronic obstructive pulmonary disease. *Chest 64*:317-322, 1973.

109. Siesjö, B.K.: *Brain Energy Metabolism*. New York, John Wiley & Sons, 1978.

110. Kurtz, D., Zenglein, J.P., Imler, M., et al.: Étude du sommeil nocturne au cours de l'encephalopathie port-cave. *Electroencephalogr Clin Neurophysiol 33*:167-178, 1972.

111. Clark, T.J.H., and Collins, J.V.: Use of benzoctamine as sedative in patients with respiratory failure. *Br Med J 1*:75-76, 1973.

112. Marneros, A., and Rieger, H.: Oneirodelir bei paroxysmaler Hypersomnie mit Periodenatmung und Atemwegsobstruktion. *Fortschr Neurol Psychiat 46*:222-228, 1978.

113. Benos, J.: Encephalopathia pancreatica. *Munch med Wschr 115*: 1842-1844, 1973.

114. Benos, J.: Funktionspsychosen und neurologische Ausfälle bei Pankreatitis. *Med Klin 69*:1185-1192, 1974.

115. Benos, J.: Zur Differentialdiagnose der deliranten Psychose bei akuter Pankreatitis vom Alkoholderlir. *Z Allgemeinmed 49*:1172-1173, 1973.

116. Johnson, D.A., and Tong, N.T.: Pancreatic encephalopathy. *South Med J 70*:165-167, 1977.

117. Schuster, M.M., and Iber, F.L.: Psychosis with pancreatitis. *Arch Intern Med 116*:228-233, 1965.

118. Sharf, B., and Bental, E.: Pancreatic encephalopathy. *J Neurol Neurosurg Psychiatry 34*:357-261, 1971.

119. Mitra, M.L.: Confusional states in relation to vitamin deficiencies in the elderly. *J Am Geriatr Soc 19*:536-545, 1971.

120. Brin, M., and Bauernfeind, J.C.: Vitamin needs of the elderly. *Postgrad Med 63*:155-163, 1978.

121. Dremick, E.J., Joven, C.B., and Swendseid, M.E.: Occurrence of acute Wernicke's encephalopathy during prolonged starvation for the treatment of obesity. *N Engl J Med 274*:937-939, 1966.

122. Faris, A.A.: Wernicke's encephalopathy in uremia. *Neurology 22*: 1293-1297, 1972.

123. Frantzen, E.: Wernicke's encephalopathy. *Acta Neurol Scand 42*: 426-441, 1966.

124. Groen, R.H., and Hoff, H.C.W.: Wernicke's disease. *Eur Neurol 15*:109-115, 1977.

125. Kramer, J., and Goodwin, J.A.: Wernicke's encephalopathy. *JAMA 238*:2176-2177, 1977.

126. Lopez, R.I., and Collins, G.H.: Wernicke's encephalopathy. A complication of chronic hemodialysis. *Arch Neurol 18*:248-259, 1968.

127. Nadel, A.M., and Burger, P.C.: Wernicke encephalopathy following prolonged intravenous therapy. *JAMA 235*:2403-2405, 1976.

128. Victor, M., Adams, R.D., and Collins, G.H.: *The Wernicke-Korsakoff Syndrome*. Philadelphia, F.A. Davis Co., 1971.

129. Gregory, I.: The role of nicotinic acid (niacin) in mental health and disease. *J Ment Sci 101*:85-109, 1955.

130. Spies, T.D., Aring, C.D., Gelperin, J., and Bean, W.B.: The mental symptoms of pellagra. *Am J Med Sci 196*:461-475, 1938.

131. Spivak, J.L., and Jackson, D.L.: Pellagra: an analysis of 18 patients and a review of the literature. *J Hopk Med J 140*:295-309, 1977.

132 Eilenberg, M.D.: Psychiatric illness and pernicious anaemia: a clinical re-evaluation. *J Ment Sci 106*:1539-1548, 1960.

133. Hart, R.J., and McCurdy, P.R.: Psychosis in vitamin B_{12} deficiency. *Arch Intern Med 128*:596-597, 1971.

134. Holmes, J.McD.: Cerebral manifestations of vitamin B_{12} deficiency. *Br Med J 2*:1394-1398, 1956.

135. Samson, D.C., Swisher, S.N., Christian, R.M., and Engel, G.L.: Cerebral metabolic disturbance and delirium in pernicious anemia. *Arch Intern Med 90*:4-14, 1952.

136. Strachan, R.W., and Henderson, J.G.: Psychiatric syndromes due to avitaminosis B_{12} with normal blood and marrow. *Q J Med 34*: 303-317, 1965.

137. Reynolds, E.H.: Neurological aspects of folate and vitamin B_{12} metabolism. *Clin Hematol 5*:661-696, 1976.

138. Roos, D., and Willanger, R.: Various degrees of dementia in a selected group of gastrectomized patients with low serum B_{12}. *Acta Neurol Scand 55*:563-576, 1977.

139. Botez, M.I., Fontaine, F., Botez, T., and Bachevalier, J.: Folate-responsive neurological and mental disorders: report of 16 cases. *Eur Neurol 16*:230-246, 1977.

140. Hoffbrand, A.V.: Pathology of folate deficiency. *Proc Roy Soc Med 70*:82-84, 1977.

141. Sapira, J.D., Tullis, S., and Mullaly, R.: Reversible dementia due to folate deficiency. *South Med J 68*:776-778, 1975.

142. Strachan, R.W., and Henderson, J.G.: Dementia and folate deficiency. *Q J Med 36*:189-204, 1967.

143. Haupt, R.: Akute symptomatische Psychose bei Vitamin A-Intoxikation. *Nervenarzt 48*:91-95, 1977.

144. Restak, R.M.: Pseudotumor cerebri, psychosis, and hypervitaminosis *J Nerv Ment Dis 155*:72-75, 1972.

145. Bradbury, M.W.: "Electrolyte Disorders and the Brain," in Maxwell, M.H., and Kleeman, C.R., Eds., *Clinical Disorders of Fluid and Electrolyte Metabolism*. New York, McGraw-Hill Book Co., 1972.

146. Snively, W.D., and Becker, B.: Body fluids and neuro-psychologic disturbances. *Psychosomatics 9*:295-305, 1968.
147. Wohlrabe, J.C., and Pitts, F.N.: Delirium and complex electrolyte disturbance. *Dis Nerv Syst 25*:44-47, 1965.
148. Maxwell, M.H., and Kleeman, C.R., Eds.: *Clinical Disorders of Fluid and Electrolyte Metabolism.* New York, McGraw-Hill Book Co., 1972.
149. Arieff, A.I., and Guisado, R.: Effects on the central nervous system of hypernatremic and hyponatremic states. *Kidney Int 10*:104-116, 1976.
150. Caron, J.C., Cappoen, J.P., Chopin, C., et al.: Les intoxications par l'eau après accès polydipsiques. *Rev Neurol (Paris) 133*:485-495, 1977.
151. Chinn, T.A.: Compulsive water drinking. *J Nerv Ment Dis 158*:78-80, 1974.
152. Fowler, R.C., Kronfol, Z.A., and Perry, P.J.: Water intoxication, psychosis, and inappropriate secretion of antidiuretic hormone. *Arch Gen Psychiatry 34*:1097-1099, 1977.
153. Goodner, D.M., Arnas, G.M., Andros, G.J., et al.: Psychogenic polydipsia causing acute water intoxication in pregnancy at term. *Obstet Gynecol 37*:873-876, 1971.
154. Mendelson, W.B., and Deza, P.C.: Polydipsia, hyponatremia, and seizures in psychotic patients. *J Nerv Ment Dis 162*:140-143, 1976.
155. Noonan, J.P.A., and Ananth, J.: Compulsive water drinking and water intoxication. *Compr Psychiatry 18*:183-187, 1977.
156. Rabiner, C.J., and Saravay, S.M.: Water intoxication and food faddism. *Psychosomatics 15*:113-114, 1974.
157. Rae, J.: Self-induced water intoxication in a schizophrenic patient. *Can Med Assoc J 114*:438-439, 1976.
158. Raskind, M.: Psychosis, polydipsia, and water intoxication. *Arch Gen Psychiatry 30*:112-114, 1974.
159. Swanson, A.G., and Iseri, O.A.: Acute encephalopathy due to water intoxication. *N Engl J Med 258*:831-834, 1958.
160. Editorial: Hyponatremia. *Lancet 1*:642-644, 1978.
161. Matuk, F., and Kalyanaramar, K.: Syndrome of inappropriate secretion of antidiuretic hormone in patients treated with psychotherapeutic drugs. *Arch Neurol 34*:374-375, 1977.
162. Dubovsky, S.L., Grabon, S., Berl, T., and Schrier, R.W.: Syndrome of inappropriate secretion of antidiuretic hormone with exacerbated psychosis. *Ann Intern Med 79*:551-554, 1973.
163. Raskind, M.A., Orenstein, H., and Christopher, T.G.: Acute psychosis, increased water ingestion, and inappropriate antidiuretic hormone secretion. *Am J Psychiatry 132*:907-910, 1975.

164. Moses, A.M., and Miller, M.: Drug-induced dilutional hyponatremia. *N Engl J Med* 291:1234-1239, 1974.
165. Lewis, N.H.: Iatrogenic psychotic depressive reaction in hypertensive patients. *Am J Psychiatry* 127:1416-1417, 1971.
166. Burnell, G.M., and Foster, T.A.: Psychosis with low sodium syndrome. *Am J Psychiatry* 128:1313-1314, 1972.
167. Mitchell, W., and Feldman, F.: Neuropsychiatric aspects of hypokalemia. *Can Med Assoc J* 98:49-51, 1968.
168. Lehrer, G.M., and Levitt, M.F.: Neuropsychiatric presentation of hypercalcemia. *Mt Sinai J Med NY* 27:10-18, 1960.
169. Mastropolo, P.L., and Grace, W.J.: Diagnostic and therapeutic considerations in hypercalcemia syndromes. *Crit Care Med* 4:20-23, 1976.
170. Samaan, N.A., Hickey, R.C., Sethi, M.R., et al.: Hypercalcemia in patients with known malignant disease. *Surgery* 80:383-388, 1976.
171. Smith, W.O., and Lindeman, R.D.: Acute hypercalcemia—a review and case report illustrating therapeutic value of mithramycin. *J Okla State Med Assoc* 70:255-261, 1977.
172. Cornette, M., and Grisar, T.: A study of clinical signs and EEG profiles in hypercalcemic encephalopathy. *Acta Neurol Belg* 77:129-143, 1977.
173. Etheridge, J.E., and Grabow, J.D.: Hypercalcemia without EEG abnormalities. *Dis Nerv Syst* 32:479-482, 1971.
174. Swash, M., and Rowan, A.J.: Electroencephalographic criteria of hypocalcemia and hypercalcemia. *Arch Neurol* 26:218-228, 1972.
175. Singer, F.R., Bethune, J.E., and Massry, S.G.: Hypercalcemia and hypocalcemia. *Clin Nephrol* 7:154-162, 1977.
176. Flink, E.B., McCollister, R., Prasad, A.S., et al.: Evidences for clinical magnesium deficiency. *Ann Intern Med* 47:956-968, 1957.
177. Hall, R.C.W., and Joffe, J.R.: Hypomagnesemia. Physical and psychiatric symptoms. *JAMA* 224:1749-1751, 1973.
178. Arieff, A.I., and Carroll, H.J.: Cerebral edema and depression of sensorium in nonketotic hyperosmolar coma. *Diabetes* 23:525-531, 1974.
179. Maccario, M.: Neurological dysfunction associated with nonketotic hyperglycemia. *Arch Neurol* 19:525-534, 1968.
180. Posner, J.B., and Plum, F.: Spinal-fluid pH and neurologic symptoms in systemic acidosis. *N Engl J Med* 277:605-613, 1967.
181. Shavelle, H.S.: Cerebral syndromes of diabetes mellitus. *Calif Med* 110:283-291, 1969.
182. Engel, G.L., Ferris, E.B., and Logan, M.: Hyperventilation: analysis of clinical symptomatology. *Ann Intern Med* 27:683-704, 1947.

183. Allen, T.E., and Agus, B.: Hyperventilation leading to hallucinations. *Am J Psychiatry 125*:632-637, 1968.

184. Cartwright, G.W.: Diagnosis of treatable Wilson's disease. *N Engl J Med 298*:1347-1350, 1978.

185. Rowland, L.P.: Acute intermittent porphyria: search for enzymatic defect with implications for neurology and psychiatry. *Dis Nerv Syst 22*:1-12, 1961.

186. Roth, N.: The psychiatric syndromes of porphyria. *J Neuropsychiatry 4*:32-44, 1968.

187. Stein, J.A., and Tschudy, D.P.: Acute intermittent porphyria. *Medicine 49*:1-16, 1970.

188. Becker, D.M., and Kramer, S.: The neurological manifestations of porphyria: a review. *Medicine 56*:411-423, 1977.

189. Major, L.F., Brown, L., and Wilson, W.P.: Carcinoid and psychiatric symptoms. *South Med J 66*:787-790, 1973.

190. Lehmann, J.: Mental disturbances followed by stupor in a patient with carcinoidosis. *Acta Psychiatr Scand 42*:153-161, 1966.

191. Southren, A. L., Warner, R.R.P., Christoff, N.I., and Weiner, H.E.: An unusual neurologic syndrome associated with hyperserotonemia. *N Engl J Med 260*:1265-1268, 1959.

192. Lehmann, J.: Mental and neuromuscular symptoms in tryptophan deficiency: pellagra, carcinoidosis, phenylketonuria, Hartnup disease and disturbances of tryptophan metabolism induced by p-chlorophenylalanine, levodopa, and alphamethyldopa. *Acta Psychiatr Scand 48* (Suppl 237), 1972.

193. Engelman, K., Lovenberg, W., and Sjoerdsma, A.: Inhibition of serotonin synthesis by para-chlorophenylalanine in patients with the carcinoid syndrome. *N Engl J Med 277*:1103-1108, 1967.

194. Gruner, W.: Exogene Psychose eines Patienten mit Karzinoidsydrom nach Behandlung mit p-Chlorophenylalanin (PCPA). *Psychiatr Clin 8*:266-276, 1975.

195. Beaumont, P.J.V.: Endocrines and psychiatry. *Br J Hosp Med 17*:485-497, 1972.

196. Smith, C.K., Barish, J., Correa, J., and Williams, R.H.: Psychiatric disturbances in endocrinologic disease. *Psychosom Med 34*:69-86, 1972.

197. Whybrow, P.C., and Hurwitz, T.: "Psychological Disturbances Associated with Endocrine Disease and Hormone Therapy," in Sachar, E.J., Ed., *Hormones, Behavior, and Psychopathology.* New York, Raven Press, 1976, pp. 125-143.

198. Court, J., and Diaz, F.: Alteraciones de conciencia en el sindrome de Sheehan. *Rev Med Chili 101*:780-783, 1976.

199. Hanna, S.M.: Hypopituitarism (Sheehan's syndrome) presenting with organic psychosis. *J Neurol Neurosurg Psychiatry 33*:192-193, 1970.

200. Parker, R.R., Isaacs, A.D., and McKerron, C.G.: Recoverable organic psychosis after hypopituitary coma. *Br Med J 1*:132-133, 1976.

201. Browning, T.B., Atkins, R.W., and Weiner, H.: Cerebral metabolic disturbances in hypothyroidism. *Arch Intern Med 93*:938-950, 1954.

202. Asher, R.: Myxoedematous madness. *Br Med J 2*:555-562, 1949.

203. Tonks, C.M.: Mental illness in hypothyroid patients. *Br J Psychiatry 110*:706-710, 1964.

204. Easson, W.M.: Myxedema with psychosis. *Arch Gen Psychiatry 14*:277-283, 1966.

205. Brewer, C.: Psychosis due to acute hypothyroidism during the administration of carbimazole. *Br J Psychiatry 115*:181-183, 1969.

206. Davidoff, F., and Gill, J.: Myxedema madness: psychosis as an early manifestation of hypothyroidism. *Conn Med 41*:618-621, 1977.

207. Jayaratna, P.S.: Hypothyroidism with episodic psychiatric and cardiac manifestations. *Proc Roy Soc Med 69*:581-582, 1976.

208. Thrush, D.C., and Boddie, H.G.: Episodic encephalopathy associated with thyroid disorders. *J Neurol Neurosurg Psychiatry 37*:696-700, 1974.

209. Royce, P.C.: Severely impaired consciousness in myxedema—a review. *Am J Med Sci 261*:46-50, 1971.

210. Hooshmand, H., and Sarhaddi, S.: Hypothyroidism in adults and children. EEG findings. *Clin Electroencephalogr 6*:61-67, 1975.

211. Burch, E.A., and Messervy, T.W.: Psychiatric symptoms in medical illness: hyperthyroidism revisited. *Psychosomatics 19*:34-40, 1978.

212. Jamieson, G.R., and Wall, J.H.: Psychoses associated with hyperthyroidism. *Psychiatr Q 10*:464-480, 1936.

213. McGee, R.R., Whittaker, R.L., and Tullis, I.F.: Apathetic thyroidism: review of the literature and report of four cases. *Ann Intern Med 50*:1418-1431, 1959.

214. Siersbaek-Nielsen, K., Hansen, J.M., Schioler, M., et al.: Electroencephalographic changes during and after treatment of hyperthyroidism. *Acta Endocrinol 70*:308-314, 1972.

215. Denko, J.D., and Kaelbling, R.: The psychiatric aspects of hypoparathyroidism: review of the literature and case reports. *Acta Psychiatr Scand (Suppl) 38*:7-70, 1962.

216. Greene, J.A., and Swanson, L.W.: Psychosis in hypoparathyroidism. *Ann Intern Med 14*:1233-1236, 1941.

217. Clark, J.A., Davidson, L.J., and Ferguson, H.C.: Psychosis in hypoparathyroidism. *J Ment Sci 108*:811-815, 1962.

218. Anderson, J.: Psychiatric aspects of primary hyperparathyroidism. *Proc Roy Soc Med 61*:1123-1124, 1968.

219. Watson, L.: Clinical aspects of hyperparathyroidism. *Proc Roy Soc Med 61*:1123, 1968.

220. Mallette, L.E., Bilezikian, J.P., Heath, D.A., and Aurbach, G.D.: Primary hyperparathyroidism: clinical and biochemical features. *Medicine* 53:127-146, 1974.
221. Gatewood, J.W., Organ, C.H., and Mead, B.T.: Mental changes associated with hyperparathyroidism. *Am J Psychiatry* 132:129-132, 1975.
222. Karpati, G., and Frame, B.: Neuropsychiatric disorders in primary hyperparathyroidism. *Arch Neurol* 10:387-397, 1964.
223. Mattson, B.: Addison's disease and psychosis. *Acta Psychiatr Scand (Suppl)* 255:203-210, 1974.
224. Regestein, Q.R., Rose, L.I., and Williams, G.H.: Psychopathology in Cushing's syndrome. *Arch Intern Med* 130:114-117, 1972.
225. Cohen, S.: Cushing's syndrome. Report of a case. *Ann West Med Surg* 4:288-293, 1950.
226. Hertz, P.E., Nadas, E., and Wojtkowski, H.: Cushing's syndrome and its management. *Am J Psychiatry* 112:144-145, 1955.
227. Tucker, R.P., Weinstein, H.E., Schteingart, D.E., and Starkman, M.: EEG changes and serum cortisol levels in Cushing's syndrome. *Clin Electroencephalogr* 9:32-37, 1978.
228. Levine, P.M., Silberfarb, P.M., and Lipowski, Z.J.: Mental disorders in cancer patients. A study of 100 psychiatric referrals. *Cancer* 42:1385-1391, 1978.
229. Davies, R.K., Quinlan, D.M., McKegney, F.P., and Kimball, C.P.: Organic factors and psychological adjustment in advanced cancer patients. *Psychosom Med* 35:464-471, 1973.
230. Holland, J., and Glass, E.: Occurrence of delirium in preterminal stages of advanced cancer. Unpublished manuscript.
231. Walther-Büel, H.: *Die Psychiatrie der Hirngeschwülste.* Wien, Springer, 1951.
232. Schmid-Wermser, I., Nagel, G.A., and Schmid, A.H.: Zur Klinischen Diagnose von Hirnmetastasen beim Bronchuskarzinom. *Schweiz Med Wschr* 104:464-468, 1974.
233. Brain (Lord), and Norris, F.H.: *The Remote Effects of Cancer on the Nervous System.* New York, Grune & Stratton, 1965.
234. Fessel, W.J.: Remote effects of benign neoplasms. *N Engl J Med* 288:323, 1973.
235. Mitchell, W.M.: Etiological factors producing neuropsychiatric syndromes in patients with malignant disease. *Intern J Neuropsychiatry* 3:464-468, 1967.
236. Posner, J.B.: Neurological complications of systemic cancer. *Med Clin N Am* 55:625-646, 1971.
237. Shapiro, W.R.: Remote effects of neoplasm on the central nervous system: encephalopathy. *Adv Neurol* 15:101-117, 1976.
238. Canning, B., Kobayshi, R.M., Kaplan, C.G., et al.: Progressive multifocal leukoencephalopathy. *West J Med* 125:364-369, 1976.

239. Charatan, F.B., and Brierley, J.B.: Mental disorder associated with primary lung carcinoma. *Br Med J 1*:765-768, 1956.
240. Alkan, M.L., Mayersdorf, A., and Dvilansky, A.: Electroencephalographic and encephalopathic findings in multiple myeloma: hyperviscosity versus hypercalcemia. *Clin Electroencephalogr 6*:16-22, 1975.
241. Reagan, T.J., and Okazaki, H.: The thrombotic syndrome associated with carcinoma. *Arch Neurol 31*:390-395, 1974.
242. Irvine, R.E.: Hypothermia in old age. *Practitioner 213*:795-800, 1974.
243. Shibolet, S., Lancaster, M.C., and Danon, Y.: Heat stroke. *Aviat Space Envir Med 47*:280-301, 1976.
244. Lindenmayer, J.P., and Pappenheim, E.: A case of accidental electrocution. *Psychiatr Q 47*:218-227, 1973.

Additional References

Alberti, K.G.M.M., and Nattrass, M. Severe diabetic ketoacidosis. *Med Clin N Am 62*:799-814, 1978.
d'Avella, D., Zuccarello, M., Scanarini, M., et al. Neurogenic hypernatremia. *Acta Neurochir 46*:151-157, 1979.
Bergonzi, P., Bianco, A., Mazza, S., and Mennuni, G. Night sleep in patients with severe hepatic failure. *Eur Neurol 17*:271-275, 1978.
Cogan, M.G., Covey, C.M., Arieff, A.I., et al. Central nervous system manifestations of hyperparathyroidism. *Am J Med 65*:963-970, 1978.
Etheridge, W.B., and O'Neill, W.M. The "dialysis encephalopathy syndrome" without dialysis. *Clin Nephrol 10*:250-252, 1978.
Geller, S.A., and Paronetto, F. Adrenal cortical carcinoma with Cushing's syndrome, organic psychosis, and aphasia in a seventy-one-year-old woman. *Mt Sinai J Med NY 45*:509-523, 1978.
Herman, T.S., Hammond, N., Jones, S.E., et al. Involvement of the central nervous system by non-Hodgkin's lymphoma. *Cancer 43*:390-397, 1979.
Hildebrand, J. *Lesions of the Nervous System in Cancer Patients.* New York, Raven Press, 1978.
Jose, C.J., Mehta, S., and Perez-Cruet, J. Th syndrome of inappropriate secretion of antidiuretic hormone (SIADH). *Can J Psychiatry 24*:225-231, 1979.
Kennedy, P.G.E., Mitchell, D.M., and Hoffbrand, B.I. Severe hyponatremia in hospital patients. *Br Med J 2*:1251-1253, 1978.
Lederman, R.J., and Henry, C.E. Progressive dialysis encephalopathy. *Ann Neurol 4*:199-204, 1978.
Lee, D.B.N., Zawada, E.T., and Kleeman, C.R. The pathophysiology and clinical aspects of hypercalcemic disorders. *West J Med 129*:278-320, 1978.
Loiudice, T.A., Tulman, A., and Buhac, I. L-dopa and hepatic encephalopathy. *New York State J Med 79*:364-366, 1979.

Mann, S.C., and Boger, W.P. Psychotropic drugs, summer heat and humidity, and hyperpyrexia: A danger restated. *Am J Psychiatry 135*: 1097-1100, 1978.

Mans, A.M., Saunders, S.J., Kirsch, R.E., and Biebuyck, J.F. Correlation of plasma and brain amino acid and putative neurotransmitter alterations during acute hepatic coma in the rat. *J Neurochem 32*:285-292, 1979.

Marshall, J.R. Neuropsychiatric aspecs of renal failure. *J Clin Psychiatry 40*:81-85, 1979.

Mordes, J.P., and Wacker, W.E.C. Excess magnesium. *Pharmacol Rev 29*:273-300, 1978.

Murray, T.M., Josse, R.G., and Heersche, J.N.M. Hypercalcemia and cancer: An update. *Can Med Assoc J 119*:915-920, 1978.

Nemoto, E.M. Pathogenesis of cerebral ischemia-anoxia. *Crit Care Med 6*:203-214, 1978.

Neill, J.F., Glew, R.H., and Peters, S.P. Familial psychosis and diverse neurologic abnormalities in adult-onset Gaucher's disease. *Arch Neurol 36*:95-99, 1979.

Noriega-Sanchez, A., Martinez-Maldonado, M., and Haiffe, R.M. Clinical and electroencephalographic changes in progressive uremic encephalopathy. *Neurology 28*:667-669, 1978.

Parkinson, I.S., Feest, T.G., Ward, M.K., et al. Fracturing dialysis osteodystrophy and dialysis encephalopathy. *Lancet 1*:406-409, 1979.

Ping, F.C., and Jenkins, L.C. Protection of the brain from hypoxia: A review. *Can Anaesth Soc J 25*:468-473, 1978.

Reuler, J.B. Hypothermia: Pathophysiology, clinical settings, and management. *Ann Intern Med 89*:519-527, 1978.

Rozas, V.V., Port, F.K., and Rutt, W.M. Progressive encephalopathy from dialysate aluminum. *Arch Intern Med 138*:1375-1377, 1978.

Shin, I., Schlagenhauff, R.E., and Strong, H.E. The value of electroencephalographic recordings in dialysis encephalopathy: Case-reports and review of literature. *Clin Electroencephanogr 9*:195-200, 1978.

Snider, W.D., De Maria, A.A., and Mann, J.D. Diazepam and dialysis encephalopathy. *Neurology 29*:414-415, 1979.

Steigman, F. Preventing portal systemic encephalopathy in the patient with cirrhosis. *Postgrad Med 65*:118-126, 1979.

Trewby, P.N., Casemore, C., and Williams, R. Continuous bipolar recording of the EEG in patients with fulminant hepatic failure. *Electroencephanogr Clin Neurophysiol 45*:107-110, 1978.

CHAPTER 13

DELIRIUM DUE TO INFECTION

INTRODUCTION

Dᴇʟɪʀɪᴜᴍ ᴡᴀs ꜰᴏʀ centuries linked inextricably with infections. Historical review in Chapter 1 highlights this intimate association as it is reflected in the medical literature from Hippocrates on. Delirium was usually defined by the medical writers of the Roman period as transient insanity associated with fever. Galen and his followers differentiated fever delirium from phrenitis, in which the brain was the primary affected organ. Probably in the seventeenth centry the idea took hold that delirium was due to fever, which resulted in increased velocity of the flow of blood to the brain and interfered with its secretions. Delirium was believed to follow such interference and represent a waking dream. This hypothesis was further developed in the eighteenth century by writers such as Erasmus Darwin and John Hunter (*see* Chapter 1).

Fordyce (1), in his famous "Five Dissertations on Fever," devotes much space to delirium. He states that the latter arises frequently in fever and results from interference with sleep. In the slightest degree of delirium "the sleep is attended with numerous and distressing dreams, which render it unrefreshing" (1, p. 39). Fordyce notes that the brain of the patient dying in febrile delirium is usually normal. He distinguishes two types of such delirium: one characterized by fullness of the vessels of the brain, the other—without any detectable pathology of the organ. At about the same time that Fordyce wrote his book, Greiner (2) published one of the most penetrating studies of delirium ever written, entitled "The Dream and the Febrile Insanity." The hypotheses linking fever, sleep, dreaming, and delirium are of great theoretical interest and address fundamental questions not only about the nature of delirium, but also of the organization of the mind.

As late as the beginning of this century the term "fever delirium" was viewed as a prototype of delirium in general. Swift (3) wrote in 1907 that the most common causes of the syndrome were acute infectious diseases, such as typhoid fever, pneumonia, and septicemia. Delirium associated with these diseases was believed to result from a combination of factors including cerebral anemia or hyperemia, toxemia, and hyperpyrexia. The latter was thought to be usually combined with cerebral hyperemia (4).

Infectious delirium used to be classified according to the timing of its onset in relation to fever. Delirium may precede the onset of fever, occur at the height of the latter, come on at the stage of defervescence, or set in at the stage of convalescence (delirium decrementi, delirium of collapse). Delirium at the height of the fever is the most common form (5-7). The delirium of collapse was thought to be due to a combination of anemia of the brain, impaired nutrition, and sleep deprivation (6).

An indication of the importance attached by physicians to delirium associated with infections may be seen in the fact that a subjective experience of delirium in the course of typhoid was the topic of the 1901 Presidential Address to the Neurological Society of London (8). This fascinating account is unique in its wealth of details. The author gives a particularly interesting discussion of the fusion of the dreams and delirious experiences, especially illusions and hallucinations.

In recent years, the frequency and importance of infectious delirium has declined, at least if one is to judge by the dwindling number of references to it in the medical and psychiatric writings. It must not be thought, however, that delirium due to systemic and intracranial infections is a thing of the past. A book on fever published in 1978 devotes several pages to delirium as one of the more prominent nervous system symptoms of infectious diseases (9). The authors discuss meningitis, encephalitis, typhoid fever, typhus, pneumonia, malaria, influenza, rheumatic fever, and puerperal fever as the most important diseases in which delirium is a common complication. In the tropical countries infectious diseases, such as meningitis, encephalitis,

typhoid fever, brucellosis, malaria, lobar pneumonia, trypanosomiasis, etc. are among the most common causes of delirium and
are ubiquitous (10-15). A survey carried out in this country
in the 1920s showed that about 25 percent of the 375 people
questioned had experienced delirium, by far most often in
association with influenza, typhoid fever, and pneumonia (16).
More recent incidence figures are lacking, yet many authors
allude to the high frequency of delirium associated with infection in the elderly persons. A special one-day census conducted
at Los Angeles County General Hospital on March 25, 1965,
showed that thirty-four patients aged over sixty years had
delirium (acute brain syndrome); infection, mostly pneumonia,
accounted for 25 percent of the cases, i.e. it was the most
frequent single cause of delirium (17).

A recent editorial in the *British Medical Journal* points out
that "The current preoccupation with non-infective causes of
organic psychosis and the successful control of infection have
diverted attention away from infective causes, yet these are
relatively common causes in Britain and very common in other
parts of the world" (18). Delirium is a common complication
of febrile illness in childhood. Kanner (19) speaks of the "great
frequency of delirium in children's infections" and underscores
the paucity of relevant literature. He states that delirium can
probably be manifested as early as sixteen months of age. It
can occur in the course of any infectious disease, especially
typhoid fever, rheumatic fever, scarlet fever, pneumonia, septicemia, and erysipelas. It is infrequent in mumps and diphtheria. Bollea (20) adds to this list influenza, salmonella infections, measles, pertussis, brucellosis, chickenpox, and various types
of meningitis and encephalitis.

In conclusion, despite medical advances, infectious diseases
remain a common cause of delirium among the very young, the
poor, and the elderly in this country; and in all age groups in the
tropical and/or underdeveloped countries.

MECHANISMS OF INFECTIOUS DELIRIUM

Old hypotheses about the mechanisms underlying delirium
in infectious diseases mentioned in the preceding section still
stand. Pyrexia and toxemia still need to be considered in the

light of current knowledge. Wallace (21) has classified the relevant pathogenetic mechanisms into three major groups: infections within the CNS giving rise to direct toxic effects, such as necrosis, cerebral inflammation, edema of the brain, and inhibition of enzyme systems; systemic infections causing CNS hypoxia, ischemia, and/or abnormal ionic or acid-base environment of CNS; and reactions to drugs used for treatment of the infection.

Certain recently reported effects of fever are relevant to delirium (9). Hyperthermia induced in animals has been shown to result in an increase in cerebral metabolic rate for oxygen by about 5 percent per 1°C increase in body temperature (22). At constant $PaCO_2$, there is a corresponding increase in cerebral blood flow. It appears that 42°C is a critical temperature level, above which enzyme inactivation occurs (22). Fever, by increasing brain energy demands, could potentially be harmful in the presence of hypoxia, hypoglycemia, or ischemia, that is, conditions of deprivation of oxygen, substrate, or both. Blood pyruvate and lactate are abnormally elevated in human febrile infections (23). This finding has been tentatively explained as being secondary to increased breakdown of glucose and glycogen. Various factors have been suggested to account for these metabolic changes. Increased turnover of cellular constituents, enhanced ionic permeability of excitable membranes, thiamine deficiency, release of adrenaline, and alkalosis have all been postulated (22, 23). Furthermore, fever seems to affect sleep and dreams and the electroencephalogram (24-26). Artificially induced hyperthermia in children, given an intravenous injection of 1 ml. of typhoid vaccine, produced high-voltage, slow waves, increased delta activity, spike-and-wave formations, and some seizure discharges (24). These changes occurred in nearly all cases before the peak of the temperature, which ranged from 102° to 105.6°F. Similar EEG changes have been found in adults during artificial hyperthermia. The EEG abnormalities tend to stay for several days after return to normal body temperature. Karacan et al. (26) have reported that artificially induced fever was accompanied by sleep changes characterized by more awakenings, reduction of stage 4 sleep and of stage 1-REM. The authors speculated that these changes might be due to the effect of fever on the arousal mechanism. These speculations were challenged by later investigators who concluded on the basis of animal experiments that no direct relationship between fever and sleep disturbance existed, and that the latter was most likely due to an action of bacterial products, such as mucopeptide, independent of fever. Thus, it appears that either fever alone, or bacterial toxins, or both can produce abnormalities in the EEG and in sleep cycle. Fever has also been demonstrated to speed up the subjective estimate of time (27). All these effects of elevated temperature may contribute to delirium complicating febrile illness.

Recent experimental work has documented decrements in work performance in subjects with induced tularemia and sandfly fever. The decrements were maximal when symptoms were greatest, did not correlate with fever, and were subject to marked individual variation (28). This interesting work may perhaps throw some light on the common observation that some individuals become delirious with slight fever, while others remain lucid even when the temperature is high. In the experiments just quoted, some subjects performed well in spite of fever. Furthermore, the decrements in performance were not thought to be related causally to the various metabolic changes accompanying fever, such as the adrenocortical response or the metabolic wasting.

In summary, our understanding of the pathophysiology of infectious delirium is negligible. A few suggestive clues, quoted above, lead to more questions rather than provide answers. It appears that the mechanisms underlying infectious delirium are complex and involve the effects of high fever as well as various metabolic and biochemical changes probably related to the organisms and organs implicated in the given infection.

INFECTIONS MORE OFTEN ASSOCIATED
WITH DELIRIUM

Every known infection can give rise to delirium in some patients. To list all infectious diseases that have ever been reported would be both impossible and pointless. Only the more important associations will be referred to. The infections in Table 13-I are relevant to the subject in this country today.

TABLE 13-I

INFECTIOUS DISEASES CAUSING DELIRIUM

1. Systemic Infections
   Pneumonia
   Typhoid
   Typhus and other rickettsial infections
   Acute rheumatic fever
   Malaria
   Influenza
   Brucellosis
   Septicemia and bacteremia
   Scarlet fever
   Infectious hepatitis
   Infective endocarditis

2. Intracranial Infections
   a. Acute bacterial infections
      Meningitis—meningococcal, pneumococcal, Hemophilus influenzae, etc.
      Abscess
      Subdural empyema
   b. Fungal infections
      Cryptococcosis
      Coccidioidomycosis
      Histoplasmosis
      Moniliasis
      Mucormycosis
   c. Acute viral infections
      Meningitis
      Encephalitis
      Poliomyelitis
   d. Postinfectious and postvaccinial encephalomyelitis
   e. Rickettsial infections
      Rocky Mountain spotted fever
   f. Parasitic infections
      Cerebral malaria
      Cysticercosis
      Schistosomiasis
      Trypanosomiasis
      Trichinosis
      Toxoplasmosis
   g. Subacute and chronic infections
      Tuberculosis meningitis
      Neurosyphilis
   h. Miscellaneous
      Sydenham's chorea
      Reye's syndrome

Systemic infections. Among the most important causes of delirium among children and the elderly are systemic infections. As mentioned earlier, children are liable to develop delirium in the course of any febrile illness. Patients over the age of sixty tend to be more ill and develop delirium more readily with infections in general than do young adults. An apparently innocuous urinary tract infection may suffice to precipitate acute brain failure in the elderly.

Pneumonia. Probably the most common infectious disease associated with delirium today is pneumonia. A study carried out in the preantibiotic era found pronounced delirium in about 20 percent of adults suffering from pneumonia (29). All the patients were relatively young, ranging in age from sixteen to fifty. Alcohol abuse and abnormal premorbid personality were stressed as predisposing factors. Alcoholism is still viewed as such a factor today (9). Old age, however, is probably more important. Dunn and Arie (30) warn that in old people, infections, such as pneumonia, may be clinically silent until they are quite advanced and delirium may be the presenting manifestation. Murphy (31) quotes Flint to the effect that lung diseases, mostly pneumonia and chronic bronchitis and emphysema, account for about 20 percent of cases of mental confusion in the elderly. In a special delirium unit, set up in a geriatric hospital, infection accounted for about 10 percent of the cases of confusion. The most common sites were lungs and the urinary tract (32). Pneumonia is the most common postoperative complication in the elderly (33).

Bacteremia. In the elderly, bacteremia may be secondary to urinary infection and catheterization, or other causes, and manifest only delirium and agitation (33). It is important to be aware of this so as to prevent the development of bacteremic shock and death.

Typhoid fever. For a long time typhoid has been known for its frequent association with delirium. A recently published study of Vietnamese adults with typhoid reports delirium in about 20 percent of the patients (34). This study indicates that circulating bacteria and endotoxin do not play a major role in the pathogenesis of this disease. Other recent reports on typhoid fever show that delirium is a very frequent complication of it, is usually severe, and may last up to three weeks after the subsidence of fever (14, 15). Delirium is not a bad prognostic sign. Its severity is not related to the height of the temperature (14).

Brucellosis. Delirium is reported to accompany brucellosis in about 10 percent of the early cases (35). *Typhus* and other rickettsial infections have been notorious for their association with delirium. Guttmann (36) has offered an excellent account of psychiatric complications of typhus personally observed in 430 cases during World War II. Delirium, of various degrees of severity, was commonly observed at all stages of the disease: the prodromal, the height, and the decrudescence. In some cases the symptoms had a very rich, dream-like character. In general, a marked variability of symptoms was striking.

Viral infections. These may give rise to delirium without apparently invading the nervous system (37). Among the earliest symptoms of many viral infections are impairment of concentration and reduction of speed of mental activity. Experimental studies with an induced viral illness, sandfly fever, showed decrements in cognitive performance even though delirium was not apparently manifest (28). These decrements may be regarded as early, prodromal symptoms of impending delirium. Loss of interest in reading, difficulty in marshalling one's thoughts, mild depression, and a tendency to withdraw from activities are additional features of an early phase of a viral infection, such as influenza. Gould (37) rightly views these manifestations as an early stage of delirium. The latter may eventually become fully manifest if the illness becomes severe and/or the patient has pronounced susceptibility to the syndrome. Published case reports often make it impossible to judge if delirium observed in a given patient was a manifestation of encephalitis due to the virus or if it represented an encephalopathy lacking focal neurological signs. Patients with *influenza,* for example, may apparently develop either of these complications and manifest delirium (38). *Acute viral hepatitis* is believed by some authors to do the same (39). It may give rise to encephalitis, meningitis, or meningoencephalitis as well as to delirium in the absence of neurologic signs indicative of direct cerebral involvement by the virus (40, 41). Neuropsychiatric complications of viral hepatitis may occur before the onset of jaundice and cause diagnostic difficulties. This development and such complications are uncommon.

INTRACRANIAL INFECTIONS

These are often accompanied by delirium (42). They should always be considered in the differential diagnosis of the syndrome, especially when its cause is not immediately apparent. Neurological signs are usually present but may be absent, and delirium may be the main presenting clinical feature. This is particularly liable to occur in the case of encephalitis.

Acute encephalitis. Commonly this is associated with delirium of some degree of severity. Acute viral encephalitis may be epidemic or sporadic. The former is most often caused by members of the arbovirus group. The sporadic cases are probably most frequently due to herpes simplex virus (43, 44). Less common causes include enteroviruses, mumps (45), varicella-zoster, rubeola, rubella, cytomegalovirus, rabies, infectious mononucleosis, etc. (46). Acute encephalitis of any etiology is commonly associated with delirium, which may be the presenting manifestation. A good deal of confusion is evident in the literature on encephalitis with regard to the nature of the psychiatric symptoms. The latter may be a strikingly variable and give the impression of a schizophrenic disorder (47-49). Catatonic behavior, marked disinhibition manifested verbally and in action, free expression of normally unconscious wishes and impulses, florid hallucinations, paranoid delusions, depersonalization, regression, and other such features have frequently resulted in the erroneous diagnosis of acute schizophrenia. Yet careful examination can as a rule elicit evidence of fluctuating global cognitive impairment which should help establish the diagnosis of delirium and spur immediate search for the cause of the cerebral disorder.

Typically, the patient presents with a history of headache, rhinorrhea, sore throat, fever, nausea, vomiting, malaise, vertigo, photophobia, and other nonspecific symptoms within preceding several days or weeks. Mental symptoms may develop acutely or subacutely and may be very dramatic in their mode of presentation (47-55). Neurological symptoms may include ataxia, facial weakness, incontinence, tremors, dysphasia, stupor, coma, seizures, etc. (50). On occasion, no neurological symptoms and signs are in evidence initially and the patient may present with delirium only (48-53). Fever is likely to be present at some stage and progress to hyperpyrexia which may respond to barbiturates but not to antipyretic drugs (48). The patient may be extremely uncooperative and thus make examination of mental status and other investigations difficult or even impossible. Intravenous sodium amytal may allow examination in a particularly difficult patient, but the drug may precipitate severe hypotension in an encephalitic patient. The EEG is usually abnormal, with diffuse or focal slowing of background activity. Such abnormalities are the rule in herpes simplex encephalitis (50, 56). In the latter condition, distinctive high-voltage periodic sharp waves may be present and are diagnostically important (56). Abnormalities of the CSF include increased number of white cells but may be absent (50). Spinal fluid cultures for bacteria, viruses, and fungi should be part of diagnostic investigations. Acute and convalescent sera should be examined for titers of viral antibodies.

Infectious mononucleosis. Since mononucleosis is relatively common, it deserves special mention. It may on occasion present with neurological symptoms, including delirium (57-60). Neurological involvement in one series of hospitalized patients occurred in 5.5 percent (60). Headache, drowsiness, diplopia, paraparesis, seizures, and other neurological signs may be found in addition to delirium. Such signs and symptoms may precede, follow, or even occur as the only manifestation of an attack of infectious mononucleosis, and they may recede completely (57). The EEG is usually abnormal and shows focal or generalized slow-wave activity. Atypical lymphocytes and heterophil agglutinins may be found in the CSF. An interesting clinical manifestation of neurological involvement in infectious mononucleosis may be metamorphopsia. The patients experience distortions of perception of size, position, and distance of objects. These symptoms have been labeled the "Alice in Wonderland Syndrome" (58). Disorientation and other features of delirium seem to be absent in these cases.

Encephalitis lethargica. There is considerable historical importance connected with encephalitis lethargica, and a recent review has highlighted features of it which are important for the student of delirium (61). Pandemic of encephalitis in the years 1916-1926 gave rise to a large body of literature that contains a wealth of clinical observations. The latter are relevant to the present theme. Three types of early manifestations were recognized: lethargic, hyperkinetic, and amyostatic. In the course of the disease one form might predominate or all three could occur in various combinations and sequences. Delirium was a feature of all three types, and that demonstrates that this syndrome may display either lethargy, hyperkinesis, or both. Bizarre behavior, restlessness, and excitement were features of the hyperkinetic type. Catatonic schizophrenia was a common diagnostic error in those cases. Furthermore, association with severe sleep disturbances was striking yet patients were reportedly oriented as soon as they became aroused.

Reye's syndrome. An encephalopathy with hepatic involvement occurring in children, Reye's syndrome, is usually associated with delirium (42, 62, 63). The patient first develops fever and upper respiratory infection, and within ten days or so shows headache, vomiting, hyperventilation, and delirium. The latter often progresses to coma. Seizures occur in about 85 percent of cases. Several viruses have been implicated as putative causes of this syndrome, among them herpes virus hominis, hepatitis, influenza viruses A and B (62), and varicella (42). The mortality is on the average at least 50 percent. About 1,000 cases have been reported to date (63). Abnormal elevation of hepatic enzymes in the serum and of blood ammonia, hypoglycemia, and increased intracranial pressure are the usual laboratory findings. Barbiturates have been tried to reverse intracranial hypertension (63).

Meningitis. Of any type, bacterial, viral, or fungal, meningitis may cause delirium (42). Mild delirium, change in personality, and low-grade fever may comprise clinical features of tuberculous or fungal meningitis. Lethargy, stupor, coma, and delirium may dominate the clinical picture of acute bacterial or viral (aseptic) meningitis, but delirium is a less prominent feature of meningitis than of encephalitis (42, 43, 46).

Brain abscess. Typically, brain abscess presents with headache, focal neurological signs, and a reduced level of awareness. In about one-half of patients the symptoms and signs of infection are absent, and the patient presents with a clinical picture suggestive of a space-occupying lesion (64). Delirium may be a manifestation of a rapidly expanding abscess or one accompanied by intracranial hypertension. Presence of a pericranial infection (ear, mastoid, sinuses) or of an infection (such as infective endocarditis) in another part of the body provides suggestive clues for the diagnosis of brain abscess.

Acute poliomyelitis. This infection may be complicated by delirium in about 15 percent of cases, as was observed during the Boston epidemic of 1955 (65). All the delirious patients were in the acute febrile phase of the disease and all had signs of bulbar or bulbospinal involvement. Most of the patients were in respirators. The delirium lasted from five days to six weeks, the average duration being about two weeks. A striking feature displayed by the patients in this study was the pleasurable and nonfrightening quality of their hallucinations. Kinesthetic illusions and hallucinations were unusually common and seemed to be suggested by the various sounds and motions produced by the respirator. The investigators speculated that lesions in the midbrain and diencephalon observed in patients dying of bulbar poliomyelitis might be responsible for delirium in this disorder.

Neurosyphilis. Delirium occurs in about ten percent of patients with neurosyphilis and associated psychiatric disorders (66). Bockner and Coltart (67) observed a confusional state of apparently rapid onset in two of nine cases of the general paralysis of the insane and advise that the latter should be considered in the differential diagnosis of every case of early dementia or confusional state.

Cerebral malaria and *infective endocarditis.* These are discussed in the section on hypoxia in Chapter 12. *Trypanosomiasis* is often accompanied by delirium as well as by disorders of the sleep-wakefulness cycle, usually diurnal somnolence and nocturnal insomnia (10). The EEG is abnormal. *Trichinosis* with central nervous system involvement is accompanied by delirium in 70 percent of cases (68, 69). It occurs in the second week of infection as a manifestation of meningoencephalitis caused by the larvae of Trichinella spiralis. Symptoms of meningitis usually accompany those of delirium. Focal paralysis or paresis, muscular weakness, and even coma may occur. The EEG shows diffuse slowing of background activity (68).

Toxoplasmosis may occasionally present as encephalitis with delirium (70). *Amebic meningoencephalitis* is another rare cause of delirium in this country (43).

Sydenham's chorea and *rheumatic fever*. Both may be accompanied by delirium, but such an association is rarely seen nowadays (71, 72). Some investigators maintain that rheumatic encephalitis may occur and feature delirium. EEG abnormalities are reported in 30 to 70 percent of patients with rheumatic fever with or without delirium or chorea (72). Sydenham's chorea has been observed to be associated with transient cognitive and behavioral disorders (71). Furthermore, complex partial seizures may complicate the course of chorea and be followed by transient delirium (72). A recent study of twenty-eight children with Sydenham's chorea found abnormal EEG's in about 60 percent of them. The most common abnormality was irregular posterior slowing, but several children had sharp epileptic spikes (72). These abnormalities indicate the presence of a diffuse cerebral disorder and suggest that delirium may occur in Sydenham's chorea more frequently than has been recognized to date.

REFERENCES

1. Fordyce, G.: *Five Dissertations on Fever.* 2nd American edition. Boston, Bedlington and Ewer, 1823.
2. Greiner, F.C.: *Der Traum und das fieberhafte Irreseyn.* Altenburg, Brockhaus, 1817.
3. Swift, H.M.: Delirium and delirious states. *Bost Med Surg J 157:* 687-692, 1907.
4. Verco: Delirium. *St Bart Hosp Rep (Lond) 13:*332-342, 1877.
5. Phillips, J.: Delirium. *Clev Med J 8:*531-542, 1909.
6. Weber, H.: On delirium or acute insanity during the decline of acute diseases, especially the delirium of collapse. *Med Chir Trans (Lond) 30:*135-159, 1865.
7. Hirsch, W.: A study of delirium. *New York Med J 70:*109-115, 1899.
8. Mickle, W.M.J.: Mental wandering. *Brain 24:*1-26, 1901.
9. Villaverde, M.M., and MacMillan, C.W.: *Fever. From Symptom to Treatment.* New York, Van Nostrand Reinhold Co., 1978.
10. Antoine, P.: Étude neurologique et psychologique des malades trypanosomes et leur évolution. *Ann Soc Belge Med Trop 57:*227-247, 1977.

11. Black, R.H.: Tropical diseases of psychiatric importance. *Papua New Guinea Med J 19*:19-23, 1976.
12. Buchan, T.: Organic confusional states. *SA Med J 46*:1340-1343, 1972.
13. Editorial: Temporary mental confusion in a medical ward. *C Afr J Med 20*:127-129, 1974.
14. Khosla, S.N., Srivastava, S.C., and Gupta, S.: Neuro-psychiatric manifestations of typhoid. *J Trop Med Hyg 80*:95-98, 1977.
15. **Osuntokun, B.O., Bademosi, O., Ogunremi, K.,** and Wright, S.G.: Neuropsychiatric manifestations of typhoid fever in 959 patients. *Arch Neurol 27*:7-13, 1972.
16. Ziegler, L.H.: A study of delirium. *Am J Psychiatry 6*:105-117, 1926-7.
17. Freedman, D.K., Troll, L., Mills, A.B., and Baker, P.: *Acute Organic Disorder Accompanied by Mental Symptoms.* Sacramento, Calif., Dept. of Mental Hygiene, 1965.
18. Editorial: Organic psychosis. *Br Med J 2*:214-215, 1974.
19. Kanner, L.: *Child Psychiatry.* Fourth edition, Springfield,Ill., Charles C Thomas, 1972, pp. 329-337.
20. Bollea, G.: "Acute Organic Psychoses of Childhood," in Howells, J.G., Ed., *Modern Perspectives in International Child Psychiatry.* New York, Brunner & Mazel, 1971, pp. 706-732.
21. Wallace, J.F.: Infectious delirium. *Southwest Med 50*:181-183, 1969.
22. Siesjö, B.K., Carlsson, C., Hagerdal, M., and Nordstrom, C.H.: Brain metabolism in the critically ill. *Crit Care Med 4*:283-294, 1976.
23. Gilbert, V.E.: Blood pyruvate and lactate during febrile human infections. *Metabolism 17*:943-951, 1968.
24. Baird, H.W., and Garfunkel, J.M.: Electroencephalographic changes in children with artificially induced hyperthermia. *J Ped 48*:28-33, 1956.
25. Kadlecova, O., Masek, K., Rotta, J., and Homma, J.Y.: Fever and sleep cycle changes caused by bacterial products. *J Hyg Epid Micr Immun 18*:472-475, 1974.
26. Karacan, I., Wolff, S.M., Williams, R.L., Hursch, C.J., and Webb, W.B.: The effects of fever on sleep and dreams. *Psychosomatics 9*:331-339, 1968.
27. Alderson, M.J.: Effect of increased body temperature on the perception of time. *Nurs Res 23*:42-49, 1974.
28. Alluisi, E.A., Beisel, W.R., Bartelloni, P.J., and Coates, G.D.: Behavioral effects of tularemia and sandfly fever in man. *J Infect Dis 128*:710-717, 1973.
29. Curtius, F., and Wallenberg, M.: Ueber die Entstehung des Pneumonie-Delirs. *Deutsch Arch Klin Med 176*:100-110, 1934.
30. Dunn, T., and Arie, T.: Mental disturbance in the ill old person. *Br Med J 2*:413-416, 1973.

31. Murphy, E.: The confused elderly patient. *J Irish Med Assoc 61*:99-103, 1968.
32. Fish, F., and Williamson, J.: A delirium unit in an acute geriatric hospital. *Gerontol Clin 6*:71-80, 1964.
33. Polly, S.M., and Sanders, W.E.: Surgical infections in the elderly: prevention, diagnosis, and treatment. *Geriatrics 32*:88-97, 1977.
34. Butler, T., Bell, W.R., Levin, J., et al.: Typhoid fever. *Arch Intern Med 138*:407-410, 1978.
35. Alapin, B.: Psychosomatic and somatopsychic aspects of brucellosis. *J Psychosom Res 20*:339-350, 1976.
36. Guttman, O.: Psychic disturbances in typhus fever. *Psychiatr Q 26*:478-491, 1952.
37. Gould, J.: Virus disease and psychiatric ill-health. *Br J Clin Pract 11*:1-5, 1975.
38. Olivarius, B. de F., and Fog, M.: Neuroinfections in Asian influenza. *Dan Med Bull 6*:248-252, 1959.
39. Liebowitz, S., and Gorman, W.F.: Neuropsychiatric complications of viral hepatitis. *N Engl J Med 246*:932-937, 1952.
40. Friedlander, W.J.: Neurologic signs and symptoms as a prodrome to viral hepatitis. *Neurology 6*:574-579, 1956.
41. Lowy, F.: The neuropsychiatric complications of viral hepatitis. *Can Med Assoc J 30*:237-239, 1965.
42. Oill, P.A., Yoshikawa, T.T., and Yamauchi, T.: Infectious disease emergencies. Part 1: Patients presenting with an altered state of consciousness. *West J Med 125*:36-46, 1976.
43. Butler, I.J., and Johnson, R.T.: Central nervous system infections. *Ped Clin N Am 21*:649-668, 1974.
44. Miller, J.R., and Harter, D.H.: Acute viral encephalitis. *Med Clin N Am 56*:1393-1404, 1972.
45. Keddie, K.M.G.: Toxic psychosis following mumps. *Br J Psychiatry 111*:691-696, 1965.
46. Rosenthal, M.S.: Viral infections of the central nervous system. *Med Clin N Am 58*:593-603, 1974.
47. Stewart, R.M., and Baldessarini, R.J.: Viral encephalopathy and psychosis. *Am J Psychiatry 133*:717, 1976.
48. Weinstein, E.A., Linn, L., and Kahn, R.L.: Encephalitis with a clinical picture of schizophrenia. *Mt Sinai J Med NY 21*:341-354, 1955.
49. Wilson, L.G.: Viral encephalopathy mimicking functional psychosis. *Am J Psychiatry 133*:165-170, 1976.
50. Nolan, D.C., Carruthers, M.M., and Lerner, A.M.: Herpesvirus hominis encephalitis in Michigan. *N Engl J Med 282*:10-13, 1970.
51. Raskin, D.E., and Frank, S.W.: Herpes encephalitis with catatonic stupor. *JAMA 231*:544-546, 1975.
52. Penn, H., Racy, J., Lapham, L., et al.: Catatonic behavior, viral

encephalopathy, and death. *Arch Gen Psychiatry* 27:758-761, 1972.

53. Sobin, A., and Ozer, M.N.: Mental disorders in acute encephalitis. *Mt Sinai J Med NY* 33:73-82, 1966.
54. Misra, P.C., and Hay, G.G.: Encephalitis presenting as acute schizophrenia. *Br Med J* 1:532-533, 1971.
55. Wagonfeld, S., and Dashef, S.S.: The return of memory and personal meaning. *J Am Acad Child Psychiatry* 12:314-332, 1973.
56. Chien, L.T., Boehn, R.M., Robinson, H., et al.: Characteristic early electroencephalographic changes in herpes simplex encephalitis. *Arch Neurol* 34:361-364, 1977.
57. Friedland, R., and Yahr, M.D.: Meningoencephalopathy secondary to infectious mononucleosis. *Arch Neurol* 34:186-188, 1977.
58. Copperman, S.M.: "Alice in Wonderland" syndrome as a presenting symptom of infectious mononucleosis in children. *Clin Pediatr* 16:143-146, 1977.
59. Schlesinger, R.D., and Crelinsten, G.L.: Infectious mononucleosis dominated by neurologic symptoms and signs. *Can Med Assoc J* 117:652-653, 1977.
60. Silverstein, A., Steinberg, G., and Nathanson, M.: Nervous system involvement in infectious mononucleosis. *Arch Neurol* 26:253-258, 1972.
61. Walters, J.H.: Encephalitis lethargica revisited. *J Oper Psychiatry* 8:37-45, 1977.
62. Hochberg, F.H., Nelson, K., and Janzen, W.: Influenza type B-related encephalopathy. *JAMA* 231:817-821, 1975.
63. Safar, P.: Brain resuscitation in metabolic-toxic-infectious encephalopathy. *Crit Care Med* 6:68-70, 1978.
64. Beller, A.J., Sahar, A., and Praiss, I.: Brain abscess. *J Neurol Neurosurg Psychiatr* 36:757-768, 1973.
65. Holland, J.C.B., and Coles, M.R.: Neuropsychiatric aspects of acute poliomyelitis. *Am J Psychiatry* 114:54-63, 1957.
66. Arieti, S., and Reiser, M.F., Eds.: *American Handbook of Psychiatry*, 2nd edition, Vol. 4. New York, Basic Books, 1975, p. 138.
67. Bockner, S., and Coltart, N.: New cases of G.P.I. *Br Med J* 1:18-20, 1961.
68. Barr, R.: Human trichinosis. *Can Med Assoc J* 95:912-916, 1966.
69. Dalessio, D.J., and Wolff, H.G.: Trichinella spiralis infection of the central nervous system. *Arch Neurol* 4:407-417, 1961.
70. Minto, A., and Roberts, F.J.: The psychiatric complications of toxoplasmosis. *Lancet* 1:1180-1182, 1959.
71. Gatti, F.M., and Rosenheim, E.: Sydenham's chorea associated with transient intellectual impairment. *Am J Dis Child* 118:915-918, 1969.
72. Chien, L.T., Economides, A.N., and Lemmi, H.: Sydenham's chorea and seizures. *Arch Neurol* 35:382-385, 1978.

Additional References

Brown, N.K., and Thompson, D.J. Non-treatment of fever in extended-care facilities. *New Engl J Med 300*:1246-1250, 1979.

Chandra, B. Treatment of disturbances of consciousness caused by measles encephalitis with levodopa. *Eur Neurol 17*:265-270, 1978.

Everett, B.A., Kusske, J.A., Rush, J.L., and Pribram, H.W. Cryptococcal infection of the central nervous system. *Surg Neurol 8*:157-163, 1979.

Lees, A.W., and Tyrrell, W.F. Severe cerebral disturbance in legionnaires' disease. *Lancet 2*:1336-1337, 1978.

Linneman, C.C., and Janson, P.J. The clinical presentations of Rocky Mountain spotted fever. *Clin Pediatr 17*:673-679, 1978.

Reding, M., Ohr, J., Quigley, H., and Lorenzo, A.S. Rocky Mountain spotted fever presenting as a generalized seizure and acute hallucinosis. *Nebr Med J 63*:179-184, 1978.

Rubin, R.L. Adolescent infectious mononucleosis with psychosis. *J Clin Psychiatry 39*:773-775, 1978.

Torres, J.R., Sanders, C.V., Strub, R.L., and Black, F.W. Cat-scratch disease causing reversible encephalopathy. *JAMA 240*:1628-1629, 1978.

Varma, V.K., Nakra, B.R.S., and Singh, S. Post-febrile "organic" psychosis. *Patna J Med 46*:153-158, 1972.

Williams, B.B., and Learner, A.M. Some previously unrecognized features of herpes simplex virus encephalitis. *Neurology 28*:1193-1196, 1978.

CHAPTER 14

DELIRIUM DUE TO TOXIC AGENTS

A GREAT MANY exogenous substances can give rise to delirium. Those agents currently being used as drugs are discussed in Chapter 10. In this chapter industrial toxic agents are dealt with. They may cause delirium either as a result of accidental exposure, mostly at work, or of intentional intake for the purpose of achieving an unusual or exciting experience. A whole range of industrial solvents have been abused by children and adolescents in recent years, and it is important to be familiar with their deliriogenic and other toxic effects.

The literature on the psychological or psychiatric effects of toxic agents is, on the whole, quite inadequate. Psychiatrists have displayed almost no interest in this aspect of psychopathology. The literature reflects this. It is marked by poor description of the mental symptoms and by inconsistent and highly ambiguous terminology. Terms such as "behavioral changes," "mental effects," "confusion," "psychosis," etc. are used by the various writers without any attempt to define them and to specify operational or diagnostic criteria ruling the application of the given term. As a result, it is often impossible to know to what type of mental phenomena the particular writer is referring. Books and monographs on toxicology, both general and industrial, are quite uneven and inconsistent in their treatment of psychopathological effects of chemical agents. Speaking specifically of delirium, some textbooks go so far as to list toxic substances that have been reported to cause it (1, 2), while texts such as the massive and authoritative work by Patty (3) do not even include the word "delirium" in the index. Von Oettingen (2) lists over sixty agents, including drugs, industrial chemicals, poisonous plants and mushrooms, and venoms, which have been reported to cause delirium. That author separately lists substances that give rise to "confusion and disorientation" and to "hallucinations," respectively. Such separation is redundant, since delirium typically features disorientation and confusion and is often associated with hallucinations.

Casarett and Doull (4) discuss delirium as one of the most common manifestations of the action of a toxic agent on the nervous system and more specifically on the reticular formation. These authors emphasize that direct evidence in support of the statement that delirium results from the action on the reticular system is lacking, but such an action may be assumed in view of the fact that the syndrome is known to be associated with generalized damage to subcortical white matter. While these statements are open to question and are probably invalid, one welcomes the authors' attempt to give delirium a fairly prominent place among the behavioral effects of toxic chemicals. Such treatment of the syndrome is fully justified in view of the published observations on the toxic effects of numerous agents which are stated to include delirium, confusion, or disorientation, or all three of these manifestations. There is little doubt that delirium is one of the most frequent symptoms of the effects on central nervous system exerted by environmental toxic agents.

The incidence of delirium due to industrial poisons is unknown. The writer has seldom encountered it during twenty years of work as a psychiatric consultant to medical and surgical wards of a general hospital. In view of the inadequate description and ambiguous terminology mentioned earlier, it should surprise nobody that reliable statistical data are lacking. Study of toxicological literature and clinical impressions lead one to believe that simple intoxication is the most common behavioral syndrome induced by chronic poisoning with many, or most, industrial poisons. This disorder features mild cognitive impairment, usually decreased alertness and ability to concentrate, reduced efficiency of performance on various psychomotor and vigilance tasks, irritability, apathy, somnolence, etc. It appears that delirium is the most common mental disorder manifested by a person who is acutely and relatively severely poisoned or by one who is chronically intoxicated but suffers acute cerebral decompensation as a result of an increase in the concentration of the toxic agent in the body, or of the exposure to some other potentially deliriogenic factor. It is conceivable that psychological stress may play such a decompensating role too. A chronically intoxicated person usually experiences some prodromal symptoms before developing delirium. It appears that, regardless of the toxic agent involved, such prodromal symptoms feature increasing disturbance of the sleep-wakefulness cycle, characterized by a combination of somnolence during the day and insomnia, with or without vivid dreams or nightmares, at night. Fleeting hallucinations, either hypnagogic or merging with dreams on awakening, tend to follow and often constitute a prelude to a full-blown delirium. The latter is always transient and may resolve spontaneously to be followed by return to a state of chronic simple intoxication with the implicated toxic chemical. Delirium may be the first event resulting in a proper evaluation of the patient and a diagnosis of chronic poisoning.

One gets the impression that severe behavioral toxicity, including delirium, has become less frequent in industry in the past thirty years or so (5). It is not known if this decline in the incidence of delirium is apparent or real. Advances in the control of industrial hazards and in occupational hygiene and medicine have likely achieved some reduction in the incidence of severe behavioral toxicity in industry. At the same time, there has been an unprecedented recent increase in the frequency of abuse of various industrial chemicals, mostly aliphatic and aromatic solvents, and of the related mental disorders, including delirium. This is added reason for discussing the syndrome in relation to its chemical causes other than medical drugs. Since no monographs on this topic seem to exist, the writer had to rely on the standard textbooks of general and industrial toxicology as guides to the relevant literature. In many cases the latter is too ambiguous and vague in its reporting of mental effects of poisons to allow reasonable judgment of whether or not a given agent can give rise to delirium and does so with any frequency. Only those toxic agents for which the deliriogenic potential has been fairly well established have been included here. No attempt has been made to cite every industrial chemical that has ever been reported or implied to give rise to delirium. In many cases the author has interpreted reports that a given agent can cause "confusion" to indicate that it is in fact deliriogenic.

METALS AND METALLOIDS

Arsenic. Hydrogen arsenide (arsine) is reported by some authors to cause delirium (2), but other writers do not indicate that arsenic or any of its compounds can give rise to this syndrome (5).

Lead. "Encephalopathia saturnina" was the name attached to the cerebral form of plumbism in 1850 (5). It is the rarest form of this disease in adults. Delirium, convulsions, and coma are among its chief manifestations. This form of lead poisoning has almost disappeared (5). An acute attack of encephalopathy is sometimes followed by dementia. The pathology is that of a meningo-encephalopathy. Lead encephalopathy is currently more often seen in children than in adults and usually results from ingestion of peeling or flaking lead-based paint. Such paint used to be applied prior to the mid-1950s and is currently found mostly in inner city areas. The onset of lead poisoning in children is usually insidious (6). Convulsions, stupor, and coma usually develop after a period of nondescript symptoms, such as fatigue, anorexia, irritability, motor unsteadiness, abdominal pain, etc.

In adults, tetraethyl lead poisoning is probably the most important cause of acute lead encephalopathy (7, 8). In milder cases, headache, anxiety, and insomnia with disturbing dreams are the usual symptoms. In more severe encephalopathy, delirium with hallucinations, excitement, and paranoid delusions is common. The severity of these symptoms is not apparently correlated with total blood-lead levels or porphyrin abnormalities (7). In one study, blood-lead levels ranged from 64.2 to 92.5 μg. per 100 g. (7). Urinary excretion of lead is increased. Tetraethyl lead is added to gasoline as an anti-knock agent. Poisoning with it has been most often reported in those who blend the chemical with gasoline, or clean tanks which had contained leaded gasoline. The agent can cause acute plumbism when inhaled or absorbed through the skin (5). The incidence of encephalopathy due to industrial exposure to tetraethyl lead is relatively low at present thanks to the precautions applied by industries involved. A new source of such encephalopathy is gasoline sniffing by children and adolescents (9). Blood levels of lead are elevated and those of erythrocytic delta-aminolevulinic acid markedly decreased in such cases. The EEG is diffusely slowed. Treatment of the acute encephalopathy in children has involved administration of BAL and EDTA, followed by penicillamine (9).

Mercury. Mercurialism is one of the oldest forms of industrial intoxication. Elemental mercury vaporizes readily at room temperature and may be inhaled. Poisoning has occurred in miners of mercury, among hatters, in makers of solder for dry batteries and employees of mercury thermometer and barometer manufacturing plants, in laboratory workers, etc. (5). Inorganic mercury can give rise to both acute and chronic intoxication. Headaches, fatigue, shyness, tremor, and irritability (erethism) are characteristic features (10). Elemental mercury is most likely to cause intoxication by inhalation of the vapor. It has a high degree of fat solubility and may affect cerebral blood vessels by altering their permeability (11). Intoxicated patients display poor concentration and recent memory deficits with well-preserved intellectual function (11, 12). Delirium does not seem to be a feature of inorganic mercurialism.

Intoxication with organic compounds of mercury, used most extensively as fungicides, is more likely to involve the nervous system than is that due to inorganic compounds and elemental mercury. Methyl mercury compounds are marked for affecting the nervous system alone. They are capable of penetrating the blood-brain barrier and have a low toxic threshold. Intoxication with methylmercury is typically of slow onset and features ataxia, dysarthria, paresthesias, weakness, tremor, visual and hearing defects, irritability, depression, delirium, stupor, and coma (13, 14). Delirium seems to be a relatively uncommon manifestation of mercurialism (5). Simple intoxication, amnestic syndrome, dementia, and organic personality disorder seem to be the more usual mental disorders in mercury poisoning.

Nickel. Acute poisoning due to inhalation exposure to nickel carbonyl is said to consist of two phases: first, headache, dizziness, nausea and vomiting; and second, chest pain, cough, mental confusion, and convulsions (5). Thus, it appears that delirium (mental confusion) may be induced by nickel carbonyl.

Thallium. Poisoning with this metal may occur as a result of ingestion of rat poison. The initial symptoms of thallotoxicosis are often neuropsychiatric in nature and may include delirium as well as ataxia, tremor, convulsions, etc. (15). Alopecia, a common manifestation of thallium intoxication, usually occurs fifteen to thirty days after ingestion and is preceded by neurologic symptoms.

ALIPHATIC HYDROCARBONS

The aliphatic series of these compounds includes the saturated and the unsaturated ones. The saturated series includes methane, ethane, propane, and butane gases as well as liquids and solids. Methane is biologically inert and exerts a toxic effect only by replacing oxygen. Saturated hydrocarbons from propane through the octanes have increasingly strong narcotic properties and may cause confusion among the various effects on the nervous system (5). Vertigo, headache, convulsions, and coma may result from exposure to vapors of these compounds.

HALOGENATED HYDROCARBONS

These compounds are widely used in industry as solvents and vehicles by which chlorine is used in the manufacture of plastics, pesticides, etc. Several of them are known to induce delirium.

Methyl chloride. Methyl chloride is a gas used mainly as a chemical intermediate and as a foaming agent in the production of foamed plastics. It is a central nervous system depressant whose toxic symptoms include drowsiness, blurred vision, dizziness, ataxia, nightmares, restlessness, and delirium (16, 17). Convulsions and coma may occur.

Methylene chloride. This is used as a solvent and extracting agent. It is highly volatile, and its inhalation is said to lead to "drunkenness" (5). Exposure to this agent results in sustained elevation of carboxyhemoglobin (18).

Ethylene dichloride. This is used as a solvent. Intoxication may feature "mental confusion" (3).

Carbon tetrachloride. Refrigerants, solvents, and aerosol propellants are synthesized by carbon tetrachloride. It is one of the most toxic of the common solvents, with deleterious effects on the nervous system, hepatic function, and kidneys (5, 19). The neurological symptoms and signs tend to appear early in cases of acute poisoning and may dominate the clinical picture. Headache, vertigo, weakness, blurring of vision, tremor, paresthesias, and drowsiness are the initial manifestations, to be followed by delirium (19). Coma and death may result, especially in alcoholics.

Trichloroethylene. This is used in large quantities as a metal degreaser and dry cleaning agent. It is readily absorbed and excreted by the lungs. Absorption of this compound results in narcosis. There may be symptoms of euphoria and excitement, dizziness, drowsiness, delirium, and loss of consciousness (5). Subjects exposed to this agent usually complain of fatigue, gastrointestinal symptoms, flushing of the face, sweating, and palpitations (20). There is often intolerance of alcohol and tobacco.

Tetrachloroethylene. The main dry cleaning solvent for clothing, which is also used for degreasing, is tetrachloroethylene. It has narcotic properties and other toxic effects which resemble closely those of trichloroethylene (5).

Methyl bromide. Methyl bromide is utilized as a fumigant and insecticide. Acute exposure produces nausea, vomiting, and headache. Neurological symptoms are common and have been observed to fall into three stages: 1. premonitory stage with headache, vertigo, gait disturbance; 2. cerebral irritation stage with *delirium*, twitching, and seizures; 3. recovery stage, which may last several years and feature hallucinations, memory impairment, aphasia, and incoordination (21). Delirium is a common feature of acute methyl bromide poisoning. Coma and death may result. Methyl bromide encephalopathy in a child may resemble Reye's syndrome (21).

AROMATIC HYDROCARBONS

The aromatic series of hydrocarbons is based upon benzene and molecules which incorporate one or more benzene rings. Their chief sources are coal and petroleum. They are mostly used as solvents and as synthetic substrates.

Benzene. This is a volatile, highly flammable liquid. It is often present in gasoline, thinners, and solvents. Inhalation of benzene vapor leads to narcosis, hepatic and renal damage, myocardial sensitization to catecholamines, and aplastic anemia (22). Acute toxicity may feature exhilaration, dizziness, headache, staggering gait, delirium, and loss of consciousness (22, 23). Shortness of breath, irritability, and unsteadiness on walking may persist for several weeks after acute intoxication. Acute benzene intoxication has been called "benzol jag" by industrial workers on account of its symptoms resembling drunken behavior with confusion (5).

Toluene, xylene, and *styrene.* These are less toxic than benzene. Acute toxicity involves central nervous system depression. The whole range of manifestations of narcosis may be produced. They range in severity from euphoria, reduced psychomotor performance and fatigue, to delirium and loss of consciousness upon high-level exposure. Brain damage may occur as a result of deliberate abuse of toluene (23). Sudden death, apparently due to cardiac arrhythmias, has occurred among glue sniffers.

MIXED ALIPHATIC-AROMATIC HYDROCARBONS

Gasoline (petrol). Gasoline is a mixture of C_4 to C_{12} hydrocarbons, including parafins, olefins, naphthenes, and aromatics. Inhalation of gasoline vapors may result in narcosis. Deliberate inhalation or sniffing has become a serious health problem (24-27). It has induced an "inhalation psychosis" or delirium (24). The toxicity of gasoline depends on its composition. Abusers of it have reported that fifteen to twenty breaths of the vapor may produce intoxication for five to six hours (25). Symptoms come on within five minutes and include a pleasant euphoria. Visual hallucinations and illusions, which are sometimes very rich and vivid, tend to follow (26). Other reported perceptual disturbances have included kinesthetic hallucinations of spinning, floating, moving, etc.; illusion of physical lightness; metamorphopsia; micropsia; hyperacusis; altered colors; and auditory and tactile hallucinations (26). Some degree of disorientation, memory impairment, and other cognitive deficits are found depending on the severity of intoxication. Thus, the "inhalation psychosis" is, strictly speaking, nothing but delirium (24). High gasoline concentration may cause coma and death. Repeated intoxication may lead to progressive dementia and cerebellar ataxia (27). Lead encephalopathy may follow sniffing of leaded gasoline (8).

Physical signs and symptoms accompany progressive stages of acute gasoline intoxication. They include dizziness, nausea, sneezing, coughing, and flushed skin in the induction state; tinnitus, blurred vision, diplopia, cramps, headache, and pallor in the early CNS depression stage; drowsiness, ataxia, slurred speech, and nystagmus in the medium CNS depression stage; and stupor, epileptiform seizures and coma in the late CNS depression stage (28). The EEG showed diffuse slowing of the background activity in some of the reported cases (24, 26).

AROMATIC NITRO COMPOUNDS

Dinitrophenols. These have been used as herbicides, insecticides, and other pesticides. Acute poisoning is manifested by restlessness, anxiety, flushed skin, tachycardia, hyperthermia, headache, weakness, vertigo, insomnia, and delirium. Tremors, convulsions, and coma may occur (29). Fatal hyperpyrexia may develop.

Trinitrotoluene, or *TNT.* This compound, a powerful explosive, has been occasionally reported to cause delirium. Its more common toxic effects include headache, insomnia, and generalized weakness.

ESTERS

Dimethyl sulphate. An important alkylating agent, dimethyl sulphate is primarily an irritant which produces inflammation of the eyes, upper airway, and skin. It has been reported to cause delirium (3).

Glyceryl trinitrate. Hypotension, tachycardia, nausea, vomiting, and headache ("powder head") are produced by glyceryl trinitrate. More intense exposure has given rise to confusion, especially in conjunction with alcohol (5).

Amyl nitrite. Commonly used for the treatment of angina

pectoris, amyl nitrite has recently become abused by sensation seekers. It is reportedly inhaled during sexual intercourse just before orgasm so as to intensify and prolong it (23). Its side effects include dizziness, headache, hypotension, and syncope. Methemoglobinemia may be produced. The drug may cause confusion and hallucinations.

ALCOHOLS

Methyl alcohol (methanol) is extensively used in industry as a solvent, etc. Intoxication is usually the result of intentional ingestion. The onset of symptoms is typically delayed by as many as seventy-two hours. Severe acidosis is produced. Symptoms include visual disturbances, such as blurred vision, spots and flashes before the eyes, photophobia, etc.; headache; paresthesias; nausea and vomiting; and dyspnea. Confusion, amnesia, lethargy, delirium, stupor, and coma may all develop in the acidotic patients (5, 30). Death may occur. Prompt alkalinization has been lifesaving and is the mainstay of treatment. Peritoneal dialysis may have to be carried out.

HYDROGEN SULFIDE

This highly poisonous gas is formed by the decay of organic matter containing sulphur, such as sewage and industrial waste water in tanneries, abattoirs, glue factories, etc. It is also present in natural gas from some fields. Production and refining of high-sulfur-petroleum is said to be the greatest source of danger from hydrogen sulphide in the United States at the present time (5). The gas has rapid action and causes severe histotoxic anoxia by inhibition of cytochrome oxidase. In lower concentrations (50 to 500 ppm) it acts primarily as a respiratory irritant. It also irritates the conjunctiva and produces severe conjunctivitis with keratitis. Photophobia is a common symptom of the mildest form of poisoning. Exposure to 1,000 ppm results in rapid collapse and imminent central respiratory paralysis, which is the cause of death. Exposure to concentration insufficient to result in loss of consciousness may cause delirium and polyneuritis.

CARBON DISULFIDE (CS₂)

This colorless, transparent fluid of sweetish, aromatic odor is a major industrial toxic agent. It is currently used mostly in the manufacture of viscose rayon, cold vulcanization of rubber, etc. Reports of severe mental symptoms in workers poisoned with CS_2 appeared as early as the 1860s and were labeled "carbon disulfide neurosis" (31). In 1892, Peterson reported on three cases of what he called "acute mania from inhaling carbon bisulfide," in what was the first American paper on the psychiatric toxicity of CS_2. This disorder was nothing but delirium. Subsequent reports from Italy indicated that about one-half of the CS_2 poisoned workers suffered from "psychoses," which apparently represented cases of delirium (5). Following months or even years of exposure, some workers would suddenly become delirious and display excitement and hallucinations. A whole range of mental symptoms have been described: irritability, depression, delirium, dementia, loss of memory, changes in personality, insomnia, bad dreams, impotence and loss of libido, and temper outbursts (5, 31). In addition to the mental disturbances, the workers were reported to suffer from a whole gamut of physical symptoms, such as visual disturbances, gastric complaints, ataxia, tremors, etc. It has gradually become apparent that chronic exposure to CS_2 has atherogenic effect, with evidence of coronary heart disease (31).

Studies, mostly by European workers, have clarified to some extent the bewildering medley of psychiatric symptoms reported by the earlier observers. Hanninen (32) carried out psychological tests among viscose rayon workers and concluded that the psychological changes in those poisoned by CS_2 consist of slowly developing intellectual decline accompanied by depression. The patients show disturbances in motor functions, decreased alertness and vigilance, impaired general intellectual performance, and low productivity. As a result, occupational and social performance of the poisoned worker suffers. Mancuso and Locke (33) studied viscose rayon workers in the United States and found a higher suicide rate among them. It is hypothesized that chronic exposure to CS_2 may lead to latent effects which predispose the person to the development of a mental disorder and/or suicide.

Thus, it appears that acute CS_2 poisoning, which is rare in the United States, may feature delirium. The much more common and important chronic poisoning results in mild or moderate dementia, or an organic personality or affective (depressive) disorder, on which an episode of full-blown delirium may be superimposed due to increased intoxication or some other factor. In addition, chronic impairment of cognitive and other psychological functions is likely to induce a depressive response in at least some of the affected individuals.

The pathophysiology underlying the mental changes in CS_2 poisoning is not fully understood. The agent is believed to interfere with certain respiratory enzymes in the brain and thus with cellular metabolism. Inhibition of cerebral monoamine oxidase has been reported. A decrease in the number of cortical ganglion cells has been observed in some cases of CS_2 poisoning (31, 33).

FLUOROHYDROCARBONS

These compounds have narcotic properties at high concentrations. A syndrome called "polymer-fume fever" has been described in those exposed to decomposition products of fluoroplastics (5). Fluorohydrocarbons of the Freon type are used as propellants for deodorant sprays. Inhalation of the latter has resulted in confusion, hallucinations, excitement, general impairment of mental activity, and muscular incoordination (34). These reported mental symptoms seem to amount to delirium.

SOLVENT ABUSE

Solvent abuse has been defined as the deliberate inhalation of volatile organic substances other than the conventional anesthetic gases (35). The chemicals involved fall into three groups: 1. organic solvents; 2. hydrocarbon mixtures such as gasoline and lighter fuel; and 3. aerosol propellants. Gasoline sniffing and toxicity have been discussed. Abuse of other organic solvents remains to be briefly reviewed.

Prior to the current epidemic of solvent abuse there had been outbreaks of illicit inhalation of anesthetic gases, such as nitrous oxide and ether. During the past fifteen years a dramatic increase in the abuse of volatile solvents has occurred. A wide range of products have been abused: various cements, fingernail polish remover, ink, lacquer thinners, lighter fluid, cleaning fluid, gasoline, antifreeze, virtually all products packaged in aerosol cans, and pure solvents (toluene, acetone, ethyl ether) (28, 35). The chemical constituents of the abused products include a variety of aliphatic, aromatic, and halogenated hydrocarbons; ketones; esters, such as amyl acetate; alcohols, such as butyl and propyl alcohols; glycols, for example methyl Cellosolve acetate; and ethers (35). Toxic effects of these assorted agents encompass those on the kidney and liver function, blood, and the nervous system (23, 28, 35). The nature and incidence of the induced behavioral abnormalities have been discussed in many publications but remain unclear. Glasser (24) has proposed that acute intoxication from inhalation of organic solvents be called "inhalation psychosis," which, he asserts, "appears to be a toxic delirium." Some of the most frequently implicated chemicals, such as toluene, carbon tetrachloride, and methyl cellosolve acetate, have already been discussed separately as potentially deliriogenic agents. Their combinations encountered in the various abused products may be expected to induce delirium when they are inhaled in high concentrations for the deliberate purpose of achieving a euphoric or hallucinatory or delirious state. The EEG in the state of acute intoxication with some of these agents has been reported to show reduced frequency of the background activity (24). Yet, as Wyse (28) points out, the EEG abnormalities in solvent abuse tend to be transient and not always present. The pathophysiology of solvent inhalation is incompletely understood. The inhaled vapors enter the blood rapidly and pass the blood-brain barrier to exert their neurotoxic effects. Hydrocarbons in general are central nervous system depressants, but excitement tends to precede narcosis and loss of consciousness. The sniffer tends to experience initially a feeling of euphoria and excitement, followed by hallucinations and delusions. As the concentration of the inhaled vapor increases, drowsiness and progressive reduction of alertness and awareness develop and finally loss of consciousness sets in. These central nervous system effects resemble the stages of diethyl ether anesthesia (28).

Subjective experiences of the sniffers usually consist of pleasant euphoria and excitement, often with a sense of strength and personal invulnerability. It is during this stage that self-mutilation and violence may occur. The hallucinations are visual and/or auditory and said to be experienced by about 50 percent of the sniffers. They are typically pleasant and often grandiose in the sense that the inhaler figures in them as a hero. Hallucinations may also be frightening and involve fierce animals, threatening ghost-like figures, etc. (28). Illusions or hallucinations of floating or spinning are common. Distortions of space and visual perceptions often occur. It is not known to what extent cognitive impairment accompanies these affective and perceptual abnormalities, and thus how often delirium results from inhaling solvent vapors.

SYNTHETIC ORGANIC INSECTICIDES

Chlorinated cyclic hydrocarbons (such as DDT, chlordane, dieldrin, etc.), *organophosphorus compounds,* and *carbamates* represent the main classes of these pesticides. All of them can cause poisoning in man and give rise to similar neurotoxic manifestations. Biskind and Bieber (36) described thirty years ago neuropsychiatric manifestation of DDT as featuring "unbearable emotional turbulence," and symptoms such as excitement, irritability, confusion, anxiety, inability to attend, forgetfulness, and depression. These investigators stressed "extreme apprehensiveness" as a common characteristic of DDT poisoning. Many somatic symptoms were found to accompany the mental disorder, among them nausea, vomiting, diarrhea, joint pains, cough, paresthesias, tachycardia, etc. The word "delirium" is never mentioned in this context, but the mental disorder described by various authors bears some resemblance to it.

Carbamate pesticides, such as methomyl, aminocarb, and promecarb, are reversible inhibitors of cholinesterase and as such give rise to toxic effects resembling those of the organophosphate insecticides. Poisoning by anticholinesterases was already discussed in Chapter 6. It was pointed out that the nature of the psychiatric syndrome induced by cholinesterase inhibitors was unclear. Difficulty in concentration, "mental confusion," drowsiness, difficulty in thinking and in focusing attention, memory impairment, and psychomotor slowing are symptoms reported to have characterized both acute and chronic poisoning with organophosphate pesticides (37). In addition, depression, lethargy, anxiety, irritability, and increased dreaming have been frequently observed in the intoxicated subjects. Gershon and Shaw (38), referring to the effects of an organophosphorus insecticide on schizophrenics, state clearly: "This was not a form of delirium, and consciousness was not impaired." These authors state that their own results were similar in that only two forms of psychiatric illness could be observed in intoxicated persons, i.e. depressive and schizophrenic reactions. At the same time, Gershon and Shaw emphasize that their patients displayed severe memory impairment and difficulty in concentration, that is, symptoms strongly suggestive of an organic mental disorder.

In conclusion, review of the literature leaves little doubt that organophosphorus insecticides can give rise to an organic brain syndrome, the precise nature of which is unclear. Delirium, amnestic syndrome, dementia, or a syndrome for which there is currently no label in the classification of mental disorders might be the appropriate designation for the observed mental symptoms, but published reports do not allow a definite conclusion. One notes that anticholinesterases exert an excitatory action on the EEG in the sense that desynchronization is induced, and there is an increase in the frequency and a decrease in the voltage of the background activity (39). Yet it appears that when toxic doses of these agents are absorbed, then a decrease, instead of an increase, in alertness is induced, and even coma may result (40). It follows that, theoretically, delirium could be induced by organophosphorus insecticides if a sufficiently large dose of one of these compounds is absorbed. On the whole, however, behavioral effects of these agents have not been definitely clarified. As Clark (41) has pointed out, the reported observations on humans are so contradictory and inconsistent that no definite trends have emerged. The most surprising finding is the relative paucity of evidence for disturbed mental function in the presence of profound reduction of acetylcholinesterase.

REFERENCES

1. Arena, J.M.: *Poisoning.* 3rd edition. Springfield, Ill., Charles C Thomas, 1974.
2. Oettingen, W.F., von: *Poisoning. A Guide to Clinical Diagnosis and Treatment.* 2nd edition. Philadelphia, W.B. Saunders Co., 1958, pp. 89-90.
3. Patty, F.A.: *Industrial Hygiene and Toxicology.* New York, Wiley (Interscience), 1962.
4. Casarett, L.J., and Doull, J., Eds.: *Toxicology. The Basic Science of Poisons.* New York, MacMillan Publishing Co., Inc., 1975.
5. Hamilton, A., and Hardy, H.L.: *Industrial Toxicology.* 3rd edition. Acton, Mass., Publishing Sciences Group, Inc., 1974.
6. Needleman, H.L.: Lead poisoning in children: neurologic implications of widespread subclinical intoxication. *Semin Psychiatry* 5:47-53, 1973.
7. Beattie, A.D., and Moore, M.R.: Tetraethyl-lead poisoning. *Lancet* 2:12-15, 1972.
8. Kahan, V.L.: Paranoid states occurring in leaded-petrol handlers. *J Ment Sci* 96:1043-1047, 1950.
9. Boeckx, R.L., Postl, B., and Coodin, F.J.: Gasoline sniffing and tetraethyl lead poisoning. *Pediatrics* 60:140-145, 1977.
10. Felton, J.S., Kahn, E., Salick, B., et al.: Heavy metal poisoning: mercury and lead. *Ann Intern Med* 76:779-792, 1972.
11. Vroom, F.Q., and Greer, M.: Mercury vapour intoxication. *Brain* 95:305-318, 1972.
12. Ross, W.D., Gechman, A.S., Sholiton, M.C., and Paul, H.S.: Need for alertness to neuropsychiatric manifestations of inorganic mercury poisoning. *Compr Psychiatry* 18:595-598, 1977.
13. Joselow, M.M., Louria, D.B., and Browder, A.A.: Mercurialism: environmental and occupational aspects. *Ann Intern Med* 76:119-130, 1972.
14. Maghazaji, H.I.: Psychiatric aspects of methylmercury poisoning. *J Neurol Neurosurg Psychiatry* 37:954-958, 1974.
15. Bank, W.J., Pleasure, D.E., Suzuki, K., et al.: Thallium poisoning. *Arch Neurol* 26:456-464, 1972.
16. Hansen, H., Weaver, N.K., and Venable, F.S.: Methyl chloride intoxication. *Arch Industr Hyg Occup Med* 8:328-334, 1953.

17. Scharnweber, H.C., Spears, G.N., and Cowles, S.R.: Chronic methyl chloride intoxication in six industrial workers. *J Occup Med 16*: 112-113, 1974.
18. Stewart, R.D., Fisher, T.N., Hosko, M.J., et al.: Experimental human exposure to methylene chloride. *Arch Environ Health 25*:342-348, 1972.
19. Stevens, H., and Forster, F.M.: Effect of carbon tetrachloride on the nervous system. *Arch Neurol Psychiatry 70*:635-649, 1953.
20. Smith, G.F.: The investigation of the mental effects of trichlorethylene. *Ergonomics 13*:580-586, 1970.
21. Shield, L.K., Coleman, T.L., and Markesbery, W.R.: Methyl bromide intoxication: Neurologic features, including simulation of Reye syndrome. *Neurology 27*:959-962, 1977.
22. Haley, T.J.: Evaluation of the health effects of benzene inhalation. *Clin Toxicol 11*:531-548, 1977.
23. Bruckner, J.V., and Peterson, R.G.: "Toxicology of Aliphatic and Aromatic Hydrocarbons," in Sharp, C.W., and Brehm, M.L., Eds., *Review of Inhalants: Euphoria to Dysfunction*. Washington, D.C., National Institute on Drug Abuse, 1977, pp. 124-163.
24. Glaser, F.B.: Inhalation psychosis and related states. *Arch Gen Psychiatry 14*:315-322, 1966.
25. Poklis, A., and Burkett, C.D.: Gasoline sniffing: a review. *Clin Toxicol 11*:35-41, 1977.
26. Tolan, E.J., and Lingl, F.A.: "Model psychosis" produced by inhalation of gasoline fumes. *Am J Psychiatry 120*:757-761, 1964.
27. Valpey, R., Sumi, S.M., Copass, M.K., and Goble, G.J.: Acute and chronic progressive encephalopathy due to gasoline sniffing. *Neurology 28*:507-508, 1978.
28. Wyse, D.G.: Deliberate inhalation of volatile hydrocarbons: a review. *Can Med Assoc J 108*:71-74, 1973.
29. Baker, A.B., and Tichy, F.Y.: The effects of the organic solvents and industrial poisonings on the central nervous system. *Proc Assoc Res Nerv Ment Dis 32*:475-505, 1953.
30. Bennett, I.L., Freeman, H.C., Mitchell, G.L, and Cooper, M.N.: Acute methyl alcohol poisoning: a review based on experiences in an outbreak of 323 cases. *Medicine 32*:431-463, 1953.
31. Davidson, M., and Feinleib, M.: Carbon disulfide poisoning: a review. *Am Heart J 83*:100-114, 1972.
32. Hanninen, H.: Psychological picture of manifest and latent carbon disulphide poisoning. *Br J Industr Med 28*:374-381, 1971.
33. Mancuso, T.F., and Locke, B.Z.: Carbon disulfide as a cause of suicide. *J Occup Med 14*:595-606, 1972.
34. Kramer, R.A., and Pierpaoli, P.: Hallucinogenic effect of propellant components of deodorant sprays. *Pediatrics 48*:322-323, 1971.

35. Hayden, J.W., and Comstock, E.G.: The clinical toxicology of solvent abuse. *Clin Toxicol 9*:169-184, 1976.
36. Biskind, M.S., and Bieber, I.: DDT poisoning. A new syndrome with neuropsychiatric manifestations. *Am J Psychother 3*:261-270, 1949.
37. Levin, H.S., and Radnitzky, R.L.: Behavioral effects of organophosphate pesticides in man. *Clin Toxicol 9*:391-405, 1976.
38. Gershon, S., and Shaw, F.H.: Psychiatric sequelae of chronic exposure to organophosphorus insecticides. *Lancet 1*:1371-1374, 1961.
39. Karczmar, A.G., Usdin, E., and Wills, J.H.: *Anticholinesterase Agents.* New York, Pergamon Press, 1970, p. 394.
40. Heath, D.F.: *Organophosphorus Poisons.* New York, Pergamon Press, 1961.
41. Clark, G.: Organophosphorus insecticides and behavior, a review. *Aerosp Med 42*:735-740, 1971.

Additional References

Freeman, J.W., and Couch, J.R. Prolonged encephalopathy with arsenic poisoning. *Neurology 28*:853-855, 1978.

Israelstam, S., Lambert, S., and Oki, G. Poppers, a new recreational drug craze. *Can Psychiatr Assoc J 23*:493-495, 1978.

Rosenberg, H., Orkin, F.K., and Springstead, J. Abuse of nitrous oxide. *Anesth Analg 58*:104-106, 1979.

Sigell, L.T., Kapp, F.T., Fusaro, G.A., et al. Popping and snorting volatile nitrites: A current fad for getting high. *Am J Psychiatry 135*:1216-1217, 1978.

Smith, D.L. Mental effects of mercury poisoning. *South Med J 71*:904-905, 1978.

Taylor, J.R., Selhorst, J.B., Houff, S.A., and Martinez, J. Chlordecone intoxication in man. *Neurology 28*:626-630, 1978.

CHAPTER 15

DELIRIUM DUE TO HEAD INJURY, BRAIN TUMOR, EPILEPSY, AND CEREBROVASCULAR DISEASES

T HIS CHAPTER IS devoted to a discussion of delirium caused by or associated with the major classes of primary diseases of the brain. Some intracranial disorders, such as infections or fat embolism for example, are discussed in other chapters to which they logically belong. The most important and prevalent cerebral diseases are grouped in the present chapter. It should be emphasized that delirium caused by the diseases discussed here is not different in its behavioral characteristics from that caused by systemic diseases affecting the brain secondarily. Any disease, regardless of whether it originates in the brain or elsewhere in the body, which causes a diffuse disturbance of cerebral metabolism or neurotransmission, is liable to give rise to an acute failure of the higher functions of the brain or delirium.

HEAD INJURY

Trauma to the head is probably one of the most common causes of delirium, especially in young adults. Nearly a million persons present themselves to British hospitals after head injury every year (1). In the United States, there were 8 million head injuries recorded in 1971, with almost 2 million of them reportedly severe enough to be classified by the National Center for Health Statistics as concussion, contusion, skull fracture, etc. (2). The Los Angeles County Hospital alone provides treatment for about 1,000 acute head injuries annually (3). Severe head injuries are much less common than mild ones but have a mortality rate of 50 percent (1, 3). "Severe" head injury has been defined as one followed by coma lasting six hours or longer (3).

Head injuries have been classified into three types: blunt, sharp, or compression (4). Blunt injuries are further subdivided into deceleration or acceleration. They are the most common type of head injury in peace time and give rise to concussion or diffuse generalized brain injury upon which may be superimposal focal brain damage in an area distant from the site of impact. Cerebral concussion is defined as the reversible or irreversible disruption of neural function by trauma occurring in a diffuse symmetrical manner throughout the brain (4). Ommaya (5) has proposed that cerebral concussion represents a graded set of clinical syndromes which follow head trauma and which involve a disturbance in the level and content of awareness of increasing severity. Such disturbance, hypothesizes Ommaya, is caused by mechanically induced strains acting on the brain in a centripetal sequence; that is to say, in the mild cases the effects are at the surface of the brain, and with increasing severity they extend inwards to involve the diencephalic-mesencephalic areas at the most severe degrees of trauma. Confusion and disturbances of memory comprise the effects of the milder levels of trauma and can occur without loss of consciousness. The latter is invariably followed by confusion and amnesia. The lesser grades of cerebral concussion are common and in the majority of cases are confined to confusion and amnesia. The patient may be briefly "dazed," i.e. confused and disoriented for time. If coma follows injury to the head, the patient passes subsequently through stages of stupor and confusion. In the stage of confusion he or she displays defective memory and concentration, disorientation, and other cognitive and attentional deficits which allow one to equate the term "confusion" with "delirium." It is hypothesized that delirium of some degree of severity and of variable duration is an invariable manifestation of cerebral concussion.

Hooper (4) speaks of the "stage of confusion" which follows coma and stupor in a patient suffering from concussion. It should be noted that Hooper confines the term "concussion" to those injuries in which consciousness is lost (4, p. 36). He points out that this stage is marked by considerable variation, as its manifestations are influenced by the patient's personality, the environment, and the severity of the diffuse brain damage. Some patients are quiet and subdued during this stage, others display restlessness, talkativeness, and even belligerence. Lewin (6) uses slightly different terminology and talks of the stage of delirium which passes into a state of "quiet confusion." In the latter the patient tends to be cooperative and alert but is disoriented for time and place, does not know why he is in the hospital, and has little or no insight into his condition. The stages of delirium and confusion (we would use the term "delirium" for both) follow even a very brief episode of coma and may last only a minute or two (6). After more severe concussion the delirium may last hours, days, or even weeks before normal levels of awareness and orientation are regained. As a general rule, in an uncomplicated case of concussion the progress of the patient is clearly towards recovery of function. If delirium returns after a lucid period or becomes worse, one should immediately suspect a complication: intracranial, extracranial, or both.

The most important intracranial complications of concussion include hemorrhage, chronic subdural hematoma, subdural effusion, cerebral edema, epileptic seizures, and infection. Each of these complications may feature increased impairment of awareness in a patient who was improving or was already lucid. Delirium, progressing to stupor and coma, is a common manifestation of subarachnoid, subdural, extradural, and intracerebral hemorrhage in a case of head injury. Delirium, fluctuating in severity, is a typical feature of the chronic subdural hematoma (4).

Extracranial complications of head trauma which may induce and/or exacerbate delirium include respiratory acidosis or alkalosis, hypernatremia or hyponatremia, hypoxia from chest or other injuries, hypercarbia, shock, blood loss, fat embolism from long bone fracture, etc. Alcohol intake predisposes to head injury as a result of accidental falls and traffic accidents. Furthermore, alcohol tends to increase the severity of the traumatic delirium, may induce vomiting and subsequent aspiration, and may, in an alcoholic patient, result in a withdrawal delirium being added to the traumatic one.

Management of traumatic delirium should follow the principles of the treatment of this syndrome generally. Sedation should be resorted to only if the patient is restless or belligerent, and in danger of harming himself or somebody else as a result. Hooper (4) recommends intramuscular chlorpromazine but we prefer haloperidol for reasons discussed in Chapter 9.

BRAIN TUMOR

Delirium is a common manifestation of cerebral neoplasm. Walther-Büel (7) has reported on psychiatric disorders in 600 proven cases of brain tumor of various pathological types and anatomical sites. He found evidence of mental disorder in 70 percent of the patients. Twenty-six percent of the total group showed evidence of "clouding of consciousness," which seems to be equivalent to what we call delirium. This disorder was most commonly observed in patients with occipital, brain stem, frontal, and temporal tumors. It occurred least often with neoplasms in the area of the sella and cerebellum. Güvener et al. (8) found "mental changes" in about 60 percent of 326 patients with supratentorial tumors. "Confusion" was observed in about 18 percent of the cases. Friedman and Odom (9) observed "confusion" and other "mental changes" in 50 percent of patients aged sixty years or older who had an intracranial tumor. Riggs and Rupp (10) studied eighty-six patients with supratentorial glioma and found organic mental syndrome in about 45 percent. The "syndrome" was said to include confusion, disorientation, personality change, intellectual deterioration, and forgetfulness. Thus, it is unclear what proportion of the patients displayed delirium. Rapidly growing malignant lesions were reported to be more frequently associated with mental clarity. Invasion of rhinencephalic-hypothalamic structures was found in 89 percent of the patients with psychiatric disturbances. Strobos (11) has reviewed several reports on mental changes in tumors of the temporal lobe and found an incidence ranging from 33 to 94 percent. In his own series, about 70 percent of patients were observed to exhibit such changes, most often represented by a "gradual slowing of cerebration, loss of memory, and apathy." In all of these patients there was evidence of increased intra-cranial pressure. Assal et al. (12) found disturbances of consciousness (presumably delirium) in 50 percent of patients with tumors of the posterior fossa, nearly all of whom showed concurrent evidence of raised intracranial pressure. Schmid-Wermser et al. (13) observed disturbances of consciousness in about 80 percent of patients with proven cerebral metastases from bronchogenic carcinoma. Kanzer (14) found evidence of a mental disorder in almost all of 205 patients with brain tumor. Delirium was a common feature of rapidly growing tumors and those which compressed the brain stem or caused sudden transient blockage of the ventricles. Small hemorrhage into a tumor, temporary compression of blood vessels by edema or tumor tissue, or epileptic seizures could all precipitate episodes of delirium. Tumors in the area of the third ventricle and brain stem are particularly likely to cause acute intermittent episodes of delirium with a dreamlike quality and often with associated amnestic, Korsakoff syndrome-like features. Confusional episodes may accompany and follow attacks of severe headache in cases of colloid cyst of the third ventricle (15).

Generally poor quality of the reports on psychiatric disorders in patients with brain tumor allows only tentative conclusions about their nature and frequency. Between 50 and 70 percent of such patients seem to suffer from delirium, dementia, amnestic syndrome, organic personality syndrome, or hallucinosis. The commonest disorders are delirium and dementia. The former may be expected to occur at some point in 20 to 25 percent of the brain tumor cases. Delirium appears to be positively associated with fast-growing tumors causing raised intracranial pressure. Other mechanisms underlying delirium episodes include hemorrhage into the tumor; compression of blood vessels, especially veins, by swelling or tumor; acute blockage of the ventricular system; swelling and edema in and around or distant from the tumor; epileptic discharges; and systemic factors such as hypotension or electrolyte imbalance (16). It must be emphasized that transient episodes of delirium may develop in the course of the development of a brain tumor as a result of the above factors, acting singly or in various combinations. They are particularly likely to be associated with tumors of the occipital, temporal, and frontal lobes; of the corpus callosum;

of the brain stem; and of the area of the third ventricle. They are less common with infratentorial tumors in general and those of the cerebellum and the cerebellopontine angle in particular (17).

EPILEPSY

Classification and terminology of psychiatric disorders associated with epilepsy are matters of perennial controversy and confusion so typical of the whole area of organic mental disorders. Several writers have tried recently to introduce some order into this chaotic state of affairs (18-21). Bruens (18) points out that the least controversial aspect of psychopathology associated with epilepsy is that represented by transient episodes with lowered level of consciousness, that is the so-called twilight states, which bear a clearcut relationship to a seizure. Twilight state may represent either an ictal or postictal event, or a combination of both. Helmchen (19) has focused on the reversible mental disorders in epileptic patients and distinguished episodic mood disorders and episodic psychoses. The latter include "productive" psychotic episodes, stupor, and twilight states. Helmchen asserts that the reversible syndromes fall into three groups: those which are direct manifestations of an epileptic discharge; those initiated or terminated by epileptic seizures; and those having no recognizable connection with epileptic seizures. Wechsler (22) has expressed it more succinctly: "*Epileptic delirium* and other psychotic manifestations may precede, follow, or replace the convulsive attack." Köhler (20, 21) has dealt with epileptic psychoses at great length and reviewed their assorted classifications. He points out that "epileptic psychoses" represent a heterogeneous group of mental disorders observed in epileptic patients that may be classified according to psychopathological criteria, reversibility or irreversibility, episodic or chronic course, and other relevant features. Köhler stresses clouding of consciousness as a key distinguishing characteristic of these psychoses and, accordingly, divides them into those with and without such clouding, respectively. The former are classically represented by the so-called twilight states, which may be preictal, ictal, or postictal, or bear no temporal relationship to epileptic seizures. Furthermore, Köhler includes delirious states, characterized by restlessness and mostly visual hallucinations, among the group of twilight states. This writer proposes to use the term "delirium" as one equivalent to "twilight states," "confusional states," "clouded states," and similar redundant designations. Three classes of psychoses in patients with epilepsy have been distinguished: global disruption of personality; primary disturbance of mood; and organic psychosyndromes, which include delirium (23). The notorious schizophrenialike psychoses of epilepsy are assigned to the category of "global disruption of personality." Since our focus in this book is on the organic mental disorders, and specifically delirium, only this category of psychiatric syndromes in epileptics will be discussed (19-24). The following classification of epileptic delirium is proposed:

1. Ictal delirium (twilight state)
    a. complex partial status epilepticus (psychomotor status);
    b. Absence (petit mal) status;
2. Postictal delirium (clouded, twilight, or confusional state);
3. Interictal delirium (not temporally related to seizures);
4. Delirium due to antiepileptic drugs.

Ictal delirium. Ictal delirium is a term applied here to the absence or petit mal and complex partial or psychomotor status epilepticus. The absence status, first described by Lennox (25) in 1945, is believed to occur much more often than the psychomotor status. It can occur at all ages, but is most common in children and has been observed to come on in later life in persons without a past history of seizures (26). Its frequency is difficult to ascertain. Celesia (27) found status epilepticus in 2.6 percent of 2,290 patients with seizures and diagnosed absence status in thirteen patients, i.e. in about 0.5 percent of the total sample. He found psychomotor status in only two patients. The absence status features confusion, speech arrest, automatisms, and amnesia (27-30). Automatisms may be either stereotyped or reactive (27). The former consist of repetitive movements that follow a regular sequence and may feature chewing, blinking, swallowing, etc. The latter form of automatism consists of relatively complex and purposeful actions that create the impression of an appropriate response to environmental stimuli or inner motives. The patient may walk, light a cigarette, prepare food, etc. Catatonic posturing may be present. The patient usually, but not always, has a history of petit mal or grand mal epilepsy or both. The EEG shows diffuse 1.5 to 3-Hz spike or poly-spike and slow-wave complexes. Duration of an episode varies and may range from minutes to several days, occasionally longer than one week (27). One writer claims that an attack can last "years" (29). In the latter case it would make no sense to speak of delirium. An attack may be precipitated by an emotional upset, infection, menses, etc. Diagnosis depends on the EEG. Some of the patients have been mistakenly diagnosed as schizophrenics or sufferers from a dissociative state or drug intoxication. Treatment of an attack involves intravenous administration of diazepam.

The complex partial or psychomotor status has been seldom reported in English-language literature (21, 24, 28, 31, 32). Helmchen (19) has suggested that infrequent reporting of this condition may result from these patients being treated by psychiatrists who fail to associate the symptoms with epilepsy and do not order an EEG. Belafsky et al. (28) claim that the psychomotor status can be distinguished clinically from the absence status. The former is characterized by a continuous "twilight state" (delirium) with partial responsiveness and complex automatisms, and recurrent total unresponsiveness and stereotyped, simple automatisms. The EEG also displays two corresponding phases. Escueta et al. (31) have reported on a prolonged state of "mental confusion" in a patient with psychomotor status and episodic, stereotyped, repetitive automatisms for about 154 and 104 hours, respectively.

Postictal delirium. This may follow any type of epileptic seizure, partial or generalized. Helmchen (19) asserts that "twilight states" (delirium) occur most often following a seizure and subside after a few hours or days. They are most common after seizures of centrencephalic epilepsy. They are associated with generalized abnormalities in the EEG. Levin (32) reported on fifty-two patients with "epileptic clouded states" occurring most often within twenty-four hours after a series of grand mal seizures of idiopathic epilepsy. Levin emphasizes that this syndrome is nothing but delirium, characterized by confusion, excitement, hallucinations (mostly auditory), and delusions. One notes that all these patients had been admitted to a mental hospital as a result of disturbed, often assaultive, behavior. This suggests that the sample is biased in favor of more dramatic and florid psychiatric symptomatology. The delirium tended to recur in these patients. Epilepsy varied in severity but was mostly at least moderately severe. About one-third of the patients had a history of abuse of alcohol, and withdrawal of the latter seemed to be responsible for both seizures and delirium in several cases. Levin notes that even though the patients were often combative, they were not dangerous since their disorganized mental functions practically precluded planned aggression. There is no clearcut demarcation between postictal delirium lasting several days or even weeks, as in Levin's cases, and that which immediately follows an epileptic seizure and typically lasts for some minutes or a few hours.

Following a complex partial seizure some patients display postictal automatism, which may be regarded as a transient confusional state, or delirium, for which the patient is subsequently amnesic (21). These postictal automatisms may merge with the ictal ones and the distinction between them without an EEG recording may be impossible. Postictal automatisms generally last longer, however. Gastaut (33) postulates that they result from exhaustion of the neuronal systems and represent epiphenomena accompanying confusional states that follow rather commonly certain partial seizures of temporal origin. This writer believes that postictal automatisms and confusional states represent seizure-related delirious episodes.

Interictal delirium. This seems to occur in a proportion of patients with temporal lobe epilepsy. Glaser (34) describes thirty-seven patients who suffered from "psychomotor-temporal lobe seizure states" and psychotic episodes not believed to be a part of the seizure complex and lasting from one to many days. Over half of the patients are reported to have displayed fluctuating confusion with temporal disorientation, memory impairment, attention disturbance, and partial or complete amnesia subsequently. Thinking was disorganized and loose; perceptual discrimination fluctuated; hallucinations and body image disturbances were common. Flor-Henry (35) found confusional states in 18 percent of fifty patients with temporal lobe epilepsy and history of psychotic episodes. Patients who suffered from confusional states had the highest incidence of brain damage and the most disturbed social adaptation of the whole group. They also had a high proportion of deviant personality traits. Pathogenesis of these interictal confusional or delirious episodes is unknown.

Delirium due to antiepileptic drugs is discussed in Chapter 10.

CEREBROVASCULAR DISEASES (CVD)

Vascular disease of the brain is one of the commonest and most important causes of delirium. The latter is, in turn, one of the most frequent psychiatric manifestations of CVD. Peters and Gille (36) found the latter to be the second commonest cause of delirium ("acute secondary psychosis") among 562 patients diagnosed in a neuropsychiatric hospital. Alcoholism and CVD were judged to be the main causes of the syndrome in 70 percent of cases. Whether this finding has general validity is unknown, but it does highlight the frequency of the association between CVD and delirium. In the discussion to follow both acute and chronic vascular diseases of the brain are considered insofar as they pertain to delirium.

CVD has three major components: (1) decreased perfusion pressure due to a pathological process such as atherosclerosis, embolism, thrombosis, arteritis, cardiac failure, etc., and consequently the inadequate supply of the metabolic substrate necessary to sustain normal brain function; (2) pathophysiological change in the metabolism of the brain, which may be transient or may be infarction or may be hemorrhage; and (3) focal or general cerebral dysfunction, or both. Focal cerebral dysfunction includes transient ischemic attacks, progressing stroke, and completed stroke (prolonged neurological deficit) (37). "General cerebral dysfunction" refers to general ischemia of the brain resulting from reduction of its blood supply due to such conditions as cardiac arrest, for example. Delirium may be a manifestation of any of the pathological processes that lead to cerebral ischemia. The latter may involve the carotid or the vertebrobasilar arterial system, or both.

Transient ischemic attacks (TIA). These attacks are episodes of focal cerebral dysfunction of vascular origin, rapid onset (less than five minutes), and brief duration (usually two to fifteen minutes but occasionally as long as twenty-four hours) (38). They do not leave a permanent neurological deficit. An attack may involve either the carotid or the vertebrobasilar arterial system. In the former case, there may be paresis, paresthesias, visual symptoms, dysphasia, dysarthria, headache, etc. (39). Visual hallucinations and "mental change" are reported to occur in less than 3 percent of cases (39). Whether delirium occurs in association with carotid artery TIA is unclear. Vertebrobasilar TIA feature bilateral symptoms such as weakness, numbness, paresthesias, loss of vision, ataxia, vertigo, dysphagia, etc. "Mental change" is reported to occur in about 5 percent of cases (39). Delirium does not seem to be a common feature of vertebrobasilar TIA either.

Stroke. Stroke follows one or more TIAs in a large proportion of cases. Its importance is related to its frequency and mortality, and the disability to which it gives rise. About 395,000 persons have a thromboembolic stroke in the United States each year, and about 40 percent of them die within thirty days after the event (39). About one-half of the survivors, i.e. about 120,000, are said to require special care as a result. The majority of the strokes are due to cerebral infarction caused by thrombosis or cerebral embolism; subarachnoid hemorrhage and intracerebral hemorrhage account for most of the remainder. Emboli originate most often in the heart or the arteries to the brain such as the carotid, vertebral, or basilar. Thrombotic infarctions are divided into those occurring in the carotid or vertebrobasilar arterial distribution. The clinical picture is determined by the site of the brain damage. A stroke may be classified as progressing or completed (37). The latter category implies that the duration of the deficit has been more than three weeks.

Internal carotid artery. Internal carotid artery occlusion in the neck may be unilateral or, less often, bilateral. Its onset tends to be sudden and delirium may be among the presenting symptoms (40-42). Hass and Goldensohn (40) found "organic mental syndromes" characterized by depression, irritability, and confusion to be the first symptoms of carotid artery occlusion in three out of thirty-five patients. Hurwitz et al. (41) observed "impaired mentation," presumably delirium and/or dementia, in ten of fifty-seven patients. Shapiro (42) reports that mental changes occur in about 30 percent of patients with bilateral carotid artery occlusion. The most common psychiatric picture is progressive dementia; delirium occurs less often. Shapiro describes a patient who developed delirium with hallucinations and delusions as a manifestation of bilateral carotid artery occlusion.

Anterior, middle, or posterior cerebral arteries. Delirium may occasionally dominate the clinical picture in *infarctions* in the distribution of anterior, middle, or posterior cerebral arteries (43-45). Visual impairment as well as vivid visual hallucinations, occurring in a setting of agitated delirium, have been reported (45). In such cases, delirium came on from one to three days after the sudden onset of visual impairment and lasted a few days to two months. Infarctions in several anatomical sites seem capable of inducing delirium: medial temporo-occipital region unilaterally or bilaterally (45), hippocampal formation, fusiform and lingual gyri, and cingulate gyrus and orbital areas (39, 44). No ready explanation for the occurrence of delirium in such infarctions can be given.

Vertebrobasilar arterial system. Symptoms of obstruction within the vertebrobasilar arterial system depend on the site of occlusion or stenosis, its degree, and the availability of collateral flow. Complete occlusion of the main trunk of the basilar artery usually leads to death. Incomplete obstruction is more common and may result in various transient and fluctuating or permanent disorders and deficits, such as deafness, vertigo, drop attacks, etc., which reflect dysfunction of the brain stem. Visual disturbances are usually present and may include fortification spectra, blurring of vision, hemianopic field defects, and visual hallucinations. The latter may range from simple, black and white ones to highly complex and colored visions, and result from ischemia of the visual association areas (46). Occipital headaches, ataxia, bilateral paresthesias over the body, akinetic mutism, hemiplegia, etc. may occur in various combinations. Some clouding of consciousness, or delirium of some degree of severity, may accompany these symptoms. Drop attacks, without loss of consciousness, are a common feature. Impairment of consciousness is said to be uncommon early in the course of pathologic events (37). Occlusion of the subclavian artery may result in the so-called subclavian steal syndrome that may feature confusion as well as symptoms of vertebrobasilar insufficiency, either on exercising the affected arm or spontaneously.

Intracerebral hemorrhage. This is usually associated with marked hypertension. Symptoms tend to come on during activity and progress rapidly. Severe headache is common. Consciousness is impaired or lost in most cases.

Subarachnoid hemorrhage. Subarachnoid hemorrhage of the primary type is one in which initially the bleeding occurs directly into the subarachnoid space and is most often due to a ruptured intracranial aneurysm or to an angioma. Symptoms develop suddenly and severe headache is typically the first to appear. A disturbance of consciousness of some degree of severity follows. Sencer and Andiman (47) observed confusion in twenty-four of fifty-nine patients admitted for a ruptured intracranial aneurysm. Confusion may accompany headache initially and be followed by coma; loss of consciousness may be transient and confusion succeeds it. For example, some of the reported patients suddenly developed severe head pain and confusion as long as ten days before lapsing into coma. Other patients were admitted to hospital with an organic mental syndrome (presumably delirium) and a history of transient unconsciousness within preceding hours or a few days. Meningeal irritation, with or without other neurological signs or symptoms, accompanies the delirium. Okawara (48) studied warning signs occurring prior to rupture of an intracranial aneurysm. Among the signs were lethargy and visual hallucinations, that is, symptoms suggestive of delirium. Repeated minor leakage of blood and vascular disturbances are believed to underlie the warning signs.

A recent study found that 50 percent of patients with sub-arachnoid hemorrhage showed "alteration of sensorium" or focal deficit on admission to hospital (49). Delirium is a common feature of the hemorrhage and usually clears up within a week, but occasionally it may persist for weeks and gradually merge with a more chronic and stable dementia, which may be only partly reversible.

Psychiatric sequelae of subarachnoid hemorrhage include intellectual impairment of some degree of severity in about half of the survivors (50). Patients with middle cerebral artery aneurysms are particularly prone to this development.

Intracranial arteriovenous malformation. In about 5 percent of cases subarachnoid hemorrhage is caused by an intracranial arteriovenous malformation. Intellectual deterioration or "mental changes" have been reported in about 15 to 50 percent of the cases of the latter (51). Waltimo and Putkonen (51), however, found no intellectual impairment in forty patients with arterio-venous malformations. The meaning of these discrepancies in the reported incidence is obscure. In a few reported cases "mental confusion" was the reason for the patient's seeking help (52). One patient developed progressive intellectual deterioration as well as visual hallucinations and paranoid ideas. Excision of the malformation was followed by some improvement (52). Catatonic symptoms have been reported in a case of ruptured arteriovenous malformation of the left frontal lobe (53). A similar clinical picture has been observed in a case of subarachnoid hemorrhage of unknown cause (54).

Cerebral embolism. The source of cerebral embolism may be in the heart or lungs, or in one of the arteries to the brain, especially the carotid. Embolism due to a cardiac source commonly results from a cardiac arrhythmia, valvular heart disease, myocardial infarction, or subacute bacterial endocarditis. The onset of symptoms is typically rapid and the patient usually becomes confused rather than unconscious. A convulsion may occur initially. The immediate mortality is 7 to 10 percent (55). Fat and air embolism are referred to in Chapter 12. Fat embolism may be followed by delirium after a latent period of hours to days following injury.

Cerebral sinus and venous thrombosis. Most often this occurs in association with childbirth, osteomyelitis, pyogenic infections of the sinuses or the mastoids, etc. Thrombosis of the superior longitudinal sinus in particular is liable to give rise to delirium as an early manifestation (56).

Chronic subdural hematoma. CSH was already mentioned briefly in the section on head trauma. Its importance in the present context is related to the fact that delirium is an important presenting feature of this treatable condition, yet one that is characterized by serious morbidity and high mortality. Mental symptoms, usually referred to in the literature as mental changes, confusion, memory loss, disorientation, somnolence, stupor, lethargy, etc., are among the most important and readily missed presenting manifestations. Recent reports on CSH give the incidence of mental symptoms to be about 80 percent (57). Disorientation and confusion, that is to say symptoms usually signifying the presence of delirium, are the most common abnormalities of the mental status (57-60). These clinical features are especially prominent and important in the elderly patients who may not display the typical symptoms of increased intracranial pressure such as headache and papilledema (58, 59). The patients are all too often misdiagnosed as cases of stroke, senile dementia, or unspecified psychiatric disorder. Unfamiliarity with organic mental disorders on the part of physicians has probably contributed to some of these diagnostic errors. The diagnosis is often delayed or not determined until an autopsy is carried out (54). The patient will almost invariably die or suffer irreversible brain damage and dementia unless early diagnosis is made and proper operative treatment is instituted. In one of the early studies, 60 percent of patients over sixty-five years died before CSH was diagnosed (59).

The peak incidence of CSH is during the sixth and seventh decades of life (58). One-half of all cases occur in persons sixty years old or older. History of head trauma is absent in some 35 to 50 percent of patients (58). The trauma may be minor, such as a tumble out of bed. The time interval from trauma to operation averages about ten weeks but may be as long as six months (55). Symptoms tend to develop insidiously and usually include those of increased intracranial pressure and various focal neurologic deficits. Delirium or dementia may develop subacutely or in a stepwise manner. As many as 17 percent of patients studied are initially admitted with psychiatric diagnoses and up to 30 percent are said to exhibit recent personality changes. Somnolence, confusion, disorientation, and memory impairment are reported to dominate the clinical picture in about half of the elderly patients with CSH. Some patients complain of headache, blackouts, incontinence, and seizure (59). Hemiparesis, hemianopia, and aphasia are common neurologic findings. Some patients are comatose on admission to hospital. Catatonic features may be present occasionally (61). CSH has been rightly called a "great imitator" (59). Diagnosis is predicated on the recognition of a global organic mental disorder, delirium or dementia or both, and instituting proper laboratory investigations: computerized tomography, brain scan, and angiography (57, 59). Treatment may be surgical or nonsurgical, the former giving the best results. In one series, 53 percent of surgically treated patients had full recovery of function (57).

Noninfectious cerebral arteritis may give rise to symptoms of metabolic encephalopathy or cerebral infarction, or both. The following arteritides of undetermined origin have been recognized (57):

1. Cranial (temporal) arteritis
2. Systemic lupus erythematosus
3. Polyarteritis nodosa
4. Wegener's granulomatosis
5. Allergic or hypersensitivity arteritis
6. Rheumatoid arteritis
7. Neuro-Behçet's disease
8. Thrombotic microangiopathy
9. Pulseless disease

Cranial (temporal, giant-cell) arteritis. This can give rise to several types of mental syndromes: depression, delirium, dementia, and hallucinosis (62-66). Cochran et al. (63) claim that mental symptoms are common in this disorder but the validity of this claim is uncertain. Paulley and Hughes (65) report that mental symptoms were prominent in about 45 percent of their seventy-six patients, and were "predominant" in about 15 percent. These authors observe that "madness," that is confusion, depression, or dementia, may be the main mode of presentation in some patients and lead to diagnostic errors. Andrews (62) states that "confusion" (a term which is often used to signify delirium) may dominate the clinical picture and resolve with steroid therapy. It is notable, in view of the foregoing claims, that a recent report on an epidemiologic study of cranial arteritis makes no mention of psychiatric manifestations (67). Despite this curious omission, there seems to be little doubt that delirium, dementia, and/or depression do occur in association with cranial arteritis. A combination of one of these syndromes with polymyalgia rheumatica, headache, visual disturbances (amaurosis fugax, diplopia), and age over sixty years should always suggest cranial arteritis. Even more important is to remember that the latter may present with an organic mental disorder. Early diagnosis is essential if treatment is to be instituted and blindness or dementia prevented.

Systemic lupus erythematosus. SLE has spawned more neuropsychiatric studies and literature than any other disease of comparable prevalence, and out of all proportion to the latter. It is far more difficult to find usable articles on psychiatric complications of myocardial infarction, stroke, cancer, or chronic obstructive pulmonary disease, that is to say, on the most highly prevalent causes of serious morbidity and mortality in this country, than on mental disorders in SLE. One reason for this disproportionate attention paid to them may be their notoriously high incidence. As Johnson and Richardson (68) put it: "If the confusional state accompanying fever and the anxiety or despondency accompanying any chronic debilitating disease are included, certainly almost all patients with SLE would be found to have disorders of mental function." Osler (69) wrote in 1895 that fever is a frequent accompaniment of an attack of what was then called "erythema exudativum multiforme," and "at the height of the attack delirium may occur." One of Osler's patients had recurrent febrile episodes accompanied by colic, vomiting, diarrhea, "erythema multiforme," and delirium. The attacks were invariably heralded by cold feet. During his delirium this patient was said to hallucinate "all sorts of things."

The frequency and nature of the mental disorders in the course of SLE have been a subject of some controversy. Fessel and Solomon (70) have reviewed the literature until 1960 and counted 272 cases of psychosis with SLE reported over a period of sixty years. The average incidence of psychosis was found to be 22 percent; one in four cases was thought to be due to steroid therapy. The nature of the psychiatric manifestations was found to be quite variably reported. Organic, schizoaffective, schizophrenic, and depressive disorders (psychoses) are found in the earlier reports. It is of note that the earliest papers, by Kaposi and Osler, respectively, refer to delirium (68, 69). More recent studies give the incidence of neuropsychiatric manifestations in SLE as ranging between 3 and 75 percent (68, 71-73). A review of ten studies published between 1964 and 1976 reveals an average incidence of exactly 50 percent.

The nature of the reported mental disorders in SLE varies from author to author and his or her psychiatric diagnostic competence and orientation. Guze (74) diagnosed organic brain syndromes in about 37 percent of twenty-four episodes of psychiatric illness in the course of SLE. Ganz et al. (75) found mostly mixed, "organic" mental symptoms in 22 percent of a group of patients with SLE. O'Connor and Musher (76) studied 150 patients, ninety of whom exhibited symptoms of central nervous system SLE. Two-thirds of those who manifested psychiatric symptoms were diagnosed as suffering from delirium. Feinglass et al. (73) have reported on a group of 140 patients with SLE and found neuropsychiatric manifestations in 51 percent of them; twenty-four patients had a psychiatric disorder, with an "organic component" in all but two. Only nine of these psychiatric patients had no neurologic deficits concurrently or at another time in the course of the illness. The commonest association was with seizures. Johnson and Richardson (68) maintain that delirium, marked by delusions, hallucinations, and often psychomotor activity, is "remarkably frequent" in SLE, more so than in other systemic diseases. Dementia has been observed much less often. Heine (77) has reviewed some of the relevant studies and shows that four different investigators give consistently the figure of about 30 percent as the incidence of organic-toxic psychoses (presumably delirium). Sergent et al. (78) observed organic brain syndromes in nine of twenty-eight patients showing evidence of central nervous system involvement in SLE; fourteen of the patients exhibited a functional psychosis at some stage of the illness. Delirium in SLE is often modified by affective features, those mostly depressive, or by schizophrenia-like features (75). In conclusion, while the quality of psychiatric reports on the incidence and nature of mental disorders in SLE is generally poor, one may conclude that about every second patient with this disease is likely to suffer from one or more episodes of psychiatric illness at some stage in the course of the disease. Delirium is probably the commonest significant mental disorder encountered in these patients, with an incidence of about 20 to 30 percent. This means that delirium accounts for approximately 30 to 60 percent of diagnosable psychiatric disorders among SLE patients. A simplified, if not very accurate, generalization would state that every second patient will have had a psychiatric disorder that in one-half of the cases is liable to be delirium. Dementia is much less common. An affective, usually depressive, disorder may accompany or follow delirium in these patients, or occur independently. The same applies to schizophreniform disorders. A patient with SLE may experience more than one episode of psychiatric disorder and the diagnosis may be different for each episode (74). Thus, marked variability of clinical features, both cross-sectionally and longitudinally, is a hallmark of psychiatric complications of SLE.

SLE delirium may occur at any stage in the development of the disease but it appears to come on more frequently in its early phases, usually within the first year. Bennett et al. (79) state that mental symptoms can antedate the onset of other manifestations of SLE by several years, but it is not clear if this statement applies to delirium. The latter may also mark a terminal stage of the illness (77). Delirious episodes are usually relatively short-lasting, and their duration may vary from a few hours to several days or even weeks. Delirium tends to come on at times when the physical condition worsens (71). A wide range of neurologic symptoms, such as seizures, long tract involvement, cranial neuropathy, cerebellar signs, etc., may accompany delirium, but some patients exhibit no concomitant neurologic deficits (73). Association with seizures is particularly common. Fever is a frequent concomitant feature and possibly one that facilitates the onset of delirium. Hypertension and renal disease are found significantly more often in SLE patients exhibiting an organic mental disorder (77). Patients with such a disorder, especially if renal disease and hypertension co-exist, have a higher mortality rate than those suffering from one of the so-called functional psychiatric disorders, affective or schizophreniform. Neuropsychiatric disorders in SLE are reported by some to have a significantly higher association with vasculitis and thrombocytopenia (73). O'Connor and Musher (76) claim, however, that in their series of patients they could not demonstrate a relationship between the development of psychosis and involvement of another organ system or any single laboratory finding.

Laboratory abnormalities in SLE patients exhibiting neuropsychiatric symptoms are as variable as the clinical manifestations. No single procedure yields consistently abnormal results (80). The electroencephalogram is reported by some authors to be abnormal in all patients having psychiatric symptoms at the time, to be valuable for the assessment of the progress of SLE, and to help distinguish psychosis due to cerebral lupus from that caused by steroids (81). Small et al. (80) found abnormal EEG in eight out of ten patients with evidence of CNS involvement. Those with signs of "encephalopathy" showed diffuse slowing. Johnson and Richardson (68) assert that the EEG findings have been of little diagnostic and localizing value. Bilateral diffuse slowing has been the most constant finding in CNS lupus. Feinglass et al. (73) have found the EEG to be the most frequent laboratory abnormality in patients with neuropsychiatric manifestations. One would expect a diffuse slowing of the EEG background activity in patients with delirium, but the literature on SLE does not make clear the relationship between this type of EEG abnormality and the nature of the patient's concurrent mental disorder, if any. One may conclude that the EEG is the most consistently abnormal laboratory finding in patients with neuropsychiatric complications of SLE and the type of reported abnormality suggests that delirium may be more common in this disease than the literature leads one to believe.

CSF total protein is elevated in about 40 percent of patients with CNS lupus. The brain scan is inconsistently abnormal (71, 80). Oxygen-15 brain scanning has recently been reported as a test that reveals active cerebral lupus in most patients (82). In a series of forty-seven patients with active SLE, the scanning revealed abnormalities in forty-seven of fifty-one episodes (92%). Ten of the patients with abnormal oxygen-15 scan had no concurrent neuropsychiatric symptoms on clinical examination. It is suggested that abnormalities of cerebral metabolism and blood flow revealed by the scans indicate that the brain may be involved more often in the disease process than clinical findings have led one to believe. In patients studied serially, the scans improved *pari passu* with clinical improvement. The investigators claim that these findings endorse the view that the majority of acute psychiatric symptoms in patients with SLE are due to cerebral lupus and should be treated as such. Furthermore, this technique may help distinguish psychiatric manifestations due to steroids from those due to cerebral lupus. Finally, computed tomography has been applied to the diagnosis of CNS lupus with promising results (83). The most frequent finding has been perisulcal atrophy, which was found in 50 percent of SLE patients with neuropsychiatric symptoms. Such atrophy is said to reflect microinfarction of the cortex and to be the organic basis for mental symptoms in SLE.

Pathogenesis of delirium and other psychiatric manifestations in the course of SLE has been the subject of considerable debate. The following factors have been implicated:

1. Cerebral lesions consisting of destructive and proliferative changes in arterioles and capillaries with resultant microinfarcts and hemorrhages in cerebral cortex and brain stem (68);
2. uremia and related metabolic derangement;
3. hypertension;
4. infection;
5. fever;
6. treatment with steroids and antimalarial drugs;
7. combinations of the above factors and, in addition, psychological stress related to the meaning of the illness.

No single factor can account for psychopathology in CNS lupus in general, and for delirium in particular. Cerebral vasculitis and primary parenchymal disease have been suggested as the main pathogenetic mechanisms (82). Steroids are an unlikely cause in most cases (84). A growing body of evidence points to immune processes within the central nervous system (85), but other writers dispute this statement (84). Renal disease and associated electrolyte and other metabolic disturbances may account for some cases. As Petz (85) recently concluded, "The pathogenesis of neurological findings in SLE is still ill defined."

Management of delirium in the course of SLE involves treatment of the underlying disorder; this means corticosteroids (71, 73, 78, 80). Treatment with combined corticosteroid and cytotoxic drugs has been employed (71). Therapy of CNS lupus remains a controversial issue. Symptomatic treatment of delirium should follow the guidelines given in Chapter 9.

Polyarteritis nodosa. This can give rise to central nervous system dysfunction with the production of symptoms such as headache, seizures, blurred vision, hemiparesis, ataxia, etc. Involvement of the central nervous system is said to occur in between 20 and 46 percent of cases (86). Mental symptoms are the most common manifestation of brain disorder in these cases. An "organic toxic psychosis with confusion and disorientation" (presumably delirium) was observed in 23 percent of patients in one large series (86). Dementia was found in about 6 percent of cases. Gottwald (87) states in a recent review that neuropsychiatric manifestations of polyarteritis nodosa may occur as secondary cerebral effects of the involvement of kidneys, liver, and heart as well as result from the pathological change in cerebral blood vessels. In either case, the cerebral lesions may be diffuse or focal and give rise to disturbances of consciousness (delirium). The latter may be associated with increased intracranial pressure, cerebral seizures, and stroke. The EEG is usually abnormal, with diffuse or focal abnormalities (86).

Wegener's granulomatosis. Lesions of the respiratory tract, sinuses, arteries, and kidneys are featured. Central nervous system involvement is said to occur in about 30 percent of cases (86). Delirium may occur but its frequency is unknown.

Hypersensitivity vasculitis (small vessel vasculitis). Following ingestion of various drugs or after microbial infection, hypersensitivity vasculitis may involve cerebral arterioles and capillaries, and give rise to hemorrhagic lesions and microinfarcts in the brain. Delirium and diffuse EEG abnormalities may be among the manifestations of this form of cerebral arteritis (88).

Rheumatoid arteritis. Rheumatoid arteritis is a term used here to denote vasculitis associated with rheumatoid arthritis. This type of vasculopathy is relatively rare, and may occur as part of generalized vasculitis resembling polyarteritis nodosa or, more rarely still, it can be confined to the central nervous system. Gupta and Ehrlich (89) describe six patients with classic rheumatoid arthritis who had been on oral corticosteroids for at least two years and who suddenly developed delirium while steroids were being withdrawn. The patients displayed mild generalized slowing of the EEG background activity and high erythrocyte sedimentation rates. Increasing the doses of corticosteroids controlled the delirium. Within one week all six patients showed marked clinical improvement and concomitant drop in sedimentation rate. The authors considered that the delirium might have been due to hyperviscosity syndrome but rejected this hypothesis. The possibility that immune complex-mediated central nervous system vasculitis might have been responsible was offered instead. A case similar to the preceding has been reported by Skowronski and Gatter (90). Steiner and Gelbloom (91) described two patients, of whom one had displayed delirium, who died and were found to have intracranial arteritis. Cerebral vasculitis is a known complication of juvenile rheumatoid arthritis (92). It features cerebral seizures, meningismus, drowsiness, hyper-reflexia, irritability, and diffusely abnormal EEG. This clinical picture has been referred to as "acute toxic encephalopathy" (92). Delirium is not mentioned but its presence has been implied by some writers (92).

Neuro-Behçet's disease. This disease is a combination of oral and genital aphthous ulcers, ocular inflammation, and cerebral dysfunction. The latter occurs in 10 to 25 percent of cases and is believed to be due to cerebral vasculitis. Organic brain syndromes have been reported in 10 percent of patients with Behçet disease (93). Delirium has been reported, along with focal neurologic signs and abnormal EEG, brain scan, and/or CT scan (93).

Pulseless disease (aortic arch syndrome). Due to occlusion of the common carotid artery, pulseless disease may result in recurrent disturbances of consciousness (88).

Multi-infarct dementia. This results from multiple small or large infarcts and is most often associated with hypertension and/or extracerebral vascular disease (94). Most such infarcts are currently believed to be secondary to disease of extracranial arteries and the heart, and only in a minority of cases due to atherosclerosis of cerebral vessels (94). Thromboembolism from the extracranial sources is thought to be the chief cause of cerebral infarcts. Dementia results from accumulated small and larger strokes. It has a typically stepwise progression punctuated by episodes of delirium, which clears up and leaves in its wake increased intellectual deficits. Focal neurologic signs, such as weakness, dysphagia, dysarthria, brisk reflexes, etc., accompany the delirium. Vertebrobasilar insufficiency, described earlier, is often associated with dementia (95). Delirium may mask the dementia during the acute phase after a stroke, and it may accompany TIA's described earlier, especially those in the vertebrobasilar arterial system. Transient global amnesia may occur in such cases and needs to be distinguished from delirium by the disproportionate impairment of memory which justifies the diagnosis of an acute amnestic syndrome.

Subcortical arteriosclerotic encephalopathy. Binswanger's disease gives rise to progressive and profound dementia as a result of diffuse degeneration of subcortical white matter. Episodes of delirium may punctuate the initial phase of the disease (96).

Trauma due to *cardiac catheterization* or *angiography.* Trauma may occasionally result in thromboembolism and delirium (97, 98). Toxic reaction to contrast agent needs to be ruled out.

Migraine may occasionally present an acute confusion (delirium) in children (99, 100, 101) and in adults (102, 103). So-called acute confusional migraine has been observed in 5 percent of children aged five to sixteen years and suffering from migraine attacks (99). The acute confusion, or delirium, may be the initial manifestation of migraine and this may create a difficult diagnostic problem, especially since headache and aura may not be reported and the whole attack appears to consist of agitated delirium of sudden onset. Anxiety and combativeness are common features of this migraine variant. An attack may last minutes to as long as a day or so and typically ends in a deep sleep (99). Amnesia for the event follows. All patients described in the original report on this condition displayed defects of sensorium, slow responsivity to questions and painful stimuli, hyperactivity, and tendency to use obscene language (101). Plantar reflexes may be bilaterally extensor. EEG may be abnormal. Pathophysiology of this delirium is unknown. It has been speculatively ascribed to ischemia, infarction, or both, in a variety of hemispheric sites (99). Recent finding of abnormal CT scans in migraine, with areas of low sensitivity in the parenchyma of the cerebral hemispheres, ventricular enlargement, and/or cortical atrophy, makes this hypothesis plausible (104).

Delirious migraine or migraine delirium has been recognized for a long time (102, 103). Delirium may complicate an intense migraine aura, and, very rarely, last throughout an entire attack of the disorder (103). Klee (102) has studied 150 patients with severe migraine and found delirium in 8 percent of those personally investigated by him. The delirium tended to occur in conjunction with very severe attacks. Visual and auditory hallucinations, the former sometimes lilliputian, are commonly part of these episodes. Very rarely the delirium may last several days (102, 103). Delirious migraine aura may resemble a waking nightmare (103).

Ergotism. A patient abusing ergotamine tartrate taken for migraine may develop ergotism. Diffuse and focal cerebral dysfunction, and evidence of arteritis, may result and the patient can present with delirium and focal neurologic signs (105). There is intense vasoconstriction with secondary occlusion and thrombosis in bifrontal areas (105).

Scleroderma. Rarely, scleroderma is associated with delirium. Restlessness, visual, auditory and tactile hallucinations, and delusions may occur as part of the syndrome (106, 107). The pathogenesis of this neurologic involvement is unknown. An encephalopathy, "cerebritis," and steroids have all been blamed for the delirium (106, 107).

Alterations in blood, such as those in polycythemia, hypercoagulability, microglobulinemia, thrombocytopenia, cryoglobulinemia, etc., may result in cerebral ischemia and organic mental disorders. Some of these disorders are discussed in Chapter 12. Recurrent delirium has been reported in *mixed cryoglobulinemia* (108). Mental disorders, most often delirium, have been found in 42 percent of 541 patients with *polycythemia vera* (109). Delirium may come on suddenly in *hyperviscosity syndrome* most often associated with macroglobulinemia and, less often, multiple myeloma (88).

Thrombotic thrombocytopenic purpura. Frequently it features neurologic abnormalities, including delirium. Headache, paresis, seizures, and coma may occur. Delirium or coma are reported to occur in as many as 75 percent of cases (110). There is widespread involvement of small vessels of the gray matter of the hemispheres believed to be responsible for the neuropsychiatric manifestations (111).

Fabry's disease syndrome (angiokeratoma corporis diffusum). An inherited disorder of glycolipid metabolism, Fabry's disease may be associated with cerebral vasculopathy and transient psychosis, which appears to be a delirium even though it has been labelled "paranoid schizophrenia" (112).

MISCELLANEOUS CEREBRAL DISORDERS

Sarcoidosis. Sarcoidosis of the central nervous system is relatively rare, yet well over 400 cases have been reported (113). Both delirium and dementia have been described as features of sarcoid encephalopathy or meningoencephalitis (114, 115). Delirium may be on occasion a presenting manifestation (113, 115). Both structural and metabolic changes may account for the psychiatric symptoms. Space-occupying granulomas and granulomatous meningitis with increased intracranial pressure are among the structural causes. Of the metabolic abnormalities, diencephalic involvement with diabetes insipidus, hypercalcemia, hepatic encephalopathy, uremia, and pulmonary insufficiency are all potential causes of delirium (113). Generalized and partial seizures may occur and be followed by delirium. Steroids used for treatment of pulmonary sarcoidosis have been implicated in concurrent psychiatric disorders in about 4 percent of the treated patients (116). Transient ischemic attacks and strokes occur very rarely (113).

Paget's disease. This disease involves the skull and may give rise to neuropsychiatric symptoms. Dementia due to compression of the fourth ventricle and occult hydrocephalus is the commonest psychiatric disorder. Episodes of delirium may punctuate the chronic disorder (117, 118).

Multiple sclerosis. On occasion multiple sclerosis may present with an acute cerebral disorder (cerebral MS) featuring an organic brain syndrome (119). This development was observed in 2 percent of multiple sclerosis patients in Israel (119). How. often the associated organic brain syndrome represents delirium and how frequently it is just an initial episode in unremitting dementia is unclear.

Senile dementia. Senile dementia is stated to feature delirious episodes. Rothschild (120) speaks of a "delirious and confused type" of senile dementia. The status of this "type" is vague. Degenerative disease of the brain predisposes the patient to delirium due to the whole range of causes discussed in this book. Whether such disease itself ever causes delirium is an open question.

Allergic disease. Allergic disease is claimed to include cases of "cerebral allergy" which may manifest itself as "confusional states" among many other alleged clinical features (121). The status of this proposed disorder as a cause of delirium remains unclear.

Cranial irradiation. Recently cranial irradiation for meningeal leukemia has been described to induce acute encephalopathy with "depressed consciousness" (122). The latter appears to range from delirium to coma. The central nervous system is, of course, frequently involved in childhood leukemia, with such lesions as leukemic cellular infiltration of the brain or meninges, intracranial hemorrhage, or opportunistic infections (123). Currently used chemotherapeutic agents, described in Chapter 10, can produce encephalopathy and delirium.

REFERENCES

1. Editorial: Head injuries—from accident department to necropsy room. *Lancet 1*:589-591, 1978.
2. Dresser, A.C., Meirowsky, A.M., Weiss, G.H., et al.: Gainful employment following head injury. *Arch Neurol 29*:111-116, 1973.
3. Jennett, B., Teasdale, S., Galbraith, S., et al.: Severe head injuries in three countries. *J Neurol Neurosurg Psychiatry 40*:291-298, 1977.
4. Hooper, R.: *Patterns of Acute Head Injury.* Baltimore, Williams & Wilkins Co., 1969.
5. Ommaya, A.K., and Gennarelli, T.A.: Cerebral concussion and traumatic unconsciousness. *Brain 97*:633-654, 1974.
6. Levin, W.: *The Management of Head Injuries.* Baltimore, Williams & Wilkins, Co., 1966.
7. Walther-Büel, H.: *Die Psychiatrie der Hirngeschwülste.* Wien, Springer-Verlag, 1951.
8. Güvener, A., Bagchi, B.K., and Calhoun, H.D.: Mental and seizure manifestations in relation to brain tumors. A statistical study. *Epilepsia 5*:166-176, 1964.
9. Friedman, H., and Odom, G.L.: Expanding intracranial lesions in general practice. *Geriatrics 27*:105-115, 1972.
10. Riggs, H.E., and Rupp, C.: A clinicoanatomic study of personality and mood disturbances associated with gliomas of the cerebrum. *J Neuropath Exper Neurol 17*:338-345, 1958.
11. Strobos, R.R.J.: Tumors of the temporal lobe. *Neurology 3*:752-760, 1953.
12. Assal, G., Zander, E., and Hadjiantonion, J.: Les troubles mentaux au cours des tumeurs de la fosse postérieure. *Arch Suisses Neurol Neurochir Psychiatry 116*:17-27, 1975.
13. Schmid-Wermser, I., Nagel, G.A., and Schmid, A.H.: Zur klinischen Diagnose von Hirnmetastasen beim Bronchuskarzinom. *Schweiz med Wschr 104*:464-468, 1974.
14. Kanzer, M.: Personality disorders with brain tumors. *Am J Psychiatry 97*:812-830, 1941.
15. Cairns, H., and Mosberg, W.H.: Colloid cyst of the third ventricle. *Surg Gynecol Obstet 92*:545-570, 1951.
16. Netsky, M.G., and Watson, J. MacD.: The natural history of intracranial neoplasms. *Annu Intern Med 45*:275-284, 1956.
17. Scott, M.: Transitory psychotic behavior following operation for tumors of the cerebello-pontine angle. *Psychiatr Neurol Neurochir 73*:37-48, 1970.
18. Bruens, J.H.: Psychoses in epilepsy. *Psychiatr Neurol Neurochir 74*:175-192, 1971.
19. Helmchen, H.: "Reversible Psychic Disorders in Epileptic Patients," in Birkenmayer, W., Ed., *Epileptic Seizures—Behavior—Pain.* Bern, Huber, 1976, pp. 175-186.

20. Köhler, G.K.: Begriffbestimmung und Einteilung der sog. epileptischen Psychosen. *Schweiz Arch Neurol Neurochir 120*:261-281, 1977.
21. Köhler, G.K.: Epileptische Psychosen. *Fortschr Neurol Psychiatr 43*:99-153, 1975.
22. Wechsler, I.S.: *A Textbook of Clinical Neurology.* 7th edition. Philadelphia, W.B. Saunders, 1952, p. 607.
23. Laidlaw, J., and Richens, A., Eds.: *A Textbook of Epilepsy.* Edinburgh, Churchill, 1976, pp. 145-184.
24. Penry, J.K., and Daly, D.D., Eds.: *Complex Partial Seizures and Their Treatment.* New York, Raven Press, 1975.
25. Lennox, W.G.: The treatment of epilepsy. *Med Clin N Am 29*:1114-1128, 1945.
26. Ellis, J.M., and Lee, S.I.: Acute prolonged confusion in later life as an ictal state. *Epilepsia 19*:119-128, 1978.
27. Celesia, G.G.: Modern concepts of status epilepticus. *JAMA 235*: 1571-1574, 1976.
28. Belafsky, M.A., Carwille, S., Miller, P., et al.: Prolonged epileptic twilight states: continuous recordings with nasopharyngeal electrodes and video-tape analysis. *Neurology 28*:239-245, 1978.
29. Penry, J.K., and Dreifuss, F.E.: Automatisms associated with the absence of petit mal epilepsy. *Arch Neurol 21*:142-149, 1969.
30. Saper, J.R., and Lossing, J.H.: Prolonged trance-like stupor in epilepsy. *Arch Intern Med 134*:1079-1082, 1974.
31. Escueta, A.V., Boxley, J., Stubbs, N., Waddell, G., and Wilson, W.A.: Prolonged twilight state and automatisms: a case report. *Neurology 24*:331-339, 1974.
32. Levin, S.: Epileptic clouded states. *J Nerv Ment Dis 116*:215-225, 1952.
33. Gastaut, H.: *The Epilepsies. Electro-Clinical Correlations.* Springfield, Ill., Charles C Thomas, 1954.
34. Glaser, G.H.: The problem of psychosis in psychomotor temporal lobe epileptics. *Epilepsia 5*:271-278, 1964.
35. Flor-Henry, P.: Psychosis and temporal lobe epilepsy. A controlled investigation. *Epilepsia 10*:363-395, 1969.
36. Peters, U.H., and Gille, G.: Über die körperlichen Grunde körperlich begrundbaren Psychosen. *Dtsch med Wschr 98*:967-970, 1973.
37. Millikan, C.H., Bauer, R.B., Goldschmidt, J., et al.: A classification and outline of cerebrovascular diseases II. *Stroke 6*:564-616, 1975.
38. Millikan, C.H., and McDowell, F.H.: Treatment of transient ischemic attacks. *Stroke 9*:299-308, 1978.
39. Genton, E., Barnett, H.J.M., Fields, W.S., et al.: XIV. Cerebral

ischemia: the role of thrombosis and of antithrombotic therapy. *Stroke* 8:150-175, 1977.

40. Hass, W.K., and Goldensohn, E.S.: Clinical and electroencephalographic considerations in the diagnosis of carotid artery occlusion. *Neurology* 9:575-589, 1959.

41. Hurwitz, L.J., Groch, S.N., Wright, I.S., and McDowell, F.H.: Carotid artery occlusive syndrome. *Arch Neurol* 1:491-501, 1959.

42. Shapiro, S.K.: Psychosis due to bilateral carotid artery occlusion. *Minn Med* 42:25-27, 1959.

43. Medina, J.L., Rubino, F.A., and Ross, E.: Agitated delirium caused by infarctions of the hippocampal formation and fusiform and lingual gyri: a case report. *Neurology* 24:1181-1183, 1974.

44. Medina, J.L., Chokroverty, S., and Rubino, F.A.: Syndrome of agitated delirium and visual impairment: a manifestation of medial temporo-occipital infarction. *J Neurol Neurosurg Psychiatry* 40:861-864, 1977.

45. Mesulam, M.M., Waxman, S.G., Geschwind, N., and Sabin, T.D.: Acute confusional states with right middle cerebral artery infarctions. *J Neurol Neurosurg Psychiatry* 39:84-89, 1976.

46. Gillespie, J.A., Ed.: *Extracranial Cerebrovascular Disease and Its Management*. London, Butterworths, 1969.

47. Sencer, W., and Andiman, R.: A clinical study of intracranial aneurysms. *Mt Sinai J Med NY* 40:72-81, 1973.

48. Okawara, S.H.: Warning signs prior to rupture of an intracranial aneurysm. *J Neurosurg* 38:575-580, 1973.

49. Sundt, T.M., and Whisnant, J.P.: Subarachnoid hemorrhage from intracranial aneurysms. *N Engl J Med* 299:116-122, 1978.

50. Storey, P.B.: Brain damage and personality change after subarachnoid hemorrhage. *Br J Psychiatry* 117:129-142, 1970.

51. Waltimo, O., and Putkonen, A.R.: Intellectual performance of patients with intracranial arteriovenous malformations. *Brain* 97:511-520, 1974.

52. Carter, L.P., Morgan, M., and Urrea, D.: Psychological improvement following arteriovenous malformation excision. *J Neurosurg* 42:452-456, 1975.

53. Belfer, M.L., and d'Autremont, C.C.: Catatonia-like symptomatology. *Arch Gen Psychiatry* 24:119-120, 1971.

54. Hanson, G.D., and Brown, M.J.: Waxy flexibility in a postpartum woman—a case report and review of the catatonic syndrome. *Psychiatr Q* 47:1-9, 1972.

55. Walton, J.N.: *Brain's Diseases of the Nervous System*. 8th edition, Oxford, Oxford University Press, 1977, p. 343.

56. Plum, F., and Posner, J.B.: *The Diagnosis of Stupor and Coma*. 2nd edition, Philadelphia, F.A. Davis Co., 1972.

57. Mitsomoto, H., Conomy, J.P., and Regula, G.: Subdural hematoma. *Cleve Clin Q 44*:95-99, 1977.
58. Fogelholm, R., Heiskanen, O., and Waltimo, O.: Chronic subdural hematoma in adults. *J Neurosurg 42*:43-46, 1975.
59. Potter, J.F., and Fruin, A.H.: Chronic subdural hematoma—the "great imitator." *Geriatrics 32*:61-66, 1977.
60. Raskind, R., Glover, B., and Weiss, S.R.: Chronic subdural hematoma in the elderly: a challenge in diagnosis and treatment. *J Am Ger Soc 20*:330-334, 1975.
61. Micheels, L.J.: Catatonic syndrome in a case of subdural hematoma. *J Nerv Ment Dis 117*:123-129, 1953.
62. Andrews, J.M.: Giant-cell ("temporal") arteritis. *Neurology 16*: 963-971, 1966.
63. Cochran, J.W., Fox, J.H., and Kelly, M.P.: Reversible mental symptoms in temporal arteritis. *J Nerv Ment Dis 166*:446-447, 1978.
64. Hart, C.T.: Formed visual hallucinations: a symptom of cranial arteritis. *Br Med J 3*:643-644, 1967.
65. Paulley, J.W., and Hughes, J.P.: Giant-cell arteritis, or arteritis of the aged. *Br Med J 4*:1562-1567, 1960.
66. Vereker, R.: The psychiatric aspects of temporal arteritis. *J Ment Sci 98*:280-285, 1952.
67. Huston, K.A., Hunder, G.G., Lie, J.T., Kennedy, R.H., and Elvaback, L.R.: Temporal arteritis. A 25-year epidemiologic, clinical, and pathologic study. *Ann Intern Med 88*:162-167, 1978.
68. Johnson, R.T., and Richardson, E.P.: The neurological manifestations of systemic lupus erythematosus. *Medicine 47*:337-369, 1968.
69. Osler, W.: On the visceral complications of erythema exudativum multiforme. *Am J Med Sci 110*:629-646, 1895.
70. Fessel, W.J., and Solomon, G.F.: Psychosis and systemic lupus erythematosus. *Calif Med 92*:266-270, 1960.
71. Bennahum, D.A., and Messner, R.P.: Recent observations on central nervous system lupus erythematosus. *Semin Arthritis Rheum 4*:253-266, 1975.
72. Estes, D., and Christian, C.L.: The natural history of systemic lupus erythematosus by prospective analysis. *Medicine 50*:85-95, 1971.
73. Feinglass, E.J., Arnett, F.C., Dorrsch, C.A., et al.: Neuropsychiatric manifestations of systemic lupus erythematosus: diagnosis, clinical spectrum, and relationship to other features of the disease. *Medicine 55*:323-339, 1976.
74. Guze, S.B.: The occurrence of psychiatric illness in systemic lupus erythematosus. *Am J Psychiatry 123*:1562-1570, 1967.
75. Ganz, V.H., Gurland, B.J., Deming, W.E., and Fisher, B.: The study of the psychiatric symptoms of systemic lupus erythematosus. *Psychosom Med 34*:207-220, 1972.

76. O'Connor, J.F., and Musher, D.M.: Central nervous system involvement in systemic lupus erythematosus. *Arch Neurol 14*:157-164, 1966.
77. Heine, B.E.: Psychiatric aspects of systemic lupus erythematosus. *Acta Psychiatr Scand 45*:307-326, 1969.
78. Sergent, J.S., Lockshin, M.D., Klempner, M.S., and Lipsky, B.A.: Central nervous system disease in systemic lupus erythematosus. *Am J Med 58*:644-654, 1975.
79. Bennett, R., Hughes, G.R.V., Bywaters, E.G.L., and Holt, P.J.L.: Neuropsychiatric problems in systemic lupus erythematosus. *Br Med J 4*:342-345, 1972.
80. Small, P., Mass, M.F., Kohler, P.F., and Harbeck, R.J.: Central nervous system involvement in SLE. *Arthr Rheum 20*:869-878, 1977.
81. Finn, R., and Rudolf, N. de M.: The electroencephalogram in systemic lupus erythematosus. *Lancet 1*:1255, 1978.
82. Pinching, A.J., Travers, R.L., Hughes, G.R.V., et al.: Oxygen-15 brain scanning for detection of cerebral involvement in systemic lupus erythematosus. *Lancet 1*:898-900, 1978.
83. Bilaniuk, L.T., Patel, S., and Zimmerman, R.A.: Computed tomography of systemic lupus erythematosus. *Radiology 124*:119-121, 1977.
84. Baker, M., Hadler, N.M., Whitaker, J.N., et al.: Psychopathology in systemic lupus erythematosus. II. Relation to clinical observations, corticosteroid administration, and cerebrospinal fluid C4. *Semin Arthritis Rheum 3*:111-126, 1973.
85. Petz, L.D.: Neurological manifestations of systemic lupus erythematosus and thrombotic thrombocytopenic purpura. *Stroke 8*:719-722, 1977.
86. Ford, R.G., and Siekert, R.G.: Central nervous system manifestations of periarteritis nodosa. *Neurology 15*:114-122, 1965.
87. Gottwald, W.: Die neurologisch-psychiatrischen und muskularen Manifestationen der Vasculitis nodosa. *Fortschr Neurol Psychiatr 45*:475-483, 1977.
88. Wintrobe, M.M., Thorn, G.W., Adams, R.D., et al., Eds.: *Harrison's Principles of Internal Medicine.* 7th edition, New York, McGraw-Hill Book Co., 1974.
89. Gupta, V.P., and Ehrlich, G.E.: Organic brain syndrome in rheumatoid arthritis following corticosteroid withdrawal. *Arthritis Rheum 19*:1333-1338, 1976.
90. Skowronski, T., and Gatter, R.A.: Cerebral vasculitis associated with rheumatoid disease—a case report. *J Rheumatol 1*:473-475, 1974.
91. Steiner, J.W., and Gelbloom, A.J.: Intracranial manifestations in two cases of systemic rheumatoid disease. *Arthritis Rheum 2*:537-545, 1959.

92. Jan, J.E., Hill, R.H., and Low, M.D.: Cerebral complications in juvenile rheumatoid arthritis. *Can Med Assoc J* 107:623-625, 1972.

93. Kozin, F., Haughton, V., and Bernhard, G.C.: Neuro-Behçet disease: two cases and neuroradiologic findings. *Neurology* 27:1148-1152, 1977.

94. Hachinski, V.C., Lassen, N.A., and Marshall, J.: Multi-infarct dementia. A cause of mental deterioration in the elderly. *Lancet* 2:207-210, 1974.

95. Meyer, J.S., Ed.: *Modern Concepts of Cerebrovascular Disease.* New York, Spectrum Publications, 1975, pp. 135-158.

96. Burger, P.C., Burch, J.G., and Kunze, U.: Subcortical arteriosclerotic encephalopathy (Binswanger's disease). *Stroke* 7:626-631, 1976.

97. Dawson, D.M., and Fischer, E.G.: Neurologic complications of cardiac catheterization. *Neurology* 27:496-497, 1977.

98. Swanson, P.D., Calanchini, P.R., Dyken, M.L., et al.: A cooperative study of hospital frequency and character of transient ischemic attacks. II. Performance of angiography among six centers. *JAMA* 237:2202-2206, 1977.

99. Ehyai, A., and Fenichel, G.M.: The natural history of confusional migraine. *Arch Neurol* 35:368-369, 1978.

100. Emery, E.S.: Acute confusional state in children with migraine. *Pediatrics* 60:110-114, 1977.

101. Gascon, G., and Barlow, C.: Juvenile migraine, presenting as an acute confusional state. *Pediatrics* 45:628-635, 1970.

102. Klee, A.: *A Clinical Study of Migraine With Particular Reference to the Most Severe Cases.* Copenhagen, Munksgaard, 1968.

103. Sacks, O.W.: *Migraine. The Evolution of a Common Disorder.* Berkeley, University of California Press, 1970.

104. Mathew, N.T., Meyer, J.S., Welch, K.M.A., and Neblett, C.R.: Abnormal CT-scans in migraine. *Headache* 16:272-279, 1977.

105. Senter, H.J., Lieberman, A.N., and Pinto, R.: Cerebral manifestations of ergotism. *Stroke* 7:88-92, 1976.

106. Kaschkat, G.: Psychiatrische Syndrome bei Anämien, Kollagenerkrankungen, Mineralaushaltsstörungen und postinfektiösen Zustanden. *Internist* 16:15-19, 1975.

107. Wise, T.N., and Ginzler, E.M.: Scleroderma cerebritis, an unusual manifestation of progressive systemic sclerosis. *Dis Nerv Syst* 36:60-62, 1975.

108. Abramsky, O., and Slavin, S.: Neurologic manifestations in patients with mixed cryoglobulinemia. *Neurology* 24:245-249, 1974.

109. Calabresi, P., and Meyer, O.O.: Polycythemia vera. Clinical and laboratory manifestations. *Ann Intern Med* 50:118-120, 1958.

110. Silverstein, A.: Thrombotic thrombocytopenic purpura. *Arch Neurol* 18:358-362, 1968.

111. O'Brien, J.L., and Sibley, W.A.: Neurologic manifestations of thrombotic thrombocytopenic purpura. *Neurology* 8:55-64, 1958.
112. Liston, E.H., Levine, M.D., and Philippart, M.: Psychosis in Fabry disease and treatment with phenoxybenzamine. *Arch Gen Psychiat* 29:402-403, 1973.
113. Delaney, P.: Neurologic manifestations in sarcoidosis. *Ann Intern Med* 87:336-345, 1977.
114. Jefferson, M.: Sarcoidosis of the nervous system. *Brain* 80:540-556, 1957.
115. Wiederholt, W.C., and Siekert, R.G.: Neurological manifestations of sarcoidosis. *Neurology* 15:1147-1154, 1965.
116. Johns, C.J., Zachary, J.B., and Ball, W.C.: A ten-year study of corticosteroid treatment of pulmonary sarcoidosis. *Johns Hopkins Med J* 134:271-283, 1974.
117. Friedman, P., Sklaver, N., and Klawans, H.L.: Neurologic manifestations of Paget's disease of the skull. *Dis Nerv Syst* 32:809-817, 1971.
118. Kissel, P., Schmitt, J., and Barrucand, D.: Les complications neuropsychiatriques de la maladie de Paget. *L'Encephale* 2:97-111, 1967.
119. Kahana, E., Leibowitz, U., and Alter, M.: Cerebral multiple sclerosis. *Neurology* 21:1179-1185, 1971.
120. Rothschild, D.: "Senile Psychoses and Psychoses With Cerebral Arteriosclerosis," in Kaplan, O.J., Ed., *Mental Disorders in Later Life*. Stanford, Stanford Univ. Press, 1956, pp. 289-331.
121. Campbell, M.B.: Neurological allergy. *Rev Allergy* 22:80-89, 1968.
122. Oliff, A., Bleyer, W.A., and Poplack, D.G.: Acute encephalopathy after initiation of cranial irradiation for meningeal leukemia. *Lancet* 2:13-15, 1978.
123. Crosley, C.J., Rorke, L.B., Evans, A., and Nigro, M.: Central nervous system lesions in childhood leukemia. *Neurology* 28:678-685, 1978.

Additional References

Bennett, R.M., Bong, D.M., and Spargo, B.H. Neuropsychiatric problems in mixed connective tissue disease. *Am J Med* 65:955-962, 1978.
Carr, R.I., Shucard, D.W., Hoffman, S.A., et al. Neuropsychiatric involvement in systemic lupus erythematosus. *Birth Defects* 14:209-235, 1978.
Chester, E.M., Agamanolis, D.P., Banker, B.Q., and Victor, M. Hypertensive encephalopathy: A clinicopathologic study of 20 cases. *Neurology* 28:928-939, 1978.
Engel, J., Ludwig, B.I., and Fetell, M. Prolonged partial complex status epilepticus: EEG and behavioral observations. *Neurology* 28:863-869, 1978.

Futty, D.E., Conneally, P.M., Dyken, M.L., et al. Cooperative study of hospital frequency and character of transient ischemic attacks. V. Symptom analysis. *JAMA 238*:2386-2390, 1977.

Geier, S. Prolonged psychic epileptic seizures: A study of the absence status. *Epilepsia 19*:431-445, 1978.

Gonzalez-Scarano, F., Lisak, R.P., Bilaniuk, L.T., et al. Cranial computed tomography in the diagnosis of systemic lupus erythematosus. *Ann Neurol 5*:158-165, 1979.

Howell, D.A. Clinical and pathological consequences of lumps and swellings inside the cranium. *Br J Hosp Med 21*:60-66, 1979.

Kaufman, A. Medicolegal aspects of head injuries: Intellectual impairment and clinical-psychological assessment. *Med Sci Law 18*:56-62, 1978.

Levin, H.S., and Grossman, R.G. Behavioral sequelae of closed head injury. *Arch Neurol 35*:720-727, 1978.

Lishman, W.S. Psychiatric sequelae of head injuries: Problems in diagnosis. *J Irish Med Assoc 71*:306-314, 1978.

Little, J.R., Dial, B., Belanger, G., and Carpenter, S. Brain hemorrhage from intracranial tumor. *Stroke 10*:283-288, 1979.

Miller, J.D., Sweet, R.C., Narayan, R., and Becker, D.P. Early insults to the injured brain. *JAMA 240*:439-442, 1978.

Oddy, M., Humphrey, M., and Uttley, D. Subjective impairment and social recovery after closed head injury. *J Neurol Neurosurg Psychiatry 41*:611-616, 1978.

Ram, C.V.S. Hypertensive encephalopathy. *Arch Intern Med 138*:1851-1853, 1978.

Scott, D.F. Psychiatric aspects of epilepsy. *Br J Psychiatry 132*:417-430, 1978.

Selecki, B.R., Gonski, L., Gonski, A., et al. Retrospective survey of neuro-traumatic admissions to a teaching hospital. *Med J Aust 2*:232-274, 1978.

Shimizu, T., Ehrlich, G.E., Inaba, G., and Hayashi, K. Behçet disease (Behçet syndrome). *Semin Arthr Rheum 8*:223-260, 1979.

Siomopoulos, V., and Shah, N. Acute organic brain syndrome associated with rheumatoid arthritis. *J Clin Psychiatry 40*:76-82, 1979.

Steinbok, P., and Thompson, G.B. Metabolic disturbances after head injury: Abnormalities of sodium and water balance with special reference to the effects of alcohol intoxication. *Neurosurgery 3*:9-15, 1978.

CHAPTER 16

POSTPARTUM DELIRIUM

The question about the nature of postpartum psychosis remains controversial. Hamilton (1) in his monograph on the subject advocates the position that "postpartum delirium" is one of the main psychiatric syndromes occurring in temporal relation to childbirth. He asserts that this delirium has certain special characteristics: It tends to arise "out of a state of health" rather than follow the onset of an infection or other physical illness. It usually develops on about the third day postpartum and often lasts longer than infectious delirium. It is often associated with autonomic symptoms such as tachycardia, fever, and sweating, although infection cannot be demonstrated. The content of the hallucinations and delusions is liable to reflect concerns over birth, motherhood, and sex. Admixture of other psychiatric symptoms, affective and schizophreniform, is common. More recently, Hamilton (2) reiterated his view that delirium is one of the main variants of puerperal psychosis: "Confusion merging into delirium is very frequent in postpartum syndromes."

Silbermann et al. (3) point out that the first known description of a psychiatric disorder during puerperium, offered by Hippocrates, was that of delirium. Subsequently, many writers over the centuries described "puerperal insanity" bearing the features of the latter syndrome. Marcé (4), writing in 1858, speaks of acute delirium (délire aigu) as a potentially lethal complication of the puerperium. Silbermann et al. (3) state that postpartum delirium is the puerperal psychosis par excellence. It is characterized by fluctuating level of consciousness, perplexity, extreme anxiety, hallucinations, delusions, and marked psychomotor overactivity. These authors state that postpartum delirium resembles toxic delirium of the English-language literature. They report favorable results of treatment with perphenazine and lithium in combination. Arentsen (5) diagnosed delirium in thirty-two of 168 women who became psychotic in the first six months after birth. In about 60 percent of the cases the cause of delirium was uncertain.

A number of recent authors have expressed views on postpartum psychosis diametrically opposed to the preceding. Foundeur et al. (6) have not diagnosed delirium in any of 100 women hospitalized for postpartum mental illness at the New York Hospital-Westchester Division between 1944 and 1952. They comment that the illness, which used to be called toxic-exhaustive psychosis, or delirium, came to be regarded as dementia praecox.

Thomas and Gordon (7) point out that the frequency of toxic-exhaustive psychosis reported to occur in the postpartum period has declined sharply since the 1930s, probably as a result of improved obstetric practice, introduction of antibiotics, and changed diagnostic habits. The proportion of the reported toxic-exhaustive psychosis (delirium) had declined by the 1950s to between 3 and 5 percent of postpartum mental disorders.

Protheroe (8) found an equally low incidence of reported postpartum delirium among patients hospitalized for puerperal psychosis in a British hospital between 1927 and 1961. Only six out of 134 (about 4%) had received the diagnosis of "organic states." Stevens (9) maintains that with the development of modern obstetric practice preventing puerperal sepsis, toxic-exhaustive psychoses of the puerperium have almost disappeared. A similar conclusion has been reached by Wilson et al. (10), who found only two cases of acute brain syndrome among forty-four women with postpartum mental illness.

Melges (11) failed to diagnose delirium in any of 100 women suffering from postpartum psychiatric syndromes. He has taken the most explicit stand against the opinion that postpartum psychosis frequently represents delirium, a view held by Hamilton (2), among others. He argues that none of the fifteen of his patients who had an EEG taken was found to have abnormal slowing indicative of delirium. Furthermore, even though eighteen of his 100 patients displayed confusion and disorientation, there was no significant difference between their performance on the serial sevens and the digit-span test and that of other patients who had been admitted to the hospital more than two weeks after delivery. Melges concluded that none of his patients exhibited "classical delirium." His arguments are hardly compelling and conclusive. He made no attempt to use serial EEG recordings on those of his patients who displayed "confusion" and disorientation for time, and thus failed to rule out mild delirium. Serial sevens and digit span are commonly used bedside tests for delirium but can hardly be regarded as sufficient for diagnosis. The issue remains unresolved.

What is the status of "postpartum delirium" today? There is no doubt that infectious delirium in the postpartum period has almost disappeared with the advent of antibiotics and other medical advances. This fact does not, however, preclude the possibility that other causes may be operating and that some of the so-called "schizophrenic reactions" (11) could actually represent delirium. Many of them would most likely fail to satisfy the current criteria for the diagnosis of a schizophrenic disorder and would better be classified as atypical or schizophreniform or brief reactive psychoses (12). There is still a need for a prospective study of postpartum psychosis employing serial EEG recordings, other laboratory tests, and standardized mental status examinations, as well as a battery of neuropsychologic tests, in order to settle the controversy. The term "postpartum delirium" has little meaning and should not be used. It purports to convey information we do not have and is thus misleading. There is at this time no evidence that some pathophysiological factor, or factors, unique to the postpartum period gives rise to delirium, nor has it been demonstrated through comparative studies that the delirium occurring during puerperium has uniquely distinguishing clinical features. Introduction of the new classification of mental disorders and more explicit diagnostic criteria may help resolve these issues in the future. Meanwhile, one is struck by the similarity between reported postpartum psychoses and those which follow administration of corticosteroids or arise in the course of systemic lupus erythematosus. The same variability and fluidity of delirious, affective, and schizophrenia-like manifestations characterize the more severe, or psychotic, disorders occurring in those three settings. Whether this phenomenological similarity signifies common pathophysiological mechanisms is, of course, unknown.

REFERENCES

1. Hamilton, J.A.: *Postpartum Psychiatric Problems.* St. Louis, C.V. Mosby Co., 1962.
2. Hamilton, J.A.: Puerperal psychoses. *Gynecol Obstet* 2:1-8, 1977.
3. Silbermann, R.M., Beenen, F., and deJong, H.: Clinical treatment of postpartum delirium with perphenazine and lithium carbonate. *Psychiatria Clin* 8:314-326, 1975.
4. Marcé, L.V.: *Traité de la Folie des Femmes Enceintes.* Paris, J.B. Bailliere et fils, 1858.
5. Arentsen, K.: Postpartum psychoses. *Dan Med Bul* 15:97-100, 1968.
6. Foundeur, M., Fixsen, C., Triebel, W.A., and White, M.A.: Postpartum mental illness. *Arch Neurol Psychiatry* 77:503-512, 1957.
7. Thomas, C.L., and Gordon, J.E.: Psychosis after childbirth: ecological aspects of a single impact stress. *Am J Med Sci* 238:363-388, 1959.
8. Protheroe, C.: Puerperal psychoses: a long term study 1927-1961. *Br J Psychiatry* 115:9-30, 1969.
9. Stevens, B.C.: Psychoses associated with childbirth: a demographic survey since the development of community care. *Soc Sci & Med* 5:527-543, 1971.
10. Wilson, J.E., Barglow, P., and Shipman, W.: The prognosis of postpartum mental illness. *Compr Psychiatry* 13:305-316, 1972.
11. Melges, F.T.: Postpartum psychiatric syndromes. *Psychosom Med* 30:95-108, 1968.
12. Diagnostic and Statistical Manual of Mental Disorders. 3rd edition. Draft of January 15, 1978. Washington, D.C., American Psychiatric Association, 1978.

Additional References

Grundy, P.F., and Roberts, C.J. Observations on the epidemiology of post partum mental illness. *Psychol Med* 5:286-290, 1975.
Handley, S.L., Dunn, T.L., Baker, J.M., et al. Mood changes in puerperium, and plasma tryptophan and cortisol concentrations. *Br Med J* 2:18-22, 1977.
Hays, P. Taxonomic map of the schizophrenias, with special reference to puerperal psychosis. *Br Med J* 2:755-757, 1978.
Herzog, A., and Detre, T. Postpartum psychoses. *Dis Nerv Syst* 34:556-559, 1974.

Kane, F.J., Harman, W.J., Keeler, M.H., and Ewing, J.A. Emotional and cognitive disturbance in the early puerperium. *Br J Psychiatry* 114:99-102, 1968.

Martin, M.E. A maternity hospital study of psychiatric illness associated with childbirth. *Irish J Med Sci* 146:239-244, 1977.

Pitt, B. "Maternity blues." *Br J Psychiat* 122:431-433, 1973.

Robinson, D.B. Management of combined organic and emotional factors in a post-partum psychosis. *Minn Med* 49:1897-1905, 1966.

Roth, N. The mental content of puerperal psychoses. *Am J Psychother* 29:204-211, 1975.

Sandler, M., Ed. *Mental Illness in Pregnancy and the Puerperium.* New York, Oxford University Press, 1979.

Uddenberg, N., and Englesson, I. Prognosis of postpartum mental disturbance. *Acta Psychiatr Scand* 58:201-212, 1978.

Vislie, H. Puerperal mental disorders. *Acta Psychiatr Neurol Scand (Suppl 111)*:7-42, 1956.

Yalom, I.D., Lunde, D.T., Moos, R.H., and Hamburg, D.S. "Postpartum blues" syndrome. *Arch Gen Psychiatry* 18:16-27, 1968.

CHAPTER 17

DELIRIUM IN SURGERY

HISTORICAL INTRODUCTION

ACCIDENTAL TRAUMA AND severe burns as well as surgery with general anesthesia may precipitate delirium. Practically all of the factors responsible for the occurrence of this syndrome in the practice of surgery have been discussed in previous chapters. They will be mentioned here only briefly to underscore their relevance to delirium arising in surgical settings.

Delirium related to surgery has been known for centuries. Paré (1), the famous French surgeon living in the sixteenth century, discusses at some length delirium complicating surgical conditions and procedures. He refers to it as a transient disorder featuring "raving, talking idly or doting," and one liable to occur in association with fever and pain accompanying wounds, after loss of blood occasioned by an operation, and as a complication of gangrene. Delirium arising in this context came to be called "traumatic" or "nervous" (2).

Dupuytren (2), an eminent French surgeon, wrote an excellent description of this syndrome:

The delirium manifests itself by a singular confusion of things, places, and persons; the patient is deprived of sleep, and is possessed by some predominant idea, which is generally connected with his profession, habits, age, or sex. The limbs are constantly tossed about; the upper part of the body is covered with abundant sweat; the eyes are bright and injected; the face is animated and flushed; individuals affected with this species of delirium are often so extremely insensible, that patients with comminuted fracture of the lower extremity, have dragged off all the dressing, and walked about on the broken limb, without exhibiting any sign of pain; others, whose ribs were broken, tossed themselves about, and sung without seeming to suffer; finally, it has happened that a patient, who had been operated on for hernia, introduced his fingers into the wound, and amused himself by unrolling his intestines as if he were acting on a dead body.

Dupuytren observed absence of fever in these patients. The delirium, he noted, was particularly apt to occur in persons injured as a result of a suicidal attempt, and it had not been observed in children. It lasted as a rule not longer than six days but could be rapidly fatal. Treatment was often unsuccessful although Dupuytren found enemas of laudanum helpful. Some recent writers have suggested that delirium traumaticum was in fact delirium tremens (3), but such an interpretation is unwarranted.

Graves (4), speaking of traumatic delirium, points out that "an external injury reacting on the nerves may bring on high mental excitement, delirium, and a total privation of sleep, as we see exemplified in delirium traumaticum." Croft (5) wrote in 1870 an article devoted to delirium tremens in surgical patients and reported on thirty-one cases seen over a period of four years. Four of his patients had died. He postulated that withdrawal of alcohol, and mental and physical shock of surgery, were likely responsible for the onset of delirium tremens in his patients. Savage (6) focuses his attention on the role of anesthetics in producing "insanity." He quotes examples of patients who, following the use of anesthetics, developed a temporary or permanent mental illness. He claims that any factor which can give rise to delirium may also trigger a more chronic mental disorder such as acute delirious mania or even progressive dementia. He asserts that "nervous instability, especially that due to insane inheritance" constitutes the chief predisposing factor in these cases.

Haward (7), another nineteenth century writer, remarks that, apart from withdrawal of alcohol, want of food or sleep and the presence of fatigue or anxiety are needed for delirium tremens to arise in surgical patients. He stresses the seriousness and common occurrence of pneumonia in association with delirium. Furthermore, he points out that old people may, after injury, develop delirium of a different kind from delirium tremens, one marked by "subdued but constant talkativeness." Haward calls this variant "senile delirium" and claims that unless the patient is taken out of bed and mobilized, he will die; moving about improves the delirium. Haward states that since the introduction of antiseptics traumatic fever and delirium had become less frequent but could still be seen frequently with severe burns.

At the beginning of the present century several writers addressed the problem of what had come to be labelled "postoperative psychosis" or "postoperative insanity." Da Costa (8), a professor of surgery at Philadelphia, wrote one of the best accounts of delirium occurring in the postoperative period. He states that various forms of mental disorder may follow surgery, among them delirium, hysterical excitement, obsessions, confusion, hypochondria, melancholy, and "actual insanity." Da Costa points out that no mental disorder characteristic of the postoperative period exists. "Acute confusional insanity" is the commonest disorder encountered and is characterized by confusion of thought, incoherent speech, delirium, illusions, hallucinations, and delusions. The two most important causes of acute confusional insanity are fear and worry. Postoperative insanity may become manifest immediately after the operation and is presumably caused by anesthesia, but it usually comes on three to five days after an operation. Da Costa says at one point that delirium may be mistaken for "insanity" but elsewhere in the paper he states that the "analysis of the mental state of a delirious patient shows us that delirium is identical with confusional insanity"; evidently Da Costa is a bit confused on this point. Not even etiology seems to be the main distinguishing feature, since Da Costa includes "states of great emotional instability (as hysteria)" among the causes of delirium, and actually lists "hysterical delirium" as one of the subtypes of the former. It appears that all deliriumlike psychoses arising after surgery and not related to fever, alcohol withdrawal, exogenous toxins, uremia, or diabetes were lumped together as "acute confusional insanity." This terminological and conceptual muddle mars Da Costa's exemplary description of delirium, to which the bulk of his paper is actually devoted. He points out that the syndrome is most likely to arise in children and the elderly, usually makes its first appearance at the period between sleep and wakefulness, and may clear up when the patient becomes fully awake, only to return with the onset of drowsiness. In febrile delirium, he claims, the temperature is nearly always 102° or above. Delirium tremens is liable to become manifest after injury or operation. Da Costa asserts that delirium may be caused by morphine and cocaine, and states: "In every unexplained case of delirium think of the possibility of morphinism and search for the drug." He uses the term "traumatic delirium" or "delirium nervosum" for a condition without fever and occurring only in very nervous subjects at any time during the early postoperative days. Da Costa also draws attention to nocturnal delirium in the aged. He urges that in every case of postoperative mental disorder a careful history should be obtained, a thorough physical examination made, and a neurologist asked at once to see the patient. This enlightened advice coming from an eminent surgeon stands out as an unusual episode in the annals of surgery. Even more striking is Da Costa's closing remark that the "entire subject of postoperative psychoses is extremely interesting and highly important. There remains much to learn about it." Had this sentiment been shared by more surgeons (and psychiatrists), the state of our ignorance would be less pronounced.

Da Costa's pioneering paper appeared in 1910. A year earlier Kelly (9) published an article on postoperative psychoses and reported that about 37 percent of his own series of forty patients were "acute hallucinatory confusional insanities." Thus semantic muddle pervaded this area; yet a coherent clinical picture of the commonest postoperative psychosis had emerged and it bore a strong resemblance to, or was actually identical with, delirium in the present sense (10-15). As Abeles (16) declares, most observers agreed that the majority of postoperative mental disorders fall into "the same syndrome of toxic-exhaustive and infective states. There is the same combination of confusion, delusions, hallucinations, and disturbances in motility." He himself found "confusion," manifested by disorientation, memory impairment, bewilderment, hallucinations, etc., in seventeen of twenty-three patients with postoperative psychosis. The duration of this psychosis was at least twelve days. Abeles stresses the multifactorial origin of postoperative psychosis. He lists psychodynamic factors, metabolic factors, general anesthesia, infection, presence of vascular disease, vitamin deficiency, and use of sedatives among the variables that may, singly or combined, contribute to the onset of postoperative psychosis. Doyle (17) reported on twenty-eight consecutive cases of postoperative psychosis observed at the Mayo Clinic over a period of five years. All of the patients were "confused or delirious"; twenty were said to be confused, while eight were delirious. Doyle concludes that "the postoperative psychosis is best classified with delirium."

This brief historical survey shows that delirium and, possibly, deliriumlike functional psychoses constitute the most common forms of major mental disorders arising after surgery. Delirium in this context was early recognized to result from an interplay of multiple psychologic and organic predisposing and precipitating factors. It was repeatedly observed that a lucid interval, most often lasting two to five days, preceded the delirium. Savage (6) comments that some of the patients were found to exhibit "unusual depression, heaviness, drowsiness, or irritability from the first." That indicated that the disorder had its onset immediately after the operation but attracted no attention until obvious excitement set in. These various features of postoperative delirium have been largely reaffirmed by the more recent investigators. The latter have tended to ignore delirium after routine abdominal and other surgery but rather focused on that which has complicated open-heart surgery.

INCIDENCE OF POSTOPERATIVE DELIRIUM

The incidence of delirium is unknown. Absence of relevant epidemiologic studies, muddled terminology, and lack of interest in this area of psychiatry must be held responsible for our continuing ignorance. What reports of incidence do exist have often come from anesthetists concerned with what they refer to as *emergence delirium or excitement*. Bastron and Moyers (18) state that the incidence of such delirium ranges from 3 percent to 20 percent. Eckenhoff et al. (19) reviewed the records of 14,436 patients admitted to the recovery room of the Hospital of the University of Pennsylvania over a four-year period. These investigators defined emergence delirium as a state characterized by crying, sobbing, thrashing about, and disorientation upon emergence from general anesthesia. This syndrome could be mild or severe. The incidence of postanesthetic or emergence delirium in the whole sample of patients was 5.3 percent. The highest incidence was found after tonsillectomy, thyroidectomy, circumcision, and hysterectomy, in that order. The incidence was highest in childhood, in the physically healthy, in those given barbiturates for premedication, and in patients anesthetized with cyclopropane and/or ether. Emotional factors were thought to contribute to the high incidence of emergence delirium after breast and thyroid surgery. Pain makes the occurrence of the delirium more likely. Coppolino (20) has come up with an incidence figure very close to that of Eckenhoff et al. Kuhn and Savage (21) assert that delirium occurs in about 20 percent of patients premedicated with scopolamine hydrobromide. Greene (22) observed emergence delirium in 10.2 percent and 8.1 percent of two groups of patients, respectively. Only 5.5 percent and 1.1 percent of these two groups were considered to have exhibited severe delirium, i.e. one requiring physical restraint. Over 20 percent of patients who had received scopolamine became delirious, and Greene concluded that drug-induced CNS depression, usually aggravated by pain, was mainly responsible for emergence delirium. Scopolamine, used as a premedicant, seemed to be a major causative factor, a hypothesis supported by the observation that in nineteen of twenty-one patients who received physostigmine intravenously, relief of delirium occurred in less than five minutes.

Studies of patients in surgical intensive care units have reported an incidence of delirium ranging from 2 percent to 40 percent (23-25). The highest figure comes from a study of delirium in a windowless intensive care unit (25). The author does not provide information on the type of surgery performed or the method of case identification. His figures seem unusually high. Titchener et al. (26) diagnosed delirium in 7.8 percent of 200 surgical patients; the syndrome accounted for about one-third of postoperative psychoses. Knox (27) estimated the incidence of postoperative psychosis to be about 1 per 1,600 surgical procedures. This figure strikes one as improbably low. Hammes (28) quotes the incidence of 1 in 400 operations. The true incidence most likely lies between these last two figures.

Considering the vagueness of the term "postoperative psychosis," no incidence figure quoted in the literature has much meaning anyway. Current efforts to develop rather strict diagnostic criteria for mental disorders will allow epidemiologic studies to be conducted. Such studies will have to distinguish between *emergence* delirium, occurring during the first twenty-four hours after operation and lasting minutes or a few hours, and the *interval* delirium, one with an onset after twenty-four hours to one week after surgery (17, 29). The latter subtype is liable to have different etiology and clinical significance from the former.

ETIOLOGIC FACTORS

Postoperative delirium is usually the outcome of multiple factors acting synergistically. One or another of these factors may predominate in a given case, but it is important to take into account the presence of all the other factors in managing the patient. The following review of the more common causes of delirium which follows surgery should facilitate etiologic diagnosis and treatment of most patients.

Several authors have addressed the issue of etiology of postoperative delirium (16, 28-33). Hammes (28) has classified postoperative psychoses into four categories: (1) withdrawal psychoses; (2) toxic psychoses; (3) psychoses of circulatory and respiratory origin; and (4) functional psychoses. The first three of these categories are, with few exceptions, nothing but delirium; the fourth category comprises schizophrenic, affective, paranoid, and atypical psychoses triggered by psychologic stress of surgery, anesthesia, etc. Withdrawal psychosis or delirium refers to that which constitutes a manifestation of the withdrawal syndrome from alcohol, sedative-hypnotics, or, rarely, analgesic narcotics in a person addicted to one or more of these substances. "Toxic psychoses" is an imprecise and obsolete term for delirium (and occasionally other organic brain syndromes, such as hallucinosis, or organic delusional syndrome) due to drugs and other exogenous chemicals. "Psychoses of circulatory and respiratory origin" are almost without exception delirium due to cerebral hypoxia, ischemia, hypercarbia, acidosis, etc. This classification is inadequate because it leaves out many relevant etiologic factors and also because it creates the false impression that toxic, withdrawal, or circulatory psychoses or delirium differ from one another in core clinical features. Despite these flaws, however, Hammes' classification draws attention to some of the most important etiologic factors in postoperative delirium.

Scott (29) has focused on the causes of postoperative psychoses or delirium in the aged. He stresses the importance of cerebral hypoxia caused by various factors as a major predisposing and precipitating condition for delirium in the elderly surgical patient. He emphasizes that "In the presence of persistent provoking agents, irreversible mental changes may develop." Kaufer (30) reviews the causes of "consciousness disturbances," or delirium, in surgery, based on a study of 100 patients. In many cases it was impossible to pinpoint the etiology of delirium. Kaufer found the following groups of factors to be most often involved in postoperative delirium: (1) cerebral-organic; (2) respiratory; (3) hemodynamic; (4) infectious-toxic; and (5) metabolic. Cerebral disease, such as trauma, vascular occlusion, metastases, "cerebral sclerosis," fat embolism, etc., accounted for about 30 percent of the dominant causes of postoperative delirium. The next most important group of causative factors involved infectious-toxic factors. Postoperative infections such as wound infections, ileus, peritonitis, septicemia, etc. were among the most common causes of delirium. Withdrawal delirium occurred in 7 percent of the patients. Metabolic factors were third in importance and constituted the main etiology in 15 percent of the cases. Hepatic coma alone occurred in 8 percent of the patients. Electrolyte disturbances, acid-base imbalance, renal failure, and hydration disorders were contributing factors to delirium in some patients. Kaufer stresses that in from one-third to one-half of all the patients more than one causal factor is present. He makes a most crucial point stating that "Every disturbance in the state of wakefulness which occurs in the course of a surgical illness aggravates the prognosis." Fully 39 percent of Kaufer's delirious surgical patients died.

Morse and Litin (31) carried out one of the best studies of etiologic factors in postoperative delirium. Over a six-month period they studied sixty patients aged thirty years or over who developed delirium postoperatively. Unfortunately, the time dimension of the term "postoperative" is not given. A matched control group of nondelirious surgical patients was also studied. Factors which were found to distinguish delirious patients from controls included: age sixty years and over; greater proportion of abnormal laboratory findings; duration of operation of more than four hours; emergency surgery; presence of postoperative complications; taking more than five drugs after operation; preoperative disorientation; morbid expectation, i.e. conscious fear of death before surgery; alcoholism; depression, current or previous; family history of psychosis; previous episodes of delirium in the patient; preoperative insomnia; paranoid personality; current or previous functional psychosis; history of postoperative psychosis of any type; and retirement problems. Once again the multifactorial etiology of postoperative delirium has been demonstrated. Metabolic disturbances, high surgical stress, heart failure, infection, intoxication, age sixty or over, and pre-existing brain disease were all positively correlated with the incidence of delirium. Sensory and sleep deprivation appeared to play some etiologic role. Thus, organic, psychologic, and environmental factors all do contribute to delirium (34).

Etiologic factors in postoperative delirium may be summarized as follows:

A. Predisposing factors
   1. Age sixty years or over
   2. Addiction to alcohol and/or drugs
   3. Chronic cerebral, cardiac, renal, hepatic disease
   4. Past history of delirium or functional psychosis
   5. Family history of psychosis
   6. Paranoid personality

B. Contributing (facilitating) factors
   1. Unfamiliarity of environment
   2. Sensory deprivation
   3. Noise (suspected factor)
   4. Sleep deprivation
   5. Immobilization
   6. Fear

C. Precipitating organic factors
 1. Acute cerebral disorder: trauma, edema, fat embolism, stroke, metastases
 2. Infection, especially pneumonia, bacteremia
 3. Drug intoxication, including agents used for premedication, anesthesia, and analgesia
 4. Metabolic disturbance: dehydration, electrolyte imbalance, acid-base imbalance, hepatic or renal failure
 5. Hemodynamic disturbance: hypoxemia, hypotension, hypovolemia, circulatory failure due to asystole, arrhythmia
 6. Respiratory disorder: pulmonary embolism, hypoxemia, hypercapnia, decompensated respiratory acidosis and alkalosis
 7. Alcohol and/or drug withdrawal syndrome
 8. Nutritional and vitamin deficiency
 9. Cerebral seizures due to any cause

Delirium in the Elderly Surgical Patient

Cerebral hypoxia of any etiology, electrolyte imbalance, drugs, and alcohol and/or drug withdrawal syndromes are the most important causes of delirium postoperatively. Interval or postoperative delirium, that is to say, one occurring after a lucid interval of one or more days, is most frequent among the aged (patients aged sixty or over). By contrast, postanesthetic or emergence delirium, that which comes on within twenty-four hours of an operation, is most often seen in otherwise healthy children (19). This heightened susceptibility to delirium of the elderly patient is most important. Delirium in this age-group may be the most obvious manifestation of a physical illness, in the present case of a postoperative complication. The elderly patient is particularly vulnerable to cerebral hypoxia of any origin since his or her cerebral perfusion is often already precariously compensated. It appears that cerebral ischemia or hypoxia resulting from factors related to the operation and general anesthesia may lead to some degree of permanent brain damage and associated irreversible dementia. Nearly a century ago, Savage (6) observed that a "progressive dementia" may follow in the wake of surgery. More recently, Bedford (35, 36) has drawn attention to this problem. He asserts that "minor dementias and even permanent catastrophic mental impairment" may result from surgery under general anesthesia. He found 120 patients aged sixty-five years or over about whom relatives had reported that the patients "had never been the same since the operation." This stereotype comment seemed to reflect observation of various cognitive and personality deficits dating back to the postoperative period. Bedford rightly stresses that even relatively mild degrees of dementia may be incapacitating for a person whose work requires sustained intellectual effort. In his own study he focused on 18 patients with severe dementia with postoperative onset. He was able to test them for intellectual or cognitive performance both before and after operation. Following surgery they all displayed confusion (presumably delirium) and this state was supplanted by and shaded over into irreversible dementia. Bedford emphasizes that such dramatic incidents are rare but the very fact that they do occur warrants taking precautionary measures. Appearance of delirium upon recovery from an operation in elderly persons must be viewed as a warning sign that cerebral hypoxia or some other pathogenic factor is present and demands immediate diagnosis and treatment if permanent brain damage is to be prevented. Bedford (36) argues forcefully against the use of potent hypnotics and analgesics preoperatively, postoperatively, and in the management of delirium in the elderly surgical patients.

Shock. A major pathogenic factor to complicate surgery and lead to cerebral hypoxia is shock. It may result from heart failure, hypovolemia, decreased vasomotor tone, or markedly increased resistance to blood flow (37). Effective management of shock and its cause or causes in the perioperative period is of especial importance in the elderly patient. *Postoperative hypoxemia* of a severe degree is more likely to occur in the elderly (38). Impairment of distribution of ventilation in these patients is one of the main factors contributing to hypoxemia. The elderly are also excessively vulnerable to *postoperative infections* as a result of conditions related to the aging process, environmental factors, and age-related chronic diseases (39).

Poor nutritional status, diminished responsivity to stress, and deteriorating immune function have all been blamed for this vulnerability. Polly and Sanders (39) point out that bacteremia in the elderly surgical patient is liable to manifest itself only with delirium. The older patient is also very sensitive to various *drugs,* especially those which depress the central nervous system, such as sedatives and hypnotics. Bedford (35) advises that giving premedication and postoperative medication should not be a routine procedure in the elderly. *Dehydration* and *electrolyte imbalance* are common after surgery under general anesthesia and may precipitate delirium in the older patient (35).

In conclusion, delirium is a common postoperative complication in the elderly and one that ought to alert the surgeon to the likely presence of a postoperative complication, such as infection, and to the risk of impending cerebral damage. It is a manifestation of disordered brain function, a fact which seems to be largely ignored by the surgical staff unless the patient's behavior is disturbing because of belligerence, restlessness, or noisiness. Recognition that delirium is present should lead to immediate diagnostic investigations and remedial action based on knowledge of the etiology involved. Use of the Cerebral Function Monitor (40), or similar apparatus, may help draw attention to abnormal cerebral electrical activity as soon as it develops and thus allow timely therapeutic intervention even before delirium becomes manifest clinically. In this way permanent brain damage may be prevented. These remarks should not, however, obscure the fact that most elderly patients do not suffer any ill effects on psychologic and social functioning (41).

Postoperative Delirium Tremens

Alcohol withdrawal syndrome has been recognized as a serious postoperative complication for over a century (5, 7). Da Costa (8) gives a vivid account of delirium tremens occurring postoperatively. He states that an alcoholic typically experiences a sleepless night after an injury or operation, or may have brief periods of sleep filled with terrifying dreams. The next day he is liable to be tremulous, restless, and apprehensive. Bouts of hallucinations appear and the withdrawal syndrome may stop there. In other cases, fullblown delirium follows. The patient

cannot keep still, has severe tremulousness, hallucinates uncon-
trollably, is fearful, and starts to misidentify people around him.
He may fight and injure himself or other people. The delirium
lasts two to four days.

Any patient with a history of drinking at least one pint of
whisky or its equivalent for at least ten out of fourteen days
immediately prior to admission is at risk for developing delirium
tremens after surgery (42). Cirrhosis or enlargement of the
liver, history of past episodes of delirium tremens, and presence
of early withdrawal symptoms are variables associated with
increased probability of postoperative delirium tremens (42).
Patients operated for cancer of laryngopharynx and oral cavity
are often alcoholics and hence alcohol withdrawal syndrome
is a frequent postoperative complication in head and neck surgery (43). It has been claimed that an alcoholic who has stopped
drinking may develop delirium tremens after an accident or
operation even if he has abstained from alcohol for months (34).
Whether these cases represent true alcohol withdrawal delirium
is, in this writer's view, uncertain and improbable. It is more
likely that one is dealing with delirium due to metabolic or other
causes in patients more vulnerable to the development of the
syndrome on account of previous alcoholism.

Alcohol withdrawal delirium is liable to become manifest on
the second to fourth postsurgical day (43). Within the next
twenty-four hours the delirium is likely to grow in severity, and
full-blown delirium tremens follows. An occasional patient may
develop the delirium as long as a week after surgery. Symptoms
are as described in Chapter 11. When they occur postoperatively,
these symptoms involve additional hazards related to the removal
of or interference with wounds, skin flaps, dressings, needles,
tracheostomy or drainage tubes, etc. (43). Serious complications may follow. Despite this it is claimed that postoperative
delirium tremens does not have higher mortality than that
arising in other settings (42).

Prevention and management of delirium tremens in surgery
are important. While it is not necessary to delay emergency
operations because occurrence of delirium is thought to be highly
probable, postponement of surgery whenever reasonable is ad-

vised (42). If a patient is believed to be at high risk for the development of postoperative delirium tremens on account of the indicators mentioned earlier, prophylactic use of a drug such as diazepam or chlordiazepoxide is recommended (see Chapter 11). It is also good policy to administer a high-potency vitamin B-complex preparation parenterally, both before and after surgery, to avoid confounding effects of vitamin deficiency so common among chronic alcoholics. Attention to concurrent liver disease, if present, is essential if hepatic encephalopathy is to be avoided (42). Subdural hematoma should always be ruled out in an alcoholic patient, especially if there is a history of recent head injury. Finally, an alcoholic may be concurrently addicted to barbiturates or other sedatives or hypnotics and withdrawal from them may provoke seizures and/or delirium indistinguishable from the alcohol withdrawal one. The patients should be routinely asked about recent intake of any psychotropic drugs. Presence of nystagmus, tremor, and ataxia suggests chronic barbiturate, or equivalent, intoxication.

Mays et al. (44) advocate the use of sympathetic blocking agents, such as propranolol, in the treatment of surgical delirium tremens. They found that serum albumin is decreased and plasma fatty acids are elevated over a prolonged period in patients who develop the syndrome. The fatty acids, these authors argue, have not only a nutritive but also a cytotoxic role and their increase in surgical delirium tremens appears undesirable. Propranolol has actually been used by some for the treatment of patients with delirium tremens for the control of severe tremor and tachyarrhythmia (45). However, its routine use in the surgical delirious patient cannot be recommended because of possible complications related to cardiomyopathy, bronchospasm or hypoglycemia (45).

MANAGEMENT AND PROGNOSIS OF POSTOPERATIVE DELIRIUM

Treatment of delirium is discussed in detail in Chapter 9; that of delirium tremens and drug withdrawal deliria is dealt with in Chapter 11. There is nothing about delirium in surgical settings that would call for a different therapeutic approach.

The most important aspect of management that needs to be stressed here is *early recognition* of the syndrome. Severe delirium seldom arises out of the blue: prodromal symptoms of restlessness, sleeplessness, nightmares, and anxiety or lethargy are the rule and must be looked out for. They are typically most accentuated at night and ought to be observed and reported by the night nurse. This implies training nurses in the importance of recognizing delirium. The nurse's recognition, however, will make little difference if she reports her observations to a surgeon to whom they mean little or nothing. All too often a psychiatric consultation is requested by a surgeon at a point when the patient is obviously delirious, disturbed, combative, and generally difficult to manage. At that point the patient may already have harmed himself or another patient or a nurse. Almost invariably one finds on close inquiry that such a patient had shown prodromal or early symptoms of delirium for at least a day but they were ignored by the medical staff even though nurses' notes contained clear description of them. Mishaps with far-reaching medical and legal consequences may occur and ought to be prevented by early recognition and treatment of the syndrome, and this presupposes relevant knowledge.

Likely candidates for postoperative delirium should be identified prior to surgery. They include the patient aged sixty-five years or more, the brain-damaged, the alcoholic, and the drug addict. Bedside testing of spatiotemporal orientation, recent memory, and immediate recall should be the minimum cognitive testing to be performed on every conscious surgical patient prior to surgery. This information should be recorded in the patient's chart to serve as a baseline for comparison with results of postoperative testing. Disorientation and/or memory impairment before operation point to delirium, dementia, or both. They must be regarded as presumptive evidence of a transient or permanent cerebral damage whose cause should be sought. Furthermore, any patient displaying such deficits is liable to display delirium postoperatively and is thus a case at special risk. Such a patient's mental state should be routinely observed and recorded by the nurses, and any increase in cognitive impairment must be reported. The patient should not be given narcotic analgesics unless necessary. He could be given haloperidol 2 to 10 mg. by mouth at bedtime to secure tranquilization during the night. Should delirium develop despite these measures, a search should start at once for the etiologic factor, or factors, involved. If the patient is restless and anxious or angry, in addition to being disoriented and/or otherwise cognitively impaired, haloperidol should be given first parenterally and then orally, when the patient shows signs of being tranquilized. Special measures are needed with patients who have undergone special types of surgery, such as open-heart surgery, cataract operations, orthopedic procedures, etc. Some of these will be discussed in the sections to follow.

Prognosis. The prognosis of postoperative delirium is always guarded, especially in the elderly, the chronically ill, the brain-damaged, and the alcoholic. Delirium may be followed by death, dementia, or organic personality syndrome. Titchener and Levine (46) studied psychotic reactions among 200 surgical patients; forty-four of them had psychosis, twenty-two had the diagnosis of delirium. Seven of the twenty-two delirious patients failed to recover completely and displayed some apparently permanent cognitive and personality deficits. Such an unhappy outcome has also been reported by Bedford (35) and is most likely to occur in the elderly patients. Of the delirious patients studied by Morse and Litin (47), 48 percent were completely recovered by the time of discharge from the hospital, 45 percent were improved, and 7 percent were unimproved. Duration of the delirium was one to seven days for most of the recovered patients, and more than seven days for the majority of those not recovered by the time of discharge.

One may conclude on the basis of these two studies that delirium arising after surgery must not be taken lightly, since it is a manifestation of cerebral disorder which in a proportion of cases may be followed by permanent intellectual impairment or dementia. Whether the latter can be prevented by treating the condition causing delirium is a matter of conjecture, but one sufficiently plausible to urge action.

DELIRIUM IN SPECIAL SETTINGS

Heart Surgery

This type of surgery has emerged as the one associated with the highest incidence of postoperative delirium. It has also spawned more neuropsychiatric investigations and articles than any other surgical procedure. During the past several years the incidence of postcardiotomy delirium has declined and so has the number of related publications. Reduction in cardiopulmonary bypass time and improved conditions in surgical intensive care units are the two factors usually credited for the diminishing incidence of delirium (48).

The first report on psychologic disturbances following *mitral commissurotomy* appeared in 1954 and claimed that about 20 percent of patients suffered from such disturbances (49). Subsequent studies confirmed this finding and documented the clinical features of the postoperative syndromes. The latter were said to be mainly delirium and a schizophrenia-like psychosis. Some authors speculated that symbolic meaning of the heart as the organ of life was a key variable in bringing about the psychiatric disorders. Other investigators emphasized the importance of organic causative factors such as chronic heart disease, cerebral hypoxia, pre-existing brain damage due to rheumatic fever, etc. (50). As surgical technique of closed-heart surgery improved, the incidence of postoperative psychoses tended to decline (51).

The earliest reports on neuropsychiatric complications of *open-heart surgery* began to appear in 1964 (52, 53). Some twenty-one studies have been published since then and together reported on about 1,820 cases of cardiotomy, with the incidence of postoperative psychiatric disturbances ranging from 13 to 100 percent (54). Fifteen of the twenty-one studies report such incidence to be between 30 and 60 percent. The latest studies still report a frequency of 40 to 60 percent (54). Only four studies give an incidence figure of less than 30 percent. Gilberstadt and Sako (55) found an incidence of only 13 percent, but their definition of "delirium" makes it clear why their figure is so low: they included only patients with hallucinations or severe disorientation but excluded those with "mild confusion." Other investigators claim to have cut the incidence of postcardiotomy delirium to about 5 percent by administering diazepam 2.5 to 5 mg. intravenously six times a day *after* the surgery (56). In their untreated control group the incidence of delirium was 35 percent. In the treated patients delirium could have been suppressed by the drug and this result gives no valid information about its true incidence. One group of investigators has claimed that between 1965 and 1969 the frequency of delirium after open-heart surgery dropped from 38 to 24 percent (57, 58). Decreased time on the cardiopulmonary bypass has been credited with lowering the incidence of delirium (57, 58).

Psychiatric syndromes occurring after open-heart surgery include (1) *delirium;* (2) *paranoid-hallucinatory* syndrome; (3) *hallucinosis;* and (4) *affective* (mood, dysphoric) syndrome. Some authors speak only of postcardiotomy delirium and make no mention of the other syndromes (52, 57, 58). Freyhan et al. (59) describe three syndromes, including delirium, which follow open-heart surgery. According to these investigators, the majority of patients exhibit a "multisyndromatic" syndrome, that is to say one characterized by a wide range of psychiatric symptoms occurring simultaneously or in succession. This type of clinical presentation is strongly reminiscent of postpartum psychoses, as well as those induced by steroid therapy or associated with systemic lupus erythematosus. It appears clear, however, that delirium is the most common type of psychiatric disorder occurring after open-heart surgery. Its incidence is about 24 to 30 percent (58).

Delirium in this setting is of two types: (1) with an onset on the first postoperative day; and (2) with onset after a lucid interval of at least two days after operation (57). According to Kornfeld et al. (57) less than 10 percent of the cases of postcardiotomy delirium have their onset on the first postoperative day. Dahme et al. (60) have reported recently that in their experience the opposite is true: about 75 percent of the patients exhibit signs of psychopathology on the first or second postoperative day. About 50 percent of the patients remain disturbed for one or two days, about one in four has symptoms of psychiatric disorder for three to four days, and about 12 percent of the patients remain disturbed for ten or more days. Disturbances of orientation and awareness are at their peak on the second postoperative day. Hallucinations, delusions, and paranoid ideas tend to arise on the third day (60). In the series reported by Kornfeld et al. (57), the mean day of onset of delirium was 4.2 and the mean day of recovery was 5.9. A typical course of the delirium features perceptual distortions, such as a floating sensation, and some mild disorientation, followed by vivid hallucinations, paranoid delusions, and gross disorientation (58). Heller et al. (58) classified postcardiotomy delirium into early postoperative organic brain syndrome and postcardiotomy delirium proper, respectively. The former is apparent on awakening from anesthesia, features disorientation and, often, neurologic signs, and is usually free of misperceptions, i.e. illusions and hallucinations. The postcardiotomy delirium proper occurs after a lucid interval of two to five days and is characterized by misperceptions, difficulty in distinguishing dreams from reality, and nocturnal confusion. Furthermore, minor and major delirium were distinguished depending on the presence or absence of persistent vivid hallucinations and delusions. Delirium, according to these definitions, was observed in 24 percent, and an early organic brain syndrome in 9 percent of the cases. It is this writer's impression that all of the 33 percent of patients manifested delirium, albeit with somewhat different manifestations. The early form is most likely to be seen in patients sixty years old and over.

Etiology. The etiology of postcardiotomy delirium (this term will be used here to refer to all clinical manifestations of delirium regardless of their time of onset) is multifactorial and complex. A number of putative causative factors have been proposed by various investigators, only to be challenged by others. Sterile controversies over the primacy of organic versus psychologic variables or vice versa have flared up periodically but most investigators have eschewed fanatical partisanship in this respect and endorsed a holistic viewpoint. The following list sums up the range of the postulated etiologic variables:

A. Predisposing preoperative factors
    1. age over forty-five years; very low incidence in children (58)

2. evidence of cerebral disease before surgery (59)
3. acquired versus congenital heart disease
4. severe degree of cardiac functional incapacity (61)
5. marked anxiety before surgery (61)
6. personality variables: none demonstrated, except possibly dominance (61)
7. depression preoperatively (61)
8. lower body weight (62)
9. preoperative cerebral embolism in mitral valve disease (62)
10. language barrier (63)
11. use of tranquilizers before surgery (62)

B. Factors related to operation
   1. duration of cardiopulmonary bypass time (regarded as of crucial importance by most but not all authors) (61, 62)
   2. hypotension (64)
   3. multiple-valve and aortic-replacement procedures (58, 59)

C. Factors related to postoperative states
   1. low cardiac output (65)

D. Factors related to postoperative environment
   1. altered sensory environment: sensory deprivation, monotony, noise (53, 57, 66)
   2. sleep deprivation due to frequent awakening (67-70)

In summary, postcardiotomy delirium is multidetermined. Organic, psychologic, and environmental variables contribute to its occurrence. Which of these factors carries the most weight is still a matter of considerable controversy, exemplified by opposing views on the importance of the cardiopulmonary bypass time. One could hardly deny that a constellation of organic factors constitutes a necessary, if not a sufficient, condition for delirium to occur. There is no satisfactory evidence that any of the psychologic or environmental variables is either necessary or sufficient. For example, Johns et al. (67) studied sleep patterns after open-heart surgery and concluded that both sleep deprivation and disturbances existed but were not likely the cause of delirium. Thus, the psychologic and environmental factors seem to play a contributory or facilitating rather than a causative role in delirium (for further discussion see Chapter 5).

Pathophysiology. The pathophysiology of postcardiotomy delirium has been the subject of numerous investigations and articles. Extracorporeal circulation during open-heart surgery has attracted particular attention as a suspected major source of pathophysiologic factors responsible for the occurrence of neuropsychiatric complications. Electroencephalographic (EEG) studies as well as those of cerebral blood flow and metabolism during cardiopulmonary bypass have provided evidence of cerebral dysfunction related temporally to this procedure. Lee et al. (71) found that patients subjected to various cardiac operative procedures without the use of extracorporeal circulation showed neither neurologic deficits nor psychiatric complications postoperatively. By contrast, patients who underwent cardiac surgery with extracorporeal circulation exhibited neurologic deficits, psychiatric complications, or both in the postoperative period. These investigators put forth a hypothesis that a microvascular perfusion defect represents the basic pathophysiologic condition responsible for the occurrence of the neuropsychiatric complications. It was postulated that microemboli consisting of platelets or blood cells or air resulted in defective microvascular perfusion and cerebral damage. Factors such as hypotension, hypoxemia, and low cardiac output were thought to contribute to the damage. Subsequent studies by other investigators provided some support for the occurrence of "microembolic encephalopathy" (72). Cardiopulmonary bypass was found to cause significant depression of cerebral blood flow and metabolism, and widespread microemboli generated by bubble oxygenators (72). Continuous EEG monitoring during open-heart surgery has shown that abnormalities of the EEG observed during operation correlated with the development of neurologic abnormalities (73). Abnormal EEG changes occur frequently at the onset of perfusion (74). Changes in concentration of anesthetic gases, alterations in cerebral hemodynamics, and other putative causal factors, have been invoked to account for the EEG changes at the onset of perfusion (74). A heavily filtered electroencephalograph, or cerebral function monitor, has been used to monitor cerebral electrical activity during open-heart surgery (74, 75). Changes in such activity have been noticed to occur during the first few minutes of bypass in about 63 to 82 percent of patients (75). It has been hypothesized that the onset of cardiopulmonary bypass is a time when considerable risk of damage to the brain exists due to hypotension and to particulate and gaseous microemboli (75). These hazards to the integrity of the brain have been reduced by improvements in operative technique, and a measure of cerebral protection has been achieved (76). Recent reports indicate that the incidence of cerebral dysfunction after open-heart surgery has declined since the perfusion time has been shortened and measures to diminish the risk of microemboli have been taken (76). Despite these improvements, however, delirium continues to occur and the possibility of other pathophysiologic factors must be entertained. Speidel et al. (77) mention metabolic acidosis, disturbances of fluid and electrolyte balance, accumulation of normal and abnormal cerebrotoxic metabolites, and intracerebral hemorrhages as potential contributing variables. Cerebral ischemia and hypoxia are still regarded by most writers as the best documented and significant pathophysiologic factors in postcardiotomy delirium and other manifestations of cerebral dysfunction or damage.

Prognosis. The prognosis of delirium after open-heart surgery is favorable. Kaplan et al. (78) studied children who have undergone such surgery for the correction of various congenital abnormalities. Five children became delirious and all recovered without demonstrable sequelae. Tufo et al. (79) carried out a prospective study of 100 open-heart surgery patients and found confusion, disorientation, and/or delirium (or just delirium in our terminology) in about 42 percent of the survivors. At discharge, about one-fifth of these delirious subjects still exhibited nocturnal confusion and decreased intellectual performance. Branthwaite (80) found "confusion" in twenty-two patients, all of whom recovered without any gross impairment of cognitive functioning. Such impairment does, however, occur in a few patients (81). Those patients who die after open-heart surgery tend to show neuropathologic changes including emboli in small cerebral vessels; acute petechial, perivascular, and focal sub-arachnoid hemorrhages; and acute ischemic neuronal damage.

Prevention and management. Prevention and management of postcardiotomy delirium have involved measures based on the etiologic hypotheses discussed earlier. Improvements in surgical technique seem to have made more difference than any other preventive intervention (76). Other measures have included better selection of patients for the surgery; preoperative psychologic preparation (61); postoperative psychotherapy (82); reorientation technique applied by nurses after surgery (83); provision of adequate sensory input and sleep in the intensive care unit; and the use of psychotropic drugs (56, 84).

Management of postcardiotomy delirium is not different in any essential features from that recommended for delirium in general (see Chapter 9). Agitation and psychomotor over-activity in a patient recovering from open-heart surgery is a threat to the patient's life and must be dealt with rapidly and effectively. Haloperidol is the drug of choice and its intravenous use in this situation has recently been recommended (84). Single bolus doses of between 1 and 25 mg. have been used. Tranquilization should set in after ten to forty minutes; if not, further doses need to be administered by the intravenous route. As much as 185 mg. in twenty-four hours have been used without major complications (84).

Coronary artery bypass surgery. This surgery has been followed by delirium in 16 to 28 percent of patients (85, 86). Kornfeld et al. (85) have studied 100 consecutive patients who had undergone coronary artery bypass surgery at the Columbia-Presbyterian Medical Center. Twenty-eight percent of these patients developed delirium postoperatively. History of myo-cardial infarction and severity of the illness in the recovery room were two variables which correlated significantly with incidence of delirium. Age, severity of cardiac disease, and cardiopulmonary bypass time did not show significant associa-tion with such incidence. No psychologic variable attained the .05 level of significance. The investigators postulate that the presence of a lucid interval between surgery and onset of delirium suggests the operation of such variables as sensory monotony, sleep deprivation, and anxiety. Metabolic variables are, surprisingly, not taken into account. The researchers speculate that low cardiac output may be a significant variable but this hypothesis has not been tested as yet.

Cardiac transplantation. Cardiac transplantation may be followed by delirium (87, 88). Hotson and Pedley (89) reviewed eighty-three patients who had received cardiac transplants at Stanford University Medical Center. Twelve percent of these patients developed "acute psychosis," a further 12 percent suffered from metabolic encephalopathy, and 34 percent had CNS infection. As far as one can discern from an inadequate report, probably the majority of the patients exhibiting these complications, i.e. about 58 percent of the total series, experienced delirium of some severity at some stage after the transplantation. The authors state that "behavioral changes" or intellectual impairment were the most frequent neurologic manifestations in these patients. CNS infection was the most common, and sometimes unrecognized, etiology of the delirium. Ischemia of the brain appeared to be responsible for delirium arising in the immediate postoperative period. Only three patients reportedly developed delirium in this period. Subsequently, CNS infections, particularly fungal and viral, became the main cause of delirium occurring weeks or a few months after transplantation. Immunosuppression has been blamed for this life-threatening complication.

Eye Surgery

Delirium has been a recognized complication of eye surgery for a long time. Probably the first report on this association is that of Sichel (90), published in 1863. He describes what he calls "a particular variety of senile delirium" after cataract extraction. He states that he had observed seven or eight cases of such delirium occurring at long intervals, and he believes that they are due to occlusion of the eyelids. As a result of the latter procedure, the patient is unable to tell where he is or who has come to see him. He becomes restless, complains of maltreatment, and finally tears off the bandages and starts to insult and threaten people around him. The patient has no fever or any symptoms of congestion or inflammation of the brain. The delirium starts in the evening and lasts all night. Sichel links the delirium with the use of a certain type of bandage ("bandage contentif") applied after extraction of catar- act. Some of his patients, he thought, were in the early stages of delirium tremens; others were not alcoholics. He had never observed this complication in patients aged less than sixty years. Its duration was brief and it cleared up completely. Sichel advocates "moral" treatment for the delirious patient, that is to say, telling him where he is and why, and letting him open his eyes and look around so that he may orient himself in space and place.

Several other observers reported similar cases at about the same time, but the condition seemed to attract little attention until Schmidt-Rimpler (91) devoted an article to it in 1879. His paper is focused on delirium after closure of the eyes and in dark rooms and is a report on psychiatric observations in an eye hospital. The author states that every ophthalomologist must have encountered delirium after cataract extraction. He points out that similar delirium may occur, without surgery, in eye patients kept in dark rooms. He reports on a fifty-seven-year- old woman with syphilitic acute iritis who was placed in a dark room and had one eye patched. She developed delirium on the second night and became increasingly agitated and hal- lucinatory. One notes that her treatment at the onset included atropine, which may have been responsible for the delirium. The second patient suffered from iridochoroiditis and developed delirium under circumstances similar to those just described. Schmidt-Rimpler argues that sudden exclusion of visual stimuli through patching and placement in a dark room induces in some individuals hallucinations and delirium. He clearly antici- pates future theories of sensory deprivation when he explains that delirium in these situations tends to be nocturnal, by invoking the etiologic importance of reduction of auditory stimuli in addition to the visual ones. Schmidt-Rimpler concludes by saying that delirium induced by patching the eyes and by exclu- sion of light has a different etiology from both delirium tremens and the traumatic delirium. Cutting off the stimulus input that keeps man alert seems to be responsible.

These two pioneering papers introduce a sizable body of

literature on the nature, frequency, and etiology of psychiatric disturbances after eye surgery, especially cataract. Both authors drew attention to two key factors which are still considered such today: old age and patching of the eyes. It is of historical interest that in 1887 Chisolm (92) published an article "The revolution in the after-treatment of cataract operations" in which he challenged traditional methods of such treatment and advocated drastic departure from them. He announced triumphantly that "hereafter there will be no more bandaging, dark rooms, bed operations, bed restraints, diet lists, isolation or smoked glasses needed." Chisolm called these time-honored methods "cruelty kept up for days in the name of progressive surgery." He claimed to have demonstrated that abandoning them, that is to say allowing the patients to move about right after surgery and not patching the good eye, resulted in better operative results and shorter convalescence. Somehow, Chisolm's "revolution" was slow in taking root. Meanwhile, cataract delirium provided many writers with a topic worth reporting and speculating about.

Posey (93) was probably the first American writer to focus on cataract delirium, reporting on twenty-four cases. All his patients had both eyes bandaged after the operation. The delirium was similar in all of them and characterized by restlessness, hallucinations, and delusions of persecution. Posey believed the psychosis to be psychogenic and due to the patient's preoccupation with the eyes. Kipp (94) reported on twelve cases of eye surgery or injury complicated by delirium. The majority of his patients were treated in well-lighted rooms and had one or both eyes unpatched. Most had been hospitalized for more than a week when the delirium began and they remained delirious until allowed to go home. Kipp postulated that his patients had become delirious as a result of change in their environment and of homesickness or nostalgia, which "ends in a form of melancholia with homicidal and suicidal propensities."

Bruns (95) made an interesting observation that not a single patient of a group of 232 who had cataract extractions and been treated on an ambulatory basis developed delirium. On the contrary, he observed several cases of "post-operative dementia" (most likely delirium) among patients hospitalized for the same type of cataract surgery. Three of these patients had managed to kill themselves. Bruns speculated that the delirium was due to old age and the dread of the unknown. "The stranger, the darker, the stiller, the lonelier the after-treatment, the more likely is the mental disturbance to occur," he wrote. Hence, the ambulatory patients escaped delirium, having had the advantage of returning immediately to familiar surroundings.

Fisher (96) reviewed thoroughly the literature on psychiatric complications of eye surgery prior to 1920. He credits Dupuytren with being the first to report, in 1819, delirium following cataract operations. Fisher had been able to find twenty-nine other papers on this subject. He quotes Fromaget, who claimed that occlusion of the eyes put the patient into a hypnotic state and was conducive to sleep, dreams, and delirium. This interesting idea became revived in recent years. A report from the University of Michigan, quoted by Fisher, gave the incidence of cataract delirium to be 3.1 percent; 33 percent occurred in alcoholics. Etiologic factors that Fisher was able to extract from the literature included bandaging, loneliness, nervousness, exhaustion, disturbances of cerebral circulation, fear of losing eyesight, withdrawal of alcohol, atropine, and homesickness. Fisher notes that in his own four cases several postulated etiologic factors could be excluded, viz. bandaging both eyes, alcoholism, and atropine. He recommends having a patient's friend stay with him as an attendant, as well as removing the bandages to allow the patient to wake up from his dreams.

The next major paper on cataract delirium is that by Greenwood (97), who notes its overall incidence to be 2.5 to 3 percent. He singles out old age and blindfolding of both eyes as the chief etiologic factors. Anxiety over the outcome of an anticipated surgery is probably another such factor, and so Greenwood advises that "The establishment of a mutual feeling of confidence between the physician and the patient is of major importance." Phenobarbital, relief of pain, and good nursing care are useful preventive measures. If delirium does develop, however, removal of the bandage from the unoperated eye should speed up recovery from it.

Preu and Guida (98) reported on four cases of psychoses after cataract extraction and argued that three of them represented psychogenic or experiential panic. Reading their case descriptions, however, one must conclude that all their cases represented delirium. Several major studies of cataract delirium were published between 1950 and 1970 (99-104). Bartlett (99) focuses on visual hallucinations in elderly patients with bilateral cataracts and hypothesizes that deprivation of normal visual stimuli occasioned by the disease facilitates production of hallucinations. He compares this mechanism to that of phantom limbs.

Linn et al. (100) carried out a study of twenty-one patients operated on for bilateral senile cataracts and claim to have observed "some alteration of behavior" in the course of the index hospitalization in 95 percent of the cases. Closer examination of the reported disturbances suggests that this high incidence should be taken with a grain of salt. Only four patients (19%) exhibited some disorientation for time, while eight patients displayed spatial disorientation. In delirium, orientation for time is, as a rule, defective before that for place; the discrepancy reported by Linn et al. is puzzling. Only three patients reported visual hallucinations, and this again suggests that the incidence of delirium was much lower than 95 percent. The commonest symptom was restlessness. Inadequate reporting on this series of patients makes it impossible to know which symptoms clustered together and what diagnoses were represented. Eleven of the patients had abnormal EEG, a finding which suggests possible presence of an organic brain syndrome. The investigators try to account for the huge discrepancy between their incidence of 95 percent and that generally reported in the literature, i.e. about 3 percent, by claiming that their observations of all the patients had been done on a twenty-four-hour basis. Furthermore, some degree of brain disease, evidenced by the EEG and Amytal® test, was judged to be present in eighteen of the twenty-one patients and to predispose to the development of postoperative psychiatric disturbances. Patients for the study had been drawn from the population of a home for the aged and may represent a sample skewed in the direction of high prevalence of brain disease. In a later publication, Linn (105) states that as a result of advances in the postoperative care of cataract patients, especially leaving the unoperated eye uncovered and lifting restrictions on mobility, the incidence of

major psychiatric reactions had dropped to "well below 1 percent." Oddly enough, this is the incidence of the same order of
magnitude as that given by Parker (106) fifty years earlier.
It is difficult to account for the unusually discrepant findings by
Linn et al. Methodological flaws of their study are discussed at
some length by Jackson (101).

Ziskind (104) and his associates conducted a major investigation into psychiatric effects of cataract surgery and that for
repair of detached retina. Theoretical aspects of this work are
discussed in Chapter 5. Of special interest to the present theme
are some of the findings of Ziskind and his group. He observed
more mental symptoms in patients operated on for detached
retina than those who had cataract surgery. Other variables
found to increase the frequency of psychopathologic symptoms
included history of alcoholism, double eye patching, and language barrier. One of the major hypotheses put forth by Ziskind
asserts that hallucinations and other cognitive disturbances could
best be accounted for not by sensory deprivation but rather by
a reduced level of awareness. Such disturbances may be viewed
as "aberrations of half-sleep, half-wakefulness" enhanced and
prolonged by reduced sensory input. In this state, the patients
are unable to exercise optimal conscious control over their actions
and this accounts for their noncompliance exemplified by tamper-
ing with the eye-patches. The states of reduced wakefulness
and awareness were jointly to be regarded as a necessary condition for the occurrence of a cluster of symptoms consisting of
pseudohallucinations, confusion, anxiety, restlessness, and non-
compliant behavior. External stimuli or "internal urges" precipitated these symptoms. The latter varied, Ziskind claimed,
with the degree of wakefulness. This hypothesis is, in the writer's
opinion, the most plausible one even if it has not been sufficiently
tested.

Ziskind argued that reduced awareness and the related
"hypnoid syndrome" constituted the psychopathology observed
in a few patients after eye surgery. Jackson (101) focuses on
sensory deprivation as the key variable in producing these postoperative complications. He and his associates studied seventy-
eight patients undergoing eye surgery, sixty of them for cataract.
Observed or reported psychopathologic symptoms were referred

to as "experiences," sensory, motor, cognitive, or behavioral (non-compliance). Jackson concluded that "the evidence for sensory deprivation has been mixed, and the issue has not been resolved." (p. 372). His study is noted for its attention to sound methodology, a sorely neglected aspect of research in this area. Unfortunately, however, Jackson's use of the term "experiences" makes it almost impossible to compare his findings with those of other clinical investigators and to translate his terminology into that of psychiatric symptoms and syndromes.

One other published study, that by Weisman and Hackett (103), deserves mention not because it is methodologically sound but because it has relevance for the clinician looking after the eye-surgery patient. These authors rejected the term "cataract delirium" on the grounds that it is a misnomer since the disorder so designated may develop in any patient who has had both his eyes bandaged. They go on to say that the clinical features of this delirium resemble those typical of other postoperative deliria except that the precipitating variable is the "total deprivation of vision." Disorientation for time and place, restlessness, anxiety, and hyperactivity are its key features. The delirium characteristically comes on in the evening of the second postoperative day and tends to be most severe at night. These characteristics, stressed by Weisman and Hackett, are, in part, those of delirium in general. Partly, since the authors do not mention memory and thought disturbances as defining features of delirium. Their hypothesis that blindfolding results in impaired "reality testing" and delirium led them to postulate that a "reliable, personal relation" would compensate for such an impairment. They treated six patients with methods based on this premise. They tried to substitute meaningful, auditory, gustatory, tactile, and olfactory perceptual cues for the deficient or absent visual ones. These investigators advance a rather dubious thesis that "Loss of vision, temporary or permanent, actual or threatened, may evoke delirium by depriving a precariously adjusted patient of an important source of reality testing." The hypothesis that threatened loss of vision may precipitate delirium, as this term is used in this book, is without empirical foundation. On the other hand, offering the patients information, orientation, reassurance, etc., as Weisman and Hackett had done, seemed to have a beneficial effect on their patients and offers a useful therapeutic model.

One notes lack of recent studies on delirium after eye surgery. The enthusiasm for sensory deprivation has generally evaporated and interesting hypotheses were left in midair some fifteen years ago. Promising work by Ziskind, Jackson, and others clearly calls for extension, using the latest technological advances in telemetry, etc. Continuous EEG monitoring, coupled with clinical observation, could resolve the issue of the proposed hypnoid syndrome, i.e. delirium related to a reduced state of wakefulness. The role of sensory deprivation in inducing the delirium remains ambiguous. Stonecypher (102) argues that such a role does not exist in the case of psychoses after cataract extraction. He tries to refute the sensory deprivation hypothesis by quoting clinical examples purported to prove that such deprivation does not occur after the surgery. The better, un-operated eye is left unpatched in most patients, Stonecypher points out, and the patched eye is the one which had lost so much vision that it needed surgery. He proposes that the "black-patch psychosis" is merely an "acute form of senile psychosis" due to psychologic stress and the concomitant fear. The individual particularly prone to develop the delirium is one who has a history of marginal social adjustment, has a long-standing disability, is an immigrant, is a manual laborer, a retired man, and has had a previous psychotic episode in the hospital. Stonecypher's advice on how to manage the patients follows the time-honored methods of managing delirium: orient, familiarize with the environment, and support.

While most authors stress psychologic, cerebral-organic, and environmental variables as having causal input into the delirium after cataract surgery, a few invoke other factors, such as dehydration (107) or the use of sedatives and analgesics (108).

In summary, delirium is the proper designation for the psychiatric disorder occurring after eye surgery, especially cataract extraction and surgery for retinal detachment. The incidence of this complication appears to be low, about 1 percent. Many etiologic factors have been proposed to account for delirium in this setting: old age, senile or other brain damage, sensory deprivation occasioned by patching the eyes and immobilizing the patient, psychologic stress of the unknown and the unfamiliar, drugs, and dehydration. There is considerable evidence to support the contention that various constellations of these factors operate in different patients. Cataract surgery is usually performed on elderly patients who are generally more susceptible to delirium due to many organic factors, such as intake of drugs. Unfamiliarity, reduction of perceptual cues, and fear undoubtedly facilitate the onset of delirium in the aged. Sensory deprivation alone cannot account for delirium. Mobilizing the patient early, leaving one eye unpatched, and providing good nursing care are factors credited with the decline in the incidence of delirium in recent years. If it does occur, therapeutic measures discussed in Chapter 9 should be applied. It appears that the therapeutic "revolution" launched by Chisolm (92) in 1887 has finally prevailed and reduced the incidence and thus practical importance of delirium after cataract extraction.

Burns

Delirium is the main early psychiatric complication of burns of any severity. Its incidence has been variously reported to range from 14 to 57 percent (109-111). The lowest figure comes from a study of 140 children admitted to the Boston Shriners Burns Institute (109). The authors use the term "burn encephalopathy" to refer to the neurologic disturbances complicating burns. Hallucinations, personality changes, delirium, seizures, and coma are quoted as the features of burn encephalopathy. This term, introduced in 1936, has been roundly and justly criticized by Mettler (112) as one that designates neither a specific type of structural cerebral change nor a characteristic clinical state. Two studies of adults refer specifically to delirium and give its incidence as 30 percent and 57 percent, respectively (110, 111).

Delirium is more likely to occur in the older and the more severely burned patient (109, 111). It typically comes on during the first month after burn injury and in patients with burns covering more than 40 percent of the body surface area. The syndrome is said to occur only rarely after grafting has been completed. Its etiology is, as one could expect, multi-factorial. The following causal factors have been implicated (110, 111, 113):

   A. Organic factors
      1. Hypoxia due to inhalation of carbon monoxide and other toxic gases (114)
      2. Hypovolemia related to initial shock and dehydration, and resulting in cerebral hypoxia
      3. Hyponatremia due to loss of sodium from the surface of extensive burns
      4. Infection of the burned area leading to septicemia, bacterial meningitis, septic cerebral embolism, cortical vein thrombosis, etc.
      5. Acidosis
      6. Hypertensive encephalopathy (115)
      7. Direct brain damage in severe burns of the head
      8. Administration of analgesics and hypnotics

   B. Facilitating or contributory psychologic factors (109, 111)
      1. Pain
      2. Fear
      3. Premorbid psychiatric diagnosis
      4. Sleep deprivation

In the earliest stages, hypoxia and hypovolemic shock are the most important, and potentially fatal, causes of delirium. In addition, the patient is usually terrified and in pain, yet may appear calm and lucid. Many are overtly agitated and restless. Insomnia and nightmares commonly occur at this stage (109). Delirium may set in at any time. It usually has a benign course but, depending on its cause, may be followed by coma and death (116). After the first week, infection becomes the most important cause of delirium and other central nervous system complications. Delirium due to this cause tends to develop gradually over a period of several days and most often after two to three weeks following burn injury. Prompt improvement typically follows application of skin homografts.

Cerebral edema has been proposed to account for some cases of delirium, seizures, and coma, which may on occasion follow even minor burns (117). Various hypothetical mechanisms have been offered to explain the occurrence of the edema, including hyponatremia with water intoxication, hypoxia, prolonged hypotension, a toxin produced by the burned tissue, and hexachlorophene treatment of the burns. This issue remains unsettled.

In addition to the organic factors, psychologic and environmental ones have been postulated to contribute to delirium in burn patients. The burn injury itself is often the result of an accident involving negligence or child abuse, or intoxication with alcohol or drugs. Behavior disorders in burned children have been interpreted as reflecting disturbed family relationships (118). The patient, whether child or adult, first suffers terror, pain, and emotional shock, then prolonged immobilization, painful procedures, total dependence on staff, and uncertainty about the extent of future disfigurement and its social consequence (109, 111). Various coping strategies may be observed in the burned patients: at first denial, then regression, finally acceptance. Depression and/or traumatic neurosis develop in most patients hospitalized for more than a month (109, 111). Insomnia is very common and both precedes and accompanies delirium (119). Immobilization, sensory deprivation, and boredom add to the psychologic stress and, possibly, contribute to the onset and persistence of delirium. All these factors need to be taken into account in the management of the burned patient.

The electroencephalogram in burn cases has been studied by several groups of investigators (113, 120, 121). Petersen et al. (113) studied fifty-eight patients with burns of moderate severity. In the majority of the cases, the first EEG was taken on the day of the accident. In eighteen cases (31%) the EEG changes were relatively pronounced and consisted of diffuse and/or focal abnormalities and, in two cases, of a slow-wave rhythmic activity in posterior leads. The degree of EEG abnormality correlated with the extent of the burns. Eight patients were found to be delirious and all of them had EEG abnormalities to some extent. Andreasen et al. (120) studied ten consecutive patients admitted to a burn unit. Only patients burned over more than 30 percent of the total body surface were included. Seven of the ten developed delirium. Nine of the ten patients had abnormal

EEGs. The abnormalities consisted of excessive slow-wave activity, with some decrease in amplitude. Patients with more severe burns tended to have more severe delirium and more EEG abnormalities. Andreasen et al. observed three patients who seemed to suffer persistent mild cerebral deficits as sequelae of severe burns. Hughes et al. (121) report on forty burn patients with a range of total body surface burned of 3 to 72 percent (mean = 23.4%) and mean age of nineteen years. Abnormal records were observed in 88 percent of those taken, all showing slow waves and nearly 10 percent with epileptiform activity. These abnormalities tend to cluster three to eleven days after the burn.

Management of delirium after burns does not differ from that of delirium occurring in other settings.

In summary, delirium occurs in 20 to 30 percent of patients with the more severe burns. The onset of delirium has two peaks: the first, within the first week of the burn, and the second, two to three weeks after the latter. The main etiologic factors in the early phase are hypoxic-metabolic; in the later stage, infectious. Etiology of the delirium is multifactorial but is most closely correlated with the total body surface burned.

REFERENCES

1. *The Works of That Famous Chirurgion Ambrose Parey.* Translated by T. Johnson. London, Cotes and Young, 1634.
2. Dupuytren, Baron: On nervous delirium (traumatic delirium). – Successful employment of laudanum lavements. *Lancet* 2:919-923, 1834.
3. Morse, R.M.: "Psychiatry and Surgical Delirium," in *Modern Perspectives in the Psychiatric Aspects of Surgery*, Howells, J.G., Ed. New York, Bruner/Mazel, 1976, pp. 615-636.
4. Graves, R.J.: *A System of Clinical Medicine.* 3rd American edition. Philadelphia, Barrington and Haswell, 1848, p. 389.
5. Croft, J.: Delirium tremens in surgical cases. *St. Thomas Hosp Rep* 1:451-463, 1870.
6. Savage, G.H.: Insanity following the use of anaesthetics. *Br Med J* 2:1199-1200, 1887.
7. Haward, W.: Delirium tremens and other forms of surgical delirium. *Intern Clin* 4:119-127, 1893.
8. DaCosta, J.C.: The diagnosis of postoperative insanity. *Surg Gynec Obstet* 11:577-584, 1910.

9. Kelly, H.A.: Postoperative psychoses. *Am J Obstet* 59:1035-1039, 1909.
10. Gardner, W.E.: Post-operative psychosis. *Kentucky Med J* 26:537-546, 1928.
11. Kleist, K.: *Postoperative Psychosen*. Berlin, Springer, 1916.
12. McGraw, R.B.: Post-operative emotional disorders—Their prevention and management. *Bull NY Acad Med* 6:179-188, 1930.
13. Muncie, W.: Post-operative states of excitement. *Arch Neurol Psychiatry* 32:681-703, 1934.
14. Waltman, H.W.: Post-operative neurologic complications. *Wisc M J* 35:427-436, 1936.
15. Washburne, A.C., and Carns, M.L.: Post-operative psychosis. *J Nerv Ment Dis* 82:508-513, 1935.
16. Abeles, M.M.: Post-operative psychoses. *Am J Psychiatry* 94:1187-1203, 1938.
17. Doyle, J.B.: Postoperative psychosis. *Proc Mayo Clin* 3:198-199, 1928.
18. Bastron, R.D., and Moyers, J.: Emergence delirium. *JAMA* 200:179, 1967.
19. Eckenhoff, J.E., Kneale, D.H., and Dripps, R.D.: The incidence and etiology of postanesthetic excitement. *Anesthesiology* 22:667-673, 1961.
20. Coppolino, G.A.: Incidence of post-anesthetic delirium in a community hospital: A statistical study. *Milit Med* 128:238-241, 1963.
21. Kuhn, J.A., and Savage, G.J.: Belladonna alkaloid psychosis. *Delaware M J* 46:239-242, 1974.
22. Greene, L.T.: Physostigmine treatment of anticholinergic-drug depression in postoperative patients. *Anesth Analg* 50:222-226, 1971.
23. Hale, M., Koss, N., Kerstein, M., et al.: Psychiatric complications in a surgical ICU. *Crit Care Med* 5:199-203, 1977.
24. Katz, N.M., Agle, D.P., DePalma, R.G., and DeCosse, J.J.: Delirium in surgical patients under intensive care. *Arch Surg* 104:310-313, 1972.
25. Wilson, L.M.: Intensive care delirium. *Arch Intern Med* 130:225-226, 1972.
26. Titchener, J.L., Zwerling, I., Gottschalk, L., et al.: Psychosis in surgical patients. *Surg Gynecol Obstet* 102:59-65, 1956.
27. Knox, S.J.: Severe psychiatric disturbances in the post-operative period: A five-year survey of Belfast hospitals. *J Ment Sci* 107:1078-1083, 1961.
28. Hammes, E.M.: Postoperative psychoses. *Lancet* 77:55-60, 1957.
29. Scott, J.: Postoperative psychosis in the aged. *Am J Surg* 100:38-42, 1960.

30. Kaufer, C.: Etiology of consciousness disturbances in surgery. *Minn Med 51*:1509-1515, 1968.
31. Morse, R.M., and Litin, E.M.: Postoperative delirium: A study of etiologic factors. *Am J Psychiatry 126*:388-395, 1969.
32. Mesulam, M.M., and Geschwind, N.: Disordered mental states in the postoperative period. *Urol Clin N Am 3*:199-215, 1976.
33. Patkin, M.: Postoperative confusion. *Med J Aust 2*:559-561, 1973.
34. Morse, R.M.: Postoperative delirium: a syndrome of multiple causation. *Psychosomatics 11*:164-168, 1970.
35. Bedford, P.D.: Adverse cerebral effects of anaesthesia on old people. *Lancet 2*:259-263, 1955.
36. Bedford, P.D.: Cerebral damage from shock due to disease in aged people. *Lancet 2*:505-509, 1957.
37. Lappas, D.G., Powell, W.M.J., and Daggett, W.M.: Cardiac dysfunction in the perioperative period: pathophysiology, diagnosis, and treatment. *Anesthesiology 47*:117-137, 1977.
38. Kitamura, H., Sawa, T., and Ikezono, E.: Postoperative hypoxemia: the contribution of age to the maldistribution of ventilation. *Anesthesiology 3*:244-252, 1972.
39. Polly, S.M., and Sanders, W.E.: Surgical infections in the elderly: prevention, diagnosis, and treatment. *Geriatrics 32*:88-97, 1977.
40. Sechzer, P.H., and Ospina, J.: Cerebral function monitor: evaluation in anesthesia/critical care. *Curr Ther Res 22*:335-347, 1977.
41. Gilberstadt, H., Aberwald, R., Crosbie, S., et al.: Effect of surgery on psychological and social functioning in elderly patients. *Arch Intern Med 122*:109-115, 1968.
42. Glickman, L., and Herbsman, H.: Delirium tremens in surgical patients. *Surgery 64*:882-890, 1968.
43. Helmus, C., and Spahn, J.G.: Delirium tremens in head and neck surgery. *Laryngoscope 84*:1479-1488, 1974.
44. Mays, E.T., Ransdell, H.T., and deWeese, B.M.: Metabolic changes in surgical delirium tremens. *Surgery 67*:780-788, 1970.
45. Sellers, E.M., Zilm, D.H., and Degani, N.C.: Comparative efficacy of propranolol and chlordiazepoxide in alcohol withdrawal. *J Stud Alcohol 38*:2096-2108, 1977.
46. Tichener, J.L., and Levine, M.: *Surgery as a Human Experience.* New York, Oxford University Press, 1960.
47. Morse, R.M., and Litin, E.M.: The anatomy of a delirium. *Am J Psychiatry 128*:111-116, 1971.
48. Editorial: Delirium after surgery. *Br Med J 2*:702-703, 1974.
49. Fox, H.M., Rizzo, N.D., and Gifford, S.: Psychological observations of patients undergoing mitral surgery: study of stress. *J Ment Sci 107*:1078-1096, 1961.
50. Abram, H.S.: Psychological reactions to cardiac operations: an historical perspective. *Psychiatr Med 1*:277-294, 1970.

51. Knox, S.J.: Psychiatric aspects of mitral valvulotomy. *Br J Psychiatry 109*:656-668, 1963.
52. Blachly, P.H., and Starr, A.: Post-cardiotomy delirium. *Am J Psychiatry 121*:371-375, 1964.
53. Egerton, N., and Kay, J.H.: Psychological disturbances associated with open-heart surgery. *Br J Psychiatry 110*:433-439, 1964.
54. Speidel, H., Achilles, I., Dahme, B., et al.: *Die Klassifizierung psychopathologischer Auffälligkeiten nach Herzoperationen.* Paper presented at the VI World Congress of Psychiatry, Honolulu, 28.8-3.9, 1977.
55. Gilberstadt, H., and Sako, Y.: Intellectual and personality changes following open-heart surgery. *Arch Gen Psychiatr 16*:210-214, 1967.
56. McClish, A., Andrew, D., and Tetraeault, L.: Intravenous diazepam for psychiatric reactions following open-heart surgery. *Can Anaesth Soc J 15*:63-79, 1968.
57. Kornfeld, D.S., Zimberg, S., and Malm, J.R.: Psychiatric complications of open-heart surgery. *N Engl J Med 273*:287-292, 1965.
58. Heller, S.S., Frank, K.A., Malm, J.R., et al.: Psychiatric complications of open-heart surgery. *N Engl J Med 283*:1015-1020, 1970.
59. Freyhan, F.A., Giannelli, S., O'Connell, R.A., and Mayo, J.A.: Psychiatric complications following open-heart surgery. *Compr Psychiatry 12*:181-195, 1971.
60. Dahme, B., Achilles, I., Flemming, B., et al.: Klassifikation psychopathologischer Auffälligkeiten nach Herzoperationen. *Thoraxchirurgie 25*:345-349, 1977.
61. Kornfeld, D.S., Heller, S.S., Frank, K.A., Moskowitz, R.: Personality and psychological factors in postcardiotomy delirium. *Arch Gen Psychiatry 31*:249-253, 1974.
62. Huse-Kleinstoll, G., Dahme, B., Flemming, B., et al.: Einige somatische und psychologische Prädiktoren für psychopathologische Auffälligkeiten nach Herzoperationen. *Thoraxchirurgie 24*:386-389, 1976.
63. Danilowicz, D.A., and Gabriel, H.P.: Postoperative reactions in children: "normal" and abnormal responses after cardiac surgery. *Am J Psychiatry 128*:185-188, 1971.
64. Stockard, J.J., Bickford, R.G., Myers, R.R., et al.: Hypotension-induced changes in cerebral function during cardiac surgery. *Stroke 5*:730-746, 1974.
65. Blachly, P.H., and Kloster, F.E.: Relation of cardiac output to postcardiotomy delirium. *J Thorac Cardiovasc Surg 52*:422-427, 1966.
66. Ellis, R.: Unusual sensory and thought disturbances after cardiac surgery. *Am J Nurs 72*:2021-2025, 1972.
67. Johns, M.W., Large, A.A., Masterton, J.P., and Dudley, H.A.F.:

Delirium: Acute Brain Failure in Man

Sleep and delirium after open-heart surgery. *Br J Surg* 61:377-381, 1974.

68. McFadden, E.H., and Giblin, E.C.: Sleep deprivation in patients having open-heart surgery. *Nurs Res* 20:249-254, 1971.

69. Orr, W.C., and Stahl, M.L.: Sleep disturbances after open-heart surgery. *Am J Cardiol* 39:196-201, 1977.

70. Walker, B.B.: The postsurgery heart patient. *Nurs Res* 21:164-169, 1972.

71. Lee, W.H., Bhady, M.P., Rowe, J.M., and Miller, W.C.: *Ann Surg* 173:1013-1023, 1971.

72. Brennan, R.W., Patterson, R.H., and Kessler, J.: Cerebral blood flow and metabolism during cardiopulmonary bypass: evidence of microembolic encephalopathy. *Neurology* 21:665-672, 1971.

73. Witoszka, M.M., Tamura, H., Indeglia, R., et al.: Electroencephalographic changes and cerebral complications in open-heart surgery. *J Thorac Cardiovasc Surg* 66:855-864, 1973.

74. Branthwaite, M.A.: Detection of neurological damage during open-heart surgery. *Thorax* 28:464-472, 1973.

75. Kritikou, P.E., and Branthwaite, M.A.: Significance of changes in cerebral electrical activity at onset of cardiopulmonary bypass. *Thorax* 32:534-538, 1977.

76. Aberg, T., and Kihlgren, M.: Cerebral protection during open-heart surgery. *Thorax* 32:525-533, 1977.

77. Speidel, H., Dahme, B., Flemming, B., et al.: Psychische Störungen nach offenen Herzoperationen. *Nervenarzt* 50:85-91, 1979.

78. Kaplan, S., Achtel, R.A., and Callison, C.B.: Psychiatric complications following open-heart surgery. *Heart & Lung* 3:423-428, 1974.

79. Tufo, H.M., Ostfeld, A.M., and Shekelle, R.: Central nervous system dysfunction following open-heart surgery. *JAMA* 212:1333-1340, 1970.

80. Branthwaite, M.A.: Neurological damage related to open-heart surgery. *Thorax* 27:748-753, 1972.

81. Aberg, T.: Effect of open-heart surgery on intellectual function. *Scand J Thorac Cardiovasc Surg*, Suppl. 15, 1974.

82. Dlin, B.M., Fischer, H.K., and Haddell, B.: Psychologic adaptation to pacemaker and open-heart surgery. *Arch Gen Psychiatry* 19:599-610, 1968.

83. Budd, S., and Brown, W.: Effect of reorientation technique on post-cardiotomy delirium. *Nurs Res* 23:341-348, 1974.

84. Cassem, N.H., and Sos, J.: Intravenous use of haloperidol for acute delirium in intensive care settings. Paper presented at the Annual Meeting of the American Psychiatric Association, Atlanta, Georgia, May 9, 1978.

85. Kornfeld, D.S., Heller, S.S., Frank, K.A., et al.: Delirium after coronary artery bypass surgery. *J Thorac Cardiovasc Surg 76*:93-96, 1978.

86. Rabiner, C.J., Willner, A.E., and Fishman, J.: Psychiatric complications following coronary bypass surgery. *J Nerv Ment Dis 160*: 342-348, 1975.

87. Kraft, I.: Psychiatric complications of cardiac transplantation. *Sem Psychiatry 3*:58-69, 1971.

88. Lunde, D.T.: Psychiatric complications of heart transplants. *Am J Psychiatry 126*:369-372, 1969.

89. Hotson, J.R., and Pedley, T.A.: The neurological complications of cardiac transplantation. *Brain 99*:673-694, 1976.

90. Sichel: Sur une espèce particulière de délire senile, qui survient quelquefois après l'extraction de la cataracte. *L'Union Med 17*:149-150, 1863.

91. Schmidt-Rimpler, H.: Delirien nach Verschluss der Augen und in Dunkel-Zimmern. *Arch Psychiatrie 9*:233-243, 1879.

92. Chisolm, J.J.: The revolution in the after-treatment of cataract operations. *Am J Ophthalmol 4*:153-156, 1887.

93. Posey, W.C.: Mental disturbances after operations upon the eye. *Ophthalmol Rev 19*:235-237, 1900.

94. Kipp, C.J.: The mental derangement which is occasionally developed in patients in eye hospitals. *Arch Ophthalmol 32*:375-387, 1903.

95. Bruns, H.D.: On the ambulant after-treatment of cataract extraction, with a note on postoperative delirium and on striped keratitis. *Ann Ophthalmol 25*:718-723, 1916.

96. Fisher, W.A.: Delirium following cataract and other eye operations. *Am J Ophthalmol 3*:741-747, 1920.

97. Greenwood, A.: Mental disturbances following operations for cataract. *JAMA 91*:1713-1716, 1928.

98. Preu, P.W., and Guida, F.P.: Psychoses complicating recovery from extraction of cataract. *Arch Neurol Psychiatry 38*:818-832, 1937.

99. Bartlett, J.E.A.: A case of organized visual hallucinations in an old man with cataract, and their relations to the phenomena of the phantom limb. *Brain 74*:363-373, 1951.

100. Linn, L., Kahn, R.L., Coles, R., et al.: Patterns of behavior disturbance following cataract extraction. *Am J Psychiatry 110*: 281-289, 1953.

101. Jackson, C.W.: "Clinical Sensory Deprivation: A Review of Hospitalized Eye-Surgery Patients," in *Sensory Deprivation: Fifteen Years of Research*, Zubek, J.P., Ed. New York, Appleton-Century-Crofts, 1969, pp. 332-373.

102. Stonecypher, D.D.: The cause and prevention of postoperative psychoses in the elderly. *Am J Ophthalmol 55*:605-610, 1963.

103. Weisman, A.D., and Hackett, T.P.: Psychosis after eye surgery. *N Engl J Med 258*:1284-1289, 1958.
104. Ziskind, E.: An explanation of mental symptoms found in acute sensory deprivation: researches 1958-1963. *Am J Psychiatry 121*: 939-946, 1965.
105. Linn, L.: Psychiatric reactions complicating cataract surgery. *Intern Ophthalmol Clin 5*:143-154, 1965.
106. Parker, W.R.: Postcataract extraction delirium. *JAMA 61*:1174-1177, 1913.
107. Abrahamson, I.A., and Abrahamson, I.A.: Dehydration—a cause of psychosis following cataract extraction. *Eye Ear Nose Throat Mon 47*:144-146, 1968.
108. Fasanella, R.M., Ed.: *Complications in Eye Surgery.* 2nd edition. Philadelphia, W.B. Saunders, 1965.
109. Andreasen, N.J.C., Noyes, R., Hartford, C.E., et al.: Management of emotional reactions in seriously burned adults. *N Engl J Med 286*:65-69, 1972.
110. Antoon, A.Y., Volpe, J.J., and Crawford, J.D.: Burn encephalopathy in children. *Pediatrics 50*:609-616, 1972.
111. Steiner, H., and Clark, W.R.: Psychiatric complications of burned adults: a classification. *J Trauma 17*:134-143, 1977.
112. Mettler, F.A.: Burn encephalopathy as a "diagnosis." *J Med Soc NJ 71*:817-823, 1974.
113. Petersen, I., Sörbye, R., and Johanson, B.: Electroencephalographic and psychiatric study of burn cases. *Acta Chir Scand 129*:359-366, 1965.
114. Terrill, J.B., Montgomery, R.R., and Reinhardt, C.F.: Toxic gases from fires. *Science 200*:1343-1347, 1978.
115. Berliner, B.C., Shenker, I.R., and Weinstock, M.S: Hypercalcemia associated with hypertension due to prolonged immobilization. *Pediatrics 49*:92-96, 1972.
116. Haynes, B.W., and Bright, R.: Burn coma: a syndrome associated with severe burn wound infection. *J Trauma 7*:464-475, 1967.
117. Hughes, J.R., and Cayaffa, J.J.: Seizures following burns of the skin. *Dis Nerv Syst 34*:203-211, 1973.
118. Breslin, P.W.: The psychological reaction of children to burn traumata: a review. *Ill Med J 148*:519-524, 1975.
119. Miller, W.C., Gardner, N., and Mlott, S.R.: Psychosocial support in the treatment of severely burned patients. *J Trauma 15*:722-725, 1976.
120. Andreasen, N.J.C., Hartford, C.E., Knott, J.R., and Canter, A.: EEG changes associated with burn delirium. *Dis Nerv Syst 38*:27-31, 1977.

121. Hughes, J.R., Cayaffa, J.J., and Boswick, J.A.: Seizures following burns of the skin. III. Electroencephalographic recordings. *Dis Nerv Syst* 36:443-447, 1975.

Additional References

Barash, P.G., Katz, J.D., Kopriva, C.J., et al. Assessment of cerebral function during cardiopulmonary bypass. *Heart & Lung* 8:280-287, 1979.

Eltringham, R.J., Coates, M.B., and Hudson, R.B.S. Observations on 10,000 patients in the immediate postoperative period. *Resuscitation* 6:45-52, 1979.

Heller, S.S., Kornfeld, D.S., Frank, K.A., and Hoar, P.F. Postcardiotomy delirium and cardiac output. *Am J Psychiatry* 136:337-339, 1979.

Hunziker, T., and Michel, K. Acute mental disturbances following gynaecological operations. *Schweiz Arch Neurol Neurochir Psychiatr* 122:271-283, 1978.

Korttila, K., and Levänen, J. Untoward effects of ketamine combined with diazepam for supplementing conduction anaesthesia in young and middle-aged adults. *Acta Anaesthesiol Scand* 22:640-648, 1978.

Paiement, B., Boulanger, M., Jones, C.W., and Roy, M. Intubation and other experiences in cardiac surgery: The consumer's view. *Can Anaesth Soc J* 26:173-180, 1979.

Salerno, T.A., Lince, D.P., White, D.N., et al. Monitoring of electroencephalogram during open-heart surgery. *J Thorac Cardiovasc Surg* 76:97-100, 1978.

Savage, G.J., and Metzger, J.T. The prevention of postanesthetic delirium. *Plast Reconstr Surg* 62:81-83, 1978.

Summers, W.K., and Reich, T.C. Delirium after cataract surgery: Review and two cases. *Am J Psychiatry* 136:386-391, 1979.

West, D.A., and Shuck, J.M. Emotional problems of the severely burned patient. *Surg Clin North Am* 58:1189-1204, 1978.

Whitwam, J.G. Adverse reactions to I.V. induction agents. *Br J Anaesth* 50:677-687, 1978.

CHAPTER 18

DELIRIUM IN GERIATRICS

INTRODUCTION

Delirium is one of the most frequently encountered, if not the most common, mental disorders among people aged sixty-five years and older. If one considers that such persons constitute about 10 percent of the population of the United States, or some 23 million people, then one cannot fail to view delirium as a major medical and psychiatric problem, one seriously neglected by researchers (1). Delirium, or "mental confusion," has been called "the very stuff of geriatric medicine" on account of its high prevalence, socially disruptive effects, and diagnostic significance as a cerebral manifestation of numerous diseases and toxic agents (2). The syndrome has been referred to as equivalent in the elderly to a convulsion in an infant, an acute event calling for a thorough diagnostic assessment (3). Indeed, almost any physical illness in an older person may, and often does, present as delirium. The latter, also referred to in the literature as "acute brain syndrome" or "acute brain failure" or "mental confusion" or "acute confusional state," is one of the four most common reasons for a patient's being referred to a geriatrician (4). It is most important to diagnose delirium in the elderly because its occurrence usually points to the presence of an acute and potentially treatable somatic disorder. Failure to diagnose and treat the latter promptly may result in some degree of irreversible brain damage and its associated cognitive deficits. In a minority of patients, delirium is the first manifestation of a cerebral degenerative process. The latter, in turn, favors the development of delirium. Not only physical illness but also social and psychologic stress may induce delirium in the elderly, especially those whose brain function is precariously compensated (5-7).

TERMINOLOGY: CONFUSION ABOUT CONFUSION

Terminology of mental disorders in the aged is muddled. Terms like delirium, mental confusion, organic or acute confusional state, acute brain syndrome, acute brain failure, and pseudosenility are used more or less synonymously. Many writers on the subject do not bother to define these terms. "Acute confusional state" appears to be the most commonly used designation for what is called "delirium" in this book. "Confusion," an ambiguous term, has taken a tenacious hold in psychogeriatrics. Godber (8) rightly complains that this word is "often used far too loosely of the elderly." Adams (9) is even more explicit in his criticism: "Elderly patients who are disorientated are often referred to as being 'confused.' This overworked term covers a wide range of eccentricities of speech and behavior and should not be applied as if it were a diagnosis." This writer strongly agrees.

"Confusion" has been variously defined as inability to think with one's accustomed clarity and coherence (10), as tenuous contact with reality and reduced awareness of one's relation to the environment (11), as spatiotemporal disorientation (12), as "incoherence in the train of thought" (13), and so forth. One has to agree with Lishman (10) that it is deplorable that as vague a term as "confusion" has been made by some writers the hallmark of acute organic mental disorders and incorporated into designations for the latter.

Furthermore, "confusion" is often linked in the literature with another ambiguous term, namely, "clouding of consciousness." Some authors use these two terms synonymously, while others either state that confusion is characterized by some degree of clouding of consciousness, or assert that the latter causes the former (13-15). This conceptual and semantic muddle pervades psychogeriatric literature. The word "confusion" is not a scientific term at all but a colloquial word synonymous with perplexity or the state of being mixed up in the mind (16). The writer proposes that "confusion" be used informally to mean just that and without any implied pretense that it has any precise and operationally defined meaning. If one wants to state that a patient thinks incoherently, cannot grasp the situation, or is disoriented, one should state so clearly, using relevant words and quoting the patient verbatim. Woolly statements commonly found in the literature and medical records, such as "the patient is confused" or "this patient has clouding of consciousness," should be avoided and replaced by descriptive statements detailing the patient's cognitive functioning.

The term "acute confusional state" is as clumsy as it is vague. It offers no advantage over "delirium" and has the disadvantage of alluding to "confusion." The term will be used here, synonymously with delirium, only because its use is so widespread in geriatric literature.

A term which has found some favor among British geriatricians is that of "brain failure," defined as a "syndrome characterized by impaired social functioning due to an inability to learn because of a decline of intellect" (17). Delirium in this terminology would be equivalent to acute brain failure. This designation is cogent since it draws attention to the functional decompensation of the brain as the organ subserving highest integrative functions. This writer prefers the term "delirium" as being shorter and endowed with a rich history but he has no objection to using "acute brain failure" as an otherwise strikingly apt synonym. It is a designation that places the emphasis squarely and rather dramatically on the brain and has the merit of bringing home to doctors that its onset calls for as much attention as does the occurrence of heart or liver or kidney failure.

INCIDENCE AND PREVALENCE

Given the semantic muddle discussed in the preceding section and the lack of diagnostic criteria, reported incidence figures on delirium (or confusional states) in the aged must be taken with a grain of salt. Robinson (18) quotes an incidence of 40 percent among patients over sixty years of age admitted to a neurological hospital. Bedford (11) found "confusional states" (delirium) in 80 percent of the 5,000 patients aged sixty-five years or over, admitted to the Oxford Geriatric Unit, a general medical facility serving the aged. Simon and Cahan (19) found acute brain syndrome, alone or associated with chronic brain disorder, in about 46 percent of 534 patients aged sixty or older, admitted to San Francisco General Hospital in 1959; 13 percent exhibited only acute brain syndrome. Anderson (20) claims that about 8 percent of mental disorders seen among mental hospital patients aged sixty or older are represented by acute confusional states. An epidemiological study carried out in California resulted in estimated incidence rate for acute brain syndrome in people over sixty years of age of about fifty-three per 100,000 general population in San Francisco County, or some 400 patients annually (21).

Thus, it appears that nearly one-half of patients sixty years old or older admitted to general hospitals are liable to exhibit symptoms of delirium. Epidemiological studies of delirium in general, and among the aged in particular, are badly needed.

CLINICAL FEATURES

Essential features of delirium are not different in the aged. On the other hand, some of the associated clinical manifestations are reported to be more or less common in the elderly than in the younger patients. Hallucinations and dream-like (oneiric) experiences are said to be on the whole less common in older patients who may only exhibit disorientation, memory impairment, and some type of abnormal psychomotor behavior (18). In one reported series only about 40 percent of elderly delirious patients were believed to experience hallucinations (19). Depression is said to occur in some 60 percent of the patients, a higher frequency than that observed in younger adults. The fact that delirium in the aged is often superimposed on dementia is likely to color the clinical picture. Thus, a younger or non-demented delirious patient is more likely to exhibit rich fantasy in hallucinations and dreams, and to display capacity for intact abstract thinking during the lucid intervals punctuating delirium. On the contrary, a demented patient is liable to strike one as relatively unimaginative, dull, and lacking in general information. A delirious patient who, when accessible, cannot tell the names of the recent presidents of the country or the dates of World War II, for example, is likely to be demented, mentally retarded, or uneducated. Physical symptoms often found in the elderly delirious patient include indistinct or slurred speech, tremor, incoordination, and urinary incontinence. These symptoms may, of course, be seen in a younger delirious person but seem to be more common in the older one. Focal neurologic signs are also more likely to be found in the latter since cerebrovascular disease is so highly prevalent among the aged. The EEG in elderly delirious patients may be less reliable than in the younger subject since slowing of the background activity is not an uncommon finding in nondelirious old people displaying some degree of intellectual deterioration.

The natural history and prognosis of delirium in the elderly have hardly been touched by research. Bedford (11), who studied 4,000 patients aged sixty-five or more who exhibited symptoms of delirium, states that 33 percent of them died within a month of the date of their admission to hospital. Of the survivors, nearly 80 percent had recovered within one month, and the majority actually cleared up in less than two weeks. All but 6 percent of Bedford's patients had been free of symptoms of delirium by the end of six months. It is unknown how often delirium in the elderly is the initial event in permanent dementia, due to degenerative or cerebrovascular disease. The mortality of 33 percent quoted by Bedford is quite high and one wonders how many of his patients were moribund when admitted and examined. An important aspect of delirium in the elderly is their often fragile, malnourished, and dehydrated state which, if not corrected, may readily progress to terminal illness. Furthermore, an agitated, restless, frightened, and belligerent older delirious patient is at considerable risk of cardiovascular collapse from exhaustion, of falls and fractures, of head injury and subdural hematoma, and of complications due to noncompliance with intravenous infusions, etc. Finally, delirium in the elderly commonly occurs at home rather than in a hospital and may result in the patient's wandering off, getting into a fight, and provoking retaliatory actions on the part of others. The common occurrence or exacerbation of delirium at night increases the probability of these social and medical complications.

Thus, the prognosis of delirium in the elderly is generally much more serious than in those under the age of sixty years. Mortality is high, risk of life-threatening complications is considerable, and frequent association with terminal illness ominous. All these factors highlight the importance of delirium in the aged as an often diagnostically crucial and prognostically alarming manifestation of physical illness.

ETIOLOGIC FACTORS

Delirium is said to be about four times more frequent in patients forty years and older than in those under forty (22). Furthermore, even though proper epidemiologic studies have yet to be carried out, there is accrued clinical evidence that the elderly, those older than sixty years, are especially vulnerable to delirium. This observation has been generally interpreted as reflecting the following three sets of factors operating in the aged: first, impairment of cerebral circulation and thus greater vulnerability to *hypoxia;* second, higher prevalence and incidence of *chronic diseases,* cardiovascular, metabolic, etc., and associated functional decompensation of various vital organs; and third, *increased frequency of episodes of illness,* especially respiratory and urinary infection (11, 22). Acute mental confusion, or what in this book is referred to as delirium, is said to be a more frequent presenting manifestation of physical illness in the elderly than such commonplace symptoms as fever, pain, or tachycardia (6).

The high incidence of delirium in the elderly seems to reflect changes in the susceptibility of the aging organism to disease on the one hand, and the increased vulnerability of the aging brain to ischemia, anoxia, electrolyte imbalance, drugs, and other pathogenic factors on the other. Homeostatic and immune mechanisms of the older person's body are generally less efficient and the dynamic steady state of the latter readily becomes deranged as a result of a whole range of stressors, physical, biologic, social, and psychologic. The brain of an elderly person is often damaged, or its circulation is compromised, or both. There is progressive decline of weight and blood flow of cerebral gray matter with advancing age in normal people, and even more so in those suffering from hypertension and cerebrovascular disease. Function of the brain is often already either manifestly impaired or marginally compensated. Derangement of homeostasis, and especially ischemia-hypoxia, brought about by any of a wide range of diseases, toxic agents, and external physical conditions, as well as by such factors as sensory deprivation or psychologic stress, may result in cerebral functional decompensation. Psychologic and behavioral manifestations of the latter constitute what we call delirium or acute brain failure.

Several studies provide data on the relative frequency of the various organic etiologic factors operating in delirium of the aged individual. Doty (22) found cardiac disease, postoperative states, pneumonia, liver disease, malignancy, bone fractures, uremia, and hypertensive encephalopathy to be the conditions most often associated with delirium in the older patients. In a series of 288 delirious subjects aged sixty years or older, malnutrition, heart failure, alcohol, and cerebrovascular accidents accounted for over 70 percent of etiologic factors believed to be implicated (23). In thirty-four elderly delirious patients examined in the course of a special one-day census carried out at the Los Angeles County General Hospital in 1965, infection, cerebrovascular disease, and diabetes accounted for 56 percent of the relevant medical diagnoses (21). In another study, alcohol, drug ingestion, malnutrition, and cardiac failure accounted for almost 80 percent of the etiologic factors (19).

The above studies provide some information about the frequency of the various etiologic factors in the delirium among people aged sixty years and over. These factors are among those discussed in the preceding chapters but they occupy a relatively more prominent position in the aged. Various writers have singled out certain physical illnesses or other factors as being particularly frequently associated with delirium in geriatric patients (7, 9, 12, 20, 24-26). Table 18-1 summarizes the most consistently quoted diseases and agents.

The most common and important etiologic factors listed in Table 18-1 deserve brief comment relevant to their occurrence in the aged.

Adverse Drug Reactions

These are said to be about 2.5 times more common in patients over sixty than in those under sixty years of age (27). In patients over seventy, undesirable side effects may occur in 20 to 25

TABLE 18-I

ETIOLOGY OF DELIRIUM IN THE AGED

1. Drugs: sedatives-hypnotics; phenothiazines; tricyclic antidepressants; lithium; narcotics; propoxyphene; pentazocine; antihypertensives; anticholinergics (other than psychotropic ones); diuretics; digitalis; antiparkinsonian drugs; chlorpropamide; cimetidine; steroids; indomethacin; cancer chemotherapeutics; L-dopa.
2. Alcohol intoxication and withdrawal.
3. Metabolic disorders: especially electrolyte imbalance; hepatic encephalopathy; renal failure; respiratory failure; endocrinopathies; hypothermia and hyperthermia; hypoglycemia and hyperglycemia.
4. Cardiac failure; arrhythmia; myocardial infarction; pulmonary embolism.
5. Cerebrovascular disorders: stroke; transient ischemic attack; subdural hematoma; cranial arteritis; cerebral vasculitis.
6. Infection, especially pulmonary or renal; bacteremia; meningitis, encephalitis.
7. Neoplasm: intracranial, extracranial.
8. Vitamin B-complex deficiency.
9. Head trauma, burns, surgery.
10. Epilepsy.

percent of those treated. A number of factors related to various aspects of the aging process have been proposed to account for adverse drug reactions, including delirium, in the aged. The following are the more important variables:

1. Impairment of hepatic detoxification, especially of oxidation. This mechanism is responsible for increased proneness to delirium in elderly patients taking tricyclic antidepressants, benzodiazepines, anticonvulsants, and oral hypoglycemic agents
2. Reduced renal excretion due to decreased glomerular filtration with age has the effect of prolonging half-life of such drugs as digoxin, streptomycin, gentamicin, etc.
3. Reduction in protein binding of drugs in plasma may enhance the effects of narcotics, certain diuretics, etc.
4. Tendency to postural hypotension, hypothermia, and hyperthermia as a result of deficient homeostatic protective mechanisms
5. Loss of thirst appreciation and thus tendency to hypovolemia
6. Increased drug sensitivity or target organ response
7. Errors of intake, compounded by delirium

8. Polypharmacy and related drug interactions as a consequence of multiple pathological processes each requiring drug therapy

As a result of various constellations of the above factors the elderly are highly prone to the development of drug-induced delirium (24, 27-29). Considering that the elderly receive more drugs than the general population and that about one-quarter of them receive four to six drugs concurrently, the incidence of adverse drug effects, including delirium, must be high (29). In one series, diuretics, analgesics, psychotropics, hypnotic-sedatives, and digitalis preparations accounted for the bulk of the prescribed drugs (29). Diuretics, as one might expect, topped the list of drugs with the largest number of adverse reactions, followed closely by psychotropic drugs and digitalis. It has been stressed lately that the elderly receive diuretics more often than is indicated (30). Resulting hypokalemia, hyponatremia, dehydration, hypotension, and hyperkalemia may all contribute to delirium (31).

Psychotropic drugs. Antidepressants, lithium, phenothiazines, and benzodiazepines tend to induce delirium far more readily in the aged than in the younger adult patient (28, 29, 32-36). *Benzodiazepines* are the most frequently prescribed drugs in this age-group and they are liable to cause symptoms of intoxication or delirium in the elderly patient (32, 36). It has been recommended that patients more than seventy years old should receive initially one-half of the usual dose of a benzodiazepine drug (36). Oxazepam, a benzodiazepine with a relatively low mean half-life (seven hours), is generally preferable as an anxiolytic agent for the elderly patient (36). Mental disorders attributed to psychoactive drugs have been reported as the main reason for admission to a psychogeriatric service in 16 percent of cases (28). Reports that *tricyclic antidepressants* readily induce delirium in the aged (32) seem to have discouraged the use of these drugs even when they are indicated (32). Delirium caused by these agents may be due to their direct cerebral effects, or to arrhythmias or hypotension to which they may give rise, especially in the elderly (36). Doses of maximum 75 to 100 mg. per day are recommended. *Lithium* is liable to induce severe adverse reactions in the elderly, sometimes as early as fifteen minutes after an initial dose (36). Half-life of this drug is prolonged in these patients from thirty-six to forty-eight hours. A test dose of 50 to 75 mg. of lithium carbonate and gradual increase of the total daily dosage to 600 mg. have been recommended (33). *Phenothiazines,* like all drugs with anticholinergic properties, induce delirium more readily in the older patient (35). For more discussion of deliriogenic potential of all these drugs, the reader is referred to Chapter 10.

Alcohol Intoxication and Withdrawal

Problems related to alcohol are at the top of the list of etiologic factors in one study of delirium among patients aged sixty or older, admitted to psychiatric receiving wards of a general hospital (19). In another study, 100 patients sixty years and older consecutively admitted to a county psychiatric screening ward were assessed for the presence of alcoholism (37). Forty-four of these patients were diagnosed as alcoholics; 23 percent of the total sample exhibited confusion, disorientation, and memory impairment indicative of delirium. The investigators point out that alcoholism in the elderly psychiatric patients is more prevalent than one might expect. Sixty percent of the alcoholics were judged to be brain-damaged, and this factor is liable to predispose them to delirium. The elderly alcoholic is more likely to have a very long history of excessive drinking and such a history is typically found in patients suffering from delirium tremens (see Chapter 11). Furthermore, the elderly are particularly vulnerable to vitamin deficiencies, which may be associated with excessive drinking and cause or contribute to delirium (38, 39).

Metabolic Disorders

Among the more common causes of delirium in general, and among the aged in particular are metabolic disorders (see Chapter 10).

Dehydration. Dehydration is common in the elderly sick patient and may be one of the presenting features in a delirious one. It tends to occur frequently since such a patient often exhibits reduced urinary concentrating power, depends heavily on adequate and consistent water intake, and becomes dehydrated when the latter is curtailed as a result of illness, for example. Electrolyte imbalance occurs frequently as a side effect of drugs, inadequate fluid intake, neoplasms, cerebrovascular accidents, hepatic encephalopathy, and uremia.

Respiratory failure. In one series, lung disease such as pneumonia, chronic bronchitis, and emphysema accounted for 20 percent of cases of mental confusion (26).

Diabetes. Diabetes accounted for nearly 15 percent of etiologic factors in one small group of delirious elderly patients screened in a general hospital (21). Elderly diabetics can develop ketoacidosis and are especially vulnerable to hypoglycemic reactions in response to insulin, or sulfonylurea drugs, or neoplasm (40). Typical of the older diabetic is the appearance of hyperosmolar nonketotic hyperglycemic coma. The patient is likely to have mild diabetes and a recent history of inadequate fluid intake, increasing somnolence, and polyuria. Delirium rather than coma may be the presenting mental state in these patients and its severity parallels the degree of hyperosmolarity. Intracellular dehydration involving brain cells is mainly responsible for delirium and coma. The patient may exhibit various neurologic signs, including generalized convulsions, along with delirium. Correction of dehydration and hyperglycemia is usually followed by clearing of delirium, but the latter may occasionally persist for days after therapy has been initiated (40).

Hyperthyroidism and hypothyroidism. These are said to occur in 3 to 4 percent of elderly people (41). Either may feature delirium. The former may present in its apathetic form in the aged.

Vitamin deficiencies. Vitamin deficiencies, especially of the B complex series, are present in over 10 percent of the elderly and are liable to be manifested by delirium (25, 28, 29).

Hypothermia and heat stroke. These reflect impaired temperature regulation in old people and are important causes of delirium among them (42, 43). All these and many other metabolic disorders are discussed in considerable detail in Chapter 12.

Cardiovascular Disorders

Cardiovascular disorders are highly prevalent in old age and constitute one of the most important etiologic factors in delirium among the elderly. Diseases of circulation account for between 25 and 33 percent of medical problems or diagnoses in patients over sixty (44). Heart disease is the most important single cause of death in old age, and its prevalence, especially that of ischemic heart disease, is very high (45). The incidence of cardiac failure rises with age. The most often encountered arrhythmia is frequent ectopic beats. Atrial fibrillation is reportedly present in 1.7 percent of persons aged sixty-five to seventy-four years, and in 4.8 percent of those older than seventy-five years (45). Delirium or "mental confusion" may be a manifestation of myocardial infarction, cardiac failure, various arrhythmias, aortic stenosis, or subacute bacterial endocarditis. All these conditions may result in cerebral ischemia-anoxia and hence in acute brain failure. It has been suggested that these various disorders of heart action may give rise not only to delirium but also to "cardiogenic dementia" (46).

Myocardial infarction. In the elderly, this often occurs without pain and with "confusion" as the chief presenting feature. In one series of patients sixty-five years of age and over, "acute confusion" was the third most frequent mode of presentation, having occurred in 11.6 percent of cases (45). Sudden development of delirium with agitation, restlessness, and noisy behavior may constitute the only symptom of myocardial infarction. Such symptoms may pass unnoticed in an already demented patient. Cerebral embolization, pulmonary embolism, cardiac arrhythmias, cardiogenic shock, and heart failure may complicate myocardial infarction and result in reduced cerebral blood flow and delirium.

Cardiac arrhythmias. These may manifest themselves clinically as episodes of delirium. It has been demonstrated that extrasystoles, atrial fibrillation, bradycardia, and the paroxysmal tachycardias can all bring about considerable fall in cerebral blood flow. Mental clearing has been observed on pacing cases of heart-block to a normal rate (45). Ectopic tachycardias in the elderly have been reported to present with "confusion" in about 25 percent of cases (47). All arrhythmias in the elderly require treatment (45). Antiarrhythmic drugs, however, are liable to induce delirium in some of the patients. Digoxin lidocaine, procainamide, propranolol, quinidine, and Dilantin® may all precipitate the syndrome. Holter monitoring has been recommended for patients presenting with intermittent dizziness, blackout or both (48). In one series of such patients, about 9 percent were found to have arrhythmias known to be associated with cerebral symptoms. Holter monitoring is recommended for elderly patients presenting with unexplained transient episodes of delirium.

Pulmonary heart disease. Pulmonary heart disease may be associated with episodes of delirium related to fluctuating levels of hypercapnia. Delirium, excitement, and wandering may appear in the evening or during the night (45).

Congestive heart failure. This is a common problem in geriatrics and may give rise to hypoxemia and delirium (see Chapter 12). Elderly patients with *aortic stenosis* may suffer from syncopal attacks, especially on exertion, and also from delirium (45). *Subacute and acute bacterial endocarditis* are said to be increasingly common in the elderly. Delirium may dominate the clinical picture in as many as one-half of the cases (45).

Orthostatic hypotension. This occurs more readily in the aged than in younger persons. Its causes are many and include cerebrovascular disease and drug reactions (45, 49). Symptoms range from lightheadedness, through varying degrees of delirium or "confusion," to syncope or convulsions (49). Treatment of hypertension in the elderly with antihypertensive drugs may result in inadequate cerebral perfusion and acute brain failure (50). *Hypertension* is said to cause mental confusion on occasion, but apart from hypertensive encephalopathy this complication is not likely to be caused by raised blood pressure alone (26).

Infection

Especially in the respiratory or urinary tract, infection often presents with delirium in the elderly. Fever, tachycardia, leucocytosis, cough, dyspnea, and tachypnea may be absent and delirium may be the only manifestation of broncho-pneumonia, for example (26). Most infections are more severe in the aged than in the younger patient. Various factors have been implicated in this increased susceptibility to infection, such as deteriorated function of B lymphocytes and T lymphocytes, and coexisting immunosuppressive disease (such as cancer, diabetes mellitus, renal insufficiency, and malnutrition) (51). Cholecystitis, diverticulitis, tuberculosis, septicemia, or bacteremia may all present with delirium as the only or the most prominent feature. Catheterization is a common source of bladder infections. Gram-negative bacteremia may follow the latter, and delirium may be its only manifestation. Urinary tract infections and pneumonia are relatively common post-operative complications in the elderly (51).

Intracranial Space-Occupying Lesions

Relatively frequent in the aged, these lesions may give rise to delirium. *Subdural hematoma* accounts for about 20 percent of all intracranial masses in the elderly, may follow minor head trauma, and often presents with delirium (25, 52). Maximum incidence of *brain tumors* occurs between ages sixty and seventy (53). Metastatic tumors account for 20 to 50 percent of cerebral neoplasms (25). Increased intracranial pressure is usually the main pathogenic factor in delirium occurring as a manifestation of brain tumor.

DELIRIUM VERSUS DEMENTIA

Delirium may be viewed as one of the cardinal manifestations of physical illness in the elderly, one that is reversible but may be followed by death or by chronic organic mental disorder. The latter often antedates delirium, which then becomes super-imposed on it as a result of an acute intracranial or systemic disease, or of exposure to a drug or toxic agent. In a study quoted earlier, about 46 percent of 534 patients aged sixty or older admitted to San Francisco General Hospital had evidence of delirium (acute brain syndrome), and the latter was associated with a chronic brain syndrome in nearly 70 percent of the cases (19). This suggests that the chronic syndrome (dementia) predisposes a person to the development of delirium and that the two syndromes often coexist.

Bedford (11) states emphatically that mental confusion or delirium must be clearly separated from dementia and that these two conditions must not be equated. The fact that delirium and dementia often coexist in the same person should not obscure the observation that a demented individual need not be confused or delirious, and a confused patient is by no means necessarily demented. Bedford bemoans the tendency on the part of some physicians to use the terms "mental confusion" and "dementia" synonymously and thus to imply that both of them carry equally hopeless prognosis. This is, of course, an obvious and dangerous fallacy. Despite these cogent arguments, however, one still encounters that vague term "senile delirium," favored by medical writers of a century ago (54). Post (55), for example, speaks of 'acute senile confusional state (senile delirium)" and defines it as "the acute mental reaction (acute brain syndrome) as seen in old age." Post goes on to say that many of these senile deliria differ little as regards etiology, course, and therapy from those occurring in younger people. He mentions bereavement and removal from home among the many possible causes of senile delirium and claims that when no adequate physical cause can be found on thorough investigation, one may assume the presence of an early, if mild, "senile deteriorative process." The present writer is not aware of any evidence supporting the hypothesis that Alzheimer's disease-senile dementia complex can cause delirium in the absence of any additional etiologic factors. This question is still unresolved. In any case, the term "senile delirium" is misleading and redundant and should not be used. It tends to mislead doctors and others into viewing delirium in the elderly as a condition equivalent to senile dementia, or as a manifestation of the latter. Such misconceptions are likely to result in failure to investigate and treat delirium in the aged.

Roth (15) points out that only a small minority of cases of delirium are caused by an infarct or other cerebral disease. Furthermore, he asserts that transition from a delirious to a demented state is very rare, and that the brains of patients with delirium show measurable brain damage to be equal to that found in mentally well-functioning subjects. Elsewhere, Roth (56) states that the distinction between delirium and dementia is mainly quantitative and thus not sharp. One syndrome may merge into or overlap with the other. Nevertheless, Roth urges that the two syndromes be differentiated clinically since delirium tends to be associated with relatively acute and potentially reversible physical disease, and treatment of the latter is of crucial importance.

Virtual lack of studies on the natural history of delirium in the aged, especially in its relation to the main dementing diseases, namely Alzheimer's disease-senile dementia and multi-infarct dementia, does not allow any definitive statements at this time. Delirium has been observed to usher in dementia due to cerebrovascular disease, probably reflecting transient cerebral ischemia-anoxia (57). Association of delirium with the Alzheimer's-senile disease is less well documented. The most common form of delirium encountered in the demented patient appears to be the so-called nocturnal confusion, a condition often encountered in the senile patients. Cameron (58) found that delirium could be induced in the latter by placing them in a dark room during the day. He hypothesized that the delirium might be based on an inability of the senile patient to maintain a spatial image without the aid of repeated visual sensory input. Feinberg (59) offers a different hypothetical explanation for nocturnal delirium in the demented. He postulates that intrusion of REM sleep or dreaming activity into wakefulness in patients waking up from REM sleep may account for delirium. This interesting hypothesis remains to be tested. Thus, Cameron postulated the causal role of sensory deprivation, while Feinberg hypothesizes that disorders of the sleep-wakefulness cycle may have etiologic significance in delirium of the elderly demented person. There is obvious need for more experimental research in this area.

The only firmly established relationship between dementia and delirium is their frequent coexistence. It is easy to predict that any patient with cerebrovascular disease is especially vulnerable to anything that induces cerebral ischemia-hypoxia and is thus susceptible to delirium. It is still unclear, however,

whether delirium ever arises as a manifestation of degenerative
cerebral disease with manifest dementia, or as an antecedent of
the latter syndrome. It is not known if nocturnal confusion in a
patient with senile dementia really represents delirium or a
similar syndrome, possibly with a different pathophysiology. Only
research can settle these issues in the future.

Whatever the relation of delirium to the dementias of old
age may prove to be, there is practical merit in suspecting
delirium in every elderly patient who develops global cognitive
impairment acutely and *de novo,* or whose cognitive deficits
suddenly become worse, especially if such abnormalities fluctuate
over twenty-four hours and are most pronounced at night. An
EEG showing diffuse slow activity of high voltage supports the
diagnosis of delirium. The following clinical features help distinguish the latter from dementia, although none of them is
pathognomonic of either condition.

TABLE 18-II

Essential Features	*Delirium*	*Dementia*
1. Onset	Acute, often at night.	Usually gradual.
2. Duration	Days to weeks; usually less than one month.	At least a month, usually much longer.
3. Disorientation	Present, at least for time; fluctuates. Tendency to mistake unfamiliar for familiar persons, place.	May be absent in mild cases.
4. Thinking	Slow or accelerated; may be oneiric or dreamlike, or impoverished.	Impoverished. Poor abstracting ability.
5. Memory	Recent impaired.	Recent impaired. Remote may be affected.
6. Attention	Invariably disturbed, hard to fix, tends to fluctuate.	May be intact.
7. Alertness	Reduced or increased but awareness always defective.	May be normal or reduced.
8. Perception	Invariably impaired, if only at night. Hallucinations often present.	May be intact. Hallucinations often absent.
9. Sleep	Always disrupted sleep-wakefulness cycle.	Usually normal for age.
10. Course	Typically fluctuates, with lucid intervals and nocturnal exacerbation.	Relatively stable over course of day.

The differences listed in Table 18-2 are obviously *relative* and the two syndromes merge with each other. Whenever doubt arises about which of them is present, it is safer to assume that delirium is present and plan investigations accordingly. The delirious patient tends to be either lethargic, or agitated and restless, or to shift between psychomotor underactivity and reduced alertness and wakefulness and the opposite state. Such a patient is particularly likely to be disturbing to other people on account of his or her noisiness, aggressiveness, tendency to stay awake and wander at night, paranoid delusions of a fleeting kind, and visual hallucinations. When such behavior appears suddenly either in a previously well-compensated old person or in one displaying marked intellectual deficits, delirium must be presumptively diagnosed, viewed as a manifestation of acute change in patient's physical health, and immediately investigated. In some cases no physical illness can be found and only some evidence of a degenerative cerebral process is present. In such cases delirium may apparently be precipitated by such factors as bereavement, separation from personally significant others, or transfer to an unfamiliar environment such as a hospital (60). As a general rule, however, the onset of delirium should lead to investigations aimed at identifying its presumed cause, or causes. One should never assume that psychologic or social factors alone are responsible for a given patient's delirium, since such an assumption could result in potentially disastrous omission to diagnose and treat a reversible physical disease, or to remove a toxic agent implicated in the case. It is possible, however, that just as occasional cases of fever prove to be "psychogenic," so some cases of delirium may prove to be the result of psychosocial stress and its pathophysiologic concomitants.

MANAGEMENT

Treatment of delirium in the aged does not differ in its general principles from that discussed in Chapter 9. The highest priority belongs to a search for organic etiologic factors. Prevention of injury to the patient or other people as a result of the patient's restlessness, fear, combativeness, etc., is important.

Sedation must be so adjusted that the patient neither becomes even more delirious and prone to falls and other complications as a result of it nor is pushed into stupor and coma by over-sedation. In the latter case, the patient may die, or develop venous thrombosis, dehydration, or pressure sores (25). Thus, the choice of the tranquilizer or hypnotic and its dosage are important. The dose may have to be adjusted after response to an initial one has been assessed.

Various tranquilizers, sedatives, and hypnotics have been used for treatment of delirium in the elderly. A review of these drugs will not be attempted here and the reader is referred to other sources (35). No major tranquilizer tried to date has been found to be superior to the others either in effectiveness or freedom from side effects (35). In Europe, chlormethiazole enjoys considerable popularity for the treatment of delirium in the elderly, but the drug is unavailable in the United States (61). The present writer favors *haloperidol* as the drug of choice for the treatment of delirium in most categories of patients. It is effective, has a wide margin of safety, and is relatively free from cardiovascular, hepatotoxic, deliriogenic, and other undesirable side effects. The drug can be used as drops, tablets, or parenterally (8). The dosage is discussed in Chapter 9. As a rule, it is advisable to use a small test dose initially and then increase it gradually to a level that is clinically effective and relatively free of side effects. It is important for the patient to remain alert during daytime and to be sound asleep during the night. Haloperidol, or equivalent tranquilizer, should best be given in the early evening and repeated, if necessary, after several hours (62). In this way, maximum sedation, as well as such side effects as hypotension or urinary retention, will be largely confined to the night, leaving the patient relatively alert and free from these adverse effects during the day.

REFERENCES

1. Lipowski, Z.J.: Organic brain syndromes: a reformulation. *Compr Psychiatry* 19:309-322, 1978.
2. Brocklehurst, J.C., and Hanley, T.: *Geriatric Medicine for Students.* Edinburgh, Churchill Livingstone, 1976, p. 59.

3. Anderson, W.F.: "The Inter-relationship Between Physical and Mental Disease in the Elderly," in *Recent Developments in Psychogeriatrics*, Kay, D.W.K., and Walk, A., Eds. Ashford, Kent, Headley Brothers Ltd., 1971, pp. 19-24.

4. Brocklehurst, J.C.: Psychogeriatric care as a specialized discipline in medicine. *Bull NY Acad Med 53*:702-709, 1977.

5. Psychogeriatrics. *Report of a WHO Scientific Group*. Geneva, World Health Organization, 1972.

6. Hodkinson, H.M.: *Common Symptoms of Disease in the Elderly*. Oxford, Blackwell Scientific Publications, 1976.

7. Arie, T.: Dementia in the elderly: diagnosis and assessment. *Br Med J 4*:540-543, 1973.

8. Godber, C.: The physician and the confused elderly patient. *J R Coll Physicians Lond 10*:101-112, 1975.

9. Adams, G.: *Essentials of Geriatric Medicine*. Oxford, Oxford University Press, 1977.

10. Lishman, W.A.: *Organic Psychiatry: The Psychological Consequences of Cerebral Disorder*. Oxford, Blackwell Scientific Publications, 1978, pp. 4-6.

11. Bedford, P.D.: General medical aspects of confusional states in elderly people. *Br Med J 2*:185-188, 1959.

12. Isaacs, B.: *An Introduction to Geriatrics*. London, Bailliere, Tindall & Cassell, 1965.

13. Stengel, E.: The organic confusional state and the organic dementias. *Br J Clin Pract 2*:719-724, 1969.

14. Kay, D.W.K.: "Epidemiological Aspects of Organic Brain Disease in the Aged," in *Aging and the Brain*, Gaitz, C.M., Ed. New York, Plenum Press, 1972, pp. 15-27.

15. Roth, M.: The psychiatric disorders of later life. *Psychiatr Ann 6*:417-445, 1976.

16. *The Concise Oxford Dictionary*. 3rd edition. Oxford, Oxford University Press, 1946.

17. Livesley, B.: The pathogenesis of brain failure in the aged. *Age and Ageing (Suppl) 6*:9-19, 1977.

18. Robinson, G.W.: "The Toxic Delirious Reactions of Old Age," in *Mental Disorders in Later Life*, Kaplan, O.J., Ed. Stanford, Stanford University Press, 1956, pp. 227-255.

19. Simon, A., and Cahan, R.B.: The acute brain syndrome in geriatric patients. *Psychiatr Res Rep 16*:8-21, 1963.

20. Anderson, F.: *Practical Management of the Elderly*. 3rd edition. Oxford, Blackwell Scientific Publications, 1976.

21. Freedman, D.K., Troll, L., Mills, A.B., and Baker, P.: *Acute Organic Disorder Accompanied by Mental Symptoms*. Sacramento, California Dept. of Mental Hygiene, 1965.

22. Doty, E.J.: The incidence and treatment of delirious reactions in later life. *Geriatrics 1*:21-26, 1946.
23. Simon, A., Lowenthal, M.F., and Epstein, L.J.: *Crisis and Intervention.* San Francisco, Jossey-Bass Inc., Publishers, 1970.
24. Dunn, T., and Arie, T.: Mental disturbances in the ill old person. *Br Med J 2*:413-416, 1973.
25. Libow, L.S.: Pseudo-senility: acute and reversible organic brain syndromes. *J Am Geriatrics Soc 21*:112-120, 1973.
26. Murphy, E.: The confused elderly patient. *J Irish Med Assoc 61*:99-103, 1968.
27. Editorial: Medication in the elderly. *J Irish Med Assoc 71*:136-137, 1978.
28. Kayne, R.C.: Acute brain syndrome in an elderly patient. *Drug Intel Clin Pharm 8*:476-482, 1974.
29. Williamson, J.: Prescribing problems in the elderly. *Practitioner 220*:749-755, 1978.
30. Editorial: Diuretics in the elderly. *Br Med J 1*:1092-1093, 1978.
31. Spino, M., Sellers, E.M., Kaplan, H.L., et al.: Adverse biochemical and clinical consequences of furosemide administration. *Can Med Assoc J 118*:1513-1518, 1978.
32. Achong, M.R., Bayne, J.R.D., Gerson, L.W., and Golshani, S.: Prescribing of psychoactive drugs for chronically ill elderly patients. *Can Med Assoc J 118*:1503-1508, 1978.
33. Foster, J.R., Gershell, W.J., and Goldfarb, A.I.: Lithium treatment in the elderly. 1. Clinical usage. *J Gerontol 32*:299-302, 1977.
34. Kramer, M.: Delirium as a complication of imipramine therapy in the aged. *Am J Psychiatry 120*:502-503, 1961.
35. Gershon, S., and Raskin, A.: *Genesis and Treatment of Psychologic Disorders in the Elderly.* New York, Raven Press, 1975.
36. Sellers, E.M.: Clinical pharmacology and therapeutics of benzodiazepines.*Can Med Assoc J 118*:1533-1538, 1978.
37. Gaitz, C.M., and Baer, P.E.: Characteristics of elderly patients with alcoholism. *Arch Gen Psychiatry 24*:372-378, 1971.
38. Mitra, M.L.: Confusional states in relation to vitamin deficiencies in the elderly. *J Am Geriatrics Soc 19*:536-545, 1971.
39. Brin, M., and Bauernfeind, J.C.: Vitamin needs of the elderly. *Postgrad Med 63*:155-163, 1978.
40. Podolsky, S.: Hyperosmolar nonketotic coma in the elderly diabetic. *Med Clin N Am 62*:815-828, 1978.
41. Morrow, L.B.: How thyroid disease presents in the elderly. *Geriatrics 31*:42-45, 1978.
42. Irvine, R.E.: Hypothermia in old age. *Practitioner 213*:795-800, 1974.
43. Levine, J.A.: Heat stroke in the aged. *Am J Med 47*:251-258, 1969.

44. Sivertson, S.E.: Common problems of ambulatory geriatric patients. *Postgrad Med 64*:83-89, 1978.
45. Caird, F.I., Dall, J.L.C., and Kennedy, R.D.: *Cardiology in Old Age.* New York, Plenum Press, 1976.
46. Editorial: Cardiogenic dementia. *Lancet 1*:27-28, 1977.
47. Clark, A.N.G.: Ectopic tachycardias in the elderly. *Geront Clin 12*:203-212, 1970.
48. Jonas, S., Klein, I., and Dimant, J.: Importance of Holter monitoring in patients with periodic cerebral symptoms. *Ann Neurol 1*:470-474, 1977.
49. Fine, W.: Postural hypotension. *Practitioner 220*:698-701, 1978.
50. Jones, J.V., and Graham, D.I.: Hypertension and the cerebral circulation—its relevance to the elderly. *Am Heart J 96*:270-271, 1978.
51. Polly, S.M., and Sanders, W.E.: Surgical infections in the elderly: prevention, diagnosis, and treatment. *Geriatrics 32*:88-97, 1977.
52. Raskind, R., Glover, B., and Weiss, S.R.: Chronic subdural hematoma in the elderly: a challenge in diagnosis and treatment. *J Am Geriatrics Soc 20*:330-334, 1972.
53. Schoenberg, B.C., Christine, B.W., and Whisnant, J.P.: The resolution of discrepancies in the reported incidence of primary brain tumors. *Neurology 28*:817-823, 1978.
54. Hood, P.: On senile delirium. *Practitioner 5*:278-289, 1870.
55. Post, F.: *The Clinical Psychiatry of Late Life.* Oxford, Pergamon Press, 1965.
56. Roth, M.: "Some Problems of Geriatrics Common to Medicine and Psychiatry," in *Medicine in Old Age*, Agate, J.N., Ed. Philadelphia, J.B. Lippincott Co., 1965, pp. 99-112.
57. Nemoto, E.M.: Pathogenesis of cerebral ischemia-anoxia. *Crit Care Med 6*:203-214, 1978.
58. Cameron, D.C.: Studies in senile nocturnal delirium. *Psychiatr Q 15*:47-53, 1941.
59. Feinberg, I.: "Sleep in Organic Brain Conditions," in *Sleep. Physiology and Pathology*, Kales, A., Ed. Philadelphia, J.B. Lippincott Co., 1969, pp. 131-147.
60. Litin, E.M.: Mental reaction to trauma and hospitalization in the aged. *JAMA 162*:1522-1524, 1956.
61. Haar, H.W. ter: A comparison of chlormethiazole and haloperidol in the treatment of elderly patients with confusion of organic and psychogenic origin: a double-blind crossover study. *Pharmatherapeutica 1*:563-569, 1977.
62. Bayne, J.R.D.: Management of confusion in elderly persons. *Can Med Assoc J 118*:139-141, 1978.

548 *Delirium: Acute Brain Failure in Man*

Additional References

Arie, T. Confusion in old age. *Age Ageing 7 (Suppl)*:72-76, 1978.

Bayne, J.R.D. Assessing confusion in the elderly. *Psychosomatics 20*:43-51, 1979.

Beauchene, R.E., and Davis, T.A. The nutritional status of the aged in the U.S.A. *Age 2*:23-28, 1979.

Brink, T.L., Capri, D., De Neeve, V., et al. Senile confusion: Limitations of assessment by the face-hand test, mental status questionnaire, and staff ratings. *J Am Geriatr Soc 26*:380-382, 1978.

Dimant, J., Ginzler, E.M., Schlesinger, M., et al. Systemic lupus erythematosus in the older age group: Computer analysis. *J Am Geriatr Soc 27*:58-61, 1979.

Levenson, A.J., Ed. *Neuropsychiatric Side-Effects of Drugs in the Elderly.* New York, Raven Press, 1979.

Lundin, D.V. Medication taking behavior of the elderly. *Drug Intel Clin Pharm 12*:518-522, 1978.

Myers, M.G., Kearns, P.M., Kennedy, D.S., and Fisher, R.H. Postural hypotension and diuretic therapy in the elderly. *Can Med Assoc J 119*:581-585, 1978.

Phair, J.P., Kauffman, C.A., Bjornson, A., et al. Host defenses in the aged: Evaluation of components of the inflammatory and immune responses. *J. Infect Dis 138*:67-73, 1978.

Vestal, R.E. Drug use in the elderly: A review of problems and special considerations. *Drugs 16*:358-382, 1978.

Wahl, P.R. Psychosocial implications of disorientation in the elderly. *Nurs Clin North Am 11*:145-155, 1976.

Weymouth, L.T. Nursing care of the so-called confused patient. *Nurs Clin North Am 3*:709-715, 1968.

Williams, M.A., Holloway, J.R., Winn, M.C., et al. Nursing activities and acute confusional states in elderly hip-fractured patients. *Nurs Res 28*:25-35, 1979.

Wolanin, M.O. *A Study of Confused Elderly Persons in a Long Term Care Unit.* Unpublished manuscript.

Wollner, L., McCarthy, S.T., Soper, N.D.W., and Macy, D.J. Failure of cerebral autoregulation as a cause of brain dysfunction in the elderly. *Br Med J 1*:1117-1118, 1979.

NAME INDEX

A

Abeles, M.M., 487
Abood, L.G., 174
Abrams, J., 329
Abrams, R., 222
Adams, G., 527
Adams, R.D., 36, 171
Addison, T., 360
Agulnik, P.L., 293
Allen, R.P., 257
Allison, R.S., 98
Anderson, F., 529
Andiman, R., 456
Andreasen, N.J.C., 517-18
Andrews, J.M., 460
Angst, J., 261-62
Arentsen, K., 480
Aretaeus of Cappadocia, 10, 227,
  255-56
Arie, T., 415
Arieff, A.I., 364
Aserinsky, E., 125
Assal, G., 447
Avicenna, 12, 228
Ayd, F.J., 237

B

Bachelard, H.S., 159
Bademosi, O., 350
Baker, A.B., 360
Baldessarini, R.J., 258, 264, 293
Barr, A.N., 296
Barrough, P., 13, 71
Barten, H.H., 337
Bartholomeus Anglicus, 12
Bartlett, J.E.A., 511
Bastron, R.D., 488
Bedford, P.D., 494-95, 499, 528, 530,
  540

Belafsky, M.A., 451
Bell, L., 50-51
Bender, L., 57
Bennett, R., 462
Benos, J., 371
Benton, A.L., 91
Berglund, M., 165
Betz, E., 161
Bieber, I., 439
Billiard, M., 132
Biskind, M.S., 439
Bleuler, M., 24, 36, 385
Bockner, S., 420
Bollea, G., 57, 411
Bonhoeffer, K., 23-24, 117
Bowers, M.B., 178
Branthwaite, M.A., 505
Bremer, F., 184
Brierly, J.B., 391
Brierre de Boismont, 50
Browning, T.B., 386
Bruens, J.H., 449
Bruns, H.D., 509
Buchanan, D.C., 368

C

Cadilhac, J., 172
Cadoret, R.J., 219
Cahan, R.B., 528
Calmeil, 51
Cameron, D.C., 541
Cameron, D.E., 138-39
Carlsson, C., 166
Cartwright, R.D., 123-24, 176
Casarett, L.J., 427
Cassius Felix, 11
Cay, E.L., 347
Celesia, G.G., 296, 450
Celsus, 5, 9-10, 36
Chadwick, J., 8

549

SUBJECT INDEX

A

Abstract thought testing, 204
Acetaminophen, 279
Acetylcholine, 186
Acidosis, 380-81
Acute confusional insanity, 19, 35-36, 220, 486
Addison's disease, 389
Adenosine triphosphate (ATP), 156-57
Adolescent delirium, 206-207
Affective disorders, 216, 222-27
Air embolism, 350
Alcohol
    consumption and intoxication, 17-18, 110, 114, 169-70, 232, 325-26, 446
    withdrawal syndrome, 110, 126-30, 133-34, 232, 495-97, 535.
    See also Delirium tremens
Alienation theory, 15
Alkalosis, 381
Altitude sickness, 350-51
Alzheimer's disease, 165, 431
Amanita muscaria, 263-64
Amebic meningoencephalitis, 421
Aminophylline, 299
Amitriptyline, 262-63
Amnesia, 216, 223-24
Amobarbital, 230
Amphetamines, 110, 338
Amyl nitrate, 434-35
Analgesic delirium, 275-80.
    See also names of specific analgesics
Anemia, 351, 392
"Angel dust." See Phencyclidine
Angel's trumpet, 256, 263
Angiographic trauma, 467
"Anima brutorum, De" (Willis), 14
Anoxia
    cerebral, 166, 170

decompression, 170.
    See also Hypoxia
Antibiotics, 284-86
Anticholinergic drugs
    deliriogenic effects of, 173-77, 179, 255-68
    experimental administration of, 84-85, 123-24
    as premedicants, 260-61.
    See also names of specific drugs, e.g. Scopolamine; Serotonin
Anticholinesterase compounds
    EEG and behavioral impact of, 177-78
    poisoning by, 439-41.
    See also specific drug names, e.g. Physostigmine
Anticonvulsants, 283-84
Antihistamines, 260, 330
Antimalarial drugs, 286-87
Antiparkinsonian agents, 260, 295-96
Antipsychotic drugs.
    See names of specific drugs and drugs families, e.g.
        Benzodiazepines;
        Butyrophenones; Lithium;
        Phenothiazines
Antispasmodic drugs, 260.
Antituberculosis drugs, 287-88
Anxiety and stress, 116-18, 161
Aortic stenosis, 538
Arteritis
    cerebral, 459
    cranial, 459-60
    (poly-) nodosa, 465
    rheumatoid, 466
Aspirin, 277-79
Asthma medications.
    See Belladonna alkaloids
Atabrine.
    See Quinacrine

557

Stress.
  See Anxiety and stress
Stroke, 454
Styrene, 433
Subarachnoid hemorrhage, 456-57
Subcortical arteriosclerotic
    encephalopathy, 467
Subdural hematoma, 458-59, 539
Subjective experiences of delirium.
  See Personal accounts and
      experiences
Suicide, 436
Surgery.
  See Post-operative delirium
Sydenham's chorea, 421
Systemic lupus erythematosus, 460-65

T

Tacrine, 260
Talmud, 11
Tartar emetic, 230
Tetrachloroethylene, 432
Tetrahydroaminacrine, 177-78
Thalamic projection system, 183-89
    passim
Thallium poisoning, 431
Thiamine deficiencies, 372-73
Thiothixene, 338
Thought
  associative vs. directive, 71-72
  disorders, 71-75, 84 (*see also*
      Delusions; Hallucinations)
  dynamics, 204
Thrombosis, 457-58
Thrombotic thrombocytopenic purpura,
    351-52, 392, 469
Toluene, 433
Toxic psychoses, 38
Toxoplasmosis, 421
Transient ischemic attacks, 454
Treatment
  of bromide delirium, 273-74
  of CO poisoning, 353
  of delirium tremens, 329-31
  of etiological conditions, 227, 229,
      231-32

historical evolution of, 7-21 passim,
    227-31
with sedatives, 227, 229-30, 233-39
  (*see also* names of specific
      drugs)
of steroid delirium, 292-93.
  See also Environmental and nursing
      support
Trichinosis, 420
Trichloroethylene, 432
Tricyclic antidepressants, 262-63, 534
Trihexyphenidyl, 260
Trinitrotoluene, 434
Trypanosomiasis, 420
Tularemia, 413
Twilight consciousness, 449-51
Typhoid fever, 415-16
"Typho-mania," 50-51
Typhus, 96

U

Uremia and uremic encephalopathy,
    95, 360-68

V

Vasculitis of small vessels, 465-66
Venesection.
  See Bloodletting
Verbalizations, 47, 97-98
Vertebrobasilar arterial obstructions,
    455-56
Vinblastine, 289
Vincristine, 289
Viral infections, 416.
  See also Infectious delirium
Visual distortions, 77
Vitamin deficiencies and overload,
    373-75, 536

W

Water intoxication, 392
Wegener's granulomatosis, 465
Wernicke's encephalopathy, 373
Wilson's disease, 382